Chronic Pain Management in General and Hospital Practice

Koki Shimoji • Antoun Nader
Wolfgang Hamann
Editors

Chronic Pain Management in General and Hospital Practice

Springer

Editors
Koki Shimoji
Pain Control Institute
Shinjyuku
Tokyo
Japan

Wolfgang Hamann
Guy's and St Thomas' Hospital,
Pain Management Centre
London
UK

Antoun Nader
Feinberg School of Medicine
Northwestern University Feinberg
School of Medicine
Chicago
IL
USA

ISBN 978-981-15-2932-0 ISBN 978-981-15-2933-7 (eBook)
https://doi.org/10.1007/978-981-15-2933-7

This Springer imprint is published by the registered company Springer Nature Singapore Pte Ltd.
The registered company address is: 152 Beach Road, #21-01/04 Gateway East, Singapore 189721, Singapore

Contents

Part II Pain Management Techniques

Part I
Basic Considerations

Chapter 1
History of Pain

W. Hamann

This summary of the history of pain focusses on its relevance to pain management. It is self-restricting, aiming to tease out the development of the subject pain towards the present situation of the history of medicine.

At the beginning, it is worthwhile to summarize our current understanding of the pain pathway, and then go through history bearing in mind what research tools were actually available to clinicians and researchers at particular points in times, and what relevant religious faiths and philosophies influenced the thinking about the nature of pain. One also needs to be aware that pathology can occur at any level of the pain pathway from peripheral receptors right up to relevant connections in the brain. Central pain, e.g., which may be excruciatingly debilitating, occurs without any peripheral origin but may be projected to peripheral parts of the body.

Rey [1] emphasizes the importance of discriminating between perception of pain and the ensuing suffering. Both aspects are of course therapeutic targets for the pain physician. Without alleviation of suffering there can be no effective pain management. It is therefore now generally accepted that pain management has to be holistic.

Historically, pain medicine concentrated on acute pain conditions. This may partially be due to the much shorter life expectancy in historic times. Many people did not live long enough to experience the full effects of degenerative diseases. Among the Graeco-Roman minor deities there are many gods specifically concerned with acute pain conditions and hardly any focussed on chronic pain. Similarly, among the catholic saints, there are only Milian, Saint Marcus and James the Great, whose remit is rheumatism. There are many more saints one can appeal to for help with acute pain.

Every civilization does have its own medicine experts with specific views on the significance of pain and how to deal with it. Commonly, sophisticated systems of

W. Hamann (✉)
Guy's and St Thomas' Hospital, Pain Management Centre, London, UK
e-mail: wolfgang.hamann@doctors.org.uk

K. Shimoji et al. (eds.), *Chronic Pain Management in General and Hospital Practice*, https://doi.org/10.1007/978-981-15-2933-7_1

herbal medicine were part of the treatments employed, and frequently, the same plants were used for similar indications.

This summary focusses on a few major instalments in the history of medicine preceding and during the recent scientific approach to pain and its management of pain.

The earliest written records mentioning opium date back 3000 years, on Sumerian clay tablets [2]. It is not clear whether this document refers to the use of the drug for pain control or as a narcotic. Thompson [2] also reported on Assyrian clay tablets recommending the use of ointments containing mandrake together with the use of charms for the control of toothache.

In parallel, medicine developed separately in Egypt, China, the Indian subcontinent in the form of Ayurvedic medicine and later further west in the Greco-Roman-Arabic sphere. Many aspects of pain management originating from these cultures have survived either in mainstream practice or in the form of alternative medicine.

Egyptian pain treatment was often combined with a Charm [3]. The Ebers Papyrus [3] reports use of the yeast of the opium drink, the willow tree, poppy plant, berries and seeds accompanied by chanting of a charm for pain control.

In Indian (Ayurveda) and Chinese (Tao) medicines an individual's good health was dependent on complying with conditions maintaining well-balanced relationship and heaven and earth.

The authoritative historical reference to Chinese medicine is the Yellow emperors Huang Ti's Classic of Internal Medicine (Nei Ching) dated 2697 B.C. which catalogues the knowledge current at his time. However, over the years the original information will have been added to. Analysis of style of the text available now indicates that the present text was written approximately at 1000 B.C.

The Nei Ching is a Chinese philosophical compendium on preventative medicine. It is not a medical textbook in the modern sense. It quotes the old sages [4] as saying that "they will not treat those who were already ill; they instructed those who were not ill".

Tao, which means "the way", expresses itself in the human body through the opposing concepts of Yin and Yang, which need to be kept in balance for good health and longevity. Diagnosis and treatment is based on a structured system around the five viscera, five elements as well as the seasons. Severe pain ensues when the spirit is hurt [4].

Acupuncture was introduced as a technique that can control the flow of vital forces including Yin and Yang.

It is surprising that surgical techniques do not figure highly in the Nei Ching. For this, Veith [4] gives two reasons. Firstly, the very high esteem for Chinese internal medicine hindered the development of surgery. Secondly, because of the Confucian tenet of the sacredness of the human body surgery appeared an inappropriate form of treatment.

However, two surgeons Pien Ch'iao and Hua T'o achieved prominence around 190 A.D. [4]. Apart from excellent surgical skills their success was based on the introduction of effective anaesthesia. All Hua T'o's records were unfortunately burned, and no record exists today of either his or Pien's methods of pain control.

Four Sanskrit Vedas (Rigveda, Samaveda, Yajurveda and Atharvaveda) date back to between 4500 and 1600 B.C. [5]. They form the basis of the Indian Ayurveda medical practice.

The Egyptian compendium of medicine, the Ebers Papyrus [6] was written about 1500 B.C. and refers back to data collected as early as 3500 B.C.

Historic approaches to medicine and by implication pain management were often holistic in one way or another. They went beyond solely targeting the assumed somatic mechanism. Treatment of the assumed pathology was complemented by a psychological or spiritual component. Plato [7] succinctly expressed this as follows "For this is the greatest error of our day; in the treatment of the human body the physicians first separate the soul from the body".

During Antiquity important strives were made in the development of medicine. The Hippocratic collection [1], mostly written between 430 and 380 B.C. is a collection of medical knowledge and thought available at that time. It drew both on practices at the Cosian as well as Cnidian school. Although it subscribed to the concept of humorism (black bile, yellow bile, phlegm and blood), it introduced the concept of rationalization in medicine. Hippocrates furthermore postulated the separation of medical doctrine from philosophy. At his time, medical doctrines were most or part based on philosophy about nature's origin and composition. Pain itself had no utility, but nevertheless needed to be controlled.

In the text of Epidermis V it is recommended to match like with like. One pain may calm another simultaneous one, anticipating the diffuse non-specific inhibitory control (DNIC) described by Le Bar in 1979 [8].

For gynaecological pains, the use of mandrake, a nightshade and poppy is recommended.

Alexandria with its large library was a centre for medical research in the third century B.C. Eristrasus [1] described motor and sensory nerves using vivisection on criminals, which was later forbidden by the authorities.

Roman medicine was built on the foundation of Greek knowledge and experience. In his book De Re Medicinae written about 30 A.D., Celsus [9] who was probably not a doctor himself, stated that pain was mainly useful for prognostic purposes, and that seasonal aspects, different periods in life, individual temperament and gender were important factors affecting the presentation of pain. Pain itself had no conceivable positive value. In terms of medical methodology, he discriminated between *diagnosticians* who tried to understand the pathophysiology of a condition, *empiricists* who relied on their clinical experience and *methodists* who were relying on common traits evident between specific disorders.

The most prominent physician during Roman times living in the second century was Galen [vide ref 1] a real celebrity physician. The emperors Marcus Aurelius, Commodus and Septimius Severus were among his patients. He published some 500 titles. For him, pain was important as a symptom to be treated, but also helpful for the understanding of the pathophysiology and prognosis of a condition. Dissection was for him an important tool for the understanding of underlying mechanisms of a disease. Pain was regarded as excessive mechanical stimulation in analogy to excessive brightness harming vision and sound that is too loud damaging hearing. Galen's pathophysiological model about good health depending on balance between black bile, yellow bile, phlegm and blood was finally abandoned only during the nineteenth century.

Galen's writings, the Hippocratic corpus and De Materia Medica by Dioscorides [10] have remained required reading for doctors until the mid-nineteenth century. The Materia Medica is a compendium of 800 plants described to very high botanical standards. Side effects and efficacy are described in detailed terms. The book mentions opium poppy, field poppy, lettuce, belladonna, hyoscine and black nightshade for pain control.

As part of these developments, herbal medicine advanced on an empirical basis with the detailed Materia Medica by Dioscorides surviving [10]. Willow bark as an analgesic reminds us that the first known non-steroidal anti-inflammatory has been in use for a very long time.

During medieval times in Europe, the understanding of medical matters was strongly interwoven with religious thought.

The concept of pain as punishment by God for the original sin or other sins often entailed that pain had to be endured. Consequently, there was little advance in pain management during this time. The power of a strong faith in controlling the sensation of pain is well documented by the absence of signs of suffering in artwork of the time depicting torture of saints.

Many of the Greek manuscripts only survived in Arabic translation.

With the advent of the age of Enlightenment in Europe, modern scientific method established itself gradually, and has since remained the driving force for development.

Based on anatomical knowledge, Descartes [11] proposed a dualistic system for the perception of pain that separated the sensing of pain from its emotive component. This deviated from the holistic approach towards pain management that had prevailed hitherto. The impact of his model of pain perception on the one hand had a stimulating effect on further scientific research. On the other hand, it engendered a somewhat mechanistic approach towards perception and control of pain, which has only been overcome recently with the introduction of cognitive behavioural treatment into pain management and more recently with the emphasis on mindfulness. It is significant that early modern pain centres often called themselves pain relief clinics. Unfortunately, pain relief is not always attainable in chronic pain conditions. Most pain clinics have since redefined themselves as pain management establishments.

In conclusion, over the centuries and millennia pain management has been shaped by the prevailing understanding of the underlying mechanisms as well as by culture and religion.

During the middle ages, between 500 and 1500 A.D., the concepts about the meaning and control of pain understanding of pain diverged between Europe on one side and Arabia and Persia on the other. The latter two areas became centres of high learning, building on the knowledge of Greek and Roman experts and translations of their writings.

In Europe, the largely scholastic approach towards medicine precluded any further development in the understanding of the physiology of pain. In addition, religion had a profound effect on the appreciation and contemporary meaning of pain. Either as a divine punishment by God or as redemption by suffering in a way Christ did were probably important ways to accept pain as deserving. Pain was sanctified, because it brought sufferers closer to the pain experienced by Christ [1]. For non-believers this type of reasoning is difficult to agree with. Indirectly, the religious understanding of pain amplified the inhibition of development inherent in the scholastic approach.

Renaissance and the age of enlightenment brought a change towards a more scientific approach towards medicine and biology.

In 1586 Fernel [vide Rey 1] applied Galen's concept of overstimulation to the understanding of pain. He introduced tissue damage as the common denominator for the sensation of pain. However, perception of pain was only caused by the subsequent appreciation of the injury.

During the middle of the seventeenth century, Descartes developed the dualistic system of sensory perception [12]. He accepted phantom limb pain in an arm amputee as a real phenomenon and not as an aberration of the mind. His model of nervous conduction was that of a mechanical pulley, which could be tugged at any position on its course to the brain. Interpretation of the message took place in the soul, which was supposed to reside in the pineal gland.

During the eighteenth and nineteenth century, although not universally accepted, views were held that the sentience for pain was a function of the perceived level of civilization as well as cultural and intellectual development of an individual. It was this type of thinking that led to the appalling conditions associated with slavery [13].

During the nineteenth century, there were major advances in anaesthesia and analgesia. In parallel, hypotheses and theories and factual observations about the organization of the pain pathway became increasingly detailed. Perl has provided a comprehensive time line of the development during the nineteenth and twentieth centuries [14].

Based on the study of cross-sectional spinal lesions in patients, Brown-Sequard [15] established the contralateral anterolateral tract in man as essential for the transmission of nociceptive information.

Anatomically, Edinger [16] identified the spinothalamic tract in 1890.

At the beginning of the nineteenth century Johannes Mueller [17] developed the concept of specific peripheral receptors for each individual sense, a concept previously held by Avicenna. Muellers law of "law of specific nerve energies" stated that there were specific receptors for each of the senses. However, he attributed their sensitivity to unique Vitalism based qualities of energy in the afferent nerve fibres. He came to this conclusion, because specific sensory experiences could be elicited by non-physiological excitation with electrical stimuli or, e.g., excessive pressure on the eyeball. It was Adrian's discovery of the action potential as the uniform mode of nervous conduction which disproved the hypothesis of a unique sense specific to nervous energy in primary afferent fibres.

On the basis of finely discriminating sensory testing of the skin in combination with histological investigations, von Frey [18] developed the specificity hypothesis of the senses. The test of this theory ultimately depended on electrophysiological primary afferent and postsynaptic single unit recordings. Initially only few nociceptor primary afferents were identified by Zottermann [19] the A delta fibres and by Iggo [20] among C-fibres.

During the nineteenth and twentieth century, several hypotheses were proposed discussing the issue whether pain is a specific or non-specific sensation gaining its unique properties not on the basis of specific receptors in the periphery, but solely by central nervous processing.

The debate became even more intense after it became possible to record from single postsynaptic cells in the spinal cord. Initially, only wide dynamic range units were encountered, receiving excitatory input from a wide range of nociceptive as well as non-nociceptive primary afferents. It was not clear, how the nervous system could disentangle such messages. On the basis of the electrophysiological evidence available in 1965, Melzack and Wall [21] developed the gate theory, postulating that the gate to the perception of pain was opened by discharge in primary afferent C-fibres and that it was under control of descending and segmental modulation.

Since then electrophysiological recording techniques have improved. A large proportion of primary afferent C-fibres does not subserve nociception [22], however, many do. Postsynaptically, there are neurones solely responsive to noxious stimuli [23].

In 1897, Sherrington [24] introduced the concept of the synapse into neurophysiology, allowing for modulation of information along the pathway from the periphery to the brain. The concept of integration along sensory pathways from the periphery to the ultimate termination in the brain was a considerable advancement on Descartes' "bell pulley" mechanism eliciting the sensation of pain in the soul. It was also more specific than the forces of vitalism to which Mueller still subscribed. In modern medicine, artificial activation of segmental and descending inhibition is activated by transcutaneous nerve stimulators, acupuncture, spinal cord stimulators and peripheral nerve stimulators.

Mersky's 1979 [25] definition of "Pain as an unpleasant sensory and emotional experience associated with actual or potential tissue damage, or described in terms of such damage" was adopted by the International Association for the study of pain. This definition clearly differentiates between the perceived sensory event and its emotional impact.

Until sometime during the nineteenth century, Western clinicians still discriminated between personality types on the basis of the Hippocratic philosophy of the predominant effect of one of the four humours (phlegm, black bile, yellow bile and blood). According to this classification, there were phlegmatics, cholerics, melancholics and sanguins. Pain was experienced according to one's type of personality.

Since the nineteenth century, in parallel with sensory neurophysiology, clinical and behavioural observations have served as influential tools investigating the whole breadth of pain perception as outlined in Mersky's definition.

Clinical and behavioural hypotheses and theories were reported in depth by Bourke [13]. Observations by Leriche [vide 13] during World War 1 and Beecher [26] during World War 2 described substantial injuries being sustained by soldiers without any pain being reported.

Among civilians, pain sentience was said to depend on race, personal characteristics or traits shared by individuals grouped according to class or occupation [13]. Phrenology was also of some importance. Organs of destructiveness, and an organ for fighting were supposedly identified, the location of these centres can still be found in phrenology maps sometimes sold in curiosity shops.

Whilst much of this evidence is anecdotal or of prejudicial nature, it points towards differences between individuals in central nervous processing of painful events. In other words, it became clear that there must be modulation on the passage of messages along the pain pathway.

During the second half of the twentieth century, psychological techniques of pain management became increasingly Important. In the first wave, operant conditioning based on the concept of Pavlovian reflexes were tried for a variety of medical conditions. The second wave in the form of cognitive behavioural treatment (CBT) was introduced to many pain management establishments. Courses were either residential or on an out- patient basis. They consisted of a combination between explanations of the current medical understanding of patient's pain conditions, reduction in medication and fitness training, often resulting in improvement in quality of life that mattered. More recently, the third phase has become widely accepted in the form of mindfulness training Kabat-Zinn [27], which is in essence a form of meditation without the teachings of Buddhism.

References

1. Rey R. History of pain. Paris: Editions La Decouverte; 1993. p. 11. ISBN 2-7071-2256-4, Ibid pp. 26–32, Ibid pp. 32–35, Ibid pp. 60–66, Ibid p. 72, ref 27.
2. Thompson. Proc. Roy. Soc. Med. Sect. Hist. Med. 1926;19:69–78. Quoted from Sigchrist HE. Primitive and archaic medicine. Oxford Univ. Press; 1967.
3. Ebers G. The Papyrus Ebers: translated from the German version by Cyril P. Brian. London: Geoffrey Bles; 1930. p. 24–30.
4. Veith I. The Yellow Emperor's classic of internal medicine. Berkeley: University of California Press; 1970. p. 2–3. ISBN 0-520-01296-8, p.53, Ibid p 117, Ibid p 3, Ibid.
5. Mishra LC. Scientific basis for Ayurvedic therapies. Boca Raton: CRC Press; 2004. 0-8493-1366-X. Introduction.
6. The Ebers Papyrus (trans: Ryan CP). Letchworth: The Garden City Press LTD; 1930. Royal Soc Med.
7. Stempsey WE. Plato and holistic medicine. Med Health Care Philos. 2001;4(2):201–9.
8. Le Bars D, Dickenson AH, Besson JM. Diffuse noxious inhibitory controls (DNIC). I. Effects on dorsal horn convergent neurones in the rat. Pain. 1979;6:283–304.
9. Celsus De Re Medicinae AD. 30 (quoted from Douglas Guthrie. Edinburgh: Thomas Nelson and Sons LTD; 1958. p. 72–75). Ibid pp. 74–82.
10. De Materia Medica D. Being an herbal with many other medicinal materials (trans: Osbaldeston TA). Johannesburg: Ibidis Press; 2000.
11. Descartes R. Dioptrique, Discourse Quatrieme. In: Oevres et lettres. Paris, Gallimard; 1637. [La Pleiade (1953) p. 203].
12. Descartes R. Principia Philosophica. Amsterdam: Lois Elzevir; 1644.
13. Bourke J. The story of pain. Oxford: Oxford University Press; 2014. p. 195. ISBN978-0-19-96843-9. Ibid pp. 193–268, Ibid p. 224, Ibid. p. 209.

14. Perl E. Ideas about pain, a historical view. Nat Rev Neurosci. 2007;8:71–80.
15. Brown-Sequard CE. Course of lectures on the physiology and pathology of the central nervous system. Philadelphia: Collins; 1860.
16. Edinger L. Zwolf Vorlesungen uber den Bau der Nervosen Centralorgane Fur Arzte and Studierende. Leipzig: F.C.W. Vogel; 1892. p. 150–3.
17. Müller J. Handbuch der Physiologie des Menschen fur Vorlesungen, vol. 2. Coblenz: Verlag von J. Holscher; 1837–1840.
18. von Frey M. Beitrage zur Sinnesphysiologie der Haut. Dritte Mitteilung, Konigl Sachs Ges Wiss Math Phys, Classe 48; 1895. p. 166–184.
19. Zottermann Y. Touch Pain and Tickling and electrophysiological investigation on cutaneous sensory nerves. J Physiol. 1939;95:1–28.
20. Iggo A. Cutaneous heat and cold receptors with slowly conducting © afferent fibres. Quart J Exp Physiol. 1959;44:362–70.
21. Melzack R, Wall PD. Pain mechanisms a new theory. Science. 1965;150:971–9.
22. Walker SC, Trotter PD, Swaney WT, Marshall A, Mcglone FP. C-tactile afferents: cutaneous mediators of oxytocin release during affiliative tactile interactions? Neuropeptides. 2017;64:27–38.
23. Christensen BN, Perl ER. Spinal neurons specifically excited noxious or thermal stimuli: marginal zone of the dorsal horn. J Neurophysiol. 1970;33:293–307.
24. Sherrington CS. The integrative action of the nervous system. New York: Charles Scribner's Sons; 1906.
25. Mersky H, Bogduk N. Classification of chronic pain. Seattle: IASP Press; 1994.
26. Beecher HK. Pain in man wounded in battle. Ann Surg. 1946;123(1):96–105.
27. Kabat-Zinn J. Mindfulness with Jon Kabat-Zinn. 2007. YouTube. https://www.youtube.com/watch?v=3nwwKbM_vJc.

Chapter 2
Theories of Pain

Koki Shimoji and Yoshiyuki Yokota

2.1 Specificity Theory

Specific theory of pain states that each modality of sense, touch or pain, is encoded in separate pathways. For instance, touch and pain stimuli are received by specialized sense organs. Impulses of each sensory modality are conducted along the distinct pathways and projected to the touch and pain centers in the brain, respectively. Thus, its fundamental thought is that each sense of modality has a specific receptor and associated sensory fiber sensitive to only one specific stimulus [1].

Aelius Galen, a prominent Greek physician, demonstrated that spinal cord section caused sensory (including pain) as well as motor deficits cited by Ochs [2, 3]. Vesalius, Belgium anatomist, in the middle of seventeenth century, also confirmed the findings by Galen [2, 3].

Descartes was believed to be the first philosopher who described the hypothesis on pain pathway in man in 1662 (Fig. 2.1). He described pain as a perception that exists in the brain and is distinct difference between neuronal phenomenon of sensory transduction and the perception of pain. Descartes perceived the nerves as hollow tubules that conduct both sensory and motor activities.

Descartes claimed that the heat of flame near the foot activates a fiber within the nerve tubule that travels up to the leg, to the spinal cord, and finally to the brain center. Descartes postulated proverbial bells which are the pores lining along the cord and brain ventricles. When pores open in response to the sensory stimulus "the

K. Shimoji (✉)
Niigata University Graduate School of Medicine, Niigata, Japan

Pain Control Institute, Tokyo, Japan
e-mail: koki-shimoji@nifty.com

Y. Yokota
Department of Anesthesiology, Ariake Hospital, Cancer Foundation, Koto City, Japan
e-mail: yokota@jfcr.or.jp

K. Shimoji et al. (eds.), *Chronic Pain Management in General and Hospital Practice*, https://doi.org/10.1007/978-981-15-2933-7_2

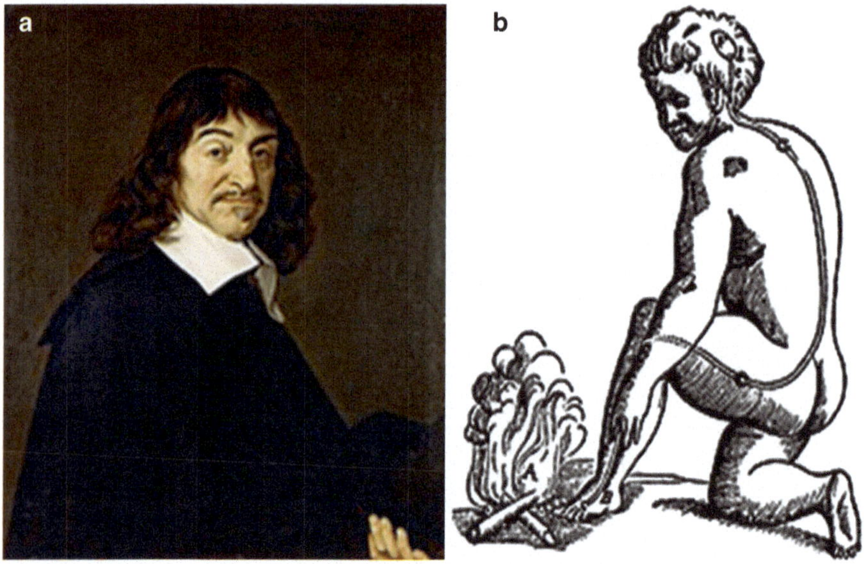

Fig. 2.1 (**a**) Portrait of René Descartes (**b**) Descartes' pain pathway: "Particles of heat" (A) activate a spot of skin (B) attached by a fine thread (cc) to a valve in the brain (de) where this activity opens the valve, allowing the animal spirits to flow from a cavity (F) into the muscles causing them to flinch from the stimulus, turn the head and eyes toward the affected body part, and move the hand and turn the body protectively [2, 3]. [Descartes et al. (1664), out of copyright; translated by M. Moayedi]

animal spirits" were thought to flow through the tubule and elicit the motor responses.

Like turning the head and eyes to recognize the flame, raising the hands and moving the body away from the flame occur to protect from burn (Fig. 2.1).

Modern concept of pain pathway was described by Bell and Shaw in 1868 [4]. They postulated that the brain is not the common sensorium as suggested by Descartes, but the brain is a heterogeneous structure as suggested by Willis in the seventeenth century [5, 6]. They suggested that nerves are constructed by heterogeneous neurons playing specialized functions. Thus, Bell and Shaw believed that different sensory neurons play for different types of motor neurons and "vital neurons" that are connected to the mind rather than the brain.

Thus, fundamental idea of specific theory of pain suggests that a pathway specific to pain exists (Fig. 2.2).

Bernard and Magendie in 1856 [7] reiterated Bell's findings and described the motor and sensory nerves having separate paths to and from the spinal cord (cited by Stahnisch [8].

The discovery of cutaneous touch receptors, such as Pacinian corpuscles [9], Meissner's corpuscles [10], Merkel's discs [11], and Ruffini's end-organs [12] gave further evidence that each specific sense is encoded by specific nerve fibers (cited by Ochs) [2, 3]. However, a specific end organ dedicated to pain sense had not yet been found.

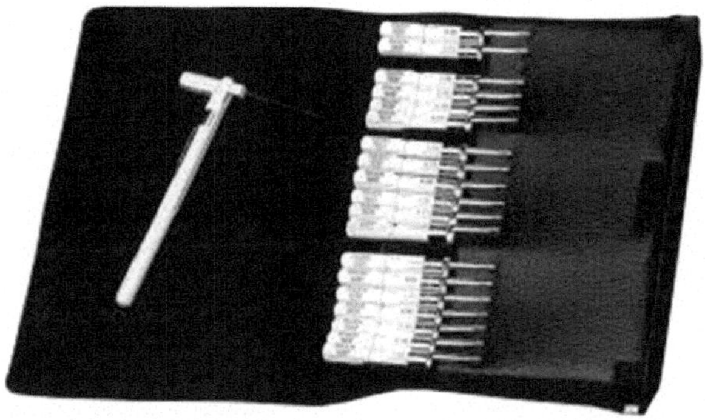

Fig. 2.2 A set of von Frey hair, a type of esthesiometer designed in 1896 by Maximilian von Frey. Von Frey filaments rely on the principle that an elastic column, in compression, will buckle elastically at a specific force, dependent on the length, diameter, and modulus of the material. Once buckled, the force imparted by the column is fairly constant, irrespective of the degree of buckling. The filaments may therefore be used to provide a range of forces to the skin of a test subject, in order to find the force at which the subject reacts because the sensation is painful. This type of test is called a mechanical nociceptive threshold test. Sets of filaments are normally made of nylon hairs, all the same length, but of varying diameter so as to provide a range of forces, typically from 0.008 g force up to 300 g force. Von Frey filaments are, therefore a diagnostic, research, and screening tool, used both in human and animal medicine

On the other hand, there were arguments that pain was different from other senses in the way that it causes unpleasantness [13, 14].

Further evidence of specific theory was reflected on Charles-Edouard Brown-Sequard's observations that sensory fibers decussate in the spinal cord [14–16]. Further, Schiff and Woroschiroff established the presence of two pathways by observations of effect of incisions at different levels of the spinal cord, anterolateral pathway for pain and temperature and the posterior bundles for tactile sense (cited by Ray) [5]. Goldscheider in1894 reported the sensory spots which elicit a specific sense such as warmth, cold, pressure, or pain, and supported the specific theory [5, 16, 17].

Max von Frey further advanced the specific theory by carrying out the experiments by developing the well-known von Frey's hairs to measure the pressure required to elicit a sensation at each skin spot identified by Blix and Goldscheider (cited by Forster and Handwerker) [18] (Fig. 2.2). Von Frey found that the distribution of pressure points was related to the distribution of Meissner's corpuscles, whereas the pain points were related to the distribution of the free nerve endings in the skin (Fig. 2.3).

Although Sherrington [19] supported the specificity theory addressed by von Frey, he also found that the behaviors of animals showed the temporal and spatial pattern of activity resulting from these four specific neurons demonstrated by von Frey. Burgess and Perl [20] discovered the primary afferent fibers that responded only to noxious mechanical stimulations, and then Besson and Perl [21] discovered nociceptive unmyelinated afferent fibers, polymodal nociceptors, and high-threshold mechanoreceptors.

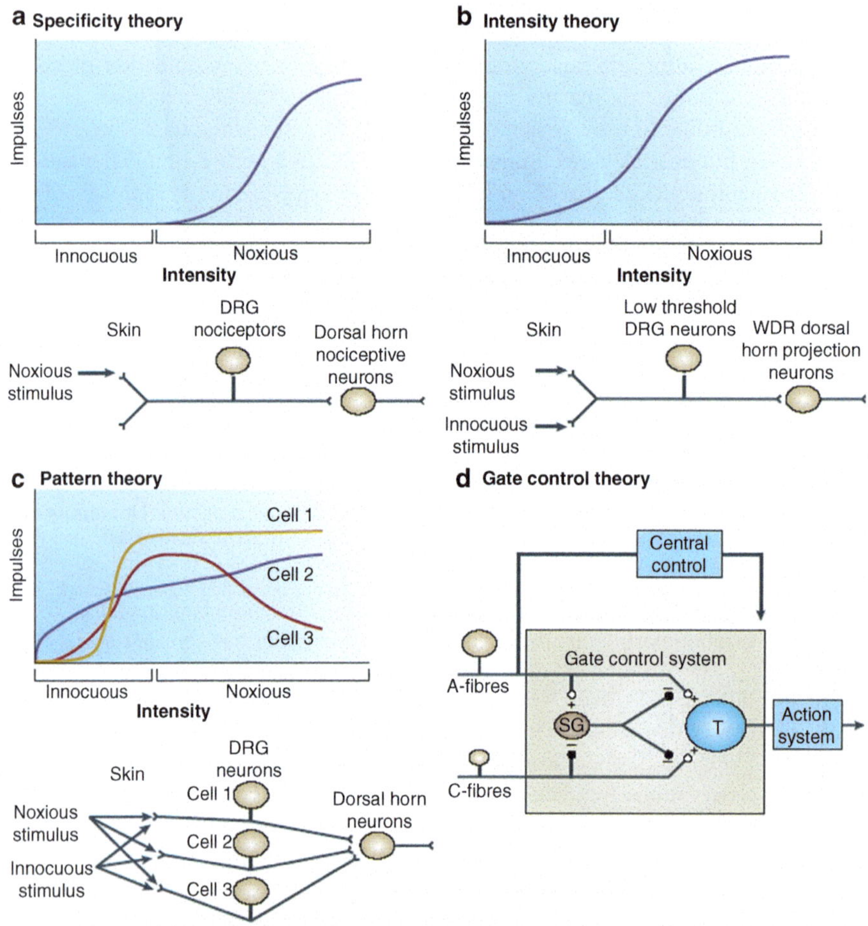

Fig. 2.3 Schematic diagrams of pain theories. (**a**) Based on the Specificity Theory of Pain; each modality (touch and pain) is encoded in separate pathways. Touch and pain stimuli are encoded by specialized sense organs. Impulses for each modality are transmitted along distinct pathways, which project to touch and pain centers in the brain, respectively. DRG, dorsal root ganglion. (**b**) based on the Intensity Theory of Pain; there are no distinct pathways for low- and high-threshold stimuli. Rather, the number of impulses in neurons determines the intensity of a stimulus. The primary afferent neurons synapse onto wide-dynamic range (WDR) second-order neurons in the dorsal horn of the spinal cord, where low levels of activity encode innocuous stimuli, and higher levels of activity encode noxious stimuli. (**c**) The Pattern Theory of Pain posits that somatic sense organs respond to a dynamic range of stimulus intensities. Different sense organs have different levels of responsivity to stimuli. A population code or the pattern of activity of different neurons encodes the modality and location of the stimulus. (**d**) The Gate Control Theory of Pain proposes that both large (A-fibers) and small (C-fibers) synapse onto cells in the substantia gelatinosa (SG) and the first central transmission (T) cells. The inhibitory effect exerted by SG cells onto the primary afferent fiber terminals at the T cells is increased by activity in A-fibers and decreased by activity in C-fibers. The central control trigger is represented by a line running from the A-fiber system to the central control mechanisms; these mechanisms, in turn, project back to the Gate Control system. The T cells project to the entry cells of the action system. +, excitation; –, inhibition. (Figure is reproduced with permission from Dr. Perl ER: Ideas about pain, a historical view, Nature Reviews Neuroscience, 2007)

Recently, Hu et al. reported that chronic post-surgical pain is related to the hepatocyte growth factor [22]. This report may support in part the specific theory in terms of gene encoding.

2.2 Intensity Theory

On the other hand, intensity theory of pain claims that there are no distinct pathways for touch or pain perception. The theory defines pain not as a unique sensory experience but as an emotion that occurs when stimulus is too strong.

Erasmus Darwin supported the idea advanced in Plato's *Timaeus* that pain is not a unique sensory modality, but an emotional state produced by stronger than normal stimuli such as intense light, pressure, or temperature [23]. Wilhelm Erb, a German neurologist also argued in 1874 that pain can be generated by any sensory stimulus, provided it is intense enough, and his formulation of the hypothesis became known as the intensive theory (cited by Moayedi and Davis, and Jost) [6, 23].

Naunyn in 1889 [24] found that repeated innocuous stimulations including electrical stimulations produced unbearable pain in patients with syphilis, and concluded that some form of summation occurs in these pathological conditions.

William Kenneth Livingston advanced a summation theory in 1943, proposing that high intensity signals, arriving at the spinal cord from damage to nerve or tissue, set up a reverberating, self-exciting loop of activity in a pool of interneurons, and once a threshold of activity is crossed, these interneurons then activate "transmission" cells which carry the signal to the brain's pain mechanism; that the reverberating interneuron activity also spreads to spinal cord cells that trigger a sympathetic nervous system and somatic motor system response; and these responses, as well as fear and other emotions elicited by pain, feed into and perpetuate the reverberating interneuron activity (cited by Moayedi and Davis [6].

Thus, the number of impulses of other neurons determines the intensity of stimuli. The primary afferent neurons synapse onto the wide-dynamic range second neurons (WDR) in the dorsal horn of the spinal cord.

The low threshold or low intensity impulses encode innocuous stimuli, whereas high levels of impulses encode noxious or pain stimuli (Fig. 2.3b) [6].

2.3 Pattern Theory

Pattern theory of pain postulates that sense organs respond to wide and dynamic range of stimuli. Different sense organs have different levels for responsivity to stimuli. The pattern of activity of different neurons encodes the modality and location of the stimuli. (Fig. 2.3c).

Pattern theory proposes that there is no separate system for perceiving pain, and the receptors for pain are shared with other senses, such as of touch. This theory considers that peripheral sensory receptors, responding to touch, warmth, and other non-damaging as well as to damaging stimuli, give rise to non-painful or painful experiences as a result of differences in the patterns and in time of the signals sent through the nervous system [6].

Thus, according to this theory, people feel pain when certain patterns of neural activity occur, such as when appropriate types of activity reach excessively high levels in the brain. These patterns occur only with intense stimulation. Because strong and mild stimuli of the same sense modality produce different patterns of neural activity, being hit hard feels painful, but being caressed does not. It suggested that all cutaneous qualities are produced by spatial and temporal patterns of nerve impulses rather than by separate, modality specific transmission routes.

Central summation theory by Livingstone [25], the fourth theory of pain [26], and sensory interaction theory [27] might be all involved in this category [6].

Central summation theory proposed that the intense stimulation resulting from the nerve and tissue damage activates fibers that project to internuncial neuron pools within the spinal cord creating abnormal reverberating circuits with self-activating neurons. Prolonged abnormal activity bombards cells in the spinal cord, and information is projected to the brain for pain perception.

The fourth theory of pain stated that pain was composed of two components: the perception of pain and the reaction one has towards it. The reaction was described as a complex physiopsychological process involving cognition, past experience, culture, and various psychological factors which influence pain perception.

Sensory interaction theory describes two systems involving transmission of pain: fast and slow system. The latter presumed to conduct somatic and visceral afferents whereas the former was considered to inhibit transmission of the small fibers [5, 6, 28].

2.4 Gate Control Theory

Melzack and Wall in 1965 [29] proposed a new theory, gate control theory of pain, which supported in part both specificity and pattern theories of pain.

The gate control theory of pain proposes that large A-fibers and small C-fibers synapse onto the substance gelatinosa cells (SG cells) and the first central transmission cells (T cells) in the dorsal horn of the spinal cord. Their model proposed that the signals in the primary afferents by stimulation of skin were transmitted to the three regions in the spinal cord, (1) the substance gelatinosa (SG), (2) the dorsal column, (3) a groups of cells which they called transmission cells (Fig. 2.3d). They proposed that the gate in the spinal cord situates in the SG which modulates the sensory transmission of sensory information from the primary afferent neurons to transmission cells (T cells) in the cord. This gating mechanism is controlled by activity of both large and small fibers. Large fiber activity inhibits (or closes) the gate, whereas small fiber activity facilitates (opens) the gate. Activity from descending fibers from supraspinal structures could also modulate this gate. The inhibitory activity exerted by the SG cells on to the primary afferent fiber terminals (both A-fibers and C-fibers) which synapse onto the T cells is increased by activity of A-fibers and decreased by activity of C-fibers. The inhibitory activity exerted by the SG cells or other interneurons onto the primary afferent terminals can be recorded as primary afferent depolarization (PAD) from the dorsal part of the spinal cord in animals [30] and even in human [31]. The T cells enter to the action system of central nervous system (CNS) including brain, and the impulses from A-fibers also activate the CNS where, in turn, impulses project back to the gate control system. Thus, the gate control theory in fact may help to reconcile the differences between the specificity and pattern theories of pain (Fig. 2.3d).

2.5 Consideration for Chronic Pain

Although the specificity theory appropriately described sensory receptors which respond only to suprathreshold stimuli, there have been no neurons in the brain which respond to both non-nociceptive and nociceptive stimuli such as wide-dynamic range neurons (WDR neurons). Although WDR neurons are well documented, their detailed functions in pain perception have to be determined.

Thus, none of these theories adequately explains the complexity of the pain system. Further, these theories focus on cutaneous pain but do not address deep-tissue, visceral, or muscular pains. Additionally, these models are focused on acute pain and may not explain mechanisms of persistent pain or chronic pain. Although the mechanisms of persistent and chronic pain are still not fully understood, it is now clear that peripheral and central plasticity can develop following repeated nociceptive stimulation even in healthy subjects [32] and in chronic pain [33]. Recent work has also demonstrated that plasticity is not only limited to changes in neurons but can also involve changes in glial cells [34]. Glial cells are thought to be related to the maintenance of persistent and chronic pain [35].

For instance, underlying mechanisms of complex regional pain syndrome (CRPS) are so complex, involving significant autonomic features. Both peripheral and central nervous system mechanisms are involved for its etiology. These include peripheral and central sensitization, inflammation, altered sympathetic and catecholaminergic function, altered somatosensory representation in the brain, genetic factors, and psychophysiological interactions [36]. Relative contributions of the mechanisms underlying CRPS may even differ across patients and even within a patient over time, particularly in the transition from "acute CRPS" to "chronic CRPS." Recently, even sex differences have been advocated in pathogenesis for development of CRPS [37]. Although nociceptive hypersensitivity in CRPS has been studied in different pain models, the underlying molecular and cellular mechanisms remain elusive.

Although there have been a variety of treatments with demonstrated effectiveness for the management of CRPS, pain clinicians are unsure what treatments would be most effective for individual clients [38].

Enhanced knowledge regarding the pathophysiology of CRPS increases the possibility of eventually achieving the goal of mechanism-based CRPS diagnosis and treatment [39].

References

1. Dubner R, Sessle BJ, Storey AT. The neural basis of oral and facial function. New York: Plenum; 1978.
2. Descartes R. De Homine Figuris et Latinitate Donatus a Florentio Schuyl. Leiden: Franciscum Moyardum & Petrum Leffen; 1662.
3. Ochs S. A history of nerve functions: from animal spirits to molecular mechanisms. Cambridge: Cambridge University Press; 2004.
4. Bell C, Shaw A. Reprint of the "idea of a new anatomy of the brain," with letters, & c. J Anat Physiol. 1868;3:147–82.
5. Rey R. The history of pain. Cambridge: Harvard University Press; 1995.
6. Moayedi M, Davis KD. Theories of pain: from specificity to gate control. J Neurophysiol. 2013;109:5–12.
7. Bernard C, Magendie F. Leçon d'ouverture du Cours de Médecine du Collège de France. Paris: Baillière; 1856.
8. Stahnisch FW. Francois Magendie (1783–1855). J Neurol. 2009;256:1950–2.
9. Pacini F. Sopra un Particolar Genere di Piccoli Corpi Globulosi Scoperti Nel Corpo Umano da Filippo Pacini Alunno Interno Degli Spedali Riunti di Pistoia. (Letter to Accademia Medico-Fisica di Firenze.); 1835.
10. Meissner G. Beitraege zur Anatomie und Physiologie der Haut. Leipzig: Leopold Voss; 1853.
11. Merkel F. Tastzellen und Tastkörperchen bei den Hausthieren und beim Menschen. Arch Mikr Anat EntwMech. 1875;11:636–52.
12. Ruffini A. Sur un nouvel organe nerveux terminal et sur la presence des corpuscules Golgi-Mazzoni dens le conjonctif souscutané de la pulpe des doigts de l'homme. Mémoires de l'Academie Royale. Roma: LAccademia Nazionale dei Lincei Lincei; 1893. p. 249–65.
13. Boring EG. Sensation and perception in the history of experimental psychology. New York: D. Appleton-Century; 1942.
14. Dallenbach KM. Pain: history and present status. Am J Psychol. 1939;52:331–47.
15. Aminoff MJ. Historical perspective Brown-Sequard and his work on the spinal cord. Spine (Phila Pa 1976). 1996;21:133–40.
16. Goldscheider A. Ueber den Schmerz in Physiologischer und Klinischer Hinsicht: Nach einem Vortrage in der Berliner Militärärztlichen Gesellschaft. Ann Arbor: University of Michigan Library; 1894.
17. Norrsell U, Finger S, Lajonchere C. Cutaneous sensory spots and the "law of specific nerve energies": history and development of ideas. Brain Res Bull. 1999;15(48):457–65.
18. Forster C, Handwerker HO. Central nervous processing of itch and pain. In: Carstens E, Akiyama T, editors. Itch: mechanisms and treatment. Boca Raton: CRC Press/Taylor & Francis; 2014. Chapter 24.
19. Sherrington CS. The integrative action of the nervous system. Cambridge: Cambridge University Press; 1947.
20. Burgess PR, Perl ER. Myelinated afferent fibres responding specifically to noxious stimulation of the skin. J Physiol. 1967;190:541–62.

21. Bessou P, Perl ER. Response of cutaneous sensory units with unmyelinated fibers to noxious stimuli. J Neurophysiol. 1969;32:1025–43.
22. Hu C, Lu Y, Chen X, Wu Z, Zhang Q. Gene transfer of a naked plasmid (pUDK-HGF) encoding human hepatocyte growth factor attenuates skin/muscle incision and retraction-induced chronic post-surgical pain in rats. Eur J Pain. 2018;22(5):961–72.
23. Jost WH. A tribute to Wilhelm H. Erb. J Neurol. 2006;253(Suppl 1):I1–2.
24. Naunyn B. Ueber die Auslösung von Schmerzempfindung durch Summation sich zeitlich folgender sensibler Erregungen. Naunyn Schmiedeberg's Arch Pharmacol. 1889;25:272–305. Access Volume 45, Issue 1 January 2001, pp. 134–135
25. Livingston WK. In: Fields HL, editor. Pain and suffering. Seattle: IASP Press; 1998. p. xvii, 250.
26. Noordenbos W. On the specificity of sensory events. Psichiatr Neurol Neurochir. 1960;63: 298–306.
27. Hardy JD, Wolf HG, Goodell H. Studies on pain. A new method for measuring pain threshold: observations of spatial summation of pain. J Clin Invest. 1940;19:649–57.
28. Perl ER. Ideas about pain, a historical view. Nat Rev Neurosci. 2007;8:71–80.
29. Melzack R, Wall PD. Pain mechanisms: a new theory. Science. 1965;150:971–9.
30. Lidierth M, Wall PD. Dorsal horn cells connected to the Lissauer tract and their relation to the dorsal root potential in the rat. J Neurophysiol. 1998;80:667–79.
31. Shimoji K, Higashi H, Kano T. Epidural recording of spinal electrogram in man. Electroencephalogr Clin Neurophysiol. 1971;30:236–9.
32. Bingel U, Herken W, Teutsch S, May A. Habituation to painful stimulation involves the antinociceptive system—a 1-year follow-up of 10 participants. Pain. 2008;140:393–4.
33. Davis KD, Moayedi M. Central mechanisms of pain revealed through functional and structural MRI. J Neuroimmune Pharmacol. 2013;8:518–34.
34. Eroglu C, Barres BA. Regulation of synaptic connectivity by glia. Nature. 2010;468:223–31.
35. Zhuo M, Wu G, Wu LJ. Neuronal and microglial mechanisms of neuropathic pain. Mol Brain. 2011;4:31.
36. Bäckryd E. Pain as the perception of someone: an analysis of the interface between pain medicine and philosophy. Health Care Anal. 2019;27:13–25.
37. Tang C, Li J, Tai WL, et al. Sex differences in complex regional pain syndrome type I (CRPS-I) in mice. J Pain Res. 2017;10:1811–9.
38. Packham T, Holly J. Mechanism-specific rehabilitation management of complex regional pain syndrome: proposed recommendations from evidence synthesis. J Hand Ther. 2018;31(2):238–49.
39. Bruehl S. An update on the pathophysiology of complex regional pain syndrome. Anesthesiology. 2010;113:713–25.

Chapter 3
Anatomical Physiology of Pain

Koki Shimoji and Satoshi Kurokawa

3.1 What Is Pain?

The widely accepted definition of pain was addressed by a taxonomy task force of the International Association for the Study of Pain: *Pain is an unpleasant sensory and emotional experience that is associated with actual or potential tissue damage or described in such terms* [1]. Thus, a key feature of this definition is that pain is a subjective sensation. When we observe the patients with pain, we should always be cautious about the patient's complaints modified by their own past and recent experiences to interpret and comment on what they perceive as pain, discomfort, distress, and anxiety. Training and experience in studying and observing patient's behavior are required to interpret what the patients are complaining of and how severe the patient's pain is.

3.2 Peripheral Mechanisms

Skin, muscle, bone, and other tissues have thousands of nerve endings within a single millimeter. When stimulated these nerves generate electrical signals, action potentials, which travel at various speeds along (afferents) nerve fibers to the spinal cord and brain. It can take from a few milliseconds to a few seconds for these signals to generate an experience of pain or to produce an appropriate physiological and/or behavioral response.

K. Shimoji (✉)
Niigata University Graduate School of Medicine, Niigata, Japan

Pain Control Institute, Tokyo, Japan
e-mail: koki-shimoji@nifty.com

S. Kurokawa
Department of Anesthesiology, Tokyo Women's Medical School, Tokyo, Japan
e-mail: satokuro@sea.plala.or.jp

K. Shimoji et al. (eds.), *Chronic Pain Management in General and Hospital Practice*, https://doi.org/10.1007/978-981-15-2933-7_3

Noxious stimulation is detected by nociceptors, which are located on free nerve endings of thin, myelinated (Aδ) and unmyelinated (C) nerve fibers, in various tissues.

Pain receptors, nociceptors, respond to high intensity mechanical (pricking, stretching), high intensity thermal (heat, cold), and intense chemical stimuli (K+, H+, prostaglandins, cytokines, etc.). These chemicals may be released as a result of damage to tissues by trauma, inflammation, or ischemia. Nociceptors are also stimulated and/or sensitized by chemicals released during inflammatory responses to infectious, toxic, or allergenic agents. The release or action of some of these chemicals can be reduced or stopped by common analgesic and anti-inflammatory treatments such as non-steroidal anti-inflammatory drugs (NSAIDS) and/or steroids.

When a nociceptor fiber detects a pain stimulus on the skin or in an internal organ, the pain signal is transmitted to the spinal cord and then on to the brain by neural pathways different from those of other skin sense (Fig. 3.1).

At each of the synapses along this pain pathway, several neurotransmitters are involved in carrying the nociceptive message. Two major groups are identified: classical neurotransmitters and neuropeptides [2, 3].

Examples of classical neurotransmitters include glutamate, aspartate, and serotonin. At least 20 neuropeptides involved in transmitting pain impulses have been identified, including substance P, vasoactive intestinal peptide, calcitonin gene-related peptide, somatostatin, and cholecystokinin. By contrast, ACTH, the enkephalins, a large family of peptides, exert an inhibitory effect on the descending control pathways.

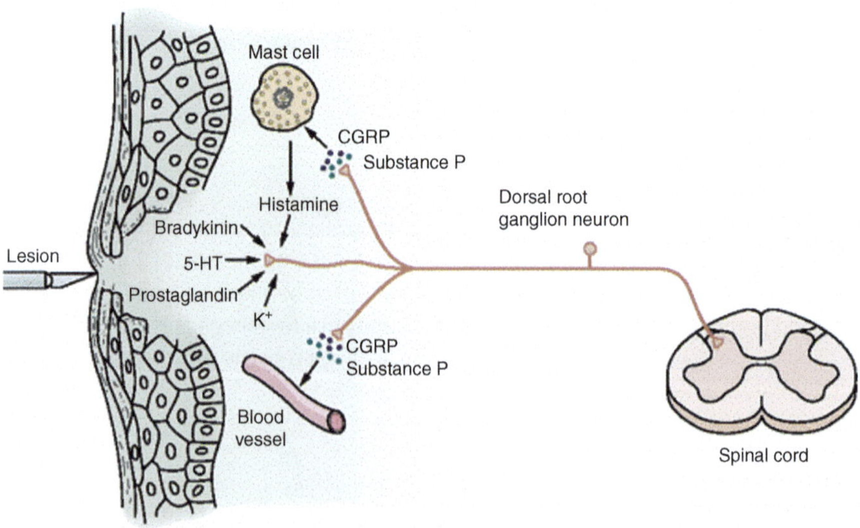

Fig. 3.1 Chemicals produced by damaged tissues and/or mast cells (K+, bradykinine,5-HT, prostaglandin, histamine, etc.) and neuropeptides (substance P, calcitonin gene-related peptide, neuropeptide-Y, etc.) are attached to the free nerve terminals to produce the signals which are sent to the spinal cord by A-delta or C fibers and then the brain through the spinal tract (Barrett KE et al.: Ganong's Review of Medical Physiology,25th Ed. www.accessmedicine.com Copyright McGraw-Hill Education)

A single nociceptive fiber can contain a variety of different peptides and neurotransmitters, and their respective roles remain largely undetermined. It is also hard to establish any correlations between the kinds of peptides that the various nociceptive pathways contain and their electrophysiological properties.

It is known, however, that glutamate and substance P are thought to be the substances most involved in the transmission of pain. For example, substance P binds to specific receptors, called neurokinine-1 (NK1) receptors, that are located on the nociceptive neurons of the dorsal horn of the spinal cord.

In general, substance P has been associated with relatively slow excitatory connections, and hence with the persistent, chronic pain sensations transmitted by C fibers, whereas glutamate is involved in the rapid neurotransmission of acute pain associated with A-delta fibers. The receptors for glutamate and substance P can be distributed in different populations of neurons that preserve their own specific characteristics. But the two types of receptors can also coexist on the same neurons, as has been observed in several different parts of the central nervous system.

3.2.1 Transduction of Pain

Transduction begins when the nociceptors of C fibers and A-delta fibers of primary afferent neurons respond to noxious stimuli. Nociceptors are exposed to noxious stimuli when tissue damage and inflammation occurs as a result of trauma, surgery, inflammation, infection, and/or ischemia.

The nociceptors are distributed in the somatic structures (skin, muscles, connective tissue, bones, joints) and visceral structures (visceral organs such as liver, gastro-intestinal tract).

There are three principal kinds of nociceptors: (1) Aδ mechanical nociceptors, (2) C-polymodal nociceptors, and (3) silent nociceptors.

The A-delta and C fibers are associated with different qualities of pain as listed in Table 3.1.

3.2.2 Noxious Stimuli and Responses

Harmful stimuli to the skin or subcutaneous tissue, such as joints or muscle, activate several classes of nociceptor terminals, the peripheral endings of primary sensory neurons whose cell bodies are located in the dorsal root ganglia and trigeminal ganglia. Three major classes of nociceptors are considered: thermal, mechanical, and polymodal as well as a class termed silent nociceptors.

Thermal nociceptors are activated by extreme temperatures (>45 °C or <5 °C). They have small-diameter, thinly myelinated Aδ fibers that conduct signals at about 5–30 m/s. Mechanical nociceptors are activated by intensive pressure applied to the skin. They also have thinly myelinated Aδ fibers conducting at 5–30 m/s. Polymodal nociceptors are activated by high intensity mechanical, chemical, or thermal (both

Table 3.1 Characteristics and functions of A-delta and C fibers

A-delta fibers	C fibers
Characteristics	
• Primary afferent fibers	• Primary afferent fibers
• Larger diameter	• Small diameter
• Myelinated	• Unmyelinated
• Fast conducting	• Slow conducting
Receptor type	
• High-threshold mechanoreceptors responding to mechanical stimuli over a certain intensity	• Polymodal receptor responding to more than one type of noxious stimuli:
	• Thermal
	• Chemical
	• Mechanical
Pain quality	
• Well-localized	• Diffuse
• Sharp	• Dull
• Stinging	• Burning
• Pricking	• Aching
• Referred to as fast or first pain	• Referred to as slow or second pain

hot and cold) stimuli. These nociceptors have small-diameter, nonmyelinated C fibers that conduct slowly, generally at velocities of 0.5–2.0 m/s (Table 3.1).

The cause of stimulation may be internal, such as pressure exerted by a tumor or external excessive stimuli such as trauma or burn. These noxious stimulations cause a release of chemical mediators from the damaged cells including: prostaglandin, bradykinin, serotonin, substance P, potassium, histamine, etc. (Fig. 3.1).

These chemical mediators activate and/or sensitize the nociceptors to the noxious stimuli. In order for a pain impulse to be generated, an exchange of sodium and potassium ions (depolarization and repolarization) occurs at the cell membranes. This results in an action potential and generation of a pain impulse (Fig. 3.2).

Fig. 3.2 Propagation of action potentials in sensory fibers results in the perception of pain. (Modified from Fields HL, Basbaum AI, Heinricher MM, 2005) [3]. (**a**) This electrical recording from a whole nerve shows a compound action potential representing the summated action potentials of all the component axons in the nerve. Even though the nerve contains mostly nonmyelinated axons, the major voltage deflections are produced by the relatively small number of myelinated axons. This is because action potentials in the population of more slowly conducting axons are dispersed in time, and the extracellular current generated by an action potential in a nonmyelinated axon is smaller than the current generated in myelinated axons. (**b**) First and second pain are carried by two different primary afferent axons. First pain is abolished by selective blockade of Aδ myelinated axons (middle) and second pain by blocking C fibers (bottom)

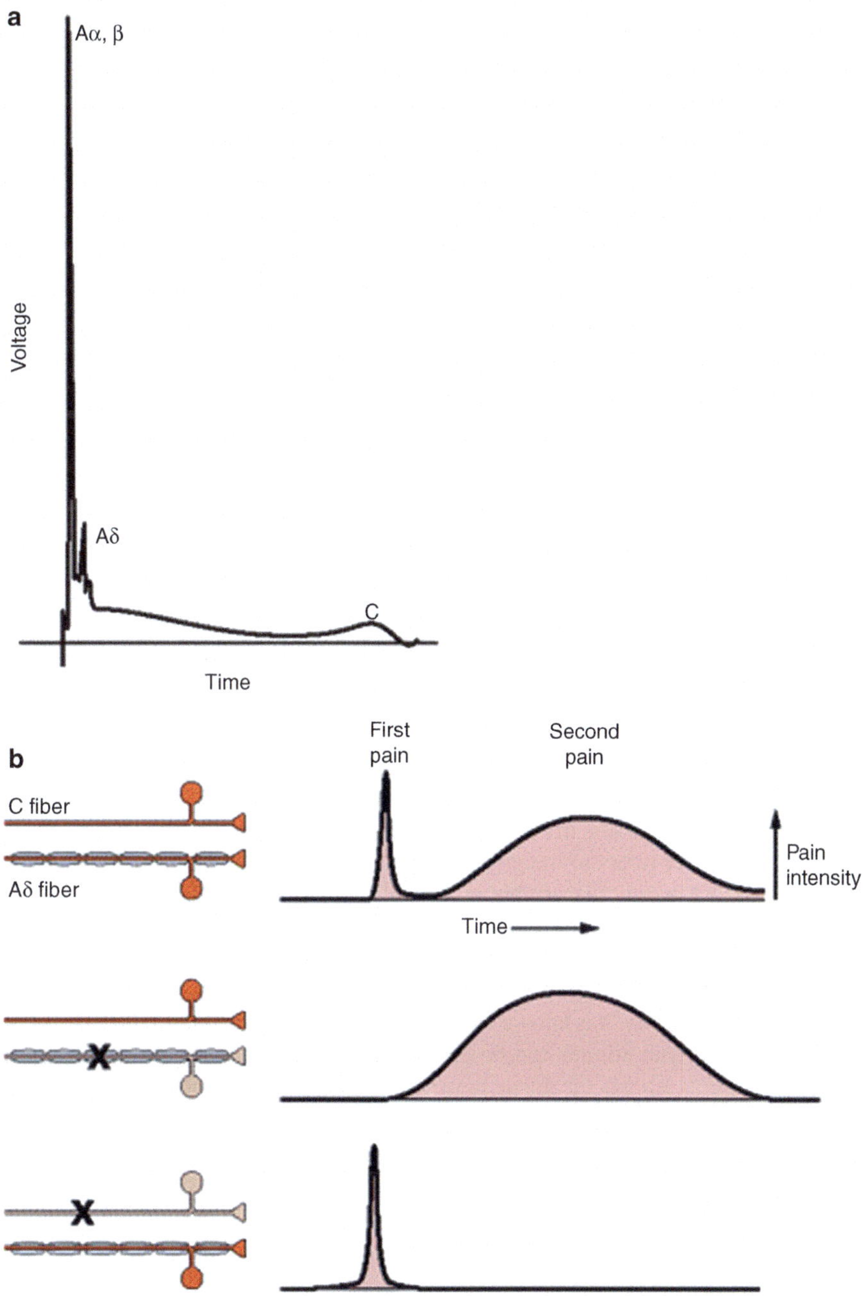
a
Aα, β
Voltage
Aδ
C
Time
b
C fiber
Aδ fiber
First pain
Second pain
Pain intensity
Time

3.3 Transmission of Pain at the Spinal Cord

The transmission process occurs in three stages. The pain impulse is transmitted: (1) from the site of transduction along the nociceptor fibers to the dorsal horn in the spinal cord, carried by the primary afferent fibers; (2) from the spinal cord to the brain stem such as thalamus, reticular formation, carried by the second neurons; (3) through connections between the thalamus, cortex, and higher levels of the brain, the third neurons.

The A-delta fiber and C fibers terminate in the dorsal horn of the spinal cord. There is a synaptic cleft between the terminal ends of the A-delta fiber and C fibers and the nociceptive dorsal horn neurons (NDHN). In order for the pain impulses to be transmitted across the synaptic cleft to the NDHN, excitatory neurotransmitters are released, which bind to specific receptors in the NDHN.

These neurotransmitters in the spinal cord are: adenosine triphosphate (ATP), glutamate, calcitonin gene-related peptide, bradykinin, nitric oxide, substance P.

Each A-delta and C fiber sends dendrites rostrally (toward the brain) and caudally (toward the feet) for two to four spinal segments. One fiber can communicate with neurons in as many as nine spinal segments. Lamina I projection neurons are predominately excited by nociceptive input directly from A-delta fibers and indirectly from C fibers. Wide dynamic range (WDR) neurons receive input from low-threshold A-beta fibers as well as direct and indirect input from nociceptive afferents. Dendrites of the WDR neurons also receive input from nociceptive (Lamina II) and non-noxious (Lamina III) cells.

The gray matter of the spinal cord is divided into ten laminae. The dorsal part is divided into five laminae (I to V), components of which mostly receive incoming pain fibers (Fig. 3.3). VII is in between these laminae and the more ventral laminae VIII and IX, and X refers to the gray matter around the central canal of the spinal cord. Lamina VI is only discernible in the bulges in the cord related to where the innervation of the limbs originates [4, 5].

Varieties of augments have been generated after the gate control theory of pain was first described. Although this mechanism has now been well documented, and has some clinical utility, it is known to be a gross over-simplification. The basic idea is that incoming pain stimuli can be gated by other stimuli, because many nerve cells talk to one another in the dorsal horn. Important fibers coming from the periphery into the dorsal horn include:

Relatively thin myelinated A-delta fibers, concerned with more accurate localization of pain, and terminating mostly laterally in laminae I and V.

Rather large A beta fibers that carry information about vibration and position sense from the periphery to the cord.

Small unmyelinated C fibers that are important carriers of the long-lasting burning pain that makes a surgical wound (for example) such an unpleasant experience. There is controversy about where these fibers terminate—according to Willis and Westlund, in primates many terminate in the deep dorsal horn and even the ventral horn, although conventionally lamina II has been said to be their destination [4, 5].

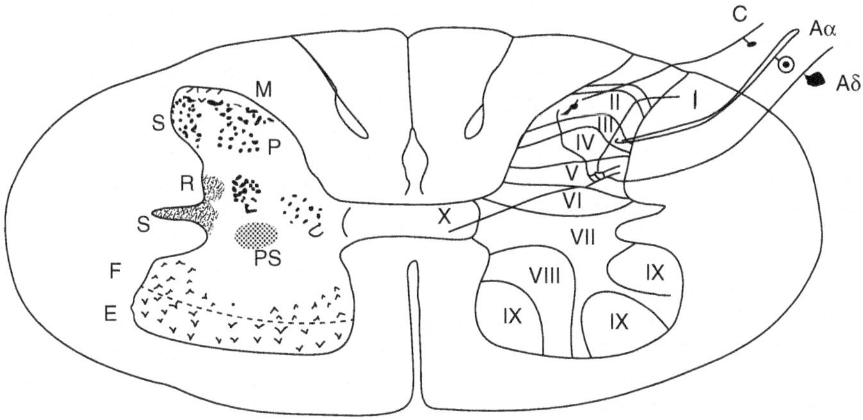

Fig. 3.3 Schematic presentation of laminae of the spinal cord (right side) and its cell groups (left side). Right side Lamina I (I): Tip of the dorsal horn; Cells respond to noxious or thermal stimuli; Sends information to the brain by the contralateral spinothalamic tract. Corresponds to the marginal zone. Lamina II (II): Involved in sensation of noxious and non-noxious stimuli, and modulating sensory input to contribute to the brain's interpretation of incoming signals as painful, or not. Sends information to Lamina III and IV; Corresponds to substantia gelatinosa. Lamina III (III): Involved in proprioception and sensation of light touch; Cells in this layer connects with cells in layers IV, V, and VI; Partially corresponds to nucleus proprius. Lamina IV (IV): Involved in non-noxious sensory information relay and processing; Cells connect with those in lamina II; Partially corresponds to nucleus proprius. Lamina V (V): Relays sensory, including nociceptive (potentially painful), information to the brain via the contralateral and spinothalamic tracts; Receives descending information from the brain via the corticospinal and rubrospinal tracts. Lamina VI (VI): Contains many small interneurons involved in spinal reflexes; Receives sensory information from muscle spindles (involved in proprioception); Sends information to the brain via ipsilateral spinocerebellar pathways. Lamina VII (VII): Large, heterogenous zone that varies through the length of the spinal cord; Receives information from Lamina II to VI, and from viscera; Relays motor information to the viscera; Gives rise to cells involved in the autonomic system; Dorsal nucleus of Clarke is part of Lamina VII. Lamina VIII (VIII): Varies depending on spinal cord level, but is most prominent in cervical and lumbar enlargements; Cells are involved in modulating motor output to skeletal muscle. Lamina IX (IX): Size and shape varies between spinal cord levels; Distinct groups of motor neurons that innervate skeletal muscle. Lamina X (X): Surrounds the central canal—the gray commissure; Axons decussate (cross over) from one side of the spinal cord to the other. Aαfibers (Aα) enter into the dorsal spinal cord and synaptically connect to wide dynamic neurons (W neurons); Aδfibers (Aδ) also synaptically connect to W neurons at Lamina V; C fibers also connect with W neurons at Lamina II through interneurons; Left side. *M* Marginal cells (Nucleus posterior marginalis), *S* Substance gelatinosa cells (Lamina II), *P* Nucleus proprius of dorsal horn, *R* Spinal reticular zone, *L* Lateral basal nucleus, *C* Clark's column (Nucleus dorsalis) (T1-L3), *S* Sympathetic preganglionic cell group (Intermediolateral cell column)(T1-L2), *PS* parasympathetic preganglionic cell groups (Intermediomedial cell column)(S2–S4), *F* Motor neuron groups for flexors, *E* Motor neuron groups for extensors

Unpleasant stimuli entering via the C fibers can be suppressed by concurrent stimulation of A-delta fibers (high amplitude low frequency stimulation, for example, by acupuncture) or by impulses passing through A-beta fibers. Examples of the latter include TENS (transcutaneous electrical nerve stimulation) and the simple expedient of rubbing the skin, which is well known by people to decrease perception of pain (Refer to Gate Control Theory).

3.4 Ascending Pathways of Pain

The pain impulse is then transmitted from the spinal cord to the brain stem and thalamus via three main nociceptive ascending pathways. These are the spinothalamic, the spinoreticular, and spinomesencephalic pathways [5–7] (Fig. 3.4).

The brain does not have a discrete pain center, so when impulses arrive in the thalamus they are directed to multiple areas in the brain where they are processed.

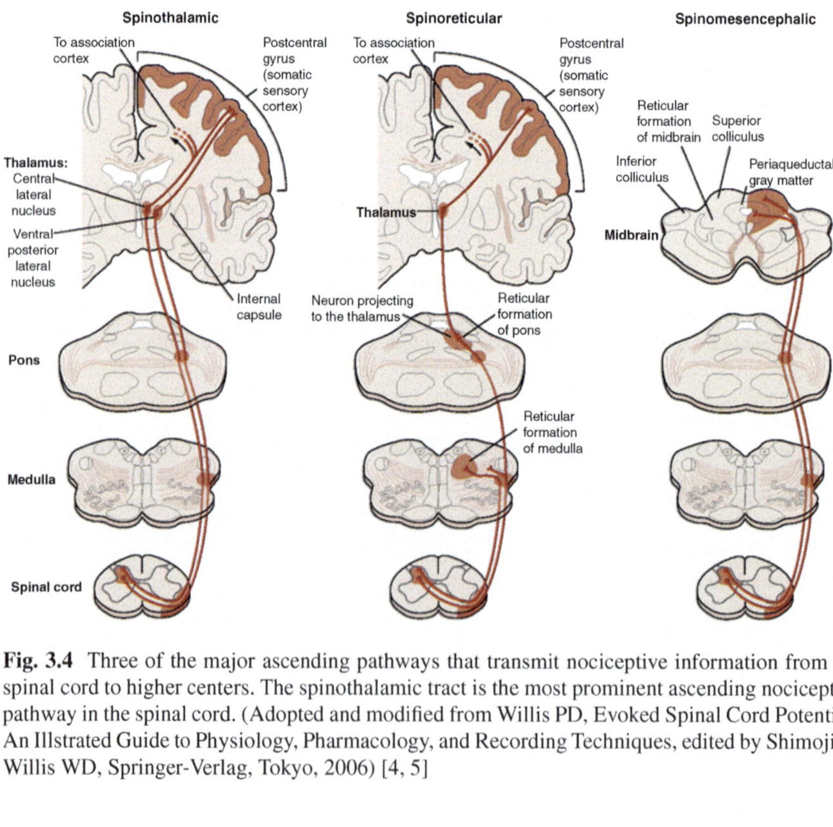

Fig. 3.4 Three of the major ascending pathways that transmit nociceptive information from the spinal cord to higher centers. The spinothalamic tract is the most prominent ascending nociceptive pathway in the spinal cord. (Adopted and modified from Willis PD, Evoked Spinal Cord Potentials An Illstrated Guide to Physiology, Pharmacology, and Recording Techniques, edited by Shimoji K, Willis WD, Springer-Verlag, Tokyo, 2006) [4, 5]

3.5 Perception of Pain

Perception of pain is the end result of the neuronal activity of pain transmission and where pain becomes a conscious multidimensional experience. The multidimensional experience of pain has affective-motivational, sensory-discriminative, emotional, and behavioral components.

When the painful stimuli are transmitted to the brain stem and thalamus, multiple cortical areas are activated, and responses are elicited.

These areas are:

1. The reticular system: This system is responsible for the autonomic and motor response to pain and for warning the individual to do something, for example, automatically removing a hand when it touches a hot saucepan. It also has a role in the affective-motivational response to pain such as looking at and assessing the injury to the hand once it has been removed from the hot saucepan.
2. Somatosensory cortex: This area is involved with the perception and interpretation of sensations. It identifies the intensity, type, and location of the pain sensation and relates the sensation to past experiences, memory, and cognitive activities. It identifies the nature of the stimulus before it triggers a response, for example, where the pain is, how strong it is, and what it feels like.
3. Limbic system: This system is responsible for the emotional and behavioral responses to pain, for example, attention, mood, and motivation, and also with processing pain and past experiences of pain [4–7].

3.5.1 Nociception Vs. Pain

The important distinction between pain and nociception should be made. Nociception is the term introduced almost 100 years ago by the great physiologist Sherrington (1906) to make clear the distinction between detection of a noxious event or a potentially harmful event and the psychological and other responses to it, that is, pain. Sherrington and others before him understood that pain was not a simple sensation, but rather was a complex experience, only a part of which was sensory in nature. Accordingly, it is most accurate to describe what we study as pain in nonhuman animals as nociception. However, although nonhuman animals cannot express in words the psychological and emotional consequences of a noxious stimulus or event, the term nociception should be applied instead of pain to that circumstance [8, 9].

The trauma or surgical procedures may be associated with longer lasting pain that may cause distress. A piece of skin that is innervated by a variety of sensory receptors called nociceptors. Nociceptors respond only to stimuli that damage tissue or have the potential to damage tissue, and there are several kinds of nociceptors identified (Fig. 3.1). When a nociceptor is activated by a mechanical, thermal, or chemical stimulus, the stimulus energy is transduced by the nociceptor to an electrical event (action potential) and the information is conveyed along nerve axons to the spinal cord, a part of the central nervous system. Input from nociceptors is transferred in the spinal cord dorsal horn to spinal neuron cell bodies whose axons ascend to supraspinal nuclei. Nociceptive information is thus distributed to multiple brain nuclei that give rise to both simple and complex responses to the peripheral noxious event [9, 10].

3.5.2 *Normal Vs. Abnormal Responses to Pain*

Pain normally evokes appropriate protective reflexes and/or behaviors, withdrawing fingers from a heated obstacle. One actually removes his fingers from the heated surface before he perceives the event as painful. Another more common type of normal or protective pain is that associated with tissue inflammation and tissue repair. One common example is post-surgical pain, which is longer lasting than the pain produced when one touches a heated surface (Fig. 3.5).

3.5.3 *Pain Sensitization*

Sensitization may occur as the consequences of tissue injury associated with a trauma or surgical procedure. By sensitization, the nociceptors change their behavior. They become more sensitive to stimuli. This factor contributes to what is termed hyperalgesia.

There is also an awakening of so-called silent or sleeping nociceptors. Silent nociceptors are thought to exist in tissues of human body. These silent nociceptors apparently play no normal physiological role in nociception or pain.

When tissue is injured, or damaged, silent nociceptors become active and begin to contribute information to the nervous system, not previously contributed [8–11].

These two events, nociceptor sensitization and awakening of silent nociceptors, exaggerate sensations provoked when applying a stimulus to or near the site of injury.

Pain stimuli →

A. Normal response→protective response→①acute response→reflexes
②If prolonged→Inflammation and repair

B. Abnormal response→Non-protective→Chronic→①Peripheral plastic changes ②Central plastic changes

Fig. 3.5 Pain that might be considered "normal" typically serves a protective function. Acute noxious stimulation, such as unexpectedly touching a hot surface or pricking a finger with a needle, evokes a nociceptive withdrawal reflex. When pain stimuli continue to exist, abnormal responses are produced in peripheral and central nervous structures

3.5.4 Hyperalgesia

As the intensity of the stimulus is increased, one would report increasing pain sensation associated with increasing intensity of stimulation. This stimulus-response function can be shown to exist for individual central nervous system neurons [12].

When tissue is injured or insulted in some way, the normal psychophysical function shifts to the left in the stimulus intensity relationship. The extent to which it shifts is dependent on the magnitude of the insult or the injury. In the normal individual, the noxious stimulus intensity is identified by some amount of pain, whereas in the presence of tissue insult or injury, the same intensity of noxious stimulation produces greater pain (Fig. 3.6).

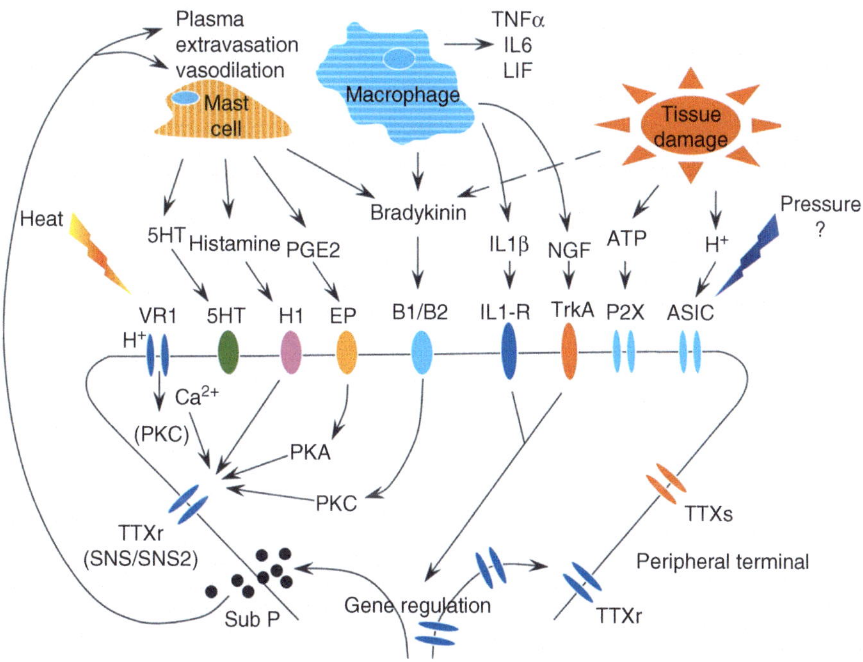

Fig. 3.6 Peripheral mechanisms of nerve fiber sensitization. Understanding the ability of peripheral neurons to sensitize is complex given the number of known ligand- and voltage-gated ion channels. However, many of these receptors use protein kinases A and C (PKA, PKC) signaling pathways. Vanilloid type 1 receptor (VR1), 5-hydroxytryptamine receptors (5HT), histamine type 1 (H1), prostaglandin E2 (PGE2), prostanoid receptor EP subtype (EP), bradykinin receptors (B1/B2), interleukin-1 beta (IL-1β), interleukin-1 receptor (IL1-R), nerve growth factor (NGF), tyrosine kinase A receptor (TrkA), adenosine triphosphate (ATP), purinergic receptor subtype P2X (P2X), hydrogen ion (H+), calcium (Ca2+), protein tetrodotoxin-resistant voltage-gated sodium channel (TTXr), tetrodotoxin-sensitive voltage-gated sodium channel (TTXs), substance P (Sub P), acid-sensing channel (ASIC). Used with Permission by Elsevier Limited. (Permission was from Drs. Costigan M, Woolf CJ: Pain: molecular mechanisms. J Pain 2000 (Suppl. 3):35–44)

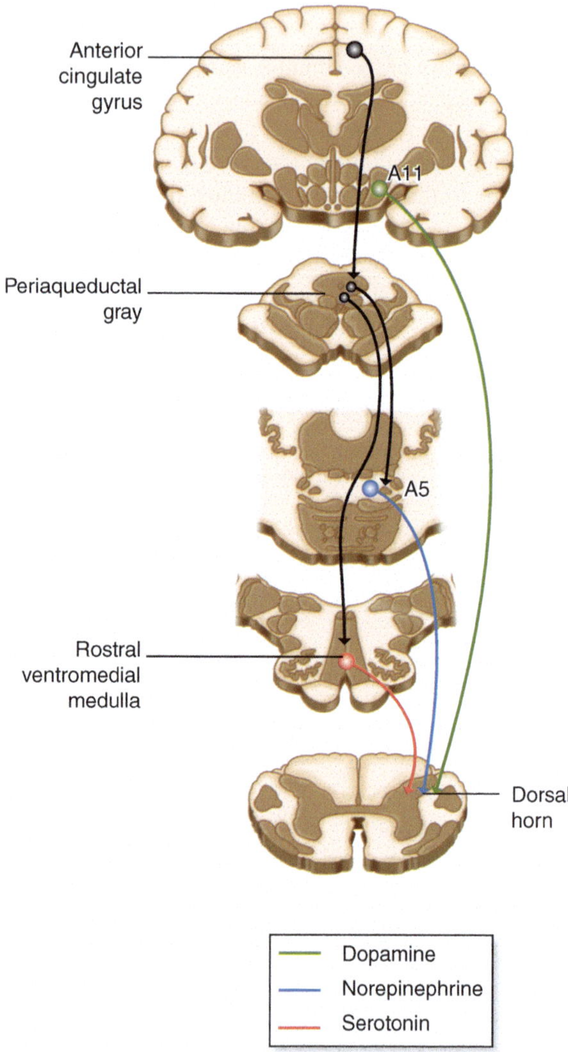

Fig. 3.7 Descending pain modulation pathways. The central pain modulatory network includes the cingulate gyrus, periaqueductal gray, dorsolateral pontine tegmentum, and ventromedial medulla. These areas exert either antinociceptive or pronociceptive effects via descending pathways that utilize serotonin, norepinephrine, or dopamine as their primary neurotransmitters. (Reproduced with permission from Dr. Eduardo E. Benarroch, Mayo Foundation for Medical Education and Research, Wolters Kluwer Health, Inc.)

How tissue insult affects responses to applied stimuli is illustrated in Fig. 3.7. Normally, there is a predictable response to stimulation that results in the sensation of pain only when the intensity of stimulation is in the noxious range [12].

The two types of hyperalgesia are termed primary and secondary and are believed to be produced by different mechanisms. Primary hyperalgesia is associated with a change in the behavior of nociceptors at the site of the injury. Secondary hyperalgesia is associated with a change in the behavior of neurons in the central nervous system. The nervous system is very dynamic and can be changed by tissue injury and insult. When one injures tissue in the periphery, a host of chemicals contribute to nociceptor sensitization and thus to primary hyperalgesia. These mediators are prostaglandins, amines, cytokines, kinins, peptides, providing targets for pharmacological intervention to prevent sensitization and the development of hyperalgesia [8–10].

When intense information from nociceptors arrives in the spinal cord, by sensitized nociceptors and awakened silent nociceptors, it increases the excitability of central neurons. This change in excitability provokes release of a variety of other mediators and modulators, excitatory amino acids and peptides, released from nociceptor terminals in the spinal cord. These mediators contribute to an increase in the excitability of central neurons and to development of secondary hyperalgesia, which is associated with chronic pain [9–11].

3.6 Development of Chronic Pain

The transition from acute to chronic pain appears to occur in discrete pathophysiological and histopathological steps. Stimuli initiating a nociceptive response vary, but receptors and endogenous defense mechanisms in the periphery interact in a similar manner regardless of the insult. Chemical, mechanical, and thermal receptors, along with leucocytes and macrophages, determine the intensity, location, and duration of noxious events.

Noxious stimuli are transduced to the dorsal horn of the spinal cord, where amino acid and peptide transmitters activate second-order neurons. Spinal neurons then transmit signals to the brain. The resultant actions by the individual involve sensory-discriminative, motivational-affective, and modulatory processes in an attempt to limit or stop the painful process.

Under normal conditions, noxious stimuli diminish as healing progresses and pain sensation lessens until minimal or no pain is detected. However, pain is persistent and intense; the secondary mechanisms are activated both at the periphery and within the central nervous system that cause allodynia, hyperalgesia, and hyperpathia that can diminish normal functioning.

These changes are thought to begin in the periphery with (1) upregulation of cyclo-oxygenase-2 and (2) interleukin-1β-sensitizing first-order neurons, which eventually sensitize second-order spinal neurons by (3) activating N-methyl-d-aspartic acid(NMDA) channels and (4) signaling microglia to alter neuronal cytoarchitecture. Throughout these processes, (5) prostaglandins, (6) endocannabinoids, (7) ion-specific channels, and (8) scavenger cells all play a key role in the transformation of acute to chronic pain [9].

Peripheral mechanisms of nerve fiber sensitization are illustrated in Fig. 3.8.

The stimuli sufficient for the activation of nociceptors appear to be tissue-specific, and tissue damage is not always required. For example, the sensitization process in the masseter muscle has been found to involve a decrease in a specific voltage-gated K+ channel. Similar mechanisms of a decrease, or increase, in specific ligand-gated or voltage-gated channels have been found in the sensitization

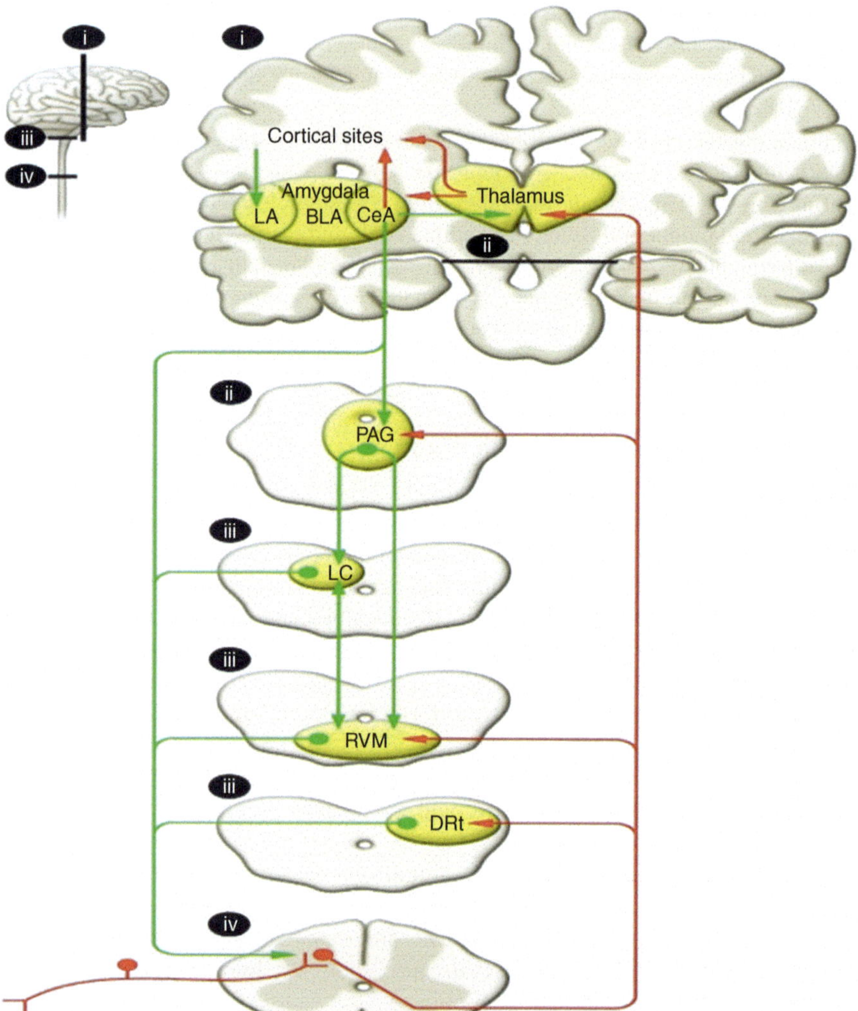

Fig. 3.8 Schematic diagram of pain modulatory circuitry. Ascending pathways are shown in red, whereas descending pathways are shown in green Ossipov et al. [55]

process of other tissues. Additionally, the so-called sleeping or silent nociceptors can become activated after exposure to inflammation and other endogenous mediators, and might represent as much as 15% of all C fibers, contributing to a significant increase in peripheral input to the CNS.(C. Voscopoulos and M. Lema∗)∗Corresponding author. E-mail: mlema@buffalo.edu

Neuroplasticity, or the physical remodeling of neuronal cytoarchitecture, occurs shortly after the onset of persistent acute pain and leads to the transition from acute pain into a chronic pain state. As a result of a peripheral lesion that persistently generates pain impulses to the spinal cord, inhibitory interneurons responsible for modulating painful nerve transmission impulses eventually die [9–11]. Furthermore, glial cells remodel neuronal synapses to intensify nociceptive transmission. Thus, these pain-transmitting neurons become more sensitive, react more intensely to stimuli, and grow more connections to second-order neurons within the CNS. This process of neuroplasticity may lead to central sensitization in which activity dependent phenotypic changes are observed in the dorsal horn neurons and other CNS structures, including higher centers [13–15].

Whereas primary hyperalgesia occurs in the periphery, secondary hyperalgesia occurs within the CNS and precedes long-term central sensitization. Most of the treatments for postoperative pain have only minimal analgesic effects on secondary hyperalgesia. As secondary hyperalgesia is felt to be a source for chronic post-surgical pain, developing agents to better treat secondary hyperalgesia might be more effective in preventing chronic post-surgical pain, and treating acute postoperative pain [16, 17].

3.6.1 Post-Surgical Pain

The factors contributing to post-surgical pain can broadly be divided between patient and surgical factors [9]. Patient factors include psychosocial status, pre-existing pain conditions, genetic predisposition to exaggerated pain response, and gender. Surgical factors include the type of anesthesia administered (general vs. regional technique) and surgical approach including the ability to identify and avoid nerve injury when possible. Additional surgical factors include the postoperative period and the type of pain treatment and duration, and full assessments of the pain, its consequences, and neurophysiological examination [18–20].

The mechanisms of acute post-surgical pain and chronic post-surgical pain are complex and poorly understood. Many of the syndromes may, at least in part, be neuropathic that result from neuroplastic changes after injury [21]. After surgical intervention, patients experience ongoing pain or are sensitive to incidental, normally non-painful stimulation.

This period of time varies, and with uncomplicated wound healing this pain progressively attenuates and disappears. The patient population with persistent post-surgical pain experiences deep pain or referred pain that lasts months or years.

The International Association for the Study of Pain defined post-procedural pain as a persistent pain state that is apparent for more than 2 months after operation and cannot be explained by other causes. The nature and properties of this pain are poorly characterized, without a distinct transition period from acute to chronic pain.

It is unclear whether the chronic condition constitutes merely an extension of perioperative pain. To give an example of the magnitude of the problem, after procedures such as thoracotomy, mastectomy, and amputation, as many as 50–70% of patients continue to experience pain for at least 6 months, with approximately 10% reporting severe pain [20, 22–24]. Post-procedural pain is also common for 1 year after lower abdominal surgery, sternotomy, hysterectomy, and herniorrhaphy with rates of 25% or greater [23, 25–30]. This problem is not restricted to major surgeries; after minor procedures, approximately 5% of patients suffer severe chronic post-surgical pain [20]. The wide variation in the incidence of chronic post-surgical pain is probably owing to differences in surgical techniques, study design, patient populations, and differing definitions of chronic pain.

3.6.2 Distress

Stress might be an unavoidable component of our life but might not produce distress unless it persists and leads to maladaptive behavior.

Distress is an aversive state in which one is unable to adapt completely to stressors and the resulting distress is manifested as a maladaptive behavior. However, we cannot objectively measure or quantify distress. We do not have reliable physiological measures that will tell us always that an animal is or is not stressed or distressed. We have no measures that provide reliable information to us about distress with the exception of the behaviors that we observe in the animals and even in human. Importantly, behavior must be assessed by individuals who are trained and knowledgeable about specific or typical behavior and who understand what is normal and what is maladaptive.

3.6.3 Preemptive Analgesia

This strategy is based on the knowledge that there will be changes in the behavior of nociceptors and central neurons when tissue is injured [31, 32]. Thus, a preemptive strategy is particularly applicable to surgeries. The strategy involves, for example, administration of opioids or epidural block before the anesthesia is started and before an incision is made in an attempt to prevent the sensitization of nociceptors [31–33]. The intent of this strategy is to prevent the development of central hyperexcitability and, as a consequence, reduce post-surgical hyperalgesia and reduce post-surgical stress and potential distress.

3.7 Descending Pain Modulation

3.7.1 Descending Serotonergic Pathways (Fig. 3.7)

Early studies with available serotonergic (5-HT) antagonists blocked stimulation produced analgesia (SPA) initiated from the rostral ventromedial medulla (RVM) [34], leading to the suggestion that descending inhibition of pain was mediated through serotonergic neurons projecting from the RVM through the dorsolateral funiculus (DLF) [6, 7]. Stimulation of the periaqueductal gray (grey) (PAG) or the RVM, including the nucleus raphe magnus (NRM) and nucleus reticularis gigantocellularis (NRG), was found to cause release of serotonin in the spinal cord [35], and intrathecal administration of 5-HT agonists elicited antinociception [36], whereas intrathecal 5-HT antagonists attenuated SPA originating from the RVM [37].

It has been argued that serotonergic RVM neurons are neither on-cells nor off-cells but that they can modulate the activities of pain-transmitting neurons [38]. However, a recent study, in which descending serotonergic RVM neurons were selectively ablated through the use of shRNA plasmids and electroporation, demonstrated that descending serotonergic projections from the RVM are important for facilitation of pain in inflammatory or neuropathic pain states, although they are not necessary for opioid-mediated inhibition of acute pain [39]. Electrophysiological studies suggested that GABAergic and glycinergic projections from the RVM mediate antinociception.

In addition to the descending serotonergic populations that are activated, the diversity of subtypes of the 5-HT receptors and the complex anatomy of the spinal dorsal horn complicates interpretation of the role of serotonin in pain modulation.

Thus, the effect of spinal serotonin can be either inhibitory or facilitatory, depending on the receptor subtype activated [40–44]. Spinal administration of an antagonist of the inhibitory 5-HT7 receptor blocked the antinociceptive effect of morphine microinjected into the RVM, whereas pharmacological antagonism of the facilitatory 5-HT3 receptor blocked hyperalgesia induced by CCK administered into the RVM [41]. Further, systemic administration of 5-HT7 agonists blocked capsaicin-induced hyperalgesia in mice, whereas 5-HT7 antagonists elicited mechanical hypersensitivity [45]. The 5-HT7 receptor has been identified in the dorsal root ganglion and on central terminals of primary afferent fibers [46–48] as well as on GABAergic interneurons in the dorsal horn of the spinal cord, which is consistent with a role in pain modulation. Although these observations indicate an important serotonergic role for pain modulation, the precise spinal mechanisms remain unclear.

3.7.2 Noradrenergic Systems and Pain Modulation

Electrical stimulation of the PAG or RVM to elicit antinociception increases measured norepinephrine levels in the cerebrospinal fluid, and this effect was blocked by spinal adrenergic antagonists [35, 49–51]. These findings suggest a strong contribution of norepinephrine in antinociception associated with descending inhibition. While neither the PAG nor the RVM contain noradrenergic neurons, both regions communicate with noradrenergic sites important to pain modulation, including the A5 (locus coeruleus), A6, and A7 (Kölliker-Füse) nuclei. These noradrenergic nuclei are a major source of direct noradrenergic projections to the spinal cord and likely may serve to ultimately inhibit the response of presynaptic and postsynaptic spinal pain transmission neurons [3].

Numerous studies have demonstrated that activation of spinal α2-adrenergic receptors exerts a strong antinociceptive effect [52–55]. PAG activation resulted in inhibition of the nociceptive responses of dorsal neurons mediated through activation of spinal α2 receptors [56]. Activation of α2-adrenergic receptors has been shown to inhibit nociceptive transmission at the level of the spinal cord through presynaptic activity, inhibiting release of excitatory neurotransmitters from primary afferent terminals, as well as through postsynaptic sites [52]. Recordings performed on spinal cord slices revealed that activation of α2-adrenergic receptors hyperpolarized neurons and was thus inhibitory. Recently, it has also been demonstrated that activation of α1-adrenergic receptors caused depolarization of GABA interneurons [56], demonstrating an additional mechanism of enhancing inhibition. On the other hand, activation of spinal α1-adrenergic receptors also enhances responses of dorsal horn neurons to noxious inputs [56] (Fig. 3.7).

Both systems, noradrenergic and serotonergic, might be included in descending nociceptive inhibitory system (DNIS) for pain. Patients with impaired DNIS were found to present an altered vagal control of the heart [57].

3.7.3 Stress-Induced Analgesia

Stress induced by brief foot shock of the forepaws of rats produces antinociception as measured in the tail-flick test [58]. Lesions of the DLF made rostral to the entry zone of the peripheral nerves of the forelimbs, which kept intact spinal tract communications between forelimb and tail, abolished stress-induced analgesia (SIA), indicating that supraspinal sites were necessary to activate a spinopetal pain inhibitory circuit. It was also found that antinociception induced by brief shock of the forepaws was abolished by systemic and intrathecal naloxone, indicating the activation of endogenous opioidergic pain inhibitory systems [58].

Stress-induced analgesia (SIA) is associated with elevated PAG levels of β-endorphin [59], and microinjection of μ-opioid receptor antagonists into the PAG or RVM abolished SIA [60, 61]. These and other studies led to the conclusion that SIA can be opioid sensitive and mediated through descending inhibitory pathways from amygdala, the PAG, and through RVM projections to the spinal cord [62].

Recent studies have revealed a role of endogenous cannabinoids in SIA and in descending modulatory pathways. Inhibition of RVM activity by microinjection of muscimol abolished antinociception induced by systemic injection of the cannabinoid agonist WIN55,212-2 [63]. Moreover, mechanisms could also underlie opioid-insensitive SIA. Opioid-insensitive SIA was abolished by systemic administration of cannabinoid 1(CB1), but not cannabinoid 2(CB2), antagonists [64]. Microinjection of the CB1 antagonist rimonabant into the dorsolateral PAG abolished such antinociception, further suggesting that SIA is mediated by endogenous cannabinoids [64]. Opioid-insensitive SIA was associated with elevated levels of endogenous cannabinoids in the PAG, and SIA was enhanced by microinjection of inhibitors of monoacylglycerol lipase, which hydrolyzes the endogenous cannabinoid 2-arachidonoylglycerol [64].

These studies indicate that endogenous cannabinoids, like opioids, regulate pain sensitivity in response to environmental conditions through descending pathways [55, 64, 65]. As SIA produces many generalized effects, including release of stress hormones, multiple physiological actions result that may contribute to antinociceptive effects.

Nociceptive inputs enter the spinal dorsal horn through primary afferent fibers that synapse onto transmission neurons. The projection fibers ascend through the contralateral spinothalamic tract. Ascending projections target the thalamus, and collateral projections also target mesencephalic nuclei, including the dorsal reticular nucleus (DRt), rostral ventromedial medulla (RVM), and the midbrain PAG. Descending projections from the DRt are a critical component of the diffuse noxious inhibitory control (DNIC) pathway.

Rostral projections from the thalamus target areas that include cortical sites and the amygdala. The lateral capsular part of the central nucleus of the amygdala (CeA) ("nociceptive amygdala") receives nociceptive inputs from the brainstem and spinal cord. Inputs from the thalamus and cortex enter through the lateral (LA) and basolateral (BLA) amygdala. The CeA sends outputs to cortical sites and the thalamus, in which cognitive and conscious perceptions of pain are integrated. Descending pain modulation is mediated through projections to the PAG, which also receives inputs from other sites, including the hypothalamus, and communicates with the RVM as well as other medullary nuclei that send descending projections to the spinal dorsal horn through the DLF.

The noradrenergic locus coeruleus (LC) receives inputs from the PAG, communicates with the RVM, and sends descending noradrenergic inhibitory projections to the spinal cord. Antinociceptive and pronociceptive spinopetal projections from the RVM positively and negatively modulate nociceptive inputs and provide for an endogenous pain regulatory system.

Ascending (red) and descending (green) tracts are shown schematically in Fig. 3.8. Areas labeled "i–iv" in the small diagram correspond with labeled details of the larger diagram [55] (Table 3.2).

Table 3.2 Naturally occurring agents that activate or sensitize nociception (modified from Fields HI et al., 2005)

Substance	Source	Enzyme involved in synthesis	Effect on primary afferent fibers
Potassium	Damaged cells		Activation
Serotonin	Platelets	Tryptophan hydroxylase	Activation
Bradykinin	Plasma kininogen	Kallikrein	Activation
Histamine	Mast cells		Activation
Prostaglandins	Arachidonic acid damaged cells	Cyclooxygenase	Sensitization
Leukotrienes	Arachidonic acid damaged cells	5-Lipoxygenase	Sensitization
Substance P	Primary afferents		Sensitization

Modified from Fields HI et al, 2005

References

1. Merskey H, Bogduk N. Part III: pain terms, a current list with definitions and notes on usage. In: Classification of chronic pain, second edition, IASP task force on taxonomy. Seattle: IASP Press; 1994. p. 209–14.
2. Bayne K. Assessing pain and distress: A veterinary behaviorist's perspective, Definition of Pain and Distress and Reporting Requirements for Laboratory Animals. In: Proceedings of the Workshop Held June 22, 2000. Washington, DC: The National Academies Press; 2000.
3. Fields HL, Basbaum AI, Heinricher MM. Central nervous system mechanisms of pain modulation. In: McMahon S, Koltzenburg M, editors. Textbook of pain. 5th ed. Burlington: Elsevier Health Sciences; 2005. p. 125–42.
4. Willis WD, Westlund KN. Neuroanatomy of the pain system and of the pathways that modulate pain. J Clin Neurophysiol. 1997;14:2–31.
5. Willis WD. Chapter 2. In: Shimoji K, Willis WD, editors. Physiology of the spinal cord, evoked spinal cord potentials. Springer; 2006. pp. 26–33.
6. Basbaum AI, Fields HL. Endogenous pain control mechanisms: review and hypothesis. Ann Neurol. 1978;4:451–62.
7. Basbaum AI, Bautista DM, Scherrer G, Julius D. Cellular and molecular mechanisms of pain. Cell. 2009;139:267–84.
8. Gebhart GF: 2000Scientific issues of pain and distress, definition of pain and distress and reporting requirements for laboratory animals, Proceedings of the Workshop held June 22, 2000,The National Academies Press. Washington, DC
9. Voscopoulos C, Lema M. When does acute pain become chronic? Brit J Anaesth. 2010;105(Suppl 1):i69–85.
10. Bérubé M, Gélinas C, Choinière M, et al. The effect of psychological interventions on the prevention of chronic pain in adults: a systematic review protocol. Syst Rev. 2017;6(1):190.
11. Jensen TS, Finnerup NB. Allodynia and hyperalgesia in neuropathic pain: clinical manifestations and mechanisms. Lancet Neurol. 2014;13:924–35.
12. Bayne K. Revised guide for the care and use of laboratory animals available. American Physiological Society. Physiologist. 1996;39(199):208–11.
13. Costigan M, Woolf CJ. Pain: molecular mechanisms. J Pain. 2000;1(3 Suppl):35–44.
14. Ueda H. Molecular mechanisms of neuropathic pain-phenotypic switch and initiation mechanisms. Pharmacol Ther. 2006;109:57–77.
15. Torebjork HE, Lundberg LE, LaMotte RH. Central changes in processing of mechanoreceptive input in capsaicin-induced secondary hyperalgesia in humans. J Physiol. 1992;448:765–80.
16. Eisenach JC. Preventing chronic pain after surgery: who, how, and when? Reg Anesth Pain Med. 2006;31:1–3.
17. Apfelbaum JL, Chen C, Mehta SS, Gan TJ. Postoperative pain experience: results from a national survey suggest postoperative pain continues to be undermanaged. Anesth Analg. 2003;97:534–40.
18. Kehlet H, Rathmell JP. Persistent postsurgical pain: the path forward through better design of clinical studies. Anesthesiology. 2010;112:514–5.
19. Granot M. Can we predict persistent postoperative pain by testing preoperative experimental pain? Curr Opin Anaesthesiol. 2009;22:425–30.
20. Kehlet H, Jensen TS, Woolf CJ. Persistent postsurgical pain: risk factors and prevention. Lancet. 2006;367:1618–25.
21. Macrae WA. Chronic post-surgical pain: 10 years on. Br J Anaesth. 2008;101:77–86.
22. Dworkin RH, McDermott MP, Raja SN. Preventing chronic postsurgical pain: how much of a difference makes a difference? Anesthesiology. 2010;112:516–8.
23. Katz J, Seltzer Z. Transition from acute to chronic postsurgical pain: risk factors and protective factors. Expert Rev Neurother. 2009;9:723–44. CrossRefMedlineGoogle Scholar.
24. Gartner R, Jensen MB, Nielsen J, Ewertz M, Kroman N, Kehlet H. Prevalence of and factors associated with persistent pain following breast cancer surgery. JAMA. 2009;302:1985–92.

25. Katz J, Cohen L. Preventive analgesia is associated with reduced pain disability 3 weeks but not 6 months after major gynecologic surgery by laparotomy. Anesthesiology. 2004;101:169–74.
26. Bruce J, Poobalan AS, Smith WC, Chambers WA. Quantitative assessment of chronic postsurgical pain using the McGill pain questionnaire. Clin J Pain. 2004;20:70–5.
27. Kalso E, Mennander S, Tasmuth T, Nilsson E. Chronic post-sternotomy pain. Acta Anaesthesiol Scand. 2001;45:935–9.
28. Bay-Nielsen M, Perkins FM, Kehlet H. Pain and functional impairment 1 year after inguinal herniorrhaphy: a nationwide questionnaire study. Ann Surg. 2001;233:1–7.
29. Haythornthwaite JA, Raja SN, Fisher B, Frank SM, Brendler CB, Shir Y. Pain and quality of life following radical retropubic prostatectomy. J Urol. 1998;160:1761–4.
30. Gottschalk A, Smith DS, Jobes DR, et al. Preemptive epidural analgesia and recovery from radical prostatectomy: a randomized controlled trial. JAMA. 1998;279:1076–82.
31. Aida S, Yamakura T, Baba H, et al. Preemptive analgesia by intravenous low-dose ketamine and epidural morphine in gastrectomy: a randomized double-blind study. Anesthesiology. 2000;92:1624–30.
32. Aida S, Fujihara H, Taga K, et al. Involvement of presurgical pain in preemptive analgesia for orthopedic surgery: a randomized double blind study. Pain. 2000;84:169–73.
33. Aida S, Baba H, Yamakura T, et al. The effectiveness of preemptive analgesia varies according to the type of surgery: a randomized, double-blind study. Anesth Analg. 1999;89:711–6.
34. Oliveras JL, Hosobuchi Y, Guilbaud G, Besson JM. Analgesic electrical stimulation of the feline nucleus raphe magnus: development of tolerance and its reversal by 5-HTP. Brain Res. 1978;146:404–9.
35. Cui M, Feng Y, McAdoo DJ, Willis WD. Periaqueductal gray stimulation-induced inhibition of nociceptive dorsal horn neurons in rats is associated with the release of norepinephrine, serotonin, and amino acids. J Pharmacol Exp Ther. 1999;289:868–76.
36. Yaksh TL, Wilson PR. Spinal serotonin terminal system mediates antinociception. J Pharmacol Exp Ther. 1979;208:446–53.
37. Jensen TS, Yaksh TL. Spinal monoamine and opiate systems partly mediate the antinociceptive effects produced by glutamate at brainstem sites. Brain Res. 1984;321:287–97.
38. Mason P. Contributions of the medullary raphe and ventromedial reticular region to pain modulation and other homeostatic functions. Annu Rev Neurosci. 2001;24:737–77.
39. Wei F, et al. Molecular depletion of descending serotonin unmasks its novel facilitatory role in the development of persistent pain. J Neurosci. 2010;30:8624–36.
40. Suzuki R, Rygh LJ, Dickenson AH. Bad news from the brain: descending 5-HT pathways that control spinal pain processing. Trends Pharmacol Sci. 2004;25:613–7.
41. Dogrul A, Ossipov MH, Porreca F. Differential mediation of descending pain facilitation and inhibition by spinal 5HT-3 and 5HT-7 receptors. Brain Res. 2009;1280:52–9.
42. Sasaki M, Obata H, Kawahara K, Saito S, Goto F. Peripheral 5-HT2A receptor antagonism attenuates primary thermal hyperalgesia and secondary mechanical allodynia after thermal injury in rats. Pain. 2006;122:130–6.
43. Green GM, Scarth J, Dickenson A. An excitatory role for 5-HT in spinal inflammatory nociceptive transmission; state-dependent actions via dorsal horn 5-HT(3) receptors in the anaesthetized rat. Pain. 2000;89:81–8.
44. Rahman W, Bauer CS, Bannister K, Vonsy JL, Dolphin AC, Dickenson AH. Descending serotonergic facilitation and the antinociceptive effects of pregabalin in a rat model of osteoarthritic pain. Mol Pain. 2009;5:45.
45. Brenchat A, et al. 5-HT7 receptor activation inhibits mechanical hypersensitivity secondary to capsaicin sensitization in mice. Pain. 2009;141:239–47.
46. Doly S, Fischer J, Brisorgueil MJ, Verge D, Conrath M. Pre- and postsynaptic localization of the 5-HT7 receptor in rat dorsal spinal cord: immunocytochemical evidence. J Comp Neurol. 2005;490:256–69.

47. Pierce PA, Xie GX, Levine JD, Peroutka SJ. 5-Hydroxytryptamine receptor subtype messenger RNAs in rat peripheral sensory and sympathetic ganglia: a polymerase chain reaction study. Neuroscience. 1996;70:553–9.
48. Cortes-Altamirano JL, Olmos-Hernandez A, Jaime HB, et al. Review: 5-HT1, 5-HT2, 5-HT3 and 5-HT7 receptors and their role in the modulation of pain response in the central nervous system. Curr Neuropharmacol. 2018;16:210–21.
49. Hammond DL, Tyce GM, Yaksh TL. Efflux of 5-hydroxytryptamine and noradrenaline into spinal cord superfusates during stimulation of the rat medulla. J Physiol. 1985;359:151–62.
50. Barbaro NM, Hammond DL, Fields HL. Effects of intrathecally administered methysergide and yohimbine on microstimulation-produced antinociception in the rat. Brain Res. 1985;343:223–9.
51. Hammond DL, Yaksh TL. Antagonism of stimulation-produced antinociception by intrathecal administration of methysergide or phentolamine. Brain Res. 1984;298:329–37.
52. Pertovaara A. Noradrenergic pain modulation. Prog Neurobiol. 2006;80:53–83.
53. Ossipov MH, Harris S, Lloyd P, Messineo E. An isobolographic analysis of the antinociceptive effect of systemically and intrathecally administered combinations of clonidine and opiates. J Pharmacol Exp Ther. 1990;255:1107–16.
54. Ossipov MH, Harris S, Lloyd P, Messineo E, Lin BS, Bagley J. Antinociceptive interaction between opioids and medetomidine: systemic additivity and spinal synergy. Anesthesiology. 1990;73:1227–35.
55. Ossipov MH, Dussor GO, Porreca J. Central modulation of pain. J Clin Invest. 2010;120:3779–87.
56. Budai D, Harasawa I, Fields HL. Midbrain periaqueductal gray (PAG) inhibits nociceptive inputs to sacral dorsal horn nociceptive neurons through alpha2-adrenergic receptors. J Neurophysiol. 1998;80:2244–54.
57. Rodrigues P, Correa L, Ribeiro M, et al. Patients with impaired descending nociceptive inhibitory system present altered cardiac vagal control at rest. Pain Physician. 2018;21:E409–18.
58. Watkins LR, Mayer DJ. Organization of endogenous opiate and nonopiate pain control systems. Science. 1982;216:1185–92.
59. Nakagawasai O, et al. Changes in beta-endorphin and stress-induced analgesia in mice after exposure to forced walking stress. Methods Find Exp Clin Pharmacol. 1999;21:471–6.
60. Wiedenmayer CP, Barr GA. Mu opioid receptors in the ventrolateral periaqueductal gray mediate stress-induced analgesia but not immobility in rat pups. Behav Neurosci. 2000;114:125–36.
61. Foo H, Helmstetter FJ. Hypoalgesia elicited by a conditioned stimulus is blocked by a mu, but not a delta or a kappa, opioid antagonist injected into the rostral ventromedial medulla. Pain. 1999;83:427–31.
62. Hopkins E, Spinella M, Pavlovic ZW, Bodnar RJ. Alterations in swim stress-induced analgesia and hypothermia following serotonergic or NMDA antagonists in the rostral ventromedial medulla of rats. Physiol Behav. 1998;64:219–25.
63. Meng ID, Manning BH, Martin WJ, Fields HL. An analgesia circuit activated by cannabinoids. Nature. 1998;395:381–3.
64. Hohmann AG, et al. An endocannabinoid mechanism for stress-induced analgesia. Nature. 2005;435:1108–12.
65. Suplita RL, Farthing JN, Gutierrez T, Hohmann AG. Inhibition of fatty-acid amide hydrolase enhances cannabinoid stress-induced analgesia: sites of action in the dorsolateral periaqueductal gray and rostral ventromedial medulla. Neuropharmacology. 2005;49:1201–9.

Chapter 4
Pathophysiology of Pain

W. Hamann

Pain has been defined by the International Association for the Study of Pain as "An unpleasant sensory and emotional experience associated with actual or potential tissue damage, or described in terms of such damage" [1].

The implication of this definition is that pain may arise from any part of the pain pathway. Frequently, however, pain is caused by trauma activating nociceptors. Conversely, the cause for a pain may be solely in the brain, even though the sufferer will project the pain onto a specific bodily location. More often and particularly in chronic pain there may be a combination of an initial and possibly ongoing peripheral stimulus which in turn will start off central sensitization in the central nervous system.

In terms of pain mechanisms, there are three different types:

1. *Nociceptive pain* after stimulation of nociceptors
2. *Neuropathic pain* caused by damage to any part of the nervous system
3. Behavioural or psychogenic pain

It is not uncommon that a patient presenting with clinical pain comprises a combination of two or even all of the above mechanisms. It is important to discriminate between each mechanism, because they require different management.

The pain pathway starts in the periphery with nociceptors in the form of free nerve endings. The afferent nerve fibres from nociceptors are either non-myelinated C-fibres or in the myelinated A-delta group [2–4]. They travel in peripheral nerves via dorsal roots to the spinal cord or via portions of the cranial nerves V, VII, IX and X to the medulla oblongata, where they synapse within the superficial layers and cross over within a few segments to ascend in the anterolateral compartment to the thalamus (spinothalamic tract) or to the brain stem (spino-tectal tract). The relatively smaller component of the spino-tectal fraction terminates in the intermediate

W. Hamann (✉)
Guy's and St Thomas' Hospital, Pain Management Centre, London, UK
e-mail: wolfgang.hamann@doctors.org.uk

K. Shimoji et al. (eds.), *Chronic Pain Management in General and Hospital Practice*, https://doi.org/10.1007/978-981-15-2933-7_4

and deep layers of the superior colliculus whereas the larger mesencephalic proportion also includes spinal projections to the periaqueductal grey substance (spino-periaqueductal fibres). The periaqueductal grey is the site of a high concentration of μ-receptors activating powerful descending inhibition on the pain pathway. The spinothalamic tract terminates in the ventroposterolateral nucleus (VPL) of the thalamus. Corresponding anatomy applies to the sensory fraction of the cranial nerves with termination in the ventroposteromedial nucleus (VPM). Third order neurones from the thalamus connect to a number of cortical and sub-cortical areas, including the somatosensory areas SI and SII, the cingulate cortex, the hypothalamus, and other areas. The somatosensory area SI is located on the postcentral gyrus where the contralateral half of the body is represented in the form of the homunculus. In chronic pain, many other areas of the brain are also involved in a complex manner that is not always fully understood.

At each synaptic level there is the potential for modulation which has been well described at the level of the dorsal horn.

Nociceptive free nerve endings are excitable by stimuli that are likely to damage tissue, resulting in the release of intracellular substances into the extracellular environment. Receptors are either modality specific like heat receptors or pressure receptors or they may respond to a variety of noxious stimuli (polymodal nociceptors). Low pH, as observed during ischaemia, is a powerful stimulus for nociceptors. A separate category contains the so-called silent nociceptors [5] which may be activated by inflammation. Distension is a powerful stimulus for nociception in hollow organs.

Heat sensitive nociceptor-neurones contain the TRPV1 receptor in their cell membranes [6]. Capsaicin binds closely to this receptor and elicits a sensation of burning pain. At sufficiently high concentration, topically applied capsaicin will, after initial strong burning sensation, inactivate TRPV1 receptors, resulting in alleviation of pain in conditions like postherpetic neuralgia, diabetic neuropathy, or neuropathic pain in HIV [7].

Repeated noxious stimulation damages cells in the vicinity of nociceptors entailing the release of intracellular material into the extracellular space. The resulting inflammation causes *peripheral sensitization*, meaning that there will be an increased number of action potentials in the primary afferent nerve fibre supplying a nociceptor in response to stimulation. Clinically, peripheral sensitization expresses itself as *Allodynia* (increased response of neurones following normally non-painful stimuli) or *Hyperalgesia* (enhanced pain response). Peripheral sensitization has been described for nociceptors in the skin as well as visceral, muscle, and joint nociceptors.

Mediators for peripheral sensitization are nerve growth factor (NGF), prostaglandins, and the release of inflammatory cytokines [8], substance P, tachykinins, and calcitonin gene related peptide (CGRP) [9]. NGF causes long-term sensitization of nociceptors [9]. CGRP is primarily found in nociceptive primary afferent neurones. It is a powerful vasodilator, but does not produce pain when injected. CGRP is highly expressed on meningeal vessels. One model of migraine describes this condition as peripheral sensitization with CGRP as a major mediator [10].

The cascade from phospholipids to arachidonic acid is therapeutically of significance. It is inhibited by steroids and the subsequent breakdown to prostaglandin is subject to inhibition by non-steroidal anti-inflammatory drugs.

Cytokines are small secreted proteins. They have specific effects on the communication between cells. Pro-inflammatory cytokines are involved with the up-regulation of inflammatory processes [11]. In particular interleukin IL-1®, IL-6, and tumour necrosis factor (TNF α) are involved in the development of pathological pain [12]. Therapeutic control of TNF α action will be discussed in the Arthritis Chapter. Algogenic cytokines may be released by monocytes, macrophages as well as by non-immune cells like fibroblasts, endothelial cells, and Schwann cells. In the central nervous system microglia can release cytokines. Cytokines are important mediators of pain following nerve injury. They play a role in the generation of several neuropathic pain states, e.g., complex regional pain syndrome, phantom limb pain, and sciatica following nucleus pulposus hernia. Cytokines may also be transported axonally in both directions and may therefore have an effect centrally after peripheral nerve injury or inflammation.

Along peripheral nerves and dorsal roots, acute and chronic pain may be caused by a variety of mechanical or ischaemic and demyelination situations. Arterial pressure on the trigeminal ganglion may cause trigeminal neuralgia. Chronic compression as in carpal tunnel syndrome and nerve entrapments in general produce combinations of pain, paraesthesia, and numbness. Transection of nerves as is necessary during amputation leads to the formation of neuromata which are responsible for *phantom limb sensation and pain*. Trauma to peripheral nerves in continuity may result in type II complex regional pain syndrome. Both these types of neuropathic pain have also a central nervous part to their pathophysiology. The importance of the action of cytokines in many of these conditions has been outlined above. Apart from gait and other sensory abnormalities, demyelinating diseases as in Tabes dorsalis may be the cause of severe burning and lancinating pains. Conceivably, an imbalance between inhibitory and excitatory mechanisms could be a contributing factor to these conditions in addition to the action of inflammatory mediators.

Compression and inflammatory irritation of dorsal roots as observed during a disc prolapse or spinal stenosis will elicit pain in the distribution pattern of the relevant neural segment. With careful sensory testing, pain can be demonstrated to be restricted to the relevant dermatome. This so called projected *nerve root pain* typically is the reason for a *positive stretch test (Lasegue sign)* needs to be differentiated from *referred pain*, e.g., from *facet joint arthropathy* which can also project into the leg right down to the ankle, but It will not follow dermatomal distribution and will not produce a positive stretch test.

Noxious stimuli to the skin typically cause *Lewis's triple response* of

1. an initial red line where the stimulus has been applied,
2. a flare which is mediated via a branch of the primary afferent axon (*Axon reflex*) and
3. the wheal caused by release of histamine.

While the axon reflex mimics autonomic vascular activity, it is in itself not an autonomic reflex.

Pain conditions are often accompanied by autonomic reflexes. This may express itself in a combination of cutaneous vasodilation or constriction and hyperhidrosis. Historically, this was regarded as a patho-physiological mechanism in its own right and the diagnosis of sympathetically maintained pain was made. For example, it was thought that the *complex regional pain syndrome* was a "*reflex sympathetic dystrophy* (RSD)". Unfortunately, sympathetic blocks are rarely effective in controlling this condition and the term RSD has been abandoned as misleading. The concept of sympathetically maintained pain in general has also become questionable. Neither in basic sciences nor in clinical medicine does convincing evidence exist to support this concept [13].

Sympathetic blocks, however, are still in use for the treatment of vasospasm and peripheral vascular disease, where the subjective effect is often striking when a previously cold leg feels warm again. This may be helpful where the underlying problem is Raynaud's disease or for the prevention of skin ulcers. It is however doubtful whether arterial vessels in an advanced state of sclerosis will benefit.

One apparently successful type of sympathetic procedure is the coeliac plexus block which can provide meaningful pain relief to patients with pancreatic pain. However, its beneficial effect may well be due to the interruption of nociceptive afferents, which run together with sympathetic nerve fibres.

Upon entering the dorsal horn, nociceptor fibres terminate in glutaminergic synapses in the superficial layers I and II in the substantia gelatinosa from where, after crossing over within a few spinal segments, postsynaptic cells project to the spinothalamic and spino-tectal tracts to the contralateral anterior funiculus. Many cells in the dorsal horn receive input from the skin, connective tissue, joints and viscera. Nociceptive information from the viscera may be interpreted erroneously as originating from the skin in the same body segment, a phenomenon called *Referred Pain*.

Primary afferent collaterals also synapse with cells in deeper layers IV and V of the dorsal horn, which are not part of the spinothalamic/spino-tectal system. Many of the cells in deeper layers are so called *wide dynamic range* neurones, because they receive excitatory input from noxious as well as non-noxious primary afferents. Much electrophysiology demonstrating *modulation* in the dorsal horn has been recorded from these, sometimes unidentified, cells. Perl [14] summed up the problem these cells posed with the following words "How this mix of cell signals and cell groups is organized to provide a sensation is unknown." As an answer to this conundrum, Melzack and Wall proposed the gate theory [15]. In a recent review Mendell [16] has analysed Melzack and Walls model where cells in the substantia gelatinosa act as gate facilitating or inhibiting transmission of nociceptive information. The gate is opened by small primary afferent and closed by large primary. In addition, the gate is also under descending control. The gate theory is the last instalment in the dispute between pattern versus specific theories advocating a non-specific pain pathway. In this context, it is important to recollect that not all primary afferent C-fibres subserve nociception and that electrophysiological recordings have been made from spinothalamic tract neurones receiving input from peripheral receptors requiring strong mechanical stimulation [17]. The important message from the concept of the gate theory is that nociceptive messages undergo modulation at synaptic relays.

Modulation in the dorsal horn is complex and operates through a number of mechanisms:

1. Descending and segmental inhibition
2. Central sensitization
3. Diffuse noxious central control (DNIC)
4. Endorphins and enkephalins
5. Active role of glia cells

1. *Segmental inhibition* was described by Sherrington in the form of antagonist inhibition. During the contraction of a muscle there was simultaneous suppression of contraction in the antagonist.

   Segmental and descending inhibition affecting second order sensory neurones has been found to be equally powerful. Conditioning electrical stimuli given to either A-fibres in peripheral nerves or descending tracts in the spinal cord can abolish the evoked discharge in postsynaptic dorsal horn neurones [18]. It is these mechanisms that are utilized with transcutaneous nerve stimulation or with dorsal column stimulators. One in three patients with neuropathic pain experience effective pain relief through medication with tricyclic antidepressant drugs [19]. These drugs exert their action through more than one mechanism. They are mono-amine reuptake inhibitors working at descending inhibitory synapses. They also block NMDA receptors as well as some sodium pumps. While they have no effect at dopaminergic transmission, this transmitter substance may also be of importance. Selective serotonin reuptake inhibitors are less effective. Gabapentin and pregabalin are two other compounds effective in the management of neuropathic pain [20]. The main analgesic mode of action appears to be attachment to the $\alpha_2 \delta$ subunit of the voltage-dependent Ca channel, thus inhibiting Ca influx via the P/Q type Ca channels.
2. The concept of *Central sensitization* has been extensively researched by Woolf et al. [21]. It means that postsynaptic nociceptive cells in the dorsal horn increase their responsiveness following excitation from primary afferent nociceptive C-fibres. Via NMDA-receptor mediated effects they respond with a higher frequency and longer lasting discharge, with an increased peripheral receptive field (*Hyperalgesia*) and they develop previously not present excitability to tactile stimuli (*Allodynia*). Figs. 4.1 and 4.2.

   Central sensitization of higher centres will be discussed below. Several chronic pain conditions, e.g., arthritis, fibromyalgia, or irritable bowel pain are now thought to be caused at least partly by central sensitization.
3. *Diffuse noxious central control (DNIC)* [22] stands for the concept that pain in one location can be suppressed by inflicting another pain to a physically remote area of the body. Historically, the DNIC was activated by barbers on market stalls when they kicked a customer on the shin just before extracting a tooth.

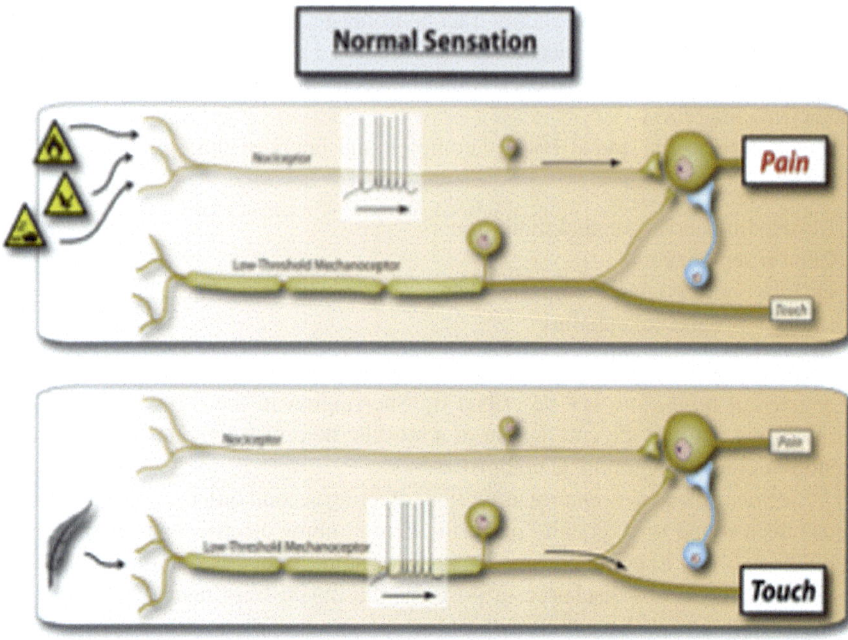

Fig. 4.1 Normal sensation. The somatosensory system is organized such that the highly specialized primary sensory neurons that encode low intensity stimuli only activate those central pathways that lead to innocuous sensations, while high intensity stimuli that activate nociceptors only activate the central pathways that lead to pain and the two parallel pathways do not functionally intersect. This is mediated by the strong synaptic inputs between the particular sensory inputs and pathways and inhibitory neurons that focus activity to these dedicated circuits [21] (permission applied for)

4. *Enkephalins* [23] are pentapeptides which are natural ligands to μ-receptors present in the central nervous system. *Endorphins* are larger peptides with similar pharmacological properties that can be found in the pituitary. These peptides constitute yet another internal system for pain control. They are released by other physical or psychological stimuli. They are well known for the "high" they evoke in long distance runners. They also fulfil another important function in that the *placebo response* is mediated through the release of enkephalins and endorphins [24]. Patients with pain following a tooth extraction were given either a placebo analgesic substance. Some patients experienced pain relief with the placebo, which could be overridden by Naloxone.

   The above ways of modulation 1–4 have so far been explained largely through results obtained from animals. Gruener et al. [25] have shown them also to be functionally important in patients with neuropathic pain following spinal cord injury.
5. *Active Role of Glia Cells*: The severe chronic pain condition complex regional pain syndrome (CRPS) is thought to be caused by an abnormal immune response

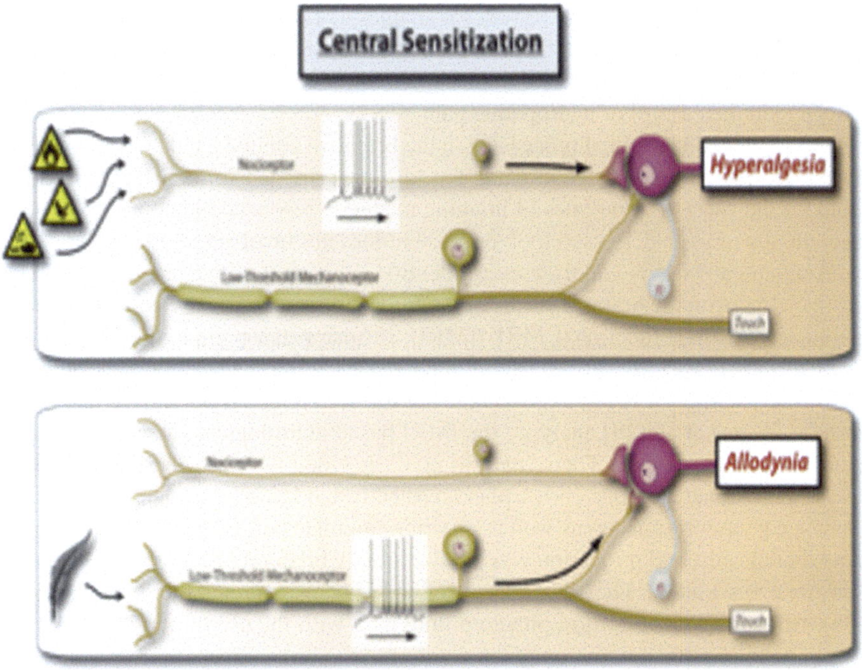

Fig. 4.2 Central sensitization. With the induction of central sensitization in somatosensory pathways with increases in synaptic efficacy and reductions in inhibition, a central amplification occurs enhancing the pain response to noxious stimuli in amplitude, duration, and spatial extent, while the strengthening of normally ineffective synapses recruits subliminal inputs such that inputs in low threshold sensory inputs can now activate the pain circuit. The two parallel sensory pathways converge [21] (permission applied for)

against substances released from injured nerve tissue. Helyes et al. [26] were able to reproduce most symptoms of CRPS in mice with a small paw injury by perfusion with human IgG from patients with the condition. During the following days, the treated mice showed characteristic behavioural, immunological, and neurochemical changes typical for the condition. The authors observed a significant increase in the density of astrocyte-related glial fibrillary acidic protein (GFAP) bilaterally as well as microglia-staining with Iba1 only on the same side in L4–L5 spinal dorsal horn, peri-aqueductal grey and somatosensory cortex.

Contrary to the meninges, central nervous tissue does not itself possess any nociceptors, and yet damage to either the spinal cord or the brain may result in the so-called *central neuropathic pain*. Gruener et al. [25] studied patients with spinal injuries including partial interruptions of the spinothalamic tract. A percentage of these patients developed intractable pain. The authors provided evidence that it was damage to the descending inhibition and the DNIC which were responsible for the development of pain following spinal injury.

Cannabis has been used in the past for analgesia. The endocannabinoid system is extended widely throughout the nervous system [27]. In a recent update by the National Academies of Sciences, Engineering and Medicine [28] it was found to be effective in the control of neuropathic pain.

Detailed mechanisms of processing in the brain are complex and not fully understood. However, noninvasive imaging has already provided some helpful information. Of the various techniques of imaging magnetic resonance imaging (MRI) has become the most widely used tool, because it does not involve radiation.

Anatomical MRI is widely used to identify either destructive lesions or degenerative effects on the brain. In terms of chronic pain mechanisms, Voxel based morphometry (VBM), functional MRI (fMRI), diffusion tensor imaging (DTI), and MRI spectroscopy have proved useful, the latter awaiting the development of more powerful machines which will provide better resolution than is possible at this point in time. Wager et al. [29] analysed the fMRI based neurological signature of acute pain in healthy subjects. Their "pain Matrix" included the ventrolateral thalamus, the second somatosensory cortex plus areas activated by many psychological processes, e.g., anterior insula as well as anterior cingulate cortex. It was interesting to note that the cerebral projection was predominantly bilateral except for the somatosensory areas 1 and 2. The bilateral projection has been exploited by Ramachandran [30], who was able to control phantom limb pain with the use of a mirror box. By placing and moving the non-amputated arm into the box, mirrors produced an illusion of the amputated limb still being present, which resulted in relief of phantom limb pain.

In terms of clinical practice, translation of current knowledge into clinical practice is still lacking. Chronic pain conditions investigated to date include back pain, fibromyalgia, temporomandibular joint pain, neuropathic pain, irritable bowel syndrome, CRPS, pelvic pain, migraine, osteoarthritis, multi-somatoform syndrome, musculo-skeletal pain, burning mouth syndrome, and Crohn's disease. In spite of numerous investigations, it has not been possible to develop diagnostic criteria for specific chronic pain conditions. However, some significant general observations have been made [31].

1. VBM and fMRI have identified objective changes in the brain signifying chronic pain.
2. Many of the structural changes caused by chronic pain are reversible once the cause for the pain has been treated effectively.

Specifically, grey matter in the neocortex has been found to be reduced between 5% and 11% volumetrically in chronic back pain. Parts of the brain involved with modulation including the dorsolateral prefrontal cortex and thalamus were equally affected. Similarly, patients with osteoarthritis show volumetric decrease in grey matter in the thalamus, the insula, and the mid-anterior cingulate cortex.

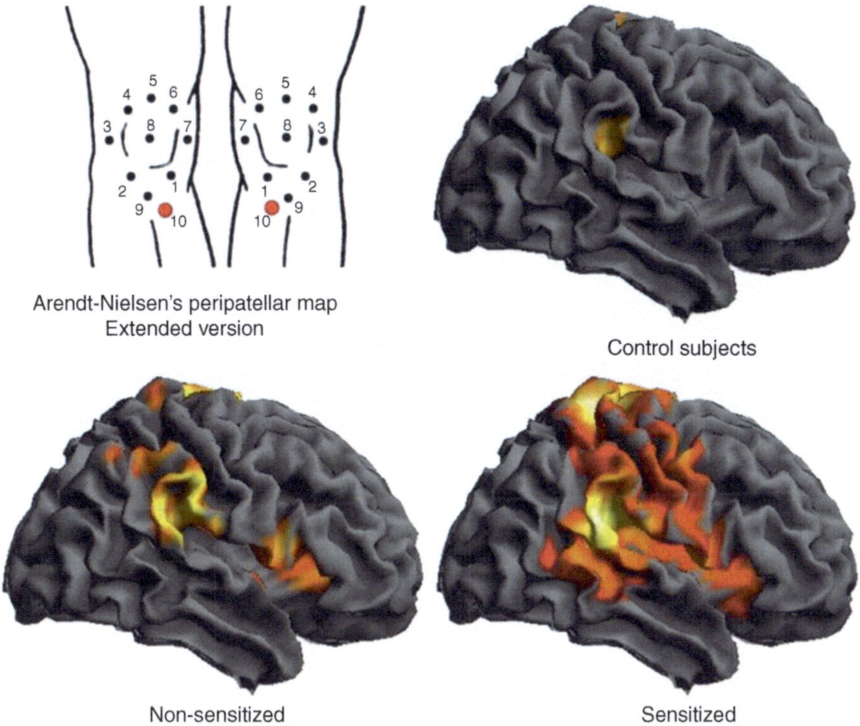

Fig. 4.3 Brain response to pressure stimulation on the anterior tibial surface (red filled circle in the Arendt-Nielsen map). Sensitized patients showed an extensive activation, whereas significant changes in nonsensitized patients involved pain-processing core areas and activation in control subjects was limited to the primary and second somatosensory areas [33] (permission applied for)

Figure 4.3 shows averaged fMRIs response from 55 patients with osteoarthritis elicited by pressure on the medial interjoint line of the knee joint. Importantly not every arthritic patient develops central sensitization. The images convincingly show the difference between patient populations with and without it [32].

Several studies on fibromyalgia showed either reduction or increase in grey matter which seemed to be age dependent. However, one study showed that when depression and anxiety were controlled there was no difference between normal controls and fibromyalgia patients (quoted from [27]).

Imaging studies have also provided substance to the saying "It is all in your mind". Cognitive behavioural treatment (CBT) has been shown to reverse volumetric signs of chronic pain. More recently mindfulness has become an important means of managing chronic pain [33]. It is likely that more refined imaging techniques of the future will shed further light on the mechanics of cerebral processing in chronic pain states.

References

1. Mersky H, Bogduk N. Classification of chronic pain. Seattle: IASP Press; 1994.
2. Iggo A. Cutaneous heat and cold receptors with slowly conducting ©afferent fibres. Quart J Exp Physiol. 1959;44:362–70.
3. Torebjörk HE, Schady W, Ochoa J. Sensory correlates of somatic afferent fibre activation. Hum Neurobiol. 1982;3(1):15–20.
4. Torebjörk HE, Ochoa J. New method to identify nociceptor units innervating glabrous skin of the human hand. Exp Brain Res. 1990;81(3):509–14.
5. Schaible HG, Grubb BD. Afferent and spinal mechanisms of joint pain. Pain. 1993;55:5–54.
6. Caterina MJ, Schumacher MA, Makoto T, Rosen TA, Levine DJ, Julius D. The capsaicin receptor: a heat activated ion channel in the pain pathway. Nature. 1997;389:816–24.
7. Derry S, Wiffen PJ, Kalso EA, Bell RF, Aldington D, Phillips T, Gaskell H, Moore RA. Topical analgesics for acute and chronic pain in adults-an overview of cochrane reviews. Cochrane Database Syst Rev. 2017;5(3):CD008609.
8. Zhang JM, An J. Cytokines, inflammation and pain. Intl Anesthesiol Clin. 2007;45(2):27–37.
9. Iyengar S, Ossipov MH, Johnson KW. The role of calcitonin-related pain mechanisms including migraine. Pain. 2017;158(4):543–59.
10. Hirth M, et al. Nerve growth factor induces sensitization of nociceptors without evidence for increased intra-epidermal nerve fibre density. Pain. 2013;154:2500–11.
11. Yuan H, Lauritsen CG, Kaiser EA, Silberstein SD. CGRP monoclonal antibodies for migraine. BioDrugs. 2017;31(6):487–501.
12. Woolf CJ, Allchorne A, Safieh-Garabedian B, Poole S. Cytokines, nerve growth factor and inflammatory hyperalgesia: the contribution of tumor necrosis factor. Br J Pharmacol. 1997;121:417–24.
13. Thacker M, Gifford L. Sympathetically maintained pain: myth or reality. 2013. https://giffordsachesandpains.files.wordpress.com/2013/06/04_chapteru.pdf.
14. Perl ED. Ideas about pain, a historical review. Nat Rev Neurosci. 2007;8:71–80.
15. Melzack R, Wall P. Pain mechanisms: a new theory. Science. 1965;150(3699):971–9.
16. Mendell LM. Constructing and deconstructing the gate theory of pain. Pain. 2014;155(2):210–6.
17. Christensen BN, Perl ER. Spinal neurones specifically excited by noxious or thermal stimuli: marginal zone of the dorsal horn. J Neurophysiol. 1970;33:293–307.
18. Brown AG, Hamann WC, Martin HF 3rd. Effects of activity in non-myelinated afferent fibres on the spinocervical tract. Brain Res. 1975;98(2):243–59.
19. Sindrup SH, Otto M, Finnerup NB, Jensen TS. Antidepressants in the treatment of neuropathic pain. Basic Clin Pharmacol Toxicol. 2005;96(6):399–409.
20. Rose MA, Kam PCA. Gabapentin: pharmacology and its use in pain management. Anaesthesia. 2002;57:451–62.
21. Woolf CJ. Central sensitization: implications for the diagnosis and treatment of pain. Pain. 2011;152:S2–S15.
22. Bannister K, Patel R, Goncalves L, Townson L, Dickenson AH. Diffuse noxious inhibitory controls and nerve injury: restoring an imbalance between descending monoamine inhibitions and facilitations. Pain. 2015;156(9):1803–11.
23. Hughes J, Smith TW, Kosterlitz HW, Fothergill LA, Morgan BA, Morris HR. Identification of two related pentapeptides from the brain with potent opiate agonist activity. Nature. 1975;258:577–9.
24. Levine JD, Newton CG, Fields HL. The mechanism of placebo analgesia. Lancet. 1978;312:654–7.
25. Gruener H, Zeilig G, Laufer Y, Blumen N, Defrin R. Differential pain modulation properties in central neuropathic pain after spinal cord injury. Pain. 2016;157:1415–25.
26. Helyes Z, Tekus V, Szentes N, Pohoczky K, Botz B, et al. Non-inflammatory autoantibody-induced glia activation in a passive transfer complex regional pain syndrome. J Neurochemistry. 2017;142(Suppl. 1):255.

27. Woodhams SG, Chapman V, Finn DP, Hohmann AG, Neugebauer W. The cannabinoid system and pain. Neuropharmacology. 2017;124:105–20.
28. Abrams DI. The therapeutic effect of Cannabis and cannabinoids: An update from the National Academies of Sciences, Engineering and Medicine report. Eur J Intern Med. 2018;49:7–11.
29. Wager TD, Atlas LY, Lindquist MA, Mathieu R, Choong WW. An fMRI-based neurologic signature of physical pain. N Engl J Med. 2013;368:1388–139.
30. Guenther K. "It's all done with mirrors" V.S. Ramachandran and the material culture of phantom limb research. Med Hist. 2016;60:342–58.
31. Kumbhare DA. Evaluation of chronic pain using magnetic resonance (MR), neuroimaging approaches, what the clinician needs to know. Clin J Pain. 2017;33(4):281–90.
32. Pujol J, Martinez-Vilavella G, Llorente-Onaindia J, Harrison BJ, Lopez-Sola M, Lopez-Ruiz M, Bianco-Hinojo L, Benito P, Deus J, Monfort J. Brain imaging of pain sensitization in patients with in patients with knee osteoarthritis. Pain. 2017;158(9):1831–8.
33. Kabat-Zinn J. Mindfulness with Jon Kabat-Zinn. YouTube. 2007. https://www.youtube.com/watch?v=3nwwKbM_vJc.

Chapter 5
Pharmacology of Analgesics

Koki Shimoji and Hitoshi Fujioka

5.1 Basic Aspect

Each analgesic drug acts under its pharmacokinetics and pharmacodynamics. Pharmacokinetics is defined how each drug is affected by the body, whereas pharmacodynamics is defined how each drug affects the body.

5.1.1 Pharmacokinetics

As mentioned above, pharmacokinetics describes how the body acts on a specific drug after administration through the absorption and distribution as well as the chemical changes of the drug in the body by metabolic enzymes such as cytochrome P450 or glucuronosyltransferase enzymes, and finally the excretion of the metabolites of the drug.

A number of different models have been developed in order to simplify many processes that take place in the interaction between the body and the drugs. The multi-compartment model gives the best approximation to real processes of drugs inside the body. However, many factors are involved in using this model.

K. Shimoji (✉)
Niigata University Graduate School of Medicine, Niigata, Japan

Pain Control Institute, Tokyo, Japan
e-mail: koki-shimoji@nifty.com

H. Fujioka
Department of Anesthesiology, Red Cross Hospital, Tokyo, Japan
e-mail: h_fujioka@medie.co.jp

K. Shimoji et al. (eds.), *Chronic Pain Management in General and Hospital Practice*, https://doi.org/10.1007/978-981-15-2933-7_5

The monocompartmental models and especially two compartmental models are the most frequently used. The various compartments are commonly referred to as the LADME scheme as followed [1]:

1. Liberation: the process of release of a drug from the pharmaceutical formulation.
2. Absorption: the process of a substance entering the blood circulation.
3. Distribution: the dispersion or dissemination of the drugs throughout the fluids and tissues of the body.
4. Metabolization (or biotransformation, or inactivation): the recognition by the body that a foreign substance is present and the irreversible transformation of parent compounds into daughter metabolites.
5. Excretion: the removal of the substances from the body. In rare cases, some drugs irreversibly accumulate in body tissue.

All these concepts can be represented through mathematical formulas that have a corresponding graphical representation. The use of these models may give an understanding of the characteristics of the compound, as well as how a particular drug will behave in the body. The effect of each analgesic is modified by its basic characteristics such as its acid dissociation constant (pKa) (See Henderson–Hasselbalch equation, page), bioavailability, solubility, absorption capacity, and distribution in the organism.

5.1.1.1 Pharmacokinetic Models

Pharmacokinetic model is performed by noncompartmental or compartmental methods. Compartmental methods estimate the concentration-time graph using kinetic models. Noncompartmental methods estimate the exposure to a drug by calculating the area under the curve of a concentration-time graph.

Single-Compartment Model

The simplest idea is to think of the body as only one homogenous compartment. This monocompartmental model presupposes that blood plasma concentrations of the drug are a true reflection of the drug's concentration in other fluids or tissues and that the elimination of the drug is directly proportional to the drug's concentration in the body (first-order kinetics) (Fig. 5.1).

Linear pharmacokinetics gives a straight line or an approximation to although the graph of the relationship between the various factors are involved (dose, blood plasma concentrations, elimination, etc.) For drugs to be effective they need to be able to move rapidly from blood plasma to other body fluids and tissues homogenously.

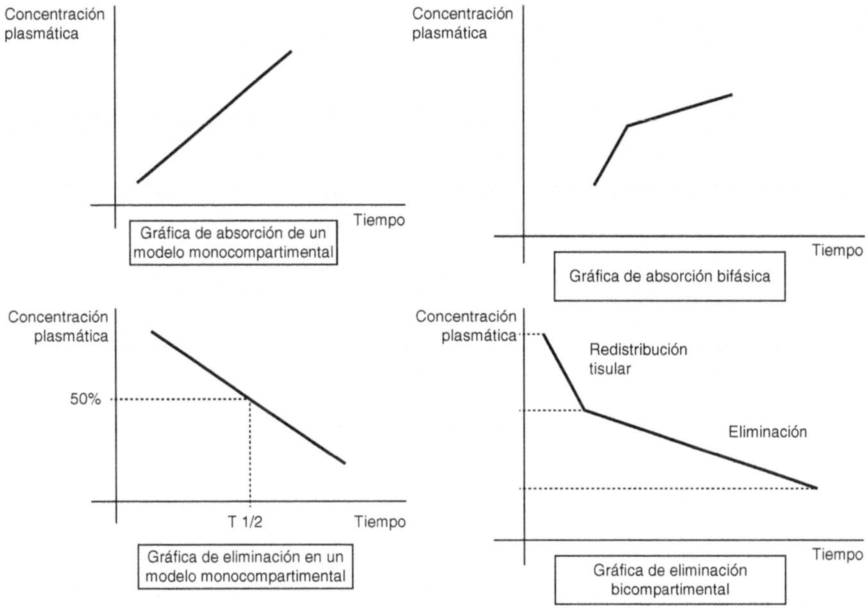

Fig. 5.1 Left graph represents the monocompartmental action model, and right graphs represent absorption and elimination for a nonlinear pharmacokinetic model (Open access, Galego: Gráfica de dous models farmacocinéticos, 28 May 2017)

For instance, after administration of a drug by intravenous injection of short duration, as a bolus, its plasma concentration is immediately maximal. It then decreases according to time. When one has a simple exponential decay, i.e., linear in semi-logarithmic scale, the elimination and the inactivation are simply dependent on the concentration. The variation of the plasma concentration is represented by the following equation:

$$C = C_0 \cdot e^{-\mathrm{Kel}T}$$

in which C represents the concentration at a given time, C_0 initial concentration, $-\mathrm{Kel}$ the constant of apparent elimination, and T time.

However, this model does not always truly reflect the real situation within an organism, since all body tissues have neither the same blood supply nor homogenous character. Therefore, the distribution of the drug will be slower in the tissues with less blood supply than in others with a better blood supply. Also, there are some tissues such as the brain which has a barrier to the distribution of drugs.

If these relative conditions for drug distribution in the different tissue types are considered along with the rate of elimination, the organism can be considered to be acting like two compartments, the central compartment that has a more rapid distribution with a well-developed blood supply and the peripheral compartment with a lower blood flow (Fig. 5.1, right). Tissues such as the brain with a high blood supply can occupy a variable position depending on a drug's ability to cross the blood–brain barrier that separates the organ from the blood supply.

Noncompartmental models are often more versatile in that they do not assume any specific compartmental model and produce accurate results also acceptable for bioequivalence studies. However, the final outcome of the transformations of a drug in an organism depends on a number of interrelated factors.

A number of functional models have been developed in order to simplify the study of pharmacokinetics. These models are based on a consideration of an organism as a number of related compartments [2].

When we consider the drug's *volume concentration* within the organism Vd_F and its volume of distribution in a tissue Vd_T, the former will be described by an equation that takes into account all the tissues that act in different ways as follows:

$$Vd_F = Vd_{T1} + Vd_{T2} + Vd_{T3} + \ldots + Vd_{Tn}$$

This formula represents the *multi-compartment model* with a number of curves that express complicated equations in order to obtain an overall curve. A number of computer programs have been developed to plot these equations [2].

Various case models were discussed in detail by Gabrielsson et al. when a drug is given by intravenous route [1, 2].

The models used in nonlinear pharmacokinetics are largely based on Michaelis–Menten kinetics (Refer to Figs. 5.2, 5.5, and 5.6).

The reaction factor of a drug depends on the route of administration, metabolism, enzymatic induction or inhibition, bioavailability, and dose.

The Rate of Absorption, Distribution

The rate at which most drugs are absorbed when given by the oral route is slower than in other routes. The time (T_{max}) at which maximum concentration (C_{max}) is achieved is modified by gastric acidity, emptying time and intestinal motor motility, etc. and also by age [3, 4].

Plasma Concentration by Intravenous Route

Drugs injected intravenously are removed from the plasma through two primary mechanisms: (1) distribution to body tissues and (2) metabolism + excretion of the drugs. The resulting decrease of the drug's plasma concentration follows a biphasic pattern (Fig. 5.1, right and Fig. 5.4).

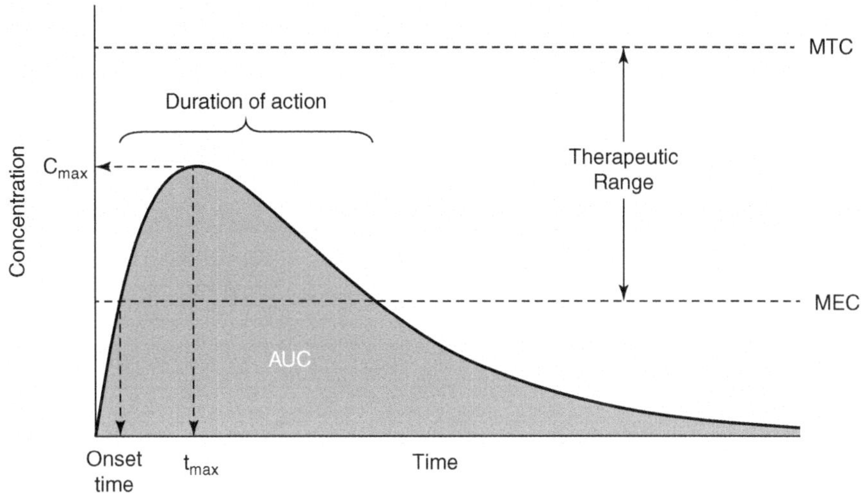

Fig. 5.2 The change in plasma drug concentration with time after administration of a single oral dose of a drug. The interrupted horizontal lines show the minimum effective concentration (MEC) and maximum toxic concentration (MTC). A therapeutic effect can be expected only when plasma level is above the MEC and below the TC basic graph for evaluating the therapeutic implications of pharmacokinetics of an analgesic drug. C_{max} = maximum concentration of an analgesic drug; t_{max} = time for reaching the maximum concentration; Onset time = time for reaching the effective concentration of an analgesic drug. The area under the plasma drug concentration-time curve (AUC) reflects the actual body exposure to drug after administration of a dose of the drug (Reproduced with permission from Mehrotra N et al: The role of pharmacokinetics and pharmacodynamics in phosphodiesterase -5 inhibitor therapy, Sexual Med, Springer Nature, 2006)

When the dose of a drug is increased above a certain threshold, the enzymes responsible for its metabolism become saturated. Then, drug's plasma concentration will increase disproportionately, and its elimination will no longer be constant (Fig. 5.3).

Enzymatic Induction or Inhibition

Some drugs have the capacity to inhibit or stimulate their own metabolism in negative or positive feedback reactions as occurs with antidepressant fluvoxamine and fluoxetine and anticonvulsant drug such as phenytoin. As larger doses of these drugs are administered the plasma concentrations of the unmetabolized increase and the elimination half-life may increase. It is therefore necessary to adjust the dose or other treatment should be considered in this regard.

Thus, nonlinearity may occur due to the whole of the pharmacokinetic sequence, absorption, distribution, metabolism, and elimination.

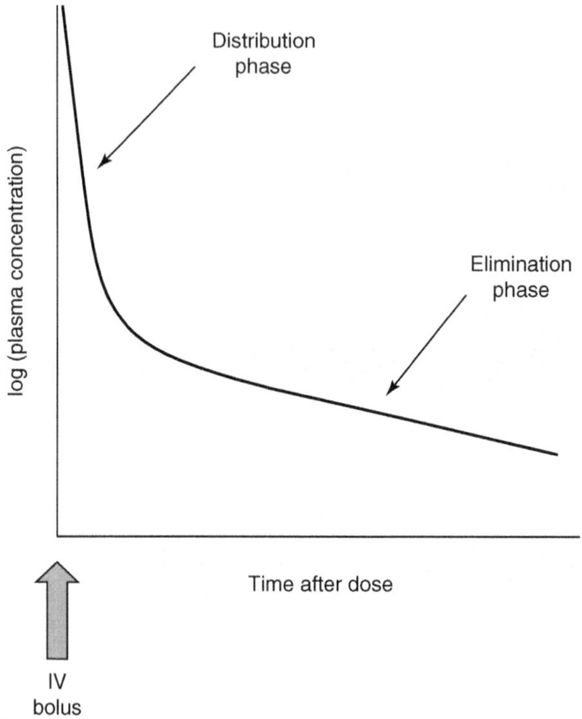

Fig. 5.3 Plasma drug concentration vs. time after an IV dose of an analgesic drug. Alpha phase (distribution phase): An initial phase of rapid decrease in plasma concentration. The decrease is primarily attributed to analgesic drug distribution from the central compartment (blood) into the peripheral compartments (body tissues). This phase ends when equilibrium of drug concentration is established between the central and peripheral compartments. Beta phase (elimination phase): A phase of gradual decrease in plasma concentration of an analgesic after the alpha phase. The decrease is primarily attributed to drug metabolism and excretion. Additional phases (gamma, delta, etc.) are sometimes seen (From Gabrielsson and Weiner, 2012) [2]

Continuous infusions of the intravenous fentanyl or propofol are commonly used to induce and maintain pain relief, sedation, or general anesthesia [5]. Infusion devices can be manually controlled (MCI) where the anesthesiologist makes each change to the infusion rate or target-controlled (TCI) where the anesthetists set a target blood or effect-site concentration and the computerized infusion device makes the necessary changes to the infusion rate.

Hughes et al. [5] proposed that context-sensitive half-times are a useful descriptor of postinfusion central compartment (plasma) kinetics (Fig. 5.4).

Bioavailability

At a practical point, an analgesic drug's bioavailability can be defined as the proportion of the drug that reaches its site of action. From this perspective the intravenous administration of a drug provides the greatest possible bioavailability, and this

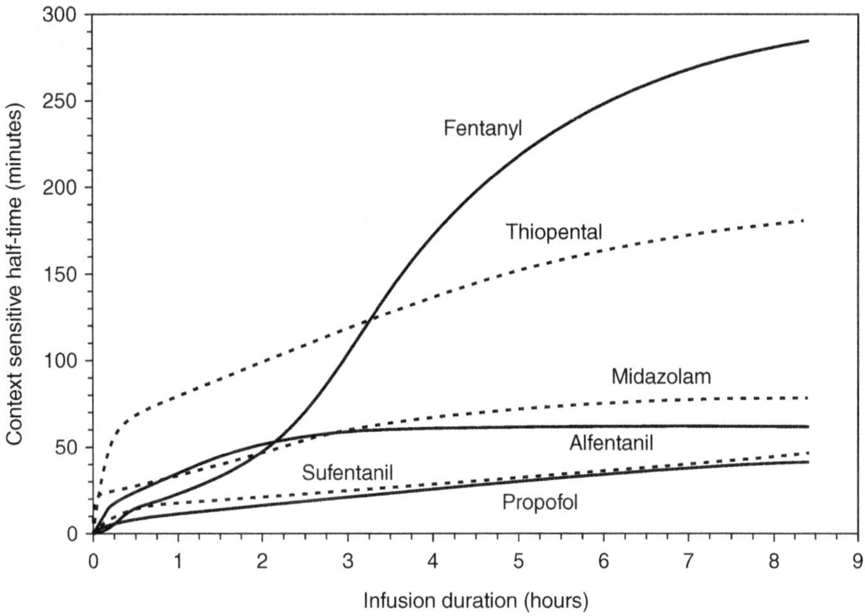

Fig. 5.4 Context-sensitive half-times as a function of infusion duration (the "context") derived from pharmacokinetic models of fentanyl, sufentanil, alfentanil, propofol, midazolam, and thiopental. These simulations demonstrate that elimination half-life is of no value in characterizing disposition of intravenous anesthetic drugs during dosing periods relevant to drug. (From Hughes et al. 1992) [5]

method is considered to yield a bioavailability of 1 (or 100%). Bioavailability of other delivery methods is compared with that of intravenous injection, absolute bioavailability, or to a standard value related to other delivery methods.

Once a drug's bioavailability has been established it is possible to calculate the changes that need to be made to its dosage in order to reach the required blood plasma levels [1, 2, 5].

Bioavailability is therefore a mathematical factor for each individual drug that influences the administered dose. It is possible to calculate the amount of a drug in the blood plasma that has a real potential to bring about its effect using the formula:

$$\text{Effective dose}\left(\text{De}\right) = \text{Bioavailability}\left(\text{B}\right) \times \text{Administered dose}\left(\text{Da}\right)$$

If a drug has a bioavailability of 0.8 (or 80%) and it is administered in a dose of 100 mg, the equation will be:

$$\text{De} = 0.8 \times 100\,\text{mg} = 80\,\text{mg}$$

That is the 100 mg administered represents a blood plasma concentration of 80 mg that has the capacity to have a pharmaceutical effect.

These concepts can be mathematically quantified and integrated to obtain an overall mathematical equation:

$$\mathrm{De} = Q \times \mathrm{Da} \times B$$

where Q is the drug's purity.

$$\mathrm{Va} = \mathrm{Da} \times B \times Q / \tau$$

where Va is defined as the drug's rate of administration and τ is the rate at which the absorbed drug reaches the circulatory system.

Finally, using the Henderson–Hasselbalch equation, and knowing the drug's pKa and pH at which there is equilibrium between its ionized (B) and non-ionized molecules (A), it is possible to calculate the non-ionized concentration of the drug and therefore the concentration that will be subject to absorption:

$$\mathrm{pH} = \mathrm{pKa} + \log B / A$$

When two drugs have the same bioavailability, they are said to be biological equivalents or bioequivalents.

Population Pharmacokinetics

Each patient's pathophysiological and therapeutic conditions as well as body weight, excretory and metabolic functions, and the presence of other drugs may alter dose-concentration relationships of an analgesic drug in the blood. For instance, blood concentrations of drugs which are eliminated mostly by the kidney may increase in patients suffering from renal failure. Population pharmacokinetics seeks to identify the measurable pathophysiologic factors that cause changes in the dose-concentration relationship and the extent of these changes. When such changes are associated with clinically significant shifts in the therapeutic index, dosage of analgesic drugs can be appropriately modified. An advantage of population pharmacokinetic modeling is its ability to analyze sparse data sets [6–8].

Software packages used in population pharmacokinetics modeling include NONMEM® (a nonlinear mixed effects modeling tool used in population pharmacokinetic/pharmacodynamics analysis), developed at the UCSF, and newer packages which incorporate the graphical user interface (GUIs) like Monolix (by Lixoft) as well as graphical model building tools, Phoenix® nonlinear mixed effects modeling (NLME) (by CERTARA).

Basic Graph for the Therapeutic Application of Pharmacokinetics

Clinical application of pharmacokinetics arises from the use of population pharmacokinetics and the characteristics of the patients' population.

Clinical monitoring is usually carried out by determination of plasma concentrations of an analgesic as this is usually the easiest and reliable way to obtain the data. Determining a drug's plasma concentration is particularly important for the drug with narrow therapeutic range and high toxicity. Drugs which pharmacokinetic monitoring is recommended include antiepileptic's (phenytoin, carbamazepine), phenobarbital, etc. (refer to Fig. 5.4).

The Michaelis–Menten model is the one of the simplest and best-known approaches to enzyme kinetics. It takes the form of an equation relating reaction velocity to substrate concentration for a system where a substrate *S* binds reversibly to an enzyme *E* to form an enzyme-substrate complex *ES*, which then reacts irreversibly to generate a product *P* and to regenerate the free enzyme *E*. This system can be represented schematically as follows:

$$E + S \rightleftharpoons ES \rightarrow E + P$$

The Michaelis–Menten equation for this system is:

$$v = \frac{V_{\max}[S]}{K_M + [S]}$$

Here, $V_{\max}$ represents the maximum velocity achieved by the system, at maximum (saturating) substrate concentrations. K_M (the Michaelis constant) is the substrate concentration at which the reaction velocity is 50% of the $V_{\max}$. $[S]$ is the concentration of the substrate *S*.

This is a plot of the Michaelis–Menten equation predicted reaction velocity as a function of substrate concentration, with the significance of the kinetic parameters $V_{\max}$ and K_M graphically depicted (Figs. 5.5 and 5.6).

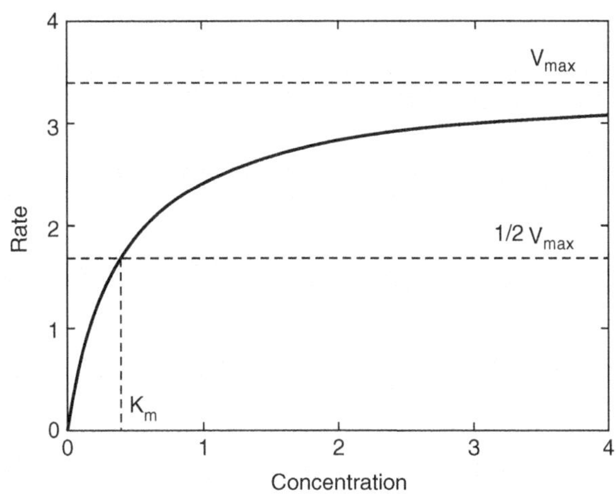

Fig. 5.5 The Michaelis–Menten kinetics model for the relationship between an enzyme and a substrate: one of the parameters studies in pharmacokinetics, where the substrate is a pharmaceutical drug

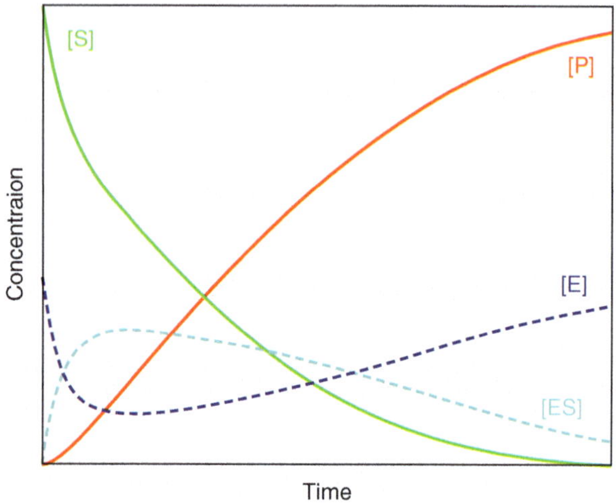

Fig. 5.6 Michaelis–Menten kinetics—change in concentrations of substrate *S*, product *P*, enzyme *E*, and complex ES over time. Following the notation at Michaelis–Menten kinetics, parameter values used were kf = 0.001, kr = 0.0001, kcat = 0.1, *S*0 = 500, *E*0 = 200, *P*0 = ES0 = 0, evaluated to *t* = 50, as in this example. (Taken from Wikipedia page, last edited on March 28, 2018)

5.2 Pharmacodynamics

Pharmacodynamics (PD) is often summarized as the study of what a drug does to the body, whereas pharmacokinetics (PK) is the study of what the body does to a drug.

Thus, pharmacodynamics is the study of the biochemical and physiological effects of drugs on the body metabolism, and the relationship between drug concentration and its effect [9]. One dominant example is drug-receptor interactions as modeled by:

$$L + R \rightleftharpoons L \cdot R$$

where L = ligand, R = receptor, reaction dynamics that can be studied mathematically through tools such as free energy maps.

The majority of drugs either activates or inhibits normal physiological and/or biochemical processes in the body or inhibits vital processes of endo- or ectoparasites and microbial organisms.

Thus, there are seven main drug actions by:

1. stimulating action through direct receptor agonist and downstream effects (agonist)
2. depressing action through direct receptor agonist and downstream effects (inverse agonist)
3. blocking/antagonizing action, where the drug binds the receptor but does not activate it (silent antagonist)
4. stabilizing action, the drug seems to act neither as a stimulant nor as a depressant but stabilize general receptor activation (buprenorphine in opioid dependent individuals, depending on the dose and the recipient)

5. exchanging/replacing substances or accumulating them to form a reserve (glycogen storage)
6. direct beneficial chemical reaction as in free radical scavenging
7. direct harmful chemical reaction which might result in damage or destruction of the cells, through induced toxic or lethal damage (cytotoxicity).

(These seven descriptions may be illustrated in a Table)

5.2.1 *Desirable Effects*

The target of the drugs is mainly to one of the following: (1) cellular membrane disruption, (2) chemical reaction with downstream effects, (3) interaction with enzyme proteins, (4) interaction with structural proteins, (5) interaction with carrier proteins, (6) interaction with ion channels, (7) ligand binding to receptors (hormone receptors, neuromodulator receptors, and neurotransmitter receptors). Analgesic drugs mostly work by (6) and (7).

In addition, enzyme-substrate binding alters the production or metabolism of key endogenous chemicals. For example, aspirin irreversibly inhibits the enzyme prostaglandin synthetase, cyclooxygenase (COX), thereby preventing inflammatory response and relieving pain. Colchicine, a drug for gout, interferes with the function of the structural protein tubulin, leading to pain relief. Digitalis, still used in heart failure, relieves chest pain by inhibiting the activity of the carrier molecule, Na-K-ATPase pump.

The widest class of analgesic drugs acts as ligands which bind to receptors which determine cellular effects. Upon drug binding, receptors can elicit their normal action (agonist), be blocked in action (antagonist), or even action opposite to normal (inverse agonist).

There are many factors affecting the pharmacodynamic effects of analgesic drugs. Pharmacokinetic factors determine peak concentrations of the analgesics in the blood and tissues where the drugs act. Genetic factors and diseases may also exist which would alter metabolism or drug action itself, and a patient's immediate status may also affect indicated dosage.

5.2.2 *Undesirable Effects*

Undesirable effects of an analgesic drug include increased probability of cell mutation (carcinogenic activity), interaction with normal metabolism, and inducing chronic condition (tolerance).

5.2.3 Therapeutic Window

The therapeutic window is the amount of a medication between the amount of an analgesic drug that gives an effect (effective dose) and the amount that gives more adverse effects than desired effects. For instance, medication with a small pharmaceutical window must be administered with care and control by frequently measuring blood concentration of the drug, since it easily loses effects or gives adverse effects.

5.2.4 Duration of Action

The duration of drug action is the length of time that the particular drug is effective. Duration of drug action depends on several factors: (1) the absolute amount of drug given, (2) the pharmaceutical preparation, (3) the reversibility of drug action, (4) the half-life of the drug, (5) the slope of the concentration-response curve, (6) the activity of metabolites, and (7) the influence of disease on drug elimination.

The duration of action of a drug with more than one effect may differ, depending on which effect is followed. Therefore, analgesic drugs with a prolonged therapeutic effect should be given once or twice daily. Analgesic drugs with a short duration of therapeutic effect are best given at regular intervals rather than by such as t.i.d. (three times a day) or q.i.d. (four times a day) regimens [10, 11].

5.2.5 Receptor Binding

The binding of ligands (analgesic drugs) to receptors is governed by the law of mass action which relates the large-scale status to the rate of numerous molecular processes. The rates of formation and back formation can be used to determine the equilibrium concentration of bound receptors. The *equilibrium dissociation constant* (Kd) is defined by:

$$L + R \leftrightarrow L \cdot R \quad K_d = \frac{[L][R]}{[L \cdot R]}$$

where L = ligand, R = receptor, square brackets [ ] denote concentration. The fraction of bound receptors is

$$\text{Fraction Bound} = \frac{[L \cdot R]}{[R] + [L \cdot R]} = \frac{1}{1 + \frac{K_d}{[L]}}$$

This expression is one way to consider the effect of a drug, in which the response is related to the fraction of bound receptors. The fraction of bound receptors is

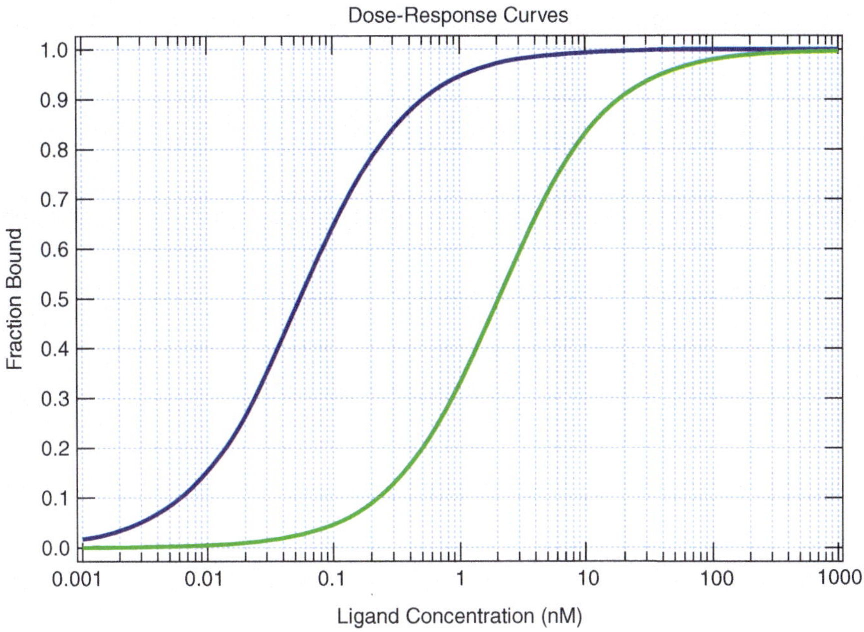

Fig. 5.7 Semi-log plots of two agonists with different Kd. The left (blue) curve represents the ligand with greater potency (permission from the author should be taken)

known as occupancy. The relationship between occupancy and pharmacological response is usually nonlinear. This explains the so-called receptor reserve phenomenon. The concentration producing 50% occupancy is typically higher than the concentration producing 50% of maximum response. The receptor reserve phenomenon is the model that states there are excess receptors on the cell surface than what is necessary for full effect (Fig. 5.7).

Often the response is determined as a function of log [L] to consider many orders of magnitude of concentration. However, there is no biological or physical theory which relates effects of analgesics to the log of concentration. It is useful to note that 50% of the receptors are bound when concentration of a ligand [L] = KD.

The graph in Fig. 5.7 represents the dose-response curves for two hypothetical receptor agonists, plotted in a semi-log fashion. The curve toward the left represents a higher potency, since lower concentrations are needed for a given response.

5.2.6 Multicellular Pharmacodynamics

The concept of pharmacodynamics has been expanded to include multicellular pharmacodynamics (MCPD). MCPD is the study of the static and dynamic properties and relationships between a set of drugs and a dynamic and diverse multicellular four-dimensional organization. It is the study of the workings of a drug on a minimal multicellular system (mMCS), both in vivo and in silico (computer

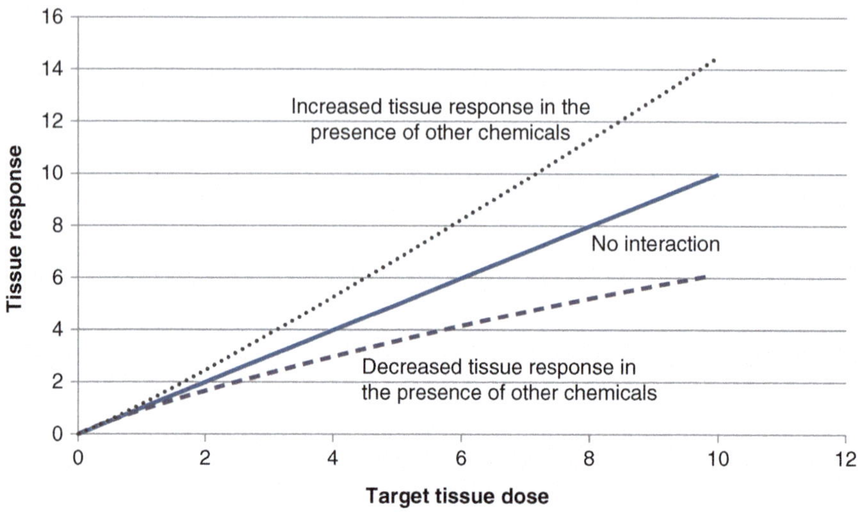

Fig. 5.8 The impact of pharmacodynamic (PD) interactions on tissue response. The term "PD interaction" refers to the case in which one unit of target tissue dose to chemical X in the presence of other chemicals leads to less (examples in Sect. 5.4.1) or more (examples in Sect. 5.4.2) than one unit of tissue response compared to exposure to chemical X by itself (Tan et al. [13])

simulation). Networked multicellular pharmacodynamics (Net-MCPD) further extends the concept of MCPD to model regulatory genomic networks together with signal transduction pathways, as part of a complex of interacting components in the cell [12].

5.2.7 *Toxicodynamics*

In the field of ecotoxicology pharmacokinetics and pharmacodynamics are termed toxicokinetics and toxicodynamics. Here, the focus is on toxic effects on a wide range of organisms. The corresponding models are called toxicokinetic and toxicodynamic models, respectively (Fig. 5.8).

5.3 Clinical Aspect

5.3.1 *Considerations in Analgesic Therapy*

NSAIDs should be considered as the first choice of treatment for superficial somatic pain, such as postsurgical pain from an incision (skin, mucosa). Deep somatic pain, following injury or extensive surgical procedures (muscle, bone), is best treated with combination analgesics, such as NSAIDs with acetaminophen or NSAIDs and/or acetaminophen with an opioid.

Adjuvant drugs may enhance the efficacy of analgesics or have analgesic activity of their own (Drugs for pain. Treat Guide Med Lett 2013) [13] For instance, caffeine in doses greater than 100 mg enhances the analgesic effect of commonly used analgesics, NSAIDs and acetaminophen. Hydroxyzine, antihistamine, in doses of 25–50 mg enhances the analgesic effect of opioids in postoperative pain, and significantly reduces the incidence of opioid-induced nausea and vomiting [13]. Corticosteroids, through their anti-inflammatory and phospholipase- inhibitory effects, can enhance analgesia in patients with pain of inflammatory origin [14, 15].

The placebo effect of analgesics and its magnitude can be modulated by psychological factors such as conditioning and expectancy. Investigators have found that the placebo response can be blocked pharmacologically by naloxone, an opioid-receptor antagonist, and psychologically by hidden injections. Consequently, the placebo effect can be harnessed to the patient's advantage. The clinician's words (attitude) relative to the therapeutic agent affect the patient's expectations and associated neurobiological changes can result in enhanced analgesia and, ultimately, can lead to a reduction in drug intake with maintenance of clinical effect [16]. In clinical practice, however, declaration of Helsinki should be kept in mind [17].

The optimal dose of an analgesic that will provide adequate pain relief must be established by titration and the drug should be administered on schedule. Timely ("by-the-clock") administration of analgesics is much more effective than waiting for pain to return before giving the next dose and may actually reduce the total dosage required for the management of a painful episode [18]. The dosage interval is predicated on the elimination half-life of the drug. Metabolism and adverse drug effects can vary widely among individuals and some patients may respond better to one NSAID or combination with opioid analgesics.

When current analgesic formulations are not optimal, further individualized approach should be taken for pain control. At times, clinicians may have to prescribe more than one type of analgesic to achieve maximal results. For example, the co-administration of ibuprofen with acetaminophen in full doses or ibuprofen and/or acetaminophen with an opioid will result in enhanced analgesia in acute or severe chronic pain.

The concurrent administration of drugs with different mechanisms of action could be effective, while the concurrent administration of drugs with similar mechanisms of action may not be rational in terms of pharmacological basis [13, 18].

5.3.2 Nonsteroidal Anti-inflammatory Agents (NSAIDs)

Nonsteroidal anti-inflammatory drugs (NSAIDs) inhibit the activity of cyclooxygenase isoenzymes COX-1 and COX-2 and, consequently, the synthesis of prostaglandins [19]. COX-1 is expressed in healthy tissues, including platelets, and it is associated primarily with homeostatic or "housekeeping" mechanisms [20]. COX-2 is expressed primarily in the brain, kidneys, female reproductive systems, and bone; and it can be induced by inflammatory cytokines in other tissues, where COX-2 is not found in platelets [20, 21]. Inhibition of COX-2 is primarily responsible for the anti-inflammatory effect of NSAIDs.

Prostaglandin PGE2 affects vascular tone and permeability, modulates inflammation, and influences pain perception [22, 23]. By reducing peripheral prostaglandin synthesis, NSAIDs decrease the recruitment of leukocytes and the synthesis of leukocyte-derived mediators of inflammation and increase the activation threshold of primary afferent sensory neurons by chemical activators. In the trigeminal nucleus or dorsal horn of the spinal cord, PGE2 acts as a pain-producing substance. NSAIDs, which cross the blood–brain barrier, also prevent the synthesis of PGE2 in the CNS.

Ibuprofen is the gold standard against which new analgesics are evaluated. Naproxen, like ibuprofen, has analgesic, anti-inflammatory, and antipyretic activity. Other available oral formulations of NSAIDs offer no apparent advantage over ibuprofen or naproxen [24].

Acetylsalicylic acid (*aspirin*) is effective in the treatment of most types of mild-to-moderate pain. However, a single dose of aspirin can irreversibly inhibit platelet function, interfere with hemostasis and cause prolonged bleeding, and precipitate asthma-like symptoms in susceptible patients. High doses and chronic use of aspirin can cause GI ulceration. Furthermore, aspirin increases the risk of Reye's syndrome in children and adolescents during viral syndromes. Because of the availability of more effective and less toxic alternatives, now aspirin in low dose is used primarily for cardiovascular [25] or potentially cancer [25, 26] prevention.

Ketorolac is available in both oral and parenteral formulations. The use of the oral formulation is restricted to those patients who have received the drug parentally during the perioperative period [27]).

COX-2 selective inhibitor is a form of non-steroidal anti-inflammatory drug (NSAID) that directly targets COX-2, an enzyme responsible for inflammation and pain. Targeting selectivity for COX-2 reduces the risk of peptic ulceration, and is the main feature of celecoxib, rofecoxib, and other members of this drug class. However, data from clinical trials revealed that COX-2 inhibitors caused a significant increase in heart attacks and strokes, with some drugs in the class having worse risks than others.

Some COX-2 inhibitors are used in a single dose to treat pain after surgery [28, 29]. Etoricoxib may be as good as other pain medications. Celecoxib appears to be also as useful as ibuprofen [30].

NSAIDs are rapidly absorbed from the stomach and the upper small intestine. They reach appreciable plasma concentrations in 30–60 min and peak values at about 2–3 h. NSAIDs are distributed throughout the body and cross the placenta. Depending on the agent and dosing, their duration of action is between 4 and 12 h. NSAIDs are metabolized in the liver by first-order kinetics. However, after larger doses, the enzymes become saturated, which leads to zero-order kinetics and increases half-lives. Metabolites are excreted primarily by the kidneys.

5.3.2.1 Precautions at Prescribing Acetaminophen and NSAIDs

In healthy people, therapeutic doses of acetaminophen, for instance, have virtually no adverse effects. In general, the occasional use of acetaminophen during pregnancy is also considered safe but may increase the risk for developing attention-deficit/hyperactivity disorder (ADHD)-like behavioral problems or hyperkinetic disorders (HKDs) in children [31–33]. It is considered as the preferred analgesic in patients with liver disease because of the absence of platelet impairment associated with NSAIDs. However, hepatotoxicity may occur with overdose and in patients with liver disease, alcoholism, and malnutrition, which may enhance acetaminophen toxicity [33]. It is also noted that the long-term use of acetaminophen may increase the anticoagulant effect of warfarin [34]. The half-life of acetaminophen may be prolonged in patients with chronic liver disease.

Overdose of acetaminophen ingestion and therapeutic misadventure may cause hepatotoxicity. Several factors, such as concomitant alcohol use or abuse, concurrent medications, genetic factors, and nutritional status, can influence the susceptibility and severity of acetaminophen hepatotoxicity.

N-acetylcysteine is a very effective antidote to acetaminophen when giving within 6–8 h, and is also recommended after a presentation of hepatotoxicity and acute liver failure. The prognosis of patients with acetaminophen-induced acute liver failure is better than other causes of acute liver failure. Liver transplantation should even be considered to those who are unlikely to survive [33].

Hepatotoxicity of acetaminophen may be related to increased mitochondrial ROS formation, which is associated with gene expression changes, suggesting disruption of the mitochondrial electron transport chain [35, 36].

Acetaminophen side effects may be treated or prevented by Crocus sativus (saffron) petals extract [37], ginger (Zingiber officinale Roscoe), vitamin E, or salvianolic acid B, a major water-soluble compound extracted from Radix Salvia miltiorrhiza have also been shown to be effective to treat acetaminophen-induced hepatotoxicity by inducing nuclear factor-erythroid-2-related factor 2 (Nrf2) expression [38, 39].

Nausea, vomiting, anorexia, diarrhea, and abdominal pain occur during the first 24 h. Clinical evidence of hepatic damage may be noted in 2–6 days, indicating avoidance of overdose and/or misuse of the drug and the early detection of the hepatotoxicity signs [40, 41].

Intolerance

Intolerance to NSAIDs is most likely to occur in individuals with a history of asthma, nasal polyps, and chronic urticarial states [42]. A history of rhinorrhea, urticaria, angioedema, or bronchospasm occurring within 3 h after exposure is an acceptable method of determining intolerance. Even a single dose of these agents can precipitate asthma in susceptible patients [43, 44]. Intolerance is not an immune phenomenon; rather it is related to the ability of NSAIDs to inhibit the enzyme cyclooxygenase and the consequent shunting of arachidonic acid down the lipoxygenase pathway, which results in increased levels of leukotrienes [45].

Gastropathy

Therapeutic doses of NSAIDs may cause nausea and vomiting and have been associated with abdominal pain, diarrhea, and dyspepsia. They can exacerbate the symptoms of peptic ulcer disease.

With chronic use of NSAIDs, gastric ulceration, perforation, and bleeding can occur [46]. The prolonged use of high doses of NSAIDs with the concomitant use of anticoagulants, aspirin, and corticosteroids, excessive alcohol intake, and advanced age increase the risk of these complications. Mucosal injury is primarily related to blockade of gastro-protective prostaglandin synthesis. Ibuprofen, in general, appears to have the lowest risk of NSAID-associated gastrointestinal toxicity [47].

Renal Toxicity

NSAIDs decrease also the synthesis of renal prostaglandins and decrease renal blood flow, leading to fluid retention and blood pressure increase, and may precipitate renal failure in susceptible patients [48, 49]. Risk factors for renal toxicity include old age, chronic renal insufficiency, congestive heart failure, hepatic cirrhosis, and the concurrent use of β-adrenergic receptor antagonists and angiotensin-converting enzyme inhibitors [50, 51].

Nephritic syndrome, acute interstitial nephritis, and an increased incidence of end-stage renal disease have been reported in patients treated chronically with NSAIDs.63 NSAIDs should be avoided in persons with preexisting renal disease.

Antithrombotic Effect

NSAIDs impair platelet adhesion to tissue components and platelet aggregation primarily through the inhibition of thromboxane A2 (TXA2) synthesis. In contrast to aspirin, platelet inhibition is reversible and short-lived with therapeutic doses of other NSAIDs. Platelet function returns to normal when most of the drug has been eliminated from the body. However, in the presence of bleeding diathesis, either hereditary, acquired, or drug induced, the antiplatelet effect of these agents may contribute to serious bleeding. NSAIDs in combination with anticoagulants can increase the International Normalized Ratio (INR) by as much as 15% [52].

Hepatotoxicity

Adverse hepatic reactions as in case of acetaminophen have been reported in association with NSAIDs, but they appear to be idiosyncratic and often dose related [53]. Predisposing factors for toxic reactions include advanced age, decreased renal function, and collagen vascular diseases. Hepatotoxicity, like most adverse drug reactions, occurs within weeks of initiation of long-term therapy [53]. Patients with cirrhosis of the liver also have impaired hemostasis and the administration of NSAIDs may further increase the risk of bleeding. Concomitant use of Chinese herbal medicines with NSIDs may alleviate NSAIDs-induced adverse effects including hepatotoxicity [54].

Renal Toxicity

NSAIDs decrease the synthesis of renal prostaglandins, leading to the decrease in renal blood flow to cause fluid retention and increase blood pressure, and may precipitate renal failure in susceptible patients [55]. Risk factors include old age, chronic renal insufficiency, congestive heart failure, hepatic cirrhosis, and the concurrent use of β-adrenergic receptor antagonists and angiotensin-converting enzyme inhibitors. Nephritic syndrome, acute interstitial nephritis, and an increased incidence of end-stage renal disease have been reported in patients treated for long time with NSAIDs [56]. NSAIDs should be avoided in persons with preexisting renal diseases.

Cardiovascular Toxicity

Selective COX-2 inhibitors are associated with a small but absolute cardiovascular risk [47]. COX-2 inhibition leads to less prostacyclin (PGI2) and more thromboxane 2 (TXA2) synthesis. PGI2 is a vasodilator and blocks platelet aggregation; TXA2 is vasoconstrictive and promotes platelet aggregation. COX-2 inhibition allows TXA2 to function unopposed. Although NSAIDs block both COX-1 and COX-2, the risk appears to be related to dose and duration of treatment. In general, NSAIDs should be used with caution in patients with a history of hypertension, ischemic heart disease, stroke, or congestive heart failure [57].

CNS Side Effects

Rarely, NSAIDs may cause tinnitus, dizziness, anxiety, drowsiness, confusion, disorientation, depression, and severe headaches. These adverse effects are noticed more commonly in older persons. Tinnitus is reversible and appears to be a signs of high blood levels of NSAIDs [58]. Aseptic meningitis has been reported in persons with systemic lupus erythematosus who were taking ibuprofen or naproxen [59].

Effects on Pregnancy and Lactation

NSAIDs at the time of conception may increase the risk of miscarriage [42]. During pregnancy, low dose intermittent administration of NSAIDs, in general, is considered to be safe. However, NSAIDs should not be prescribed during the third trimester of pregnancy [60, 61]. Potential maternal effects include prolonged gestation and labor, and increased peripartum bleeding. Potential fetal effects include premature closure of ductus arteriosus, pulmonary hypertension, renal dysfunction, reduced amniotic fluid volume, and/or increased cutaneous and intracranial bleeding [60]. In breast feeding women, ibuprofen and naproxen are considered safe.

Effects on Children

The primary concern when children are taking NSAIDs is dosage errors resulting in overdose, which may result in significant morbidity and even fatal [55]. Educating the caregivers (parents, guardians, others) about the importance of correct dosing and dosage intervals, preventing the concurrent use of other medications that may contain NSAIDs. Proper storage of analgesics in child-proof containers can minimize the risk.

Drug-Drug Interactions

Drug–drug interactions all seem to have either a pharmacodynamic or a pharmacokinetic basis. NSAIDs may decrease the antihypertensive effects of β-adrenergic blocking agents by blocking prostaglandin synthesis, angiotensin-converting enzyme inhibitors, and diuretics, and increase the toxicity of lithium and methotrexate by decreasing renal excretion, and increase the risk of peptic ulcer disease with corticosteroids by additive effect [62]. NSAIDs also increase the risk of bleeding by platelet inhibition and increase the INR (prothrombin time by international normalized ratio) with warfarin sodium [63–66].

NSAIDs can also interfere with the antiplatelet effect of low dose aspirin (81 mg per day) by blocking the access of aspirin to its active site, potentially rendering aspirin less effective when used for cardio-protection and stroke prevention [66]. To avoid significant interference, the healthcare providers should advise patients regarding the appropriate concomitant use of NSAIDs and aspirin. At least, 2 h should be elapsed after aspirin dosing before taking a NSAID and at least 8 h should be elapsed after NSAID dosing before taking an aspirin [67].

Opioid-Receptor Agonists

There are three types of opioid receptors: mu (μ), delta (δ), and kappa (K). Opioid-receptor agonists produce analgesia by acting primarily at μ-receptors found in the brain, brainstem, spinal cord, and primary afferent sensory neurons [68, 69].

Presynaptic μ-receptor activation by an opioid inhibits calcium influx into sensory neurons, which leads to decrease neurotransmitter release. Postsynaptic μ-receptor activation increases K+ conductance, which decreases postsynaptic response to excitatory neurotransmission.

Morphine is the naturally found archetypic opioid analgesic. It is a naturally existing strong, full μ-receptor agonist, which fully activates the μ-receptor displaying maximum efficacy. However, after oral administration, morphine is rapidly metabolized by hepatic Glucuronization and its bioavailability is low.

Oxycodone is a semi-synthetic strong full μ-receptor agonist. After oral administration its bioavailability is high. Oxycodone is metabolized by glucuronidation to noroxycodone and by the cytochrome P450 isoenzyme 2D6 (CYO450 2D6) to oxymorphone. Oxycodone is primarily responsible for analgesia but not its metabolites.

Codeine is a naturally occurring weak, full μ-receptor agonist. Its efficacy is less than that produced by a strong full agonist even when all the available receptors are activated. Its analgesic action is largely dependent on its hepatic demethylation to morphine, which is responsible for its analgesic activity. Demethylation by the cytochrome P450 (CYP450) isoenzyme 2D6 is subject to genetic polymorphism. Cytochrome p450 2D6 (CYP2D6) is responsible for the oxidative metabolism of up to 25% of commonly prescribed drugs such as antidepressants, antipsychotics, (opioids, antiarrhythmics, and tamoxifen besides codeine [70]. Up to 10% of patients are poor metabolizers and do not experience analgesia in response to treatment with codeine. Another 10% of the patients rapidly convert codeine to high levels of morphine, leading to severe toxicity even with therapeutic doses [71].

Codeine is a naturally occurring weak, full μ-receptor agonist. It is similar in structure to codeine but a more effective analgesic. Its bioavailability after oral administration is high. Hydrocodone is demethylated by the CYO450 isoenzyme 2D6 into hydromorphone. Since hydromorphone has a much stronger affinity for the μ-receptor than hydrocodone, it has been proposed that hydrocodone is a prodrug (bioreversible derivative of a drug molecule that undergoes an enzymatic and/or chemical transformation in vivo to release the active parent drug).

Patients who are CYP450 isoenzyme 2D6 deficient and those on CYP450 isoenzyme 2D6 inhibitors may not achieve adequate analgesia [71, 72].

Tramadol is a weak, centrally acting μ-receptor agonist with norepinephrine and serotonin reuptake inhibiting activity [72]. The drug is less effective than a strong full μ-receptor agonist and its activity appears to be limited to the CNS. After oral administration, tramadol is readily absorbed from the gastrointestinal tract. It reaches appreciable plasma concentrations in 60 minutes and peak values at about 2 h. Tramadol's bioavailability is high, and it is readily distributed from the vascular compartment to all tissues. Tramadol is extensively metabolized in the liver [72, 73] The unchanged fraction of the drug and its metabolites are excreted in the kidneys [72].

Tapentadol is a weak, centrally acting μ-receptor agonist/norepinephrine reuptake inhibitor [74, 75]. It is rapidly absorbed after oral administration, although the bioavailability of the drug is low, due to extensive first-pass metabolism. Tapentadol is readily distributed from the vascular compartment to all tissues; its plasma protein binding is about 20%. The primary metabolic pathway of tapentadol is hepatic glucuronidation[34, 35]. Tapentadol and its metabolites are rapidly and completely excreted through the kidneys [76, 77]. Tapentadol may have some advantages, as it does not require CYP450 system activation and has minimal serotonergic effects [78].

5.3.2.2 Side Effects and Precautions of Opioid-Receptor Agonists

Intolerance of Opioids

Opioid analgesic-related allergic reactions are rare. However, μ-receptor agonists are able to induce histamine release and produce pruritus and cutaneous blood vessels tend to dilate around the "blush areas," such as the face, neck, and upper thorax. Histamine release can also lead to peripheral vasodilatation and orthostatic hypotension. Opioid-receptor agonists appear to directly activate mast cells, but the release of vasoactive substances does not appear to have an immunologic action [79, 80]. Respiratory and cardiovascular support should be taken, and epinephrine and/or antihistamines such as diphenhydramine, if needed, should be given to manage symptoms [81].

Gastropathy by Opioids

Nausea and vomiting, as a result of μ-receptor activation in the medullary chemoreceptor trigger zone, are common adverse effect associated with the initiation of opioid analgesic therapy. With chronic use, constipation is the most common adverse effect. Opioid analgesics bind μ-receptors in the gastrointestinal tract, which leads to an increase in the tone of the anterior portion of the stomach and decreases gastric motility. Constipation is dose related and patients do not develop tolerance to this effect. The risk may be minimized by increasing fluid and dietary fiber intake [82]. Tablets containing the opioid agonist oxycodone and the opioid antagonist naloxone may block the action of oxycodone in the gut without compromising its analgesic effects [83].

Respiratory Effects of Opioids

Mu-receptor activation in the brain stem depresses respiratory chemoreceptor sensitivity to carbon dioxide [84]. Genetic risk predictions along with clinical risk factors effectively identify children at higher and lower risks of opioid-induced respiratory depression [85]. Concurrent administration of oxygen may cause apnea. Carbon dioxide retention produces intracranial vasodilatation and may aggravate increased intracranial pressure. Thus, opioids should be used with great caution in cases of head injury, the elderly, the debilitated, and those with pulmonary disease, particularly severe asthma because of cough reflex suppression, impairment of ciliary activity, and aggravation of bronchospasm.

CNS Side Effects of Opioids

Mu-receptor activation in the brain causes dizziness, drowsiness, sedation, and cognitive changes [79]. Cognitive chances present primarily in patients who already have cognitive dysfunction. A paradoxical reaction to the CNS effects in the elderly is not uncommon. To avoid both toxic and paradoxical effects, dosages must be reduced by as much as one-half to one-fourth. Opioid analgesics also modulate mood and behavior, causing euphoria in some and anxiety and dysphoria in others. Mu-receptor activation in the oculomotor nerve causes pupillary constriction (miosis).

As noted, before, there are not absolutely safe biologically active therapeutic agents and drugs seldom exert their beneficial effects without also causing ADEs. Opioid analgesics like other therapeutic agents, even after the administration of a single dose, may produce ADEs. However, there is also supporting evidence that opioid related ADEs are more likely to be associated with prolonged use, high doses, the presence of comorbidities, and polypharmacy [86, 87].

Tolerance of Opioids

Repeated use of a constant dose of an opioid-receptor agonist can lead to tolerance or decreased therapeutic efficacy [88]. Tolerance appears to be either genetically determined innate or acquired, which appears to have a pharmacokinetic or pharmacodynamic mechanism.

Tolerance may develop in both acute and chronic opioid users. To maintain adequate analgesia, the development of tolerance requires either an increase in the dosage or frequency of drug administration. There does not appear to be any evidence that tolerance leads to dependence. Delta opioid peptide (DOP) (δ) receptor antagonism has been shown to reduce tolerance [89].

Dependence of Opioids

Dependence is a potential hazard of opioid use. However, patients who take opioids for acute pain rarely experience euphoria and even more rarely do they develop psychological dependence or addiction. Clinically significant physical dependence is more likely to develop after several weeks of treatment with relatively large doses of an opioid [90, 91]. In these patients abrupt cessation of treatment results in withdrawal syndrome characterized by dilated pupils, rapid pulse, muscle jerks, goose flesh, flu-like symptoms, vomiting, diarrhea, tremors, yawning, and sleep.

Overdose of Opioids

Opioid overdose is a life-threatening condition. One of the essential symptoms of opioid intoxication is respiratory depression [92]. A respiratory rate less than 12 per minute in a patient who is not in physiologic sleep strongly suggests opioid intoxication, particularly when accompanied by miosis and stupor [93]. Patients with respiratory rates ≤12 breaths per minute and stupor should be ventilated with a bag-valve mask; and administered naloxone, a competitive μ-receptor antagonist, which reverses all signs of opioid intoxication [93]. Once the respiratory rate improves, the patient should be observed for 4–6 h.

Opioids in Pregnant and Nursing Women

The use of opioids in the pregnant or nursing patient is discouraged because of their general CNS depressant effects on the fetus and infant.

Prescription opioid use in pregnancy is strongly associated with neonatal complications. Antenatal cumulative prescription opioid exposure, opioid type, tobacco use, and selective serotonin reuptake inhibitor use increase the risk of neonatal abstinence syndrome [94, 95].

The short-term use of therapeutic doses of codeine in combination with acetaminophen is appropriate for the management of moderate-to-severe postoperative pain. However, if the mother is a rapid metabolizer, she may produce much more morphine than those with normal metabolic activity. This, in 2–3 days, can lead to symptoms compatible with morphine overdose [96].

Drug-Drug Interactions of Opioids

Drug–drug interactions of opioids all seem to originate from either a pharmacodynamic or a pharmacokinetic mechanism. The most serious adverse effect of opioids is respiratory depression [85]. Consequently; the risk of respiratory depression is increased (additive) with sedative-hypnotic agents such as benzodiazepines or barbiturates, tricyclic antidepressants, and other CNS depressants [97].

5.4 Prescription

5.4.1 Mild Pain

In patients with mild pain, an over-the-counter NSAID is the drug of choice (Table 5.1). Ibuprofen, 200 mg, is more effective than aspirin (acetylsalicylic acid), 650 mg; or acetaminophen, 650 mg; or naproxen 200–220 mg [99]. It is also used intravenously [100].

Table 5.1 Equianalgesia of analgesics as compared to oral morphine

Equianalgesia (morphine, PO)				
Analgesic	Strength (relative)	Equivalent dose (10 mg)	Bioavailability	Half-life of active metabolites (h)
Aspirin (non-opioid)	1/360	Impractical	100%	3.1–9
Diflunisal (NSAID, non-opioid)	1/160	1600 mg	80–90%	8–12
Dextropropoxyphene [7]	1/13–1/20	130–200 mg		
Codeine	1/10	100 mg	≈90%	2.5–3 (C6G 1.94; [8] morphine 2–3)
Tramadol	1/10	100 mg	68–72%	5.5–7 (≈9) [clarification needed]
Tapentadol	1/10	100 mg	95%	
Dihydrocodeine	1/5	50 mg	20%	4
Anileridine [9]	1/4	40 mg		
Alphaprodine	1/4–1/6	40–60 mg		
Pethidine (meperidine hydrochloride)	1/3	28 mg	50–60%	3–5
Hydrocodone	1	10 mg	≥80%	3.8–6
Metopon	1	10 mg		
Pentazocine lactate (IV) [10]	1	10 mg (6.7–13.3 mg)		
Morphine (oral)	(1)	(10 mg)	≈25%	
Oxycodone [11]	1.5	6.67 mg	≤87%	3–4.5
Morphine (IV/IM)	3	3.33 mg	100%	2–3
Clonitazene	3	3.33 mg		
Methadone (acute) [12, 98]	3–4	2.5–3.33 mg	40–90%	15–60
Diamorphine (Heroin; IV/IM) [13]	4–5	2–2.5 mg	100%	<0.6
Hydromorphone [15]	5	2 mg	30–35%	2–3
Oxymorphone [16]	7	3.33 mg	10%	7.25–9.43
Methadone (chronic) [13]	7.5	1.35 mg	40–90%	15–60
Levorphanol [16]	8	1.3 mg	70%	11–16
7-Hydroxymitragynine	17	≈0.6 mg		
Buprenorphine [7]	40	0.25 mg	35–40% (SL)	20–70, mean 37
Fentanyl	50–100	0.1–0.2 mg	33% (PO); 92% (TD)	0.04 (IV); 7 (TD)
Sufentanil	500–1000	10–20 μg		4.4
Bromadol	504	≈ 20 μg		
Etorphine	1000–3000	3.3–10 μg		
Etonitazene	2000	5.0 μg		

(continued)

Table 5.1 (continued)

Equianalgesia (morphine, PO)				
Analgesic	Strength (relative)	Equivalent dose (10 mg)	Bioavailability	Half-life of active metabolites (h)
Dihydroetorphine	1000–12,000	20–40 μg		
Carfentanil	10,000–100,000	0.1–1.0 μg		7.7

"Strength" is defined as analgesic potency relative to morphine
Tolerance, sensitization, cross-tolerance, metabolism, and hyperalgesia may be complex factors in some individuals
Interactions caused by polypharmacy, food and drink, and other factors may potentiate or inhibit the effectiveness of certain analgesics as well as drastically alter their half-life
Because some analgesics are prodrugs, individual variation in liver enzymes (e.g., cytochrome P450 enzyme CYP2D6) may result in significantly altered effects

Ibuprofen, 400 mg, is more effective than ibuprofen, 200 mg; and it is equianalgesic to naproxen, 400–440 mg [99]. A full dose of ibuprofen, and presumably naproxen, in combination with a full dose of acetaminophen is more effective than either of the two components alone [101]. A meta-analysis has also shown that this combination can also reduce postoperative opioid requirements [102].

Acetaminophen, in doses between 650 and 1000 mg, has been shown to be safe and effective for treating pain after minor surgeries like removal of lower wisdom teeth [103]. However, acetaminophen has no clinically significant anti-inflammatory effect and ibuprofen, 200 mg, is more effective than acetaminophen, 1000 mg [104]. Therefore, with notable exceptions, acetaminophen should be considered an alternative analgesic when NSAIDs are contraindicated (see NSAID-related prescription precautions).

5.4.2 *Moderate Pain*

In patients with moderate pain, full doses of ibuprofen or naproxen are the drugs of choice (Table 5.1) [47, 105, 106]. Ibuprofen, 400 mg, is more effective than codeine with aspirin, 60/650 mg; or codeine with acetaminophen, 60/600 mg [38]. Ibuprofen, 400 mg, is equianalgesic to naproxen, 400–40 mg, and naproxen 500–550 mg; but ibuprofen, 600–800 mg, is more effective [105]. Full doses of ibuprofen, and presumably naproxen, in combination with a full dose of acetaminophen is more effective than either of the two components alone [101].

Meta-analysis has shown that full doses of ibuprofen, and presumably naproxen, in combination with a full dose of acetaminophen can also reduce postoperative opioid requirements. However, if moderate pain is not controlled adequately with full doses of a NSAID/acetaminophen combination, a weak full μ-receptor agonist, e.g., codeine or hydrocodone (Table 5.1), with "add-on" doses of ibuprofen or acetaminophen to augment fixed-dose formulations may be considered.

Meta-analysis has also shown that NSAIDs have a pre-emptive effect and reduce postoperative analgesic requirements [47]. This pre-emptive effect has been shown in association with oral surgical procedures, reducing both postoperative surgical pain and the need for postoperative use of opioids. Another study suggests that there may be a window-period, and timely administration, i.e., within an hour of the surgical procedure, will provide a similar benefit. It has also been reported that the preoperative administration of ibuprofen, 1 h before the administration of local anesthesia, is an effective method for achieving deep anesthesia during the surgical procedures.

5.4.3 Severe Pain

In patients with severe postoperative pain, a strong full μ-receptor agonist, i.e., oxycodone, in combination with ibuprofen or acetaminophen (Table 5.1), with add-on doses of ibuprofen or acetaminophen to augment fixed-dose formulations should be considered. Opioid dose requirements vary widely from one patient to another; but the equivalent of oral morphine, 10 mg per 70 kg of body weight, is a reasonable staring dose [13, 106]. The dose equivalent of codeine is about 60 mg; of hydrocodone it is about 10 mg; and of oxycodone it is about 5 mg.

Hydrocodone with ibuprofen, 1 5/400 mg, is superior to ibuprofen, 400 mg [107]. Oxycodone with ibuprofen, 5/400 mg, is more effective than oxycodone with acetaminophen, 5/650 mg; or hydrocodone with acetaminophen, 7.5/500 mg [30, 108]. Oxycodone with acetaminophen, 5/500 mg, is as effective as codeine with acetaminophen, 60/1000 mg; however, ibuprofen, 600 to 800 mg, is more effective than either of the above formulations [104, 105].

Codeine, hydrocodone, and oxycodone formulations with acetaminophen are alternative drugs when NSAIDs are contraindicated.

Tramadol with acetaminophen, 75/650 mg, is as effective for the management of postsurgical pain as hydrocodone with acetaminophen, 10/650 mg (Table 5.1) [109]. However, tramadol with acetaminophen, 112/650 mg, is less effective than ibuprofen, 200 mg. Tapentadol, 200 mg, is less effective for the management of postsurgical dental pain than ibuprofen, 400 mg [110]. Clearly, neither tramadol nor tapentadol should be considered preferred analgesics for postsurgical odontogenic pain. On the other hand, the long-term effectiveness, safety and tolerability of oral tapentadol was found for the treatment of refractory chronic low back pain in a real-life clinical setting [111]. Tapentadol also has a high potential for abuse [112, 113].

Drug metabolism can differ widely among patients and effects reported should not be viewed as psychological since they generally have a pharmacological basis. Onset, peak, and duration of analgesic action and maximum safe dosages vary with drugs. To enhance analgesia when using opioid drugs, it might be recommended to add a NSAID and/or acetaminophen. Regular (around-the-clock) administration of analgesics might have positive pharmacological and psychological effects on a certain patient. Side effects such as drowsiness, nausea, and vomiting should be carefully watched for and the dosage adjusted, or other treatments initiated.

Sometimes, increasing the dosage and frequency of administration or switching to an alternate medication may be necessary to maintain analgesic effect. Dosage of analgesics should be enough, and timing of prescription should be carefully monitored.

References

1. Gabrielsson J, Meibohm B, Weiner D. Pattern recognition in pharmacokinetic data analysis. AAPS J. 2016;18:47–63.
2. Gabrielsson J, Weiner D. Non-compartmental analysis. Methods Mol Biol. 2012;929:377–89.
3. Anderson BJ, van Lingen RA, Hansen TG, Lin YC, Holford NH. Acetaminophen developmental pharmacokinetics in premature neonates and infants: a pooled population analysis. Anesthesiology. 2002;96:1336–45.
4. Haslund-Krog SS, Hertel S, Dalhoff K, et al. Interventional cohort study of prolonged use (>72 hours) of paracetamol in neonates: protocol of the PARASHUTE study. BMJ Paediatr Open. 2019;30(3):e000427.
5. Hughes MA, Glass PS, Jacobs JR. Context-sensitive half-time in multicompartment pharmacokinetic models for intravenous anesthetic drugs. Anesthesiology. 1992;76:334–41.
6. Olofsen E, Dahan A. Population pharmacokinetics/pharmacodynamics of anesthetics. AAPS J. 2005;7:E383–9.
7. Heeremans EH, Proost JH, Eleveld DJ, et al. Population pharmacokinetics and pharmacodynamics in anesthesia, intensive care and pain medicine. Curr Opin Anaesthesiol. 2010;23:479–84.
8. Martini C, Olofsen E, Yassen A, et al. Pharmacokinetic-pharmacodynamic modeling in acute and chronic pain: an overview of the recent literature. Expert Rev Clin Pharmacol. 2011;4:719–28.
9. Lees P, Cunningham FM, Elliott J. Principles of pharmacodynamics and their applications in veterinary pharmacology. J Vet Pharmacol Ther. 2004;27:397–414.
10. Carruthers SG. Duration of drug action. Am Fam Physician. 1980;21:119–26.
11. Vauquelin G, Charlton SJ. Long-lasting target binding and rebinding as mechanisms to prolong in vivo drug action. Br J Pharmacol. 2010;161:488–508.
12. Shen C, Meng Q. Prediction of cytochrome 450 mediated drug-drug interactions by three-dimensional cultured hepatocytes. Mini Rev Med Chem. 2012;12:1028–36.
13. Drugs for pain. Treat Guidel Med Lett. 2013;11:31–42.
14. Manchikanti L, Buenaventura RM, Manchikanti KN, et al. Effectiveness of therapeutic lumbar transforaminal epidural steroid injections in managing lumbar spinal pain. Pain Physician. 2012;15:E199–245.
15. Liu K, Liu P, Liu R, et al. Steroid for epidural injection in spinal stenosis: a systematic review and meta-analysis. Drug Des Devel Ther. 2015;9:707–16.
16. Finniss DG, Benedetti F. Mechanisms of the placebo response and their impact on clinical trials and clinical practice. Pain. 2005;114:3–6.
17. Puri KS, Suresh KR, Gogtay NJ, Thatte UM. Declaration of Helsinki, 2008: implications for stakeholders in research. J Postgrad Med. 2009;55:131–4.
18. Geppetti P, Benemei S. Pain treatment with opioids: achieving the minimal effective and the minimal interacting dose. Clin Drug Investig. 2009;29(Suppl 1):3–16.
19. Patrignani P, Patrono C. Cyclooxygenase inhibitors: from pharmacology to clinical read-outs. Biochim Biophys Acta. 2015;1851:422–32.
20. Hayashi S, Ueno N, Murase A, Nakagawa Y, Takada J. Novel acid-type cyclooxygenase-2 inhibitors: design, synthesis, and structure-activity relationship for anti-inflammatory drug. Eur J Med Chem. 2012;50:179–95.

21. Crofford LJ. COX-1 and COX-2 tissue expression: implications and predictions. J Rheumatol Suppl. 1997;49:15–9.
22. Kawabata A. Prostaglandin E2 and pain--an update. Biol Pharm Bull. 2011;34:1170–3.
23. Chen YF, Jobanputra P, Barton P, Bryan S, Fry-Smith A, Harris G, Taylor RS. Cyclooxygenase-2 selective non-steroidal anti-inflammatory drugs (etodolac, meloxicam, celecoxib, rofecoxib, etoricoxib, valdecoxib and lumiracoxib) for osteoarthritis and rheumatoid arthritis: a systematic review and economic evaluation. Health Technol Assess. 2008;12:1–278.
24. Monk AB, Harrison JE, Worthington HV, Teague A. Pharmacological interventions for pain relief during orthodontic treatment. Cochrane Database Syst Rev. 2017;11:CD003976.
25. Volpe M, Battistoni A, Gallo G, et al. Aspirin and the primary prevention of cardiovascular diseases: an approach based on individualized, integrated estimation of risk. High Blood Press Cardiovasc Prev. 2017;24:331–9.
26. Chubak J, Kamineni A, Buist DSM, et al. Aspirin use for the prevention of colorectal cancer: an updated systematic evidence review for the U.S. In: Preventive services task force; 2015.
27. Vacha ME, Huang W, Mando-Vandrick J. The role of subcutaneous ketorolac for pain management. Hosp Pharm. 2015;50:108–12.
28. Tirunagari SK, Derry S, Moore RA, McQuay HJ. Single dose oral etodolac for acute postoperative pain in adults. Cochrane Database Syst Rev. 2009;3:CD007357.
29. Bulley S, Derry S, Moore RA, McQuay HJ. Single dose oral rofecoxib for acute postoperative pain in adults. Cochrane Database Syst Rev. 2009;4:CD004604.
30. Derry S, Moore RA. Single dose oral celecoxib for acute postoperative pain in adults. Cochrane Database Syst Rev. 2013;10:CD004233.
31. Liew Z, Ritz B, Rebordosa C, Lee PC, Olsen J. Acetaminophen use during pregnancy, behavioral problems, and hyperkinetic disorders. JAMA Pediatr. 2014;168:313–20.
32. Aminoshariae A, Khan A. Acetaminophen old drug, new issues. J Endod. 2015;41:588–93.
33. Bunchorntavakul C, Reddy KR. Acetaminophen-related hepatotoxicity. Clin Liver Dis. 2013;17:587–607.
34. Pinson GM, Beall JW, Kyle JA. A review of warfarin dosing with concurrent acetaminophen therapy. J Pharm Pract. 2013;26:518–21.
35. Jiang J, Briedé JJ, Jennen DG, et al. Increased mitochondrial ROS formation by acetaminophen in human hepatic cells is associated with gene expression changes suggesting disruption of the mitochondrial electron transport chain. Toxicol Lett. 2015;234:139–50.
36. Lancaster EM, Hiatt JR, Zarrinpar A. Acetaminophen hepatotoxicity: an updated review. Arch Toxicol. 2015;89:193–9.
37. Omidi A, Riahinia N, Montazer Torbati MB, Behdani MA. Hepatoprotective effect of Crocus sativus (saffron) petals extract against acetaminophen toxicity in male Wistar rats. Avicenna J Phytomed. 2014;4:330–6.
38. Abdel-Azeem AS, Hegazy AM, Ibrahim KS, Farrag AR, El-Sayed EM. Hepatoprotective, antioxidant, and ameliorative effects of ginger (Zingiber officinale Roscoe) and vitamin E in acetaminophen treated rats. J Diet Suppl. 2013;10:195–209.
39. Lin M, Zhai X, Wang G, et al. Salvianolic acid B protects against acetaminophen hepatotoxicity by inducing Nrf2 and phase II detoxification gene expression via activation of the PI3K and PKC signaling pathways. J Pharmacol Sci. 2015;127:203–10.
40. Benzon HT, Kendall MC, Katz JA, et al. Prescription patterns of pain medicine physicians. Pain Pract. 2013;13:440–50.
41. Clement C, Scala-Bertola J, Javot L, et al. Misuse of acetaminophen in the management of dental pain. Pharmacoepidemiol Drug Saf. 2011;20:996–1000.
42. Risser A, Donovan D, Heintzman J, Page T. NSAID prescribing precautions. Am Fam Physician. 2009;80(1):371–1378.
43. Szczeklik A, Nizankowska E, Duplaga M. Natural history of aspirin-induced asthma. AIANE investigators. European Network on Aspirin-Induced Asthma. Eur Respir J. 2000;16:432–6.
44. Shin SW, Park BL, Chang H, et al. Exonic variants associated with development of aspirin exacerbated respiratory diseases. PLoS One. 2014;9:e111887.

45. Simon RA. Adverse respiratory reactions to aspirin and nonsteroidal anti-inflammatory drugs. Curr Allergy Asthma Rep. 2004;4:17–24.
46. Inaba T, Ishikawa S, Miyoshi M, Kurahara K. Present status of gastrointestinal damage due to non-steroidal anti-inflammatory drugs (NSAIDs). Nihon Rinsho. 2013;71:1109–15.
47. Ong CK, Lirk P, Tan CH, Seymour RA. An evidence-based update on nonsteroidal anti-inflammatory drugs. Clin Med Res. 2007;5:19–34.
48. Tufan F. Importance of acute renal failure with ibuprofen. Clin Interv Aging. 2014;9:763.
49. Hamilton DA, Ernst CC, Kramer WG, et al. Pharmacokinetics of Diclofenac and Hydroxypropyl-β-Cyclodextrin (HPβCD) following Administration of Injectable HPβCD-Diclofenac in subjects with mild to moderate renal insufficiency or mild hepatic impairment. Clin Pharmacol Drug Dev. 2018;7:110–22.
50. Waddington F, Naunton M, Thomas J. Paracetamol and analgesic nephropathy: are you kidneying me? Int Med Case Rep J. 2015;8:1–5.
51. Ejaz P, Bhojani K, Joshi VR. NSAIDs and kidney. J Assoc Physicians India. 2004;52:632–40.
52. Choi KH, Kim AJ, Son IJ, et al. Risk factors of drug interaction between warfarin and non-steroidal anti-inflammatory drugs in practical setting. J Korean Med Sci. 2010;25:337–41.
53. Aithal GP, Day CP. Nonsteroidal anti-inflammatory drug-induced hepatotoxicity. Clin Liver Dis. 2007;1(1):563–75.
54. Fong SY, Efferth TH, Zuo Z. Modulation of the pharmacokinetics, therapeutic and adverse effects of NSAIDs by Chinese herbal medicines. Expert Opin Drug Metab Toxicol. 2014;10:1711–39.
55. Risser A, Donovan D, Heintzman J, Page T. NSAID prescribing precautions. Am Fam Physician. 2009;80:1371–8.
56. Giovanni G, Giovanni P. Do non-steroidal anti-inflammatory drugs and COX-2 selective inhibitors have different renal effects? J Nephrol. 2002;15:480–8.
57. Trelle S, Reichenbach S, Wandel S, et al. Cardiovascular safety of non-steroidal anti-inflammatory drugs: network meta-analysis. BMJ. 2011;342:c7086.
58. Chen GD, Stolzberg D, Lobarinas E, et al. Salicylate-induced cochlear impairments, cortical hyperactivity and re-tuning, and tinnitus. Hear Res. 2013;295:100–13.
59. Rodriguez SC, Olguin AM, Miralles CP, Viladrich PF. Characteristics of meningitis caused by ibuprofen: report of 2 cases with recurrent episodes and review of the literature. Medicine(Baltimore). 2006;85:214–20.
60. Antonucci R, Zaffanello M, Puxeddu E, et al. Use of non-steroidal anti-inflammatory drugs in pregnancy: impact on the fetus and newborn. Curr Drug Metab. 2012;13:474–90.
61. Ostensen ME, Skomsvoll JF. Anti-inflammatory pharmacotherapy during pregnancy. Expert Opin Pharmacother. 2004;5:571–80.
62. Nalamachu S, Pergolizzi JV, Raffa RB, Lakkireddy DR, Taylor R Jr. Drug-drug interaction between NSAIDS and low-dose aspirin: a focus on cardiovascular and GI toxicity. Expert Opin Drug Saf. 2014;13:903–17.
63. Houston MC. Nonsteroidal anti-inflammatory drugs and antihypertensives. Am J Med. 1991;90:42S–7S.
64. Hersh EV, Pinto A, Moore PA. Adverse drug interactions involving common prescription and over-the-counter analgesic agents. Clin Ther. 2007;29(11):2477–97.
65. Hernandez-Diaz S, Rodriguez LA. Association between nonsteroidal anti-inflammatory drugs and upper gastrointestinal tract bleeding/perforation: an overview of epidemiologic studies published in the 1990s. Arch Intern Med. 2000;160:2093–9.
66. Meek IL, Vonkeman HE, Kasemier J, Movig KL, van de Laar MA. Interference of NSAIDs with the thrombocyte inhibitory effect of aspirin: a placebo-controlled, ex vivo, serial placebo-controlled serial crossover study. Eur J Clin Pharmacol. 2013;69:365–71.
67. Awa K, Satoh H, Hori S, Sawada Y. Prediction of time-dependent interaction of aspirin with ibuprofen using a pharmacokinetic/pharmacodynamic model. J Clin Pharm Ther. 2012;37:469–74.
68. Waldhoer M, Bartlett SE, Whistler JL. Opioid receptors. Annu Rev Biochem. 2004;73:953–90.
69. Pasternak GW, Pan YX. Mu opioids and their receptors: evolution of a concept. Pharmacol Rev. 2013;65:1257–317.

70. Samer CF, Lorenzini KI, Rollason V, Daali Y, Desmeules JA. Applications of CYP450 testing in the clinical setting. Mol Diagn Ther. 2013;17:165–84.
71. Crews KR, Gaedigk A, Dunnenberger HM, et al. Clinical Pharmacogenetics implementation consortium guidelines for cytochrome P450 2D6 genotype and codeine therapy: 2014 update. Clin Pharmacol Ther. 2014;95:376–82.
72. Grond S, Sablotzki A. Clinical pharmacology of tramadol. Clin Pharmacokinet. 2004;43:879–923.
73. Miotto K, Cho AK, Khalil MA, et al. Trends in tramadol: pharmacology, metabolism, and misuse. Anesth Analg. 2017;124:44–51.
74. Desai B, Freeman E, Huang E, Hung A, Knapp E, Breunig IM, McPherson ML. Shaya FT: clinical value of tapentadol extended-release in painful diabetic peripheral neuropathy. Expert Rev Clin Pharmacol. 2014;7:203–9.
75. Hartrick CT, Rozek RJ. Tapentadol in pain management: a μ-opioid receptor agonist and noradrenaline reuptake inhibitor. CNS Drugs. 2011;25:359–70.
76. Vadivelu N, Huang Y, Mirante B, Jacoby M, Braveman FR, Hines RL, Sinatra R. Patient considerations in the use of tapentadol for moderate to severe pain. Drug Healthc Patient Saf. 2013;5(9):151–9.
77. Kunnumpurath S, Julien N, Kodumudi G, et al. Global supply and demand of opioids for pain management. Curr Pain Headache Rep. 2018;22(5):34.
78. Faria J, Barbosa J, Moreira R, et al. Comparative pharmacology and toxicology of tramadol and tapentadol. Eur J Pain. 2018;22(5):827–44. https://doi.org/10.1002/ejp.1196.
79. McNicol E, Horowicz-Mehler N, Fisk RA, et al. Management of opioid side effects in cancer-related and chronic noncancer pain: a systematic review. J Pain. 2003;4:231–56.
80. Benyamin R, Trescot AM, Datta S, et al. Opioid complications and side effects. Pain Physician. 2008;11(2 Suppl):S105–20.
81. Cummings KC 3rd, Arnaut K. Case report: fentanyl-associated intraoperative anaphylaxis with pulmonary edema. Can J Anaesth. 2007;54:301–6.
82. Kurz A, Sessler DI. Opioid-induced bowel dysfunction: pathophysiology and potential new therapies. Drugs. 2003;63:649–71.
83. Bantel C, Tripathi SS, Molony D, et al. Prolonged-release oxycodone/naloxone reduces opioid-induced constipation and improves quality of life in laxative-refractory patients: results of an observational study. Clin Exp Gastroenterol. 2018;11:57–67.
84. Lalley PM. Opioidergic and dopaminergic modulation of respiration. Respir Physiol Neurobiol. 2008;164:160–7.
85. Biesiada J, Chidambaran V, Wagner M, Zhang X, Martin LJ, Meller J, Sadhasivam S. Genetic risk signatures of opioid-induced respiratory depression following pediatric tonsillectomy. Pharmacogenomics. 2014;15:1749–62.
86. Dela Cruz AM, Trivedi MH. Opioid addiction screening tools for patients with chronic non-cancer pain. Tex Med. 2015;111:61–5.
87. Yang Z, Wilsey B, Bohm M, Soulsby M, Roy K, Ritley D, Jones C, Melnikow J. Defining risk for prescription opioid overdose: pharmacy shopping and overlapping prescriptions among long-term opioid users in Medicaid. J Pain. 2015;16(5):445–53. pii: S1526-5900(15)00530-1
88. Whistler JL. Examining the role of mu opioid receptor endocytosis in the beneficial and side-effects of prolonged opioid use: from a symposium on new concepts in mu-opioid pharmacology. Drug Alcohol Depend. 2012;121:189–204.
89. Bird MF, Vardanyan RS, Hruby VJ, et al. Development and characterisation of novel fentanyl-delta opioid receptor antagonist based bivalent ligands. Br J Anaesth. 2015;114:646–56.
90. Sullivan MD, Howe CQ. Opioid therapy for chronic pain in the United States: promises and perils. Pain. 2013;154(Suppl 1):S94–100.
91. Nielsen S, Larance B, Lintzeris N, et al. Opioid agonist treatment for patients with dependence on prescription opioids. JAMA. 2017;317:967–8.
92. Boyer EW. Management of opioid analgesic overdose. N Engl J Med. 2012;367:146–55.
93. Barrie J, May G. Towards evidence-based emergency medicine: best BETs from the Manchester Royal Infirmary. Diagnosis of drug overdose by rapid reversal with naloxone. Emerg Med J. 2006;23:874–5.

94. Patrick SW, Dudley J, Martin PR, et al. Prescription opioid epidemic and infant outcomes. Pediatrics. 2015;135:842–50.
95. Kraft WK. Buprenorphine in neonatal abstinence syndrome. Clin Pharmacol Ther. 2018;103:112–9.
96. Fernandes K, Martins D, Juurlink D, et al. High-dose opioid prescribing and opioid-related hospitalization: a population-based study. PLoS One. 2016;11:e0167479.
97. Feng XQ, Zhu LL, Zhou Q. Opioid analgesics-related pharmacokinetic drug interactions: from the perspectives of evidence based on randomized controlled trials and clinical risk management. J Pain Res. 2017;10:1225–39.
98. Tan YM, Clewell H, Campbell J, Andersen M. Evaluating pharmacokinetic and pharmacodynamic interactions with computational models in supporting cumulative risk assessment. Int J Environ Res Public Health. 2011;8:1613–30.
99. Derry C, Derry S, Moore RA, McQuay HJ. Single dose oral ibuprofen for acute postoperative pain in adults. Cochrane Database Syst Rev. 2009;3:CD001548.
100. Koh W, Nguyen KP, Jahr JS. Intravenous non-opioid analgesia for peri- and postoperative pain management: a scientific review of intravenous acetaminophen and ibuprofen. Korean J Anesthesiol. 2015;68:3–12.
101. Hyllested M, Jones S, Pedersen JL, Kehlet H. Comparative effect of paracetamol, NSAIDs or their combination in postoperative pain management: a qualitative review. Br J Anaesth. 2002;88:199–214.
102. Elia N, Lysakowski C, Tramer MR. Does multimodal analgesia with acetaminophen, nonsteroidal anti-inflammatory drugs, or selective cyclooxygenase-2 inhibitors and patient-controlled analgesia morphine offer advantages over morphine alone? Meta-analyses of randomized trials. Anesthesiology. 2005;1(03):1296–304.
103. Weil K, Hooper L, Afzal Z, Esposito M, Worthington HV, van Wijk AJ, Coulthard P. Paracetamol for pain relief after surgical removal of lower wisdom teeth. Cochrane Database Syst Rev. 2007;3:CD004487.
104. Moore RA, Derry S, McQuay HJ, Wiffen PJ. Single dose oral analgesics for acute postoperative pain in adults. Cochrane Database Syst Rev. 2011;9:CD008659.
105. Frampton C, Quinlan J. Evidence for the use of non-steroidal anti-inflammatory drugs for acute pain in the post anaesthesia care unit. J Perioper Pract. 2009;19:418–23.
106. Toms L, McQuay HJ, Derry S, Moore RA. Single dose oral paracetamol (acetaminophen) for postoperative pain in adults. Cochrane Database Syst Rev. 2008;4:CD004602.
107. Wideman GL, Keffer M, Morris E, et al. Analgesic efficacy of a combination of hydrocodone with ibuprofen in postoperative pain. Clin Pharmacol Ther. 1999;65:66–76.
108. Litkowski LJ, Christensen SE, Adamson DN, et al. Analgesic efficacy and tolerability of oxycodone 5 mg/ibuprofen 400 mg compared with those of oxycodone 5 mg/acetaminophen 325 mg and hydrocodone 7.5 mg/acetaminophen 500 mg in patients with moderate to severe postoperative pain: a randomized, double-blind, placebo-controlled, single-dose, parallel-group study in a dental pain model. Clin Ther. 2005;27(4):418–29.
109. McClellan K, Scott LJ. Tramadol/paracetamol. Drugs. 2003;63:1079–86.
110. Kleinert R, Lange C, Steup A, et al. Single dose analgesic efficacy of tapentadol in postsurgical dental pain: the results of a randomized, double-blind, placebo-controlled study. Anesth Analg. 2008;1(07):2048–55.
111. Finco G, Mura P, Musu M, et al. Long-term, prolonged-release oral tapentadol for the treatment of refractory chronic low back pain: a single-center, observational study. Minerva Med. 2018;109:259–65.
112. McNaughton EC, Black RA, Weber SE, Butler SF. Assessing abuse potential of new analgesic medications following market release: an evaluation of internet discussion of tapentadol abuse. Pain Med. 2015;16:131–40.
113. Butler SF, McNaughton EC, Black RA. Tapentadol abuse potential: a postmarketing evaluation using a sample of individuals evaluated for substance abuse treatment. Pain Med. 2015;16:119–30.

Chapter 6
Investigation of the Chronic Pain Patient

Nicholas Padfield

6.1 To Investigate: To Seek the Cause of Pain

6.1.1 Introduction

Pain is an unpleasant physical and emotional experience, the impact of which will be the result of a combination of physical and psychological factors. The investigation of chronic pain can often be challenging as the cause is not immediately apparent, which sets it apart from acute pain when there is a readily recognizable inciting event such as trauma, infection, surgery, etc.

An understanding of the genesis of chronic pain is essential for the formulation of an appropriate treatment strategy, which may include physical, pharmacological, and psychological components.

As pain clinicians we usually start with the biological component of bio-psycho-social model of pain.

We think in terms of the familiar disease processes of congenital conditions and acquired conditions resulting from trauma, infection, inflammation, neoplasia, degeneration, metabolic and immune derived.

The starting point for investigating the cause of pain is a careful, detailed medical history which needs to elucidate the following:

- Was the onset: sudden or gradual? What factors are associated with the onset? Foreign travel might suggest an infective element such as Lyme disease, or an endemic encephalitis,
- Was it gradual, which may suggest a degenerative condition or an immune derived condition such as a collagen vascular disease.
- Where is it? Is it well localized or poorly localized? Which tissues are likely to be involved? The axial skeleton, the skin, organs of sense, the abdominal or

N. Padfield (✉)
Guys and St Thomas Hospitals, London, UK

K. Shimoji et al. (eds.), *Chronic Pain Management in General and Hospital Practice*, https://doi.org/10.1007/978-981-15-2933-7_6

pelvic viscera. Does it have a dermatomal distribution or a myofascial distribution or a non-dermatomal distribution like 'glove and stocking'?

- What is the quality of pain? Is it mechanical and nociceptive? Is it dysaesthetic, burning, allodynic?
- Is it provoked by mechanical factors such as activity, gravity, immobility, temperature, or touch?
- Is it provoked by psychological factors such as anxiety, anger, or depression?
- Does it vary in intensity during the day or night or is it constant? Does it vary with the season or menstrual period?
- What is its intensity on VAS, Likert scale, the range of best, worst, and average?
- Has it arisen as the result of a change in diet or following treatment such as radiotherapy or chemotherapy with neurotoxic agents such as cis-platins?
- Is it relieved by rest, analgesics (which ones) massage, movement, stretch altering position, relaxation techniques?
- Psychological status: anxiety, depression, borderline personality, PTSD, fears and beliefs about pain.
- Psychiatric disorder: schizophrenia, bipolar disorder, somatoform disorder.

6.2 Physical Examination

Having taken a careful medical history in most cases the cause will become apparent. However, a careful physical examination will further determine the area and tissues which are causative in most cases and will inform an appropriate treatment strategy. There will be though challenging diagnostic formulations, which will require further investigation.

So in the pain clinic we start with:

6.2.1 Inspection

- General: personal care, gait, ambulation aids (wheelchair, crutches), vocalization, emotional affect, and engagement with the consultation
- Site specific: Build, BMI, joints/deformity, skin colour (red/blue, stained, blanched)
- Appearance: skin (pitted, smooth shiny/rough, depigmented, spots/papules), oedema, hair, nails

6.2.2 Palpation

- Allodynia, painful masses, temperature, texture, sweating
- Adverse neural tension: Sciatic, femoral, brachial plexus stretch, Tinel's signs over peripheral nerves at bony prominences, reflexes
- Range of movement: active/passive, ligament/tissue laxity

6.3 By now it should be evident which pathological category the painful condition derives from and this will determine the need for elucidation by further investigation. So is the complaint arising from one or more of the following

- Congenital/Genetic: cytochrome, enzyme abnormalities, Ehlers–Danlos, Dercum's, migraine, Raynaud's disease
- Trauma: early or late complication: scarring
- Inflammation: Chronic widespread pain, chronic pancreatitis, arthritis, fibromyalgia, myofascial pain syndrome
- Autoimmune: Collagen vascular disease, CRPS, rheumatoid, lupus
- Degeneration: Intervertebral disc pathology, aneurysm
- Infection: HZ, HIV, CMV, Lyme disease
- Neoplasia: lymphoma, ependymoma, haemangioma, lipoma, Von Recklinghausen's
- Metabolic: Diabetes
- Vascular: Avascular necrosis, venous valvular insufficiency, atheroma
- Iatrogenic: Postoperative, chemotherapy, radiotherapy, medication (headache, opiate induced hyperalgesia)

This list is by no means exhaustive but is indicative of the consideration the pain physician should make.

6.4 Verbal Assessment Tools to Determine If Pain Is Nociceptive or Neuropathic

In order to plan treatment it is important to determine whether the pain is mostly mechanical and/or nociceptive or neuropathic since the response to treatment is predicated on this.

There are a number of questionnaires in use to aid determination of whether the pain is predominantly nociceptive or neuropathic. The first validated pain measure to be published was by BS Galer and MP Jensen in 1997 which they labelled the Neuropathic Pain Scale.

The sensory qualities were selected on the clinical experience of the physician involved in its development. In addition to symptom intensity and quality it also includes a question on temporal pattern (i.e., constant background pain with flairs, constant pain with fluctuation, and flairs only). It like the DN4 includes itch amongst the sensory qualities and has a score for each domain of 0–10.

One of the drawbacks is that several neuropathic pain qualities such as 'electric' or 'tingling' are not included. The neuropathic pain scale has been further modified into the Pain Quality Assessment Tool, [1].

Its use remains reserved in practice as a research tool for investigating treatment response in patients with neuropathic pain rather than a screening tool in clinic [2].

The questionniares that have common currency amongst UK pain physicians are detailed below:

6.4.1 The Leeds Assessment of Neuropathic Symptoms

This was originally devised in 2001 and further reported (2005/2006) studying a cohort of 200 patients at a time when pain was viewed very much as a dichotomy between nociceptive and neuropathic rather than as a continuum encompassing elements of both mechanisms. It consists of five questions and two sensory tests. The maximum score is 24 and any score over 12 is taken to indicate neuropathic pain. However, it is mostly focused on cutaneous sensation and is limited because many neuropathic pains do not have a cutaneous manifestation, for example, abdominal/pelvic visceral pain.

It does not quantify severity of neuropathic pain or correlate with the degree of known neurological dysfunction, i.e., nerve conduction studies in carpal tunnel syndrome.

6.4.2 These Are the Questions to Be Completed by the Patient

- Would you describe your pain as strange unpleasant sensations in your skin? (e.g., pricking, tingling, pins and needles)—Yes/No
- Does the skin in the painful areas look different to normal? (e.g., mottled, more red/pink than usual)—Yes/No
- Is the skin in the affected area abnormally sensitive to touch? (e.g., unpleasant sensations if lightly stroked, painful to wear tight clothes)—Yes/No
- Does your pain come on suddenly in bursts for no apparent reason when you are still? (e.g., like electric shocks, 'bursting' or 'jumping' sensations)—Yes/No
- Do you feel that skin temperature in the painful area has changed? (e.g., hot, burning)—Yes/No
- Does stroking the affected area of skin with a piece of cotton wool produce an unpleasant painful sensation?—Yes/No
- Does touching the affected area of skin with a sharp needle feel sharper or duller when compared to an area of normal skin?—Yes/No. [3, 4].

Back pain affects all of us at some time or other, but in about a third of the population it can be a chronic problem. In order to plan appropriate treatment it is important to differentiate between nociceptive/mechanical causes that may respond best to physiotherapy and other physical interventions, from neuropathic causes that may respond better to anti-neuropathic medication or even neuromodulation.

PainDetect is a scoring system devised and validated initially in a cohort of approximately 8000 German patients.

The study revealed that in a cohort of unselected chronic back pain sufferers 37% had predominantly neuropathic pain and this was associated with more psychological morbidity such as depression, anxiety/panic attacks, and sleep disorders. The researchers also calculated that for the given prevalence of chronic low back pain in the German LBP population, 14.5% of females and 11.4% of all male patients had predominantly neuropathic pain.

The questionnaire consists of seven questions that address the quality of neuropathic pain symptoms; it is completed by the patient and no physical examination is required. The first five questions ask about the gradation of pain, scored from 0 to 5 (never = 0, hardly noticed = 1, slightly = 2; moderately = 3, strongly = 4, very strongly = 5). Question 6 asks about the pain course pattern, scored from −1 to 2, depending on which pain course pattern diagram is selected. Question 7 asks about radiating pain, answered as yes or no, and scored as 2 or 0, respectively. The final score between −1 and 38 indicates the likelihood of a neuropathic pain component. A score of 12 indicates that pain is unlikely to have a neuropathic component (<15%), while a score of 19 suggests that pain is likely to have a neuropathic component (>90%). A score between these values indicates that the result is uncertain and a more detailed examination is required to ensure a proper diagnosis [5].

6.4.3 Douleur Neuropathique in four questions (en quatre questions)

This is an easy-to-score questionnaire consisting of seven items related to symptoms and three related to clinical examination. It was developed in 160 patients and showed 83% sensitivity and 90% specificity when compared with clinical diagnosis in the study group. It is one of the few tools that incorporate itch into the model.

A modified version of the DN4 without the clinical examination component has been devised and appears to have nearly equivalent accuracy. Like the LANSS it does not quantify the neuropathic pain [6].

There are many other scales and the reader is directed to the following article for further reading [7].

6.5 Further Investigative Tools

Continuing in the investigation of the biological causes of pain as opposed to the emotional consequences of it, the pain clinician has a range of physical investigations to call upon to help define and determine the nature of the pain complaint. These tests fall into three broad categories depending on the context of the investigation.

1. Clinical: thermography, von Frey hairs, imaging, ultrasound scan, plain X-ray, CT scan, MRI, NCC/EMG EEG.
2. Research: fMRI, QST, punch biopsy, SPECT CT, and laser speckle
3. Forensic: surveillance

6.5.1 Thermography

Measuring skin temperature is useful in situations when heat emanating from the body is expected to be abnormal: e.g., rheumatoid arthritis, Raynaud's syndrome, burning phantom limb pain, phantom body pain, CRPS, stress fractures, and tendonitis.

The technique is sensitive enough to pick up differences between painful and pain-free areas on the limbs and torsos of people having complete spinal cord injuries who report phantom body pain.

Thermography has been shown to be a valuable tool in assessing autonomic dysfunction such as differences in patterns of sweating such as found above and below the level of injury among spinal cord injured people. It can also help assess changes from interventions such as sympathectomy.

There are a variety of methods of measuring these skin temperature changes. In common use are Videothermographs, contact thermographs, infrared thermometers as well as thermistors taped to the skin.

6.5.1.1 Representative Thermography Applications

Thermography has found to be effective in assessing and tracking pain related problems with associated vascular changes. It has also been proven to be helpful in detecting and monitoring changes in burning phantom limb pain and complex regional pain syndrome and is illustrated in the following picture (Fig. 6.1).

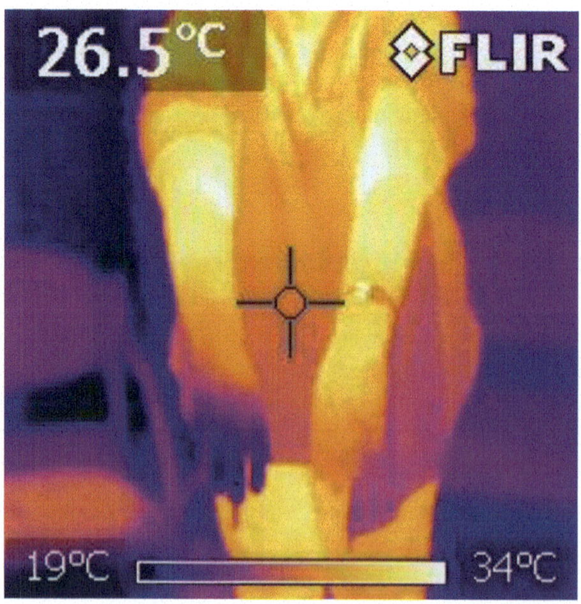

Fig. 6.1 Thermographic comparison between two distal upper limbs in a case of CRPS. The affected right hand is markedly cooler than the left. (Reproduced with kind permission from Dr. Rajesh Munglani, Guys and St Thomas Hospital, London)

6.5.2 *Von Frey Hairs*

These were originally designed by Maximillian von Frey in 1896. They are used as a diagnostic, research, and screening tool in human and animal medicine.

They consist of a set of mounted nylon columns of differing diameters that bend at different forces. This is a mechanical nociceptive test and indicates if the area tested is normally sensitive, hyperalgesic, or hypoalgesic depending on the force applied before the sensory threshold is reached. The forces range from 0.008 to 300 N.

Usually four tests at each force are employed starting at the lowest force and increasing the force until the threshold is reached. Ideally one should start near the expected population mean as starting a long way off the mean is more likely to increase the margin of error.

6.5.3 *Ultrasonography*

This is a cheap and portable effective diagnostic tool that has been available for the last few decades. It does not have the problems of the more expensive and less readily available MRI where patients can be claustrophobic or are denied the investigation because of an implanted device system as a pace maker or a spinal cord stimulator.

Ultrasonography has helped determine the changes in conditions where previously no imaging to demonstrate the pathological changes had been available. For example, the muscles of sufferers from myofascial pain where these pathological foci, which appear as 1–2-mm lesions recognized with vibration sonoelastography and the colour variance mode, can now be identified and characterized. Another example is a painful neuroma that has traditionally been diagnosed without imaging, where the clinician had relied instead on Tinel's sign as the standard indicative manoeuvre. Now ultrasonography can confirm the presence and provide an image of the swollen nerve and locate it within the soft tissues (Fig. 6.2).

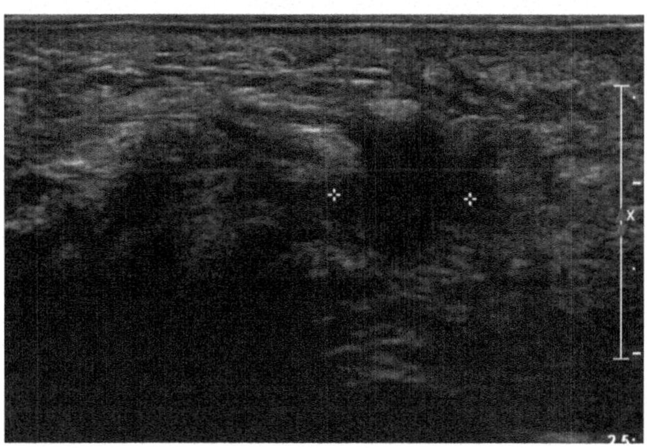

Fig. 6.2 An ultrasound scan showing a Morton's Neuroma with Measurements

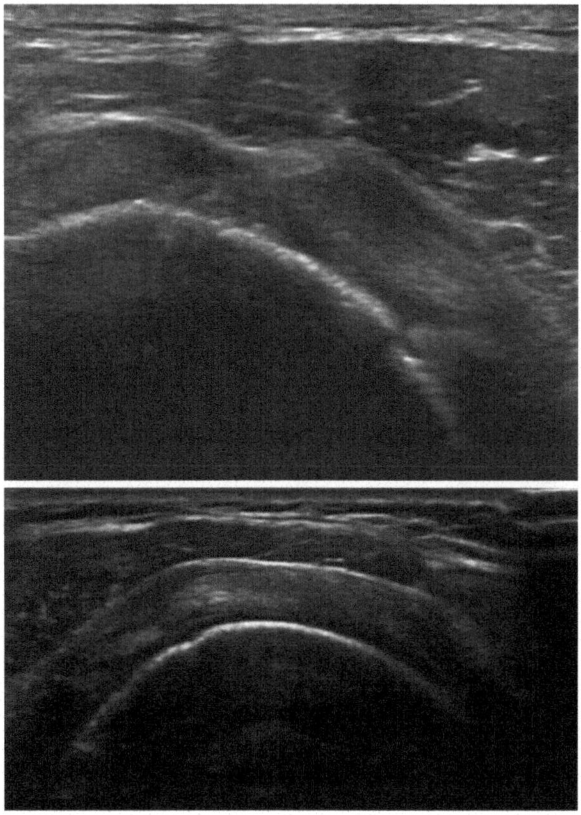

Fig. 6.3 An Ultrasound scan of a Shoulder showing a tear in the rotator cuff and a normal scan for comparison. Reproduced with kind permission of the Department of Imaging, Guys and St Thomas Hospital, London

Dynamic imaging reveals transient conditions that cannot be visualized by static scanning. Many abnormalities are not detectable when a patient is at rest. The patient may have a swelling, pain, or clicking that occurs only with a certain movement. Examples include shoulder impingement, snapping hip syndrome, subluxations, tendon gliding, and ulnar nerve dislocation. Ultrasound is an excellent imaging modality to diagnose tendinosis, tendon tears, and bursitis. Accuracy in the diagnosis of rotator cuff tears can reach 100% (full thickness tears) and 91% (partial thickness tears), depending on the experience of the individual performing the examination [8] (Fig. 6.3).

6.5.4 *Radiography*

Plain radiography has a limited place in the spectrum of available investigative tools available to the pain physician.

It is often used to image joints, vertebrae, and intervertebral discs in particular.

It can show degenerative changes and suggest (but not diagnose) osteoporosis, osteomalacia, bone marrow oedema, joint sclerosis, pathological fracture, loss of disc height, alteration in posture such as changes in lordosis, kyphosis, and scoliosis. It can image posterior instrumentation of the spine, and other joint prostheses to determine fracture, slippage, and malalignment.

6.5.5 Electromyography/Nerve Conduction Studies

These tests are commonly employed when the function of the nerves and muscles is disordered. The nerve conduction velocity studies the function of the motor and sensory nerves and are often combined with needle electromyography.

They are indicated when there is pain in the limbs and or weakness from spinal nerve compression or when there is concern about some other neurological injury or condition. They are particularly useful in investigating paraesthesia and/or weakness in the arms or legs. For example, following injury there can be apparent reduction in nerve conduction velocity due to scarring and the degree of slowing can help in the decision to decompress a nerve surgically or to treat it conservatively.

In other situations such as carpal tunnel or cubital tunnel syndromes the degree of slowing will inform surgical options.

Certain neurological conditions such as Guillain–Barré syndrome or peripheral neuropathies can be monitored with serial NCC to gauge the response to treatment and potential recovery.

In addition to measuring latency and amplitude in selected motor or sensory units, there are F wave studies that look at the conduction times from a sensory stimulus to a motor response via the spinal ventral horn. It thus looks at conduction velocity between the limb and the spine.

Further tests have been developed such as the Small Pain Fibres Method (spf) of Nerve Conduction Studies, where an electrical stimulus with a neuroselective frequency to determine the minimum voltage causing conduction using the patient as their own control. It has been shown to provide a 95% sensitivity in identifying nerve root pathology. It can be used to determine nerve impingement/pathology causing pain where EMG and standard nerve conduction studies fail.

The test uses a potentiometer to objectively measure the amplitude of the action potential at a distant site along the nerve being tested. The patient confirms a sensation when the nerve fires. Objectivity of the patient's response is confirmed by the measurement of nerve recruitment for surrounding nerves and is displayed on the instrument. The impinged nerve (pain fibres) can only report (peak) momentarily while recruiting other nerves to assist and sustain the reporting of the stimulus. Non-impinged nerves (pain fibres) do not recruit surrounding nerves and this is readily seen on the display.

The spf-NCS does not require myelin loss to detect function change, so velocity is not measured. The small-pain-fibres NCS (pf-NCS) is the preferred test with over 95% accuracy for determining the spine level(s) and side(s) for small pain fibre impingement/pathology allowing for the most accurate diagnosis and treatment procedures for patients experiencing back pain.

The interpretation is complex and requires a specialist neurophysiologist but can be very useful in diagnosing peripheral neuropathy, compression syndromes, and confirming other neurological conditions.

6.5.6 Electroencephalography

Electroencephalography (EEG) is an electrophysiological monitoring method to record electricalactivity of the brain. It is typically noninvasive, with the electrodes placed along the scalp, although invasive electrodes are sometimes used such as in electrocorticography. EEG measures voltage fluctuations resulting from ionic current within the neurons of the brain.

EEG is most often used to diagnose epilepsy, which causes abnormalities in EEG readings. It is also used to diagnose a number of conditions that can accompany chronic pain and help differentiate their contribution to the overall picture, such as sleep disorders, depth of anaesthesia, coma, encephalopathies, Alzheimer's disease.

EEG used to be a first-line method of diagnosis for tumours, stroke, and other focal brain disorders, but this use has decreased with the advent of high-resolution anatomical imaging techniques such as magnetic resonance imaging (MRI) and computed tomography (CT).

Despite limited spatial resolution, EEG continues to be a valuable tool for research and diagnosis. It is one of the few mobile techniques available and offers millisecond-range temporal resolution, which is not possible with CT, PET, or MRI. It is cheap, transportable and unlike many of the more advanced neuroimaging techniques does not lead to claustrophobia.

Derivatives of the EEG technique include evoked potentials (EP), which involves averaging the EEG activity time-locked to the presentation of a stimulus of some sort (visual, somatosensory, or auditory). Event-related potentials (ERPs) refer to averaged EEG responses that are time-locked to more complex processing of stimuli. These techniques are used in cognitive science, cognitive psychology, and psychophysiological research.

6.5.7 Nuclear Medicine/Radionuclide Scans

This is a technique whereby a radionuclide is injected intravenously or taken orally and its distribution and elimination monitored with scintigraphy. It can be used to detect cancer, trauma, infection, and inflammation. Different radionuclides are used to target different organs. Once administered, it can take several hours to reach the target organ or tissue and the scanning process itself can take from one to 5 h.

There are a number of radionuclide scans which include PET, gallium, and bone scans.

6.5.7.1 PET (Positron-Emission Tomography) Scans

A positron-emitting radionuclide (tracer) is introduced into the body on a biologically active molecule, most commonly fluorodeoxyglucose. When the nucleotide decays it emits a beta-particle which is annihilated by an oppositely charged electron to emit a pair of gamma rays which travel in diametrically opposite directions. Three-dimensional images of tracer concentration within the body are then constructed by computer analysis. In modern PET-CT scanners, three-dimensional imaging is often accomplished with the aid of a CT X-ray scan performed on the patient during the same session, in the same machine.

The concentrations of tracer imaged will indicate tissue metabolic activity as it corresponds to the regional glucose uptake.

In pain medicine the commonest use of this tracer is to explore the possibility of cancer metastasis (i.e., spreading to other sites) and diffuse brain diseases such as Parkinson's, transient ischaemic attacks, multiple sclerosis, amyotrophic lateral sclerosis, and Huntington's chorea. One of the disadvantages of PET scanners is their operating cost, currently about £800 per scan (Fig. 6.4).

6.5.7.2 Bone Densitometry

Bone densitometry, also called dual-energy X-ray absorptiometry or DEXA, uses a very small dose of ionizing radiation to produce pictures of the inside of the body (usually the lower spine and hips) to measure bone loss. It is commonly used to diagnose osteoporosis and to assess an individual's risk for developing fractures. DEXA is simple, quick, and noninvasive. It is also the most accurate method for diagnosing osteoporosis.

T Score This number shows the amount of bone you have compared with a young adult of the same gender with peak bone mass. A score above −1 is considered normal. A score between −1 and −2.5 is classified as osteopenia (low bone mass). A score below −2.5 is defined as osteoporosis. The T score is used to estimate your risk of developing a fracture.

Z Score This number reflects the amount of bone you have compared with other people in your age group and of the same size and gender. If this score is unusually high or low, it may indicate a need for further medical tests.

Small changes may normally be observed between scans due to differences in positioning and usually are not significant.

What Are the Limitations of DEXA Bone Densitometry?

- A DEXA test cannot predict who will experience a fracture but can provide indications of relative risk.

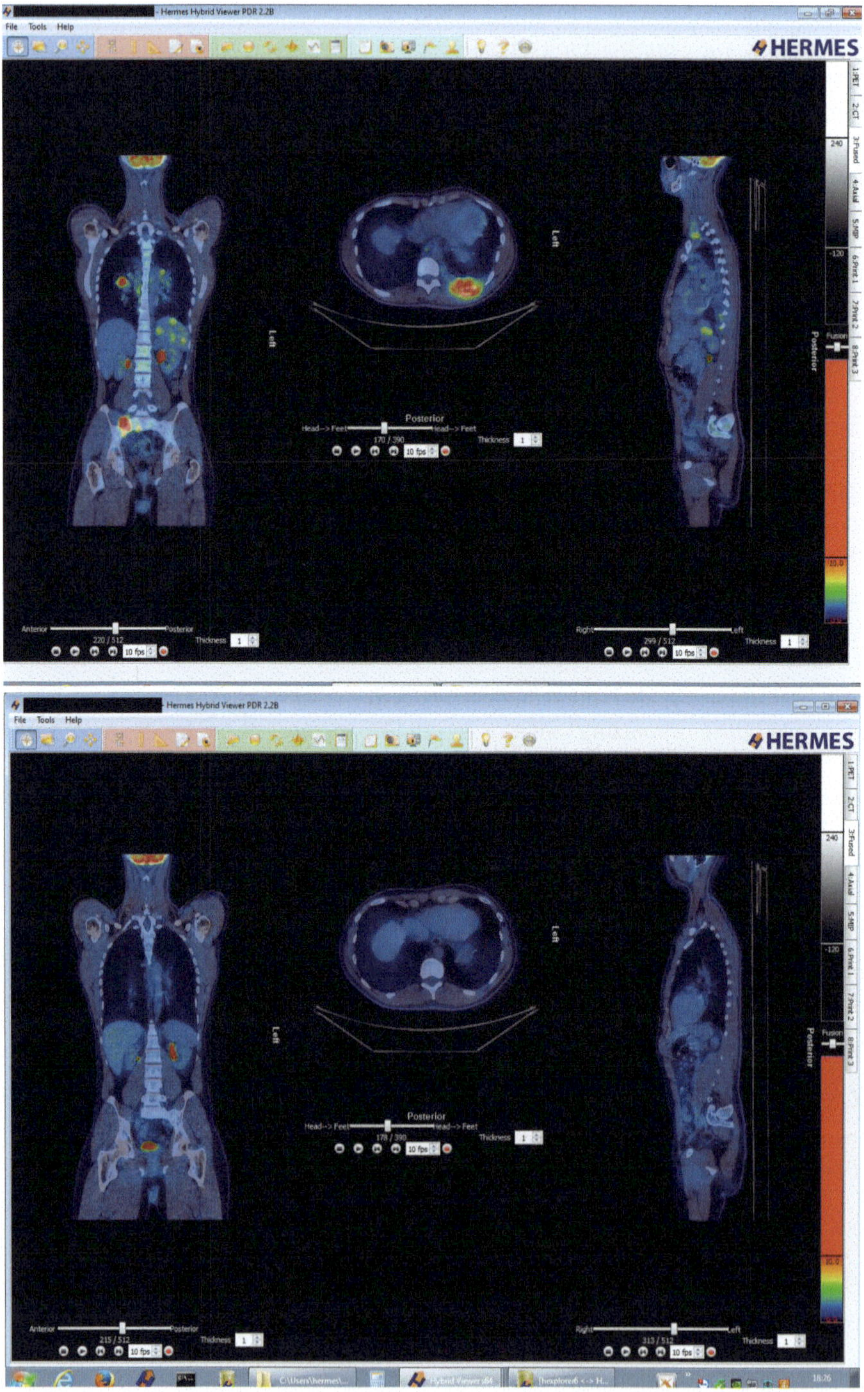

Fig. 6.4 PET scan showing metastases in a young male with Hodgkin's Lymphoma. PET scan after treatment showing the disappearance of the metastases. PET-CT images courtesy of the Clinical PET Centre at St Thomas' Hospital, School of Biomedical Engineering and Imaging Sciences, Kings College London and Guys' and St Thomas' NHS Foundation Trust

- Despite its effectiveness as a method of measuring bone density, DEXA is of limited use in people with a spinal deformity or those who have had previous spinal surgery. The presence of vertebral compression fractures or osteoarthritis may interfere with the accuracy of the test; in such instances, CT scans may be more useful.
- Central DEXA devices are more sensitive than peripheral DEXA devices but they are also somewhat more expensive.

A test done on a peripheral location, such as the heel or wrist, may help predict the risk of fracture in the spine or hip. These tests are not helpful in following response to treatment, however, and if they indicate that drug therapy is needed, a baseline central DEXA scan should be obtained.

Certain factors or conditions may interfere with bone densitometry testing. These include, but are not limited to, the following:

- Metal jewellery or other metal objects
- Body piercing
- A barium X-ray within 10 days of testing
- Calcific arthritic sclerosis of the posterior vertebrae
- Calcified abdominal aortic aneurysm
- Healed bone fractures
- Metallic clips from previous abdominal surgery
- Recent bone scans

6.5.7.3 SPECT Scans

A SPECT scan (single-photon emission computed tomography) is the technique of using nuclear medicine tomographic imaging techniques with gamma rays to provide detailed 3D images of the body.

A CT scan (computerized tomography) uses multiple X-rays; information from the X-ray beams is then processed by a computer program which determines the relative density of the tissues, creating detailed images of the body which are then processed into an image.

The SPECT CT scanner combines the framework of the CT scan with the functional information provided by nuclear medicine imaging (SPECT scan). The images from each scan are then fused together providing highly accurate anatomical detail in 3D, allowing medical specialists to more accurately pinpoint the exact location of any abnormality.

How It Works

Patients are administered a small dose of radioactive medication, this is usually via an intravenous injection into the blood stream of a radioactive tracer (a gamma emitting radioisotope). The radioactive tracers are detected by a nuclear gamma camera, these specialist cameras rotate 360 °C around the patient, allowing for the reconstruction of 3D images.

SPECT CT scanning is rarely used in practice in the UK, in the investigation of spinal pain. It is, however, used in many other countries, and perhaps the helpfulness of these scans will become recognized here in the near future. Due to the highly detailed information provided, these scans help eliminate the guesswork out of diagnosing inflammatory causes of spinal pain.

Indications for SPECT CT Scan

There are numerous indications where a SPECT CT scan can be useful in providing an accurate diagnosis, as it essentially enables a detailed analysis of internal organs, bone structures, and tissue.

In the case of spinal pain, hidden bone fractures, growths, lesions, and other abnormalities such as tumours are easily identifiable on the 3D images.

It is an especially sensitive test of intervertebral disc, facet joint, and sacro-iliac joint inflammation, illustrating precisely the areas of spinal inflammation. It can provide invaluable information when deciding on the best possible plan of treatment for the patient (Fig. 6.5).

The SPECT CT scan is predictive of the response to steroid injections; the above image shows a SPECT CT scan with an inflamed cervical facet joint. Targeting this joint alone with steroid injection and radiofrequency denervation will give excellent long-term pain relief if the joint is the cause of low back pain. If the low back pain continues afterwards, then the procedure has more than likely excluded the joint as a cause of pain (Fig. 6.6).

6.5.7.4 CT Scan

A *CT scan*, also known as *computed tomography scan*, makes use of computer-processed combinations of many X-ray measurements taken from different angles to produce cross-sectional (tomographic) images (virtual 'slices') of specific areas of a scanned object, allowing the user to see inside the object without cutting.

CT produces a volume of data that can be manipulated in order to demonstrate various bodily structures based on their ability to absorb the X-ray beam.

Since its introduction in the 1970s, CT has become an important tool in medical imaging to supplement X-rays and medical ultrasonography. It has more recently been used for preventive medicine or screening for disease, for example, CT colonography for people with a high risk of colon cancer, or full-motion heart scans for people with high risk of heart disease. A number of institutions offer full-body scans for the general population although this practice goes against the advice and official position of many professional organizations in the field primarily due to the radiation dose applied.

CT scanning of the head is typically used to detect infarction, tumours, calcifications, haemorrhage, and bone trauma. Of the above, hypodense (dark) structures can

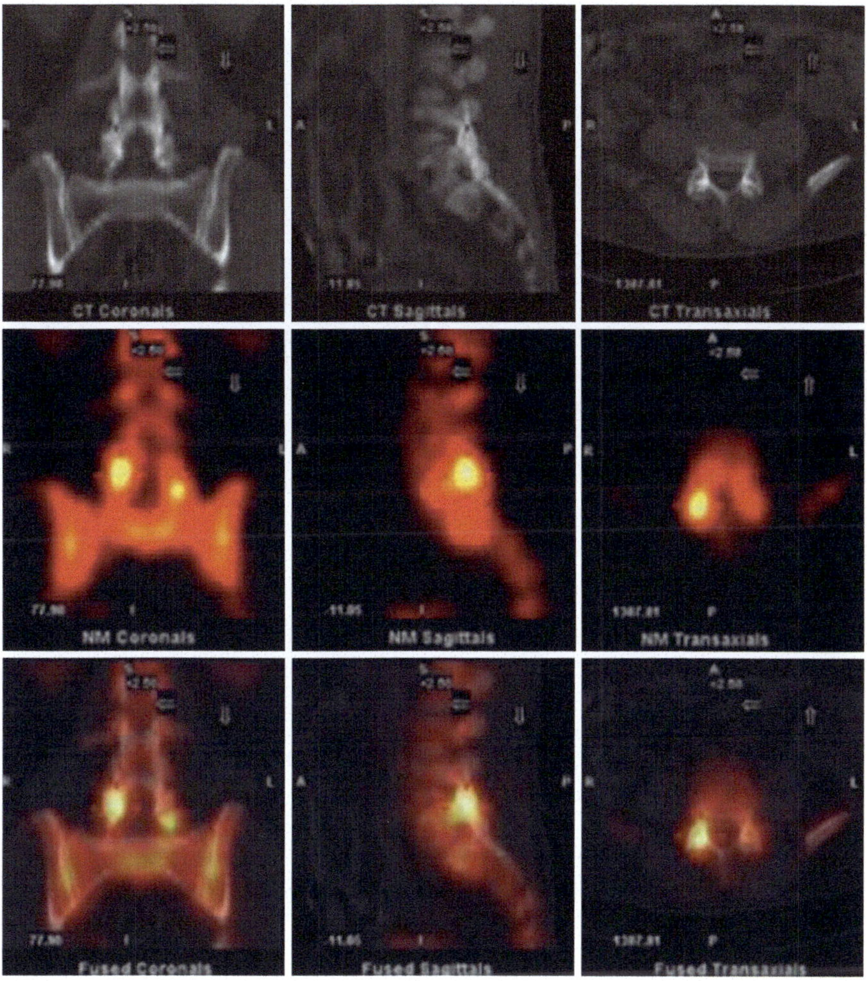

Fig. 6.5 SPECT CT scans showing areas of increased activity in the lumbar facet and sacro-iliac joints

indicate oedema and infarction, hyperdense (bright) structures indicate calcifications and haemorrhage and bone trauma can be seen as disjunction in bone windows. Tumours can be detected by the swelling and anatomical distortion they cause, or by surrounding oedema.

CT scans may be used to diagnose headache when neuroimaging is indicated and MRI is not available, or in emergency settings when haemorrhage, stroke, or traumatic brain injury are suspected.

Computed tomography (CT) scan has been shown to be more accurate than radiographs in evaluating anterior interbody fusion but may still over-read the extent of fusion.

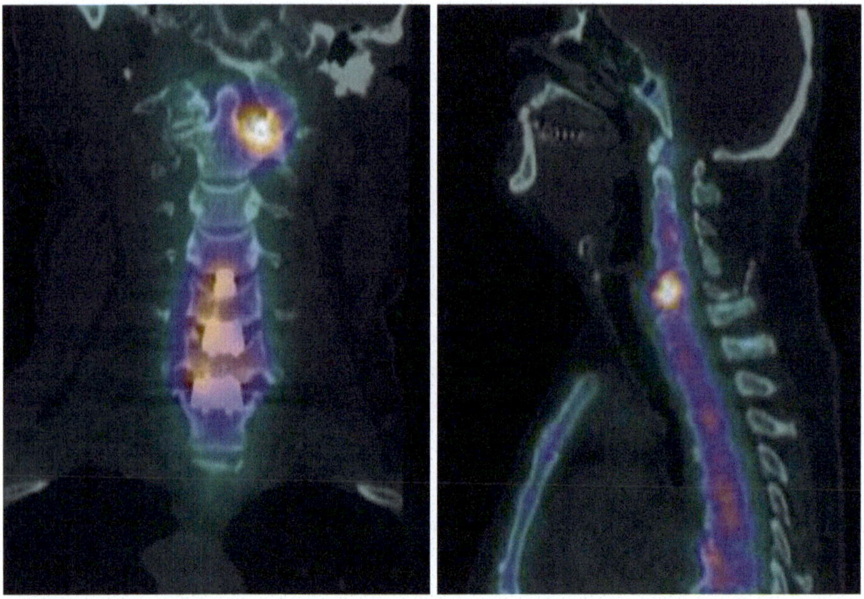

Fig. 6.6 SPECT CT scans of the cervical spine. Reproduced with kind permission from Dr. Mark Miller FRCA FFPMRCA

The radiation doses received from CT scans are variable. Compared to the lowest dose X-ray techniques, CT scans can have 100 to 1000 times higher dose than conventional X-rays. However, a lumbar spine X-ray has a similar dose as a head CT.

Prior to every CT examination, evaluate the appropriateness of the exam whether it is motivated or if another type of examination is more suitable.

6.5.7.5 MRI Scan

MRI was originally called 'NMRI' (nuclear magnetic resonance imaging). It is based upon the science of nuclear magnetic resonance (NMR). Certain atomic nuclei are able to absorb and emit radio-frequency energy when placed in an external magnetic field. In clinical and research MRI, hydrogen atoms are most often used to generate a detectable radio-frequency signal that is received by antennas in close proximity to the anatomy being examined. Hydrogen atoms exist naturally in people and other biological organisms in abundance, particularly in water and fat. For this reason, most MRI scans essentially map the location of water and fat in the body. Pulses of radio waves excite the nuclear spin energy transition, and magnetic field gradients localize the signal in space. By varying the parameters of the pulse sequence, different contrasts may be generated between tissues based on the relaxation properties of the hydrogen atoms therein.

6.5.8 *EMG/NCC Studies*

While the hazards of X-rays are now well-controlled in most medical contexts, MRI still may be seen as superior to CT in this regard. MRI is widely used in hospitals and clinics for medical diagnosis, staging of disease, and follow-up without exposing the body to ionizing radiation. MRI often may yield different diagnostic information compared with CT. There may be risks and discomfort associated with MRI scans. Compared with CT, MRI scans typically take greater time, are louder, and usually require that the subject go into a narrow, confining tube. In addition, people with some medical implants or other non-removable metal inside the body may be unable to undergo an MRI examination safely.

MRI requires a magnetic field that is both strong and uniform. The field strength of the magnet is measured in teslas——and while the majority of systems operate at 1.5 T, commercial systems are available between 0.2 and 7 T.

Two forms of image weighting are in common use: T1 (spin-Lattice) and T2 (spin-spin). Looking at each weighting in turn, T1 image weighting is useful for assessing the cerebral cortex, identifying fatty tissue, characterizing focal liver lesions, and in general for obtaining morphological information, as well as for post-contrast imaging. To create a T2-weighted image, magnetization is allowed to decay before measuring the MR signal by changing the echo time (spin-spin). This image weighting is useful for detecting oedema and inflammation, revealing white matter lesions and assessing zonal anatomy in the prostate and uterus.

A good overview article is that by Mortonet al. which considers fMRI, PET, EEG, in arthritis and fibromyalgia [9].

6.6 Physical Disability Assessment

In addition to the biological investigation of the cause of pain it is also necessary to quantify the physical disability arising from the pain in order to develop an appropriate strategy to improve physical function.

In addition to the physical examination there are two verbal rating scores in common use that can be very helpful in planning a treatment strategy. These are the Oswestry Disability Index and the Roland Morris Disability Index.

The Oswestry Disability Index arose out of the desire to quantify the disability that sufferers from chronic low back pain manifested. It was first published by Jeremy Fairbank et al. in Physiotherapy in 1980. It has subsequently been revised and the present version in common use was published in Spine in 2000. It is considered by many to be the gold standard assessment of the degree of disability and estimation of the quality of life in a patient suffering from chronic low back pain.

It consists of ten topics where each is graded from 0 to a maximum of 5 and looks at pain intensity, lifting ability, ability for self-care, ability to walk, ability to sit, sexual function, ability to stand, social life, sleep quality, and ability to travel.

Scoring is by doubling the scores to a maximum of a 100. Thus 0–20 equate with minimal disability, 21–40 Moderate disability, 41–60 Severe disability, 61–80 crippling back pain, and 81–100 these patients are either bedbound OR EXAGGERATING their symptoms. This last is the problem that bedevils all verbal rating scores in a forensic context and to the author's view makes them unreliable and therefore not helpful in formulating any opinion about the degree of disability a claimant suffers.

The index though can be very useful in showing a change induced by treatment and this is where it is mainly used [10, 11].

6.7 The Roland Morris Disability Questionnaire

This is another health status measure for chronic low back pain. It was first published in 1983.

There are 24 items that are checked by the patient. Thus the score range is from 0 to 24. If an item is not applicable it is scored as 'No' the denominator remains 24. It has been used extensively in clinical practice and research and a review of papers published on the questionnaire was published in 2000 [12, 13].

Interested readers are directed to the website www.rmdq.org/index.htm for references to published evaluations of the questionnaire.

6.8 Psychological Assessment in Chronic Pain

Pain is an unpleasant sensory and emotional experience and is described in those terms. In other words there is not just a physical/biological component to the sensation of pain but also an emotional reaction to it. The total impact of chronic pain on an individual will necessarily incorporate their emotional reaction to pain and this may be subject to many influences.

Their reaction may range from considering it a nuisance to a catastrophe.

The range of the variation of response will be predicated by previous exposure to pain in themselves, in others or what they have read, seen, or listened to in the media. This will form the basis of an individual's fears and beliefs around pain, suffering, and injury and will determine their reaction to the pain and their disability and emotional reaction from it.

Thus, for example, there is a huge difference in emotional response to chronic pain arising from torture where the pain is deliberately and maliciously inflicted in frightening circumstances, to stubbing one's toe, where the expectation is complete resolution of the pain and the circumstances were neither frightening nor malicious.

While these two examples represent extreme ends of a spectrum and continuum in pain experience, mostly commonly patient's emotional reaction will fall between them.

But pre-existing psychological upset such as post-traumatic distress disorder, say following a frightening accident, or an untreated psychiatric condition such as a depressive disorder will also influence the impact of chronic pain on an individual.

In order to formulate a comprehensive treatment strategy it is important to gauge the psychological impact of pain and also to gauge the mental health of an affected individual.

While a full psychiatric examination might be considered the gold standard, in the majority of cases it is neither practical nor warranted. However, there are a battery of psychometric tests in the form of questionnaires that have been devised in an attempt to quantify this. The tests can represent a formidable challenge in terms of reliability and validity.

Bearing in mind these will often be applied to vulnerable individuals with significantly reduced emotional reserves to cope with perceived outside stressors, the best ones need to be simple and easy to complete.

Some early ones, no doubt composed with the enthusiasm of research, were very lengthy and thus frankly doomed to failure from the outset as even psychologically robust individuals would stall because of the length of time required to complete them.

The most effective tests are short, easy to complete, and focused on the domains they are intended to measure. The following are presently in common currency, but this is a field that is constantly changing as needs and focus are in a constant state of re-evaluation.

6.8.1 *Brief Pain Inventory*

This is a self-report questionnaire that has nine questions the last being divided into seven domains. It asks the patient to rate their pain experience and record the range in a number of different situations from best to worst average and at the time of assessment and asks what treatments the sufferer has had and what benefit if any has been achieved. It also looks at the impact of the pain on the individuals general activity, mood, walking ability, work, relations with other people, sleep, and the enjoyment of life. It deals with the functional impact of pain (physical and emotional) but it does not ask any qualitative questions and thus does not consider mechanisms [14].

6.8.2 *Beck Depression Inventory*

This was first devised by Aaron Beck in 1961 and later revised in 1978. The latest version was published in 1996 as the BDI-II. It is a widely used assessment tool in both clinical and research contexts.

It consists of 21 questions scored from 0 to 3 where 0 is no impact and 3 is maximum impact in the category. The questions all deal with depressive symptoms of depression such as hopelessness and irritability, cognitions such as guilt or feelings of being punished as well as physical symptoms such as fatigue, weight loss, and lack of interest in sex.

A score of 0–10 is considered normal, 11–16 indicative of a mild mood disturbance, 17–20 indicative of a borderline clinical depression, 21–30 of a moderate clinical depression, 31–40 of a severe depression, and over 41 indicative of extreme depression.

6.8.3 Hospital Anxiety and Depression Scale

Zigmond and Snaith [15] created this measure specifically to avoid reliance on aspects of those conditions that are also common somatic symptoms of illness, for example, fatigue and insomnia or hypersomnia. The questionnaire consists of two columns containing seven questions with four possible answers scoring 0–3 that generates ordinal data. Seven of the items relate to anxiety and seven relate to depression. This, it was hoped, would create a tool for the detection of anxiety and depression in people with physical health problems. It has been widely evaluated and Bjelland et al. through a systematic review of a large number of studies identified a cut-off point of 8/21 for anxiety or depression.

However, there are mixed views over the factor structure where some support the two factor structure but others consider three or four factors. Some consider that this tool is best used as a unidimensional measure of psychological distress [15].

6.8.4 Patient Health Questionnaire 9

This consists of nine questions scoring 0–3 and has been devised to objectify depression severity. It is important to correlate the scores with clinical interview and examination in order to assess a patient's mental status, their physical state, functional impairment, and level of psychological distress. A cut-off of ten or above is considered to indicate the presence of depression. 11–14 indicates moderate depression, 15–19 indicates moderately severe depression and the advice is to prescribe prescription drugs and counselling, and if the score is above 20, thus indicating severe depression, to refer the patient to a mental health specialist for counselling in addition to prescribing drugs.

As with any psychometric questionnaire it is essential to put the assessment into context and rule out other influencing factors such as recent bereavement, bipolar disorder, and medical disorders causing depression in their own right, i.e., hypothyroidism [16].

6.8.5 *Generalized Anxiety Disorder Assessment (GAD-7)*

This is a seven question assessment tool where each question is scored from 0 to 3, with a possible maximum of 21, and is used a screening tool and severity measure for generalized anxiety disorder. It has also been found to be moderately good at screening other anxiety disorders such as panic disorder, social anxiety disorder, and post-traumatic stress disorder.

Scores of 5,10, and 15 are taken to be the cut-off points for mild, moderate, and severe anxiety [17].

6.9 Investigations that Inform Research

6.9.1 *Quantitative Sensory Testing*

Quantitative sensory testing (QST) is a term used to describe different forms of psychophysical testing of skin, mucosa, or muscle tissue that assess sensory and pain perception pathways. They typically include warm and cold perception threshold testing, heat pain, and cold pain detection threshold testing using a thermotesting device mechanical detection threshold determination using von Frey filaments and a pressure algometer; vibration detection threshold determination using a tuning fork allodynia testing using a cotton swab or paintbrush; and dynamic wind-up testing using repeated skin stimulation with a predefined force and tip size. Several additional invasive tests for the quantification of muscular pain perception using electrical stimulation or intramuscular injection of hypertonic saline also have been described. This testing is rather expensive and time consuming but provides comprehensive information on the state of peripheral sensory and pain perception as well as central sensitization.

To exclude the influence of the state of peripheral nociceptors and solely test neuronal transduction of peripheral sensory input, its processing, and its perception in the spinal cord and central nervous system, one can test the neurophysiologic response to peripheral electrical stimulation of the skin using a peripheral nerve stimulator routinely used in regional anaesthesia. Similar testing has been applied successfully to test muscle tissue sensitivity to electrical stimulation.

Specific testing of pain fibres (A-delta and C fibres) is possible using laser-evoked potentials by means of inducing heat pain without actual skin contact. To test a mechanism of endogenous analgesia, also known as *diffuse noxious inhibitory control* (DNIC), it is possible to test local or referred pain perception while providing a conditioning stimulus at the same time, based on the principle of pain inhibiting pain. Although many variations of this test have been described, the most commonly used are the induction of DNIC by immersion in ice water (so-called cold pressor test), or hot water on a different/distant body part than the one on which the pain perception testing is being performed.

QST is considered to be semi-objective because it is dependent on the patient's perception and reporting and relies on his or her cooperation and attentiveness during the testing procedure. Standardization of the experimental protocol and environmental conditions under which the testing is being performed is essential for obtaining reproducible results comparable to normative data and data from different testing laboratories/centres.

6.9.2 *Rationale for Quantitative Sensory Testing in Musculoskeletal Pain Disorders*

Musculoskeletal pain is one of the most common reasons for seeking physicians' help. The term encompasses a wide range of disease states, ranging from well-defined illnesses such as osteoarthritis, rheumatoid arthritis (RA), and gout to more unspecific regional and generalized pain syndromes such as epicondylalgia, fibromyalgia, and finally pain related to the spine such as neck and low back pain. Objective findings for abnormal central pain processing range from muscle hyperalgesia to generalized and polymodal hyperalgesia, as well as referred pain. These features in turn share many common characteristics with neuropathic pain, all of which can be detected using QST.

For that reason, various methods of QST were applied in recent years to investigate the pathophysiologic mechanisms of musculoskeletal pain, primarily using experimental muscle pain paradigms. However, many studies also have been conducted and published in which QST has been used to analyse pain pathways and mechanisms involved in musculoskeletal disease states in humans. For some of these conditions, such as fibromyalgia and myofascial pain, certain tests (e.g., pressure algometry of tender or trigger points) may contribute to the illness classification and/or diagnosis. In other diseases, the testing has been used primarily to try to elucidate potential underlying pathogenetic mechanisms, as in the case of low back pain, primary and secondary restless legs syndrome associated with small-fibre neuropathy, or temporomandibular joint pain. It is noteworthy that such testing can be performed not only locally at the site of musculoskeletal pain but also at the site of referred pain.

Most of the studies of invasive or noninvasive sensory testing of the skin or deep tissues in patients with musculoskeletal disorders have been performed primarily in an attempt to analyse the pathogenesis of the underlying illness.

6.10 Punch Biopsy

A skin punch biopsy is a sensitive and specific diagnostic test that is mainly reserved as a research tool. It has been used in CRPS to identify the mechanisms and activation of the innate immune system. It has also been used to detect a reduction in nerve fibre density, when investigating small fibre neuropathy.

For example, fibromyalgia has similar symptoms to small fibre neuropathy. Identifying small fibre neuropathy and its underlying cause in fibromyalgia patients provides them with a succinct diagnosis, increases treatment options, and facilitates more specific studies for future therapeutics.

6.11 Laser Speckle Contrast Imaging

Laser speckle contrast analysis (LASCA) is a method that visualizes tissue blood perfusion in the microcirculation instantaneously. It is an imaging technique that combines high resolution and speed.

When an object is illuminated by laser light, the backscattered light will form a random interference pattern consisting of dark and bright areas. This pattern is called a speckle pattern. If the illuminated object is static, the speckle pattern is stationary. When there is movement in the object, such as red blood cells in a tissue, the speckle pattern will change over time (Fig. 6.7).

It is very much an advanced research tool and has been used to map cerebral blood flow. It has been used in studying the cortical spreading depression implicated in migraine visual aura, and how it activates trigeminovascular afferents and evokes a series of cortical meningeal and brainstem events consistent with the development of headache [18].

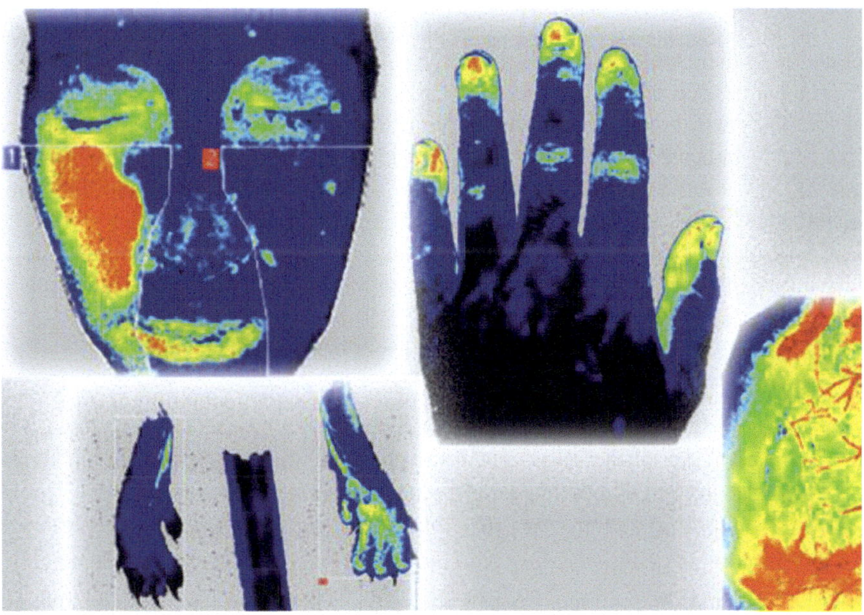

Fig. 6.7 Laser speckle images showing increased blood flow. This has been used to map changes during a migraine attack and other vascular disorders such as CRPS. Reproduced with kind permission from Perimed AB

6.12 Functional Magnetic Resonance Imaging: fMRI

fMRI is based on the same technology as *magnetic resonance imaging (MRI)*—a noninvasive test that uses a strong magnetic field and radio waves to create detailed images of the body. But instead of creating images of organs and tissues like MRI, fMRI looks at blood flow in the brain to detect areas of activity. These changes in blood flow, which are captured on a computer, help understand more about how the brain works. It is expensive and its use is still confined to research.

However, looking to the future, while it can help diagnose diseases of the brain, it might also enable doctors to get inside our mental processes to determine what we are thinking and feeling. In a forensic context fMRI might even be able to detect whether we are telling the truth! [19].

6.13 Investigation of Pain in Litigation: Covert Surveillance

6.13.1 Brief Background Information

The courts in the UK require an expert in pain medicine to determine the effect of a claimant's pain so that they can quantify general damages, special damages, and provisional damages.

This puts the pain expert in a position of considerable responsibility. The determination of pain, which is largely self-report presents a considerable challenge.

The pain expert will be instructed in cases of personal injury and clinical negligence. They will be required to determine causation. Thus the pain expert will be required to indicate to the court the effect the index event has had on the nature, quality and severity of the pain experienced by the Claimant compared with the hypothetical situation the patient would be in, absent the index event.

To do this, it is essential to consider the imaging, medical history, and self-report of pain, in order to determine pre-existing pathology and any likely degenerative processes resulting from that.

The court will want to know if the index event has caused:

1. An acceleration of the inevitable onset of the signs and symptoms reported by the claimant and found on clinical examination
2. An exacerbation of the same, where the claimant was already expressing signs and symptoms but that the index event made them materially worse
3. The signs and symptoms reported that would not have occurred absent the index event.

We have an adversarial legal system in the UK where both the claimant and the defendant are represented, so the pain expert will be instructed by either side. Their primary duty is to the court and not those instructing them, so their report must be balanced, unbiased, and truthful.

In order to achieve this the medical expert may not rely entirely on the report and witness statements of the claimant (which will usually include supportive statements from family, friends, and work colleagues) or the defence, which will include Human Resource, Occupational Health, and Department of Health, Work and Pensions records.

When there is an apparent inconsistency between report of pain and observed behaviour, taking into account the mechanism of the symptoms and signs reported, the defence will organize covert surveillance.

6.13.2 *Covert Surveillance*

The expert needs to match up movement such as bending down, reaching up, distanced walked, lifting, carrying and moving heavy objects, driving, wearing of clothes next to reported hypersensitive skin, manual dexterity, and bimanual dexterity.

The expert has to take a view on whether they consider the observed activity and the length such activity is undertaken is consistent with that reported by the claimant and the findings on clinical examination supported by other investigations.

References

1. Jensen MP, Gammaitoni AR, Olaleye DO, et al. The pain quality assessment scale: assessment of pain quality in carpal tunnel syndrome. J Pain. 2006;7:823–32.
2. Galer BS, Jensen MP. Development and preliminary validation of a pain measure specific to neuropathic pain: the neuropathic pain scale. Neurology. 1997;48:332–8.
3. Bennett M. The LANSS pain scale: the Leeds assessment of neuropathic symptoms and sign. Pain. 2001;92:147–57.
4. Bennett MI, Smith BH, Torrance N, Lee AJ. Can pain can be more or less neuropathic? Comparison of symptom assessment tools with ratings of certainty by clinicians. Pain. 2006;115:289–94.
5. Freynhagen R, Baron R, Gockel U, Tölle TR. painDETECT: a new screening questionnaire to identify neuropathic components in patients with back pain. Curr Med Res Opin. 2006;22(10):1911–20.
6. Bouhassira D, Attal N, Alchaar H, et al. Comparison of pain syndromes associated with nervous or somatic lesions and development of a new neuropathic pain questionnaire (DN4). Pain. 2005;114:29–36.
7. Jones RC 3rd, Backonja MM. Review of neuropathic pain screening and assessment tools. Curr Pain Headache Rep. 2013;363(1-8):17.
8. IASP. Clinical updates. Washington: Michael Gofeld Seattle; 2012. 20(4).
9. Morton DL, Sandhu JS, Jones AKP. Brain imaging of pain: state of the art. J Pain Res. 2016;9:613–24.
10. Fairbank JC, Couper J, Davies JB. The Oswestry low back pain questionnaire. Physiotherapy. 1980;66:271–3.
11. Fairbank JC, Pynsent PB. The Oswestry disability index. Spine. 2000;25(22):2940–52.
12. Roland MO, Morris RW. A study of the natural history of back pain. Part 1: development of a reliable and sensitive measure of disability in low back pain. Spine. 1983;8:141–4.

13. Roland M, Fairbank J. The Roland-Morris disability questionnaire and the Oswestry disability questionnaire. Spine. 2000;25:3115–24. (NB there was an error in the questionnaire reproduced in the appendix in item 18 which should read- I sleep less well because of my back)
14. Cleeland CS, Ryan KM. Pain assessment: global use of the brief pain inventory. Ann Acad Med Singap. 1994;23(2):129–38.
15. Zigmond AS, Snaith RP. The hospital anxiety and depression scale. Acta Psychiatr Scand. 1983;67(6):361–70.
16. Kroenke K, Spitzer RL. The PHQ-9: a new depression diagnostic and severity measure. Psychiatr Ann. 2002;32:1–7.
17. Spitzer RL, Kroenke K, Williams JB, et al. A brief measure for assessing generalized anxiety disorder: the GAD-7. Arch Intern Med. 2006;166(10):1092–7.
18. Bolay H, Reuter U, Dunn AK, et al. Intrinsic brain activity triggers trigeminal meningeal afferents in a migraine model. Nat Med. 2002;8(2):137–42.
19. Reardon S. The painful truth. Nature. 2015;518:474–6.

Chapter 7
Interventional Treatment of Chronic Pain

Thomas E. Smith

7.1 General Principles

Chronic pain should be assessed and treated using a holistic biopsychosocial approach—please refer to Chap. 10 for discussion of this. Interventional treatments can address nociceptive and neuropathic biological mechanisms of pain. They can be used in diagnosis (diagnostic blocks) and in treatment. They can produce dramatic benefit when used in selected patients.

7.1.1 Goals of Interventions

Desirable goals should be established prior to any intervention. The goal of all chronic pain treatment is to improve overall quality of life (QoL), physical and social functioning, and to decrease pain. The outcome of pain interventions should be judged against these criteria.

7.1.2 Recording Outcomes

Pain scores should be recorded before and following treatment, but these are less important than measures of quality of life and function. Broad outcome measures such as EQ 5D and Brief Pain Inventory, as well as condition specific measures, like (the Oswestry Disability Index for back pain), are appropriate. Medication reduction is another goal. Please refer to the chapter on Pain Measurement/Outcomes.

T. E. Smith (✉)
Guy's and St Thomas' Pain and Neuromodulation Centre, London, UK

K. Shimoji et al. (eds.), *Chronic Pain Management in General and Hospital Practice*, https://doi.org/10.1007/978-981-15-2933-7_7

7.1.3 Importance of Cost-Effectiveness and of Patient Selection

Cost-effectiveness analyses of treatments are demanded by funders of healthcare. These analyses look at degree in improvement of quality of life versus money spent on the treatment. Cost-effectiveness of any treatment is influenced greatly by "patient selection". When interventions are directed only at those most likely to benefit cost-effectiveness will be good. When interventions are performed in many patients that are not likely to benefit then cost-effectiveness will be poor. It is essential to consider patient factors that influence whether interventions are likely to be effective or not—both to avoid subjecting patients to unhelpful procedures, and to avoid effective procedures being discarded as "cost-ineffective" because of indiscriminate use.

7.1.4 When Are Interventions More Likely to Help?

(a) *Localized Pain Problem*—Interventional treatments are most likely to be effective when pain involves localized nociceptive and neuropathic mechanisms, and much less likely to be effective when pain is generalized and widespread. A patient complaining of isolated left lumbosacral back pain with muscle tenderness and tension restricted to the left paraspinal region may show long-term improvements in pain, function, and QoL from facet joint medial branch blocks and subsequent facet joint denervation. A patient with widespread chronic pain such as seen in fibromyalgia syndrome is very unlikely to benefit.
(b) *Shorter History of Pain*—Interventional treatments are more likely to benefit when used early in a pain presentation. Most interventional treatments target peripheral nociceptive and neuropathic pain drivers. In long-term pain, central sensitization becomes important and secondary dysfunctional motor and behavioural patterns accumulate—interventional treatments do not directly address these factors.
(c) *Active Social and Physical Life*—Interventional treatments are more likely to be effective in patients who are active and engaged in social and physical life. Even when clear nociceptive and neuropathic pain drivers can be addressed by interventions, it is still important to look holistically at patients' overall presentation and also target intertwining factors such as physical deconditioning, and psychological factors.
(d) *Psychological*—Depression, anxiety, and personality disorders are prevalent in the chronic pain population. Interventional treatments are less likely to be effective in the presence of these factors, and addressing these factors successfully increases the chance of good outcome with interventional treatments.
(e) *Secondary Gain*—The effect of ongoing litigation on chronic pain treatment outcomes is controversial but it is likely to impair outcomes in some cases. Some people with pain evolve a lifestyle dependent on partners, family mem-

bers, friends who take on the role as carers. This complicates their presentation and can reduce efficacy of interventional treatments. Some people with chronic pain may become financially reliant on benefits connected to their level of disability. This may reduce the probability of good functional improvements with interventions.

7.1.5 Contraindications to Interventions

The following are the most often seen contraindications to interventions:

- Presence of infection—at site of intervention or systemic
- Coagulation deficiencies
- Pregnancy (risk to foetus of X-rays and drugs)
- Comorbidities, e.g.,
  - Patients on some antiviral medications for HIV and hepatitis C should not be given corticosteroid because of slowed elimination leading to metabolic adverse events
  - Morbid obesity—many interventions less likely to help and are higher risk
- Technically not possible—e.g., patient cannot be positioned appropriately, anatomical changes/implants from previous surgery

7.1.6 Risks of Interventions

- *Of the interventional technique itself:*

  All interventions risk complications and adverse effects. Common risks are as follows:

  - Pain of procedure and flare of existing pain condition
  - Bruising/Bleeding
  - Infection

  Other risks are specific to the particular interventions and are discussed below.
- *Of interference with comorbidities and treatments:*

  It is important to be aware of patients' comorbidities and treatments before recommending an interventional treatment. For example:

  - Corticosteroid, used in many interventional treatments, can interfere with diabetic control.
  - Patients on regular anticoagulants may have an unacceptably high risk of bleeding with some interventions, but increased risk of venous thrombosis, stroke, or myocardial infarction if taken off the anticoagulant to permit a pain intervention.

7.1.7 *Other Considerations*

7.1.7.1 Inconvenience

In the consent process, emphasis is given to the risks of interventional treatment—which are usually very unlikely. Less consideration is given to the very real and common inconvenience (time, travel, fasting for sedation, need to be accompanied) involved in having interventions.

7.1.7.2 Maladaptive Focus

Some patients focus on finding a "magic bullet" solution to their complex chronic pain in the form of an intervention at the expense of accepting a need to adopt a holistic approach to their problem. In such cases, proceeding with interventions without addressing patients' understanding and behaviours is likely to be counterproductive.

7.2 Mechanisms of Action of the Most Commonly Used Drugs: Local Anaesthetics and Corticosteroids

7.2.1 *Local Anaesthetics*

Many interventional techniques involve the injection of local anaesthetics around nerves. Local anaesthetics block the influx of sodium into nerves that is required to propagate action potentials along the nerve. This effect is used to produce a block of pain nerves, but the duration of the block with conventional local anaesthetics is short—usually a few hours only. This direct effect is used in "diagnostic blocks" to see if the source of pain is from particular nerves or joints.

Sometimes pain relief following a local anaesthetic block lasts well beyond the duration of the direct block action on the nerves. Possible reasons for this include winding down of the sensitivity of peripheral nerves and/or central sensitization by the period of complete block, relaxation of muscles, and placebo.

7.2.2 *Corticosteroids*

Corticosteroids such as dexamethasone, methylprednisolone, and triamcinolone are often used in pain interventional procedures. They have a myriad of effects. They are strongly anti-inflammatory locally; this can reduce inflammation in joints and swelling of nerves. They have a localized membrane-stabilizing effect on neurones.

They are taken up by nerves and are transported to the cell nucleus where they regulate gene transcription and thus protein production. They can thereby alter nervous system function in complex ways and the duration of steroid effects can outlast the presence of the steroid.

Some of the steroid administered is inevitably taken up by the blood stream and can have systemic effects. Short-term systemic side effects may include facial flushing, suppression of immune response, and heightened mood. Hyperglycaemia in diabetics may be expected. Repeated steroid injections at short intervals are best avoided due to the risk of inducing ongoing metabolic side effects.

7.3 Specific Interventions

It is not possible to cover every possible interventional pain procedure in this chapter. Spinal pain procedures are by far the commonest so let us focus on them first.

7.3.1 The Spine

Spinal pain is the commonest chronic pain complaint. The UK Chief Medical Officer report of 2009, "Pain: Breaking through the Barrier" stated that there were 1.6 million people with chronic back pain in the UK and that the yearly cost of back pain to the economy was £12.3 billion.

Any internet search will turn up a bewildering array of treatments offered for spinal pain. The scale of the problem and the plethora of treatments offered reflect that spinal pain has many possible causes, mechanisms, and contributory factors. Interventional treatments can address only some of these.

7.3.2 Types of Spinal Pain

7.3.2.1 Axial Pain Vs Radicular Pain

A useful way to look at spinal pain is to look at whether the pain has an axial or radicular pattern.

Axial pain is adjacent to the spine and usually associated with paraspinal muscle tension and tenderness with any spread into limbs being only proximal and limited. Axial pain suggests spinal musculoskeletal drivers—facet joints, sacroiliac joints, discogenic pain (pain from degenerative discs), muscles, and ligaments.

Radicular pain travels down a limb or around the thorax in a band consistent with a nerve root and suggests nerve root irritation. Usually there are some neuropathic features.

Mixed Presentations. Some presentations have elements of axial and radicular pain. This can be due to having both axial and radicular pathology. It can also be due to severe "axial" pathology pain being referred down a limb such as in severe sacroiliac joint arthropathy. In the case of radicular pain, secondary muscle tension and guarding of the spine can cause axial pain.

Neurogenic Claudication Pain is usually seen in older patients. This occurs when spinal nerves or cauda equina blood supply is limited by stenosis (spinal canal narrowing) or fibrosis postsurgery, and cannot be increased to meet the demands of activity. A complaint of radicular symptoms in one lower limb with activity may be encountered with narrowing of one side of the spinal canal (lateral recess stenosis). In central lumbar spinal canal stenosis the typical presentation is one of low back pain and bilateral lower limb heaviness and pain with walking—especially uphill. Walking distance becomes limited and there is tendency to stoop when walking.

7.3.2.2 Interventions for Axial Pain

The Role of Facet Joint Treatments

Facet joints or "zygoapophyseal joints" are small synovial joints between vertebrae at the posterior-lateral aspect of the spine. They allow a degree of movement of the spine while stabilizing it against excessive movement. Like other synovial joints that bear a lot of loading in our lives (knees, hips) they are prone to degenerative/osteoarthritic changes. This is particularly so at the lumbar and the cervical levels.

Pain from lumbar facet joints is felt in the lumbar paraspinal area spreading into the buttocks and often into the posterior thighs. Most pain interventionalists believe that the pain driven by facet joints is worse on loading the joints—such as straightening the spine after flexion, or extension from neutral, and lateral flexion with extension. The limited studies looking at this have suggested that pain on loading of the joints is not a good discriminator and that the main positive association is localized paraspinal muscle tenderness.

Muscle tension and tenderness is seen with other drivers of axial back pain. This leads to the concept of "back pain for investigation". The only way to determine if facet joints are a major driver of low back pain is to treat them and see if the pain considerably diminishes. Interventional studies suggest that around 15% of cases of axial low back pain may have facet joint arthropathy as a main driver and therefore benefit from facet joint treatments.

Facet Joint Injections

Facet joint injections with local anaesthetic and steroid has been a popular treatment for chronic low back pain for many years. Although described as intra-articular injections, it is likely that in most cases the injections are peri-articular given the difficult anatomy of degenerative joints and the small volume of the joint. The efficacy and cost-effectiveness of facet joint injections has long been controversial. Patient selection and operator factors are likely to play important roles in determining outcomes. In general, past studies reported by interventionalists tended to report mildly positive outcomes [1], but in recent years evidence and opinion has shifted toward concluding that facet joint injections have limited efficacy and are not cost-effective in larger populations [2]. The latest NICE guidelines NICE CG59 [3] reflect this latter view and do not recommend facet joint injections for low back pain. However—there are some patients who show remarkable and prolonged benefit after traditional facet joint injections and it may be reasonable to continue to offer these injections to a select group.

Facet Joint Medial Branch Blocks and Rhizolysis: Facet Joint Denervations

An alternative to injecting the joint is to block or destroy (lesion) the nerves that supply it.

Facet joints are each supplied by two small nerves—medial branch nerves. In the cervical and lumbar levels these nerves run in relatively reliable positions as they approach the joint (Fig. 7.1). Using X-ray or ultrasound guidance these nerves can be blocked with small volumes of local anaesthetic to assess the role of the facet joints in contributing to the pain. This is known as a *diagnostic or test block* procedure. The local anaesthetic effect lasts only for hours, so one is looking for a short-lived but dramatic (75%) pain relief to occur. Patients are required to record

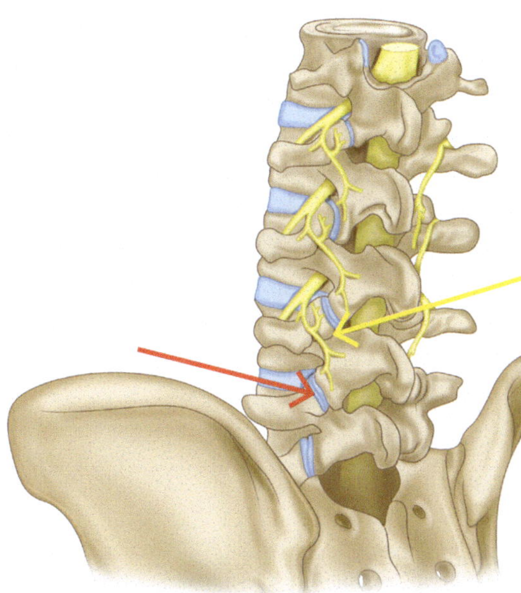

Fig. 7.1 Lumbar spine. Red arrow points to lumbar facet joint covered in liagaments. Yellow arrow points to medial branch nerve—each joint is supplied by two medial branch nerves

their pain and function before and after the blocks. If a dramatic but short-lived reduction in pain occurs, then the patients can be offered radiofrequency rhizolysis ("burning" of the nerves). This is a procedure using a radiofrequency generating machine and insulated needles with tips heated to a controlled temperature through delivery of a controlled amount of energy. This creates small ovoid burns several millimetres long and wide that "lesion" the nerves. This is a day case procedure but requires X-ray imaging and operator expertise. The burning also lesions adjacent tissue so the back tends to be painful for 2–3 weeks afterwards. However, once the acute pain settles down benefit from the resulting "denervation" of the facet joints is expected. The benefit should last 12 months more—but the nerves may grow back.

This treatment pathway—facet joint medial branch blocks for pain investigation, and, if positive, radiofrequency rhizolysis to produce facet joint denervations, is supported by current evidence [2] and the latest NICE Guidelines [3].

The Role of Sacroiliac Joint Treatments

The sacroiliac joints join the spine to the pelvis. The upper part of the joint is fibrocartilaginous, and the lower part is a synovial joint. These important joints bear heavy loads when we stand and walk. They normally have very limited movement. Their function is to combine stability with a little cushioning. They may become painful due to degenerative change or injury. Pain is then felt at the lumbosacral level in the region of the joint and typically spreads into the buttock and thigh. Where the pain is due to low-grade inflammation associated with degenerative change, intra-articular injection of corticosteroid may bring pain relief. When pain relief through intra-articular injection is short-lived, radiofrequency thermal lesioning of the sacroiliac joint's posterior innervation, known as "sacroiliac joint denervation", may bring longer lasting relief—analogous to the treatment of facet joints. Injection of the sacroiliac joint with local anaesthetic and steroid is supported by low to moderate evidence, as is radiofrequency denervation of the joint [4].

Sacroiliac joint instability/dysfunction is a condition in which there is excessive movement of the joint with loading of the joint in normal activities such as standing and walking. It is more common in women, especially those with hypermobility and tends to follow pregnancy and childbirth or trauma. Pain can be felt in the lumbosacral area but also in the groin and down the lower limb—sometimes mimicking sciatica pain. Provocative stress testing of the joint reveals the problem. This condition may respond to prolotherapy—injection of glucose solution into the joint and sacroiliac ligaments to promote fibrosis [5].

Discogenic Pain

Disc degeneration, particularly in the lumbar and cervical levels, is normal in humans. Degenerative discs sometimes irritate adjacent nerve roots to cause radicular sciatic type pain. However, the role of disc degeneration in axial spinal pain is controversial.

Sensory nerves are normally only present on the outermost layer of discs but may grow into some damaged discs. Disc degeneration may cause adjacent vertebral end-plate inflammation. A number of investigations and treatments for presumed discogenic pain have been offered through the years. Provocative discography is the injection of contrast under controlled pressure into discs to look for disc fissures and whether intradiscal pressure produces pain. Injections into the disc with corticosteroid, sclerosants, methylene blue, platelet enriched plasma, and stem cells have been offered as treatments. Heating the disc to burn invasive sensory nerves with electrical current through needles (IDET, Biacculoplasty) has been offered. Surgery has been offered—disc replacements, spacer devices (devices sited between spinous processes with the idea of holding vertebrae apart and offloading discs), and fusion surgery (removing the disc and allowing the vertebrae to fuse). None of these treatments of discogenic pain has a strong evidence base to support it and the latest NICE guidelines (NG59) to do not recommend any of them outside of a study setting. Some cases of discogenic pain may be due to a low-grade infection of the disc and that this may respond to prolonged antibiotic therapy [6] but this requires further study.

High frequency spinal cord stimulation appears to be effective in some patients [7] but this also requires further controlled studies.

Interventions for Radicular Pain

Radicular pain is that following a somatic nerve root innervation territory such as sciatica down a lower limb. Causes of radicular pain include inflammation and impingement/compression of a nerve root secondary to disc degeneration, spinal foraminal and lateral canal stenosis impinging on a nerve, scarring postsurgery, inflammation, and impingement postvertebral compression fracture [8].

Epidural injections can alleviate "irritative" radicular pain [8]. They can be particularly effective in acute sciatica from a new disc tear/protrusion. It is important to realize that epidural injections relieve radicular pain but they do not restore sensory loss or motor function loss in a nerve that is or has been physically compressed or otherwise injured. Epidural injections are not an effective treatment for axial low back pain—the commonest back pain presentation. They are not a long-term effective treatment for neurogenic claudication presentation of degenerative central spinal canal stenosis [3].

Types of Epidurals:

1. Transforaminal [9]—the needle is directed to a spinal nerve root foramen—this aim is to target a specific nerve root and achieve spread of the injectate along the nerve root into the spinal epidural space.
2. Interlaminar [9]—the needle is directed from posteriorly between the vertebral laminae into the spinal epidural. A larger volume of injectate is needed to hopefully achieve spread to the desired nerve root(s).
3. Caudal—the needle is directed into the lower end of the epidural space through the sacral hiatus. A large volume of injectate is needed to hopefully achieve spread upwards to the desired spinal nerve levels and this is only suitable for low lumbar and sacral radicular pain.

Usually corticosteroid is injected using local anaesthetic/saline as a vehicle. All epidurals for pain treatment should be performed under image guidance by a trained proceduralist.

Pulsed Radiofrequency Pain proceduralists sometime use pulsed radiofrequency treatment (see below) to a spinal nerve root/dorsal root ganglion as a treatment for radicular pain.

Racz Catheter Epidurolysis This technique involves the introduction on a steerable catheter into the epidural space to allow much greater targeting of specific nerve roots [10]. Large volumes of saline along with hyalase can be injected to promote physical freeing of low-grade fibrosis around nerve roots prior to the corticosteroid. This may resolve pain that is unresponsive to standard epidurals.

Spinal Endoscopy The lumbosacral epidural space may be examined endoscopically and fine fibrous bands tethering nerves and the dura may be lesioned. This technique is in the development and clinical research stage.

Spinal Cord Stimulation Spinal cord stimulation, see below, can be a very effective treatment for refractory radicular pain.

7.3.3 Non-Spinal Pain

7.3.3.1 Joint Injections (Non-spine)

Intra-articular joint injections may be performed for inflammatory pain secondary to low-grade degenerative changes. They are usually not effective in advanced osteoarthritis. They may be very effective in acute gout or pseudogout where inflammation is the main issue. Repeating steroid injections at intervals <6 months in the longer term is best avoided due to risk of local and systemic steroid adverse effects.

Injection of hyaluronan into painful knees joint with early osteoarthritis may provide pain relief by improving the lubrication and cushioning within the joint. It is not effective when osteoarthritis is advanced.

7.3.3.2 Peripheral Nerve Blocks

Peripheral nerve blocks with local anaesthetic and corticosteroid may alleviate neuropathic pain in the distribution of the nerve. This is more likely when the nerve has been injured by a local process (e.g., trauma/compression) and is not indicated in systemic polyneuropathy disease such as diabetic polyneuropathy. Peripheral nerve blocks may also be effective in some regional pain states—such as a suprascapular nerve block for shoulder pain or a lumbar plexus block for hip pain.

7.3.3.3 Occipital Nerve Blocks

Occipital nerve blocks deserve a special mention as they can be effective in chronic refractory migraine and status migrainosus as well as some other chronic headache conditions. Of course, they are also used to treat occipital neuralgia [11].

7.3.3.4 Trigeminal Ganglion and Nerves

The trigeminal nerve is a special peripheral nerve supplying the head and face. Some head and facial pain conditions are the most painful known. Trigeminal neuralgia and cluster headache can be devastating conditions. When these conditions prove refractory to lifestyle, medical management, and more superficial interventions, interventions targeting the trigeminal ganglion may be considered. Blocks, pulsed radiofrequency treatment [12], and in the case of trigeminal neuralgia, vascular decompression [13], and lesioning of the trigeminal ganglion with radiation (gamma knife) [14] or heat (radiofrequency needle) [15] may be considered. These are carried out in a specialist setting.

7.3.3.5 Autonomic Nervous System and Autonomic Blocks

1. Some pain nerves run alongside autonomic nerves and pass through autonomic ganglia where they may be targeted with blocks. Examples are coeliac plexus block [16] for upper gastrointestinal pain (especially pancreatic), and ganglion of impar block for pelvic pain conditions.

   Lesioning of coeliac plexus nerves with chemical agents (alcohol, phenol) can be wonderfully effective for pancreatic cancer pain. It is not recommended for non-malignant chronic pancreatitis pain as pain returns and repeat procedures result in accumulation of risk and diminishing benefit.
2. In some pain conditions the sympathetic autonomic nervous system is directly involved in the painful condition with sympathetic activity aggravating the pain and also causing undesirable symptoms including changes in blood flow to the painful region. The classic example is complex regional pain syndrome [17], another example is the autonomic cephalgia group of headaches. Blocks that may be used in these states include stellate ganglion (for upper limb), lumbar sympathetic block (lower limb) [18], and sphenopalatine (head and face) [19, 20]. These blocks require considerable expertise and imaging facilities.

7.3.3.6 Guanethidine Blocks

These are limb blocks using a venous tourniquet to limit the action of intravenously injected local anaesthetic (usually prilocaine) and guanethidine (a sympathetic nervous system modulating drug) were long practiced for complex regional pain syndrome. They have fallen out of favour due to lack of evidence of long-term efficacy.

7.3.3.7 Pulsed Radiofrequency

Pulsed radiofrequency (PRF) is the use of needles to deliver high-frequency current in bursts of 20 ms with a pause time of 480 ms to prevent temperatures exceeding 42 °C (above which tissue damage may occur). It may be used in the management of various pain syndromes [21], particularly those in which a peripheral nerve block is effective but short-lived. In these cases, PRF may provide longer term pain relief without the risks of nerve lesioning. Examples include dorsal root ganglion PRF for radicular nerve pains, ilioinguinal nerve PRF for inguinal pain, spermatic cord PRF for testicular pain [22], suprascapular nerve PRF for shoulder pain.

There is a lack of large multicentre controlled trials, but case series and sham controlled studies support PRF. The mechanism of action is unknown but altered gene expression in dorsal horn neurones has been shown to follow PRF, suggesting it may alter pain processing [23].

7.3.3.8 Nerve Ablation/Lesioning/Destruction: Radiofrequency Lesioning/Cryoablation

Usually, in pain medicine, care is taken to avoid damaging nerves during procedures—to avoid sensory and motor function loss and avoid precipitating neuropathic pain. However, in some refractory pain states, nerve destruction may be indicated.

Radiofrequency lesion of spinal medial branch nerves for facet joint pain, trigeminal ganglion radiation and radiofrequency lesioning for refractory trigeminal neuralgia, and chemical destruction of the coeliac plexus for pancreatic cancer pain have been discussed above.

Other examples include radiofrequency lesioning of genicular nerves for chronic knee pain [24] and of hip nerves for chronic hip pain. Cryoablation [25] (controlled freezing) of peripheral nerves for refractory neuropathic pain such as intercostal neuralgia can also be performed.

Spinal cord pain pathway lesioning can be performed for some severe, refractory cancer pains [26].

Botoxin Injections Botoxin has found use in a number of pain conditions [27]. It blocks the release of neurotransmitters from presynaptic terminals. It blocks acetylcholine release at neuromuscular synapses and thus blocks muscle activation—this can be used to relieve muscle dystonia.

It also blocks the release of Substance P and calcitonin gene related peptide (CGRP) from C-pain fibres which likely contributes to its efficacy in the treatment of refractory chronic migraine [28] and it may also be effective in some cases of localized neuropathic pain, especially where allodynia is present [29]. In the case of migraine, the botoxin is injected widely into the scalp and superficial neck (typically 31 injections sites) across the forehead, temporal region, occipital region, and neck at three monthly intervals.

7.3.3.9 Capsaicin Cutaneous Treatments for Neuropathic Pain

Capsaicin is the active ingredient that makes chilli "hot". It activates TRPV1 receptors. TRPV1 receptors are present in pain C nerve fibres where activation causes burning pain. After nerve injury TRPV1 receptors are up-regulated in adjacent uninjured C-fibres. This contributes to allodynia and primary hyperalgesia in neuropathic pain.

Massive activation of TRPV1 receptors results in degeneration of the terminals of pain C fibres. Capsaicin creams are available in concentrations of 0.025% and 0.075%. With this concentration, dedicated daily use is required and one must be very careful to avoid inadvertently contaminating an eye or mucosal surface with the cream.

8% Capsaicin patches have more than 100 times the concentration than the creams and have more evidence of efficacy in neuropathic pain. Studies on HIV related neuropathic pain and postherpetic neuralgia and diabetic painful peripheral neuropathy have been modestly positive [30–32]. The treatment can be painful due to the activation of the C-fibres initially. The patches are applied carefully for 30 min (feet) to 60 min (elsewhere) at three monthly intervals. Treatment is performed by a trained nurse.

7.3.4 Spinal Cord Stimulation (SCS) for Severe Refractory Neuropathic Pain and Postsurgical Back Pain

Spinal cord stimulation uses targeted, controlled delivery of low energy electrical stimulation to the posterior spinal cord and/or dorsal root ganglion to modulate pain. It developed following the publications of the gate control theory of pain by Melzack and Wall in 1965. The first SCS case was performed by Shealey in 1967. It has long been recognized that it can be an effective therapy for refractory neuropathic (nerve) pain, including radicular pain—especially that which can persist or follow spinal surgery. It was long thought that the production of paraesthesia (tingling) in the painful area was required for it to be effective. Recently it has been shown paraesthesia-free stimulation (patients do not feel the stimulation at all) has been shown to be very effective, even in some patients with spinal pain who have no history of nerve damage or spinal surgery [33, 34]. SCS therapy requires implantation of electrode leads and programmable pulse delivery devices containing a battery—similar to cardiac pacemakers. Careful patient assessment and education is required before a trial of this therapy, given its invasive and complex nature. Results can be remarkable with >50% pain relief and associated improvement in quality of life seen in 76% of patients at 2 years in the recent FDA overseen SENSA randomized controlled multicentre trial of high frequency spinal cord stimulation [35].

SCS is a therapy that demands more recognition given that it can be very effective in patients with severe pain when all else has failed to help, and that advancement in the technology is likely to widen indications and improve outcomes.

Intrathecal Pumps These systems are rare in the UK, but more widely used in the USA and some other countries. Baclofen is slowly infused into the CSF at a low spinal level to treat muscle spasticity of upper motor neurone lesion origin. Opioids, local anaesthetics, and ziconotide are used for pain indications. The evidence to support use in cancer pains is good. Use in chronic non-cancer pain other than for spasticity is less strongly evidenced [36].

The pump device is implanted into the abdominal wall where a reservoir can be refilled through an injection port at regular intervals, and the catheter runs around to the lumbar spine.

Trigger Points Trigger point injections are used in the treatment of myofascial pain characterized by trigger points or "knots" in muscles. Local anaesthetic, steroids, botulinum toxin, saline, or simply a dry needle may be injected into the trigger point with the aim of relaxing the muscle, relieving pain, and improving range of motion. There is a lack of large controlled trials for this therapy.

Summary Points
- Interventional techniques should be within a holistic biopsychosocial approach
- Interventions should be performed by trained and knowledgeable proceduralists
- The probability of benefit should be weighed against the risks in each individual case prior to any intervention
- Interventions are less likely to benefit patients with chronic widespread pain conditions and major psychosocial problems
- Interventions can produce great reduction in pain and improvements in function in patients with localized nociceptive and neuropathic pathology

References

1. Datta S, et al. Systematic assessment of diagnostic accuracy and therapeutic utility of lumbar facet joint injections. Pain Physician. 2009;12:437–60.
2. Manchikanti L, Datta S, Gupta S, Munglani R, et al. A critical review of the American pain society clinical practice guidelines for interventional techniques: part 2. Therapeutic Interventions. Pain Physician. 2010;13:E215–64.
3. Low back pain and sciatica in over 16s: assessment and management. NICE guideline [NG59]. Published date: November 2016.
4. Simopoulos T, Manchikanti L, Gupta S, et al. Systematic review of the diagnostic accuracy and therapeutic effectiveness of sacroiliac joint interventions. Pain Physician. 2015;18: E713–576.
5. Laslett M. Evidence based diagnosis and treatment of the painful sacroiliac joint. J Man Manip Ther. 2008;16(3):142–52.
6. Albert HB, Sorensen JS, Christensen BS, Manniche C. Antibiotic treatment in patients with chronic low back pain and vertebral bone edema (Modic type 1 changes): a double-blind, randomized clinical controlled trial of efficacy. Eur Spine J. 2013;22:697–707.
7. Al-Kaisy A, Palmisani P, Smith T, et al. Long-term improvements in chronic axial low back pain patients without previous spinal surgery: a cohort analysis of 10-kHz high-frequency spinal cord stimulation over 36 months. Pain Med. 2018;19(6):1219–26. https://doi.org/10.1093/pm/pnx237.

8. Bogduk N, Govind J. Medical management of acute lumbar radicular pain. An evidence-based approach. Newcastle: Newcastle Bone and Joint Institute; 1999.
9. Chang-Chien GC, Knezevic NN, McCormick Z, Chu SK, Trescot AM, Candido KD. Transforaminal versus interlaminar approaches to epidural steroid injections: a systematic review of comparative studies for lumbosacral radicular pain. Pain Physician. 2014;17(4):E509–24.
10. Helm Ii S, Benyamin RM, Chopra P, Deer TR, Justiz R. Percutaneous adhesiolysis in the management of chronic low back pain in post lumbar surgery syndrome and spinal stenosis: a systematic review. Pain Physician. 2012;15:E435–62.
11. Tobin J, Flitman S. Occipital nerve blocks: when and what to inject? Headache. 2009;49(10):1521–33.
12. Chua N, Halim W, Beems T, et al. Pulsed radiofrequency treatment for trigeminal neuralgia. Anesth Pain Med. 2012;1(4):257–61.
13. Barker FG 2nd, Jannetta PJ, Bissonette DJ, Larkins MV, Jho HD. The long-term outcome of microvascular decompression for trigeminal neuralgia. N Engl J Med. 1996;334: 1077–84.
14. Karam SD, Tai A, Wooster M, et al. Trigeminal neuralgia treatment outcomes following gamma knife radiosurgery with a minimum 3-year follow-up. J Radiat Oncol. 2014;3(2):125–1.
15. Eugene AR. Trigeminal neuralgia and radiofrequency lesioning. Brain (Bacau). 2015;6(1–2):91–6.
16. Rana MV, Candido KD, Raja O, Knezevic NN. Celiac plexus block in the management of chronic abdominal pain. Curr Pain Headache Rep. 2014;18(2):394.
17. Birklein F, Riedl B, Claus D, Neundörfer B. Pattern of autonomic dysfunction in time course of complex regional pain syndrome. Clin Auton Res. 1998;8(2):79–85.
18. Menon R, Swanepoel A. Sympathetic blocks. Contin Educ Anaesth Crit Care Pain. 2010;10(3):88–92.
19. Khan S, Schoenen J, Ashina M. Sphenopalatine ganglion neuromodulation in migraine: what is the rationale? Cephalagia. 2014;34(5):382–91.
20. Láinez MJA, Puche M, Garcia A, Gascón F. Sphenopalatine ganglion stimulation for the treatment of cluster headache. Ther Adv Neurol Disord. 2014;7(3):162–8.
21. Cahana A, Van Zundert J, Macrea L, van Kleef M, Sluijter M. Pulsed radiofrequency: current clinical and biological literature available. Pain Med. 2006;7:411–23.
22. Misra S, Ward S, Coker C. Pulsed radiofrequency for chronic testicular pain – a preliminary report. Pain Med. 2009;10(4):673–8.
23. Van Zundert J, de Louw AJ, Joosten EA, et al. Pulsed and continuous radiofrequency current adjacent to the cervical dorsal root ganglion of the rat induces late cellular activity in the dorsal horn. Anesthesiology. 2005;102:125–31.
24. Iannaccone F, Dixon S, Kaufman A. A review of long-term pain relief after genicular nerve radiofrequency ablation in chronic knee osteoarthritis. Pain Physician. 2017;20(3): E437–44.
25. Koethe Y, Mannes AJ, Wood BJ. Image-guided nerve cryoablation for post-thoracotomy pain syndrome. Cardiovasc Intervent Radiol. 2014;37(3):843–6.
26. Raslan AM, Cetas JS, McCartney S, Burchiel KJ. Destructive procedures for control of cancer pain: the case for cordotomy. J Neurosurg. 2011;114(1):155–70.
27. Sim WS. Application of botoxin in pain management. Korean J Pain. 2011;24(1):1–6.
28. Dodick DW, Turkel CC, DeGryse RE. OnabotulinumtoxinA for treatment of chronic migraine: pooled results from the double-blind, randomized, placebo-controlled phases of the PREEMPT clinical program. Headache. 2010;50(6):921–36.
29. Attal N, de Andrade DC, Adam F, et al. Safety and efficacy of repeated injections of botulinum toxin A in peripheral neuropathic pain (BOTNEP): a randomized, double-blind, placebo-controlled trial. Lancet Neurol. 2016;15(6):555–65.
30. Backonja M, et al. NGX-4010, a high-concentration capsaicin patch, for the treatment of postherpetic neuralgia: a randomized, double-blind, controlled study with an open-label extension. Pain Med. 2010;11:600–8.

31. Kennedy WR, et al. A randomized, controlled, open-label study of the long-term effects of NGX-4010, a high-concentration capsaicin patch, on epidermal nerve fiber density and sensory function in healthy volunteers. J Pain. 2010;11:579–87.
32. Vinik AI, Perrot S, Vinik EJ, et al. 8% patch repeat treatment plus standard of care (SOC) versus SOC alone in painful diabetic peripheral neuropathy: a randomised, 52-week, open-label, safety study. BMC Neurol. 2016;16:251.
33. Van Buyten JP, Al-Kaisy A, Smet I, Palmisani S, Smith T. High-frequency spinal cord stimulation for the treatment of chronic back pain patients: results of a prospective multicenter European clinical study. Neuromodulation. 2013;16(1):59–65.
34. Al-Kaisy A, Van Buyten J-P, Smet I, Palmisani S, Pang D, Smith T. Sustained effectiveness of 10 kHz high-frequency spinal cord stimulation for patients with chronic, low back pain: 24-month results of a prospective multicenter study. Pain Med. 2014;15(3):347–54.
35. Kapural L, Yu C, Doust MW, Gliner BE, Vallejo R, et al. Novel 10-kHz high-frequency therapy (HF10 therapy) is superior to traditional low-frequency spinal cord stimulation for the treatment of chronic back and leg pain: the SENZA-RCT randomized controlled trial. Anesthesiology. 2015;123:851–60.
36. Bottros M, Christo P. Current perspectives on intrathecal drug delivery. J Pain Res. 2014;7:615–26.

Chapter 8
Nerve Blocks

Ryan Zaglama and Antoun Nader

8.1 Brachial Plexus Block

Anatomy The brachial plexus is formed by nerve roots originating from the fifth cervical nerve to the first thoracic nerve (C5-T1) with occasional contribution from the fourth cervical nerve (C4) and the second thoracic nerve (T2). After exiting the corresponding foramina, the fifth (C5) and sixth cervical (C6) root join to form the upper trunk, the seventh nerve (C7) root continues as the middle trunk, the eighth cervical nerve (C8) and the first thoracic nerve (T1) join to form the lower trunk. The upper, middle, and lower trunks then divide into anterior and posterior divisions. Below the clavicle, these divisions recombine to form three cords: the lateral, the posterior, and the medial cord. The lateral cord is formed by the anterior division of the upper trunk and the superior part of the anterior division of the middle trunk. The posterior cord is formed from the posterior divisions of all the trunks (upper, middle, and lower). The medial cord is formed from the lower part of the anterior division of the middle trunk and the anterior division of the lower trunk. In the axilla, branches from these cords combine to form the distal nerves. The axillary and radial nerves are formed by branches from the posterior cord. The musculocutaneous nerve is formed by branches from the lateral cord. The median nerve is formed by branches from the lateral and medial cord. The ulnar nerve is formed by branches from the medial cord [1].

After exiting the correspondent cervical foramina, the brachial plexus lies in the fascial plane located between the anterior and middle scalene muscles. The groove between the anterior scalene and middle scalene is easily palpable by hand and identifiable by ultrasound scanning. The interscalene block is performed by injection of local anesthetic in the cephalad part of the groove,

R. Zaglama (✉) · A. Nader
Department of Anesthesiology, Feinberg School of Medicine, Northwestern University, Chicago, IL, USA
e-mail: rzaglama@nm.org

K. Shimoji et al. (eds.), *Chronic Pain Management in General and Hospital Practice*, https://doi.org/10.1007/978-981-15-2933-7_8

between the anterior and middle scalene muscles, and will result in blockade of the brachial plexus branches that innervate the shoulder [2].

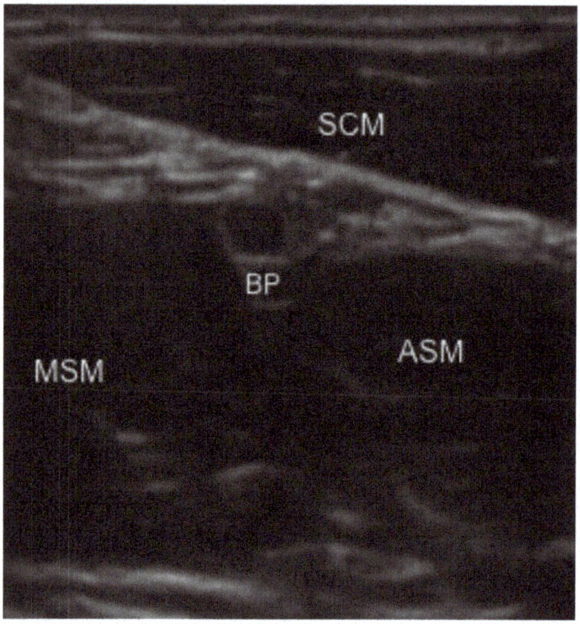

BP Brachial plexus, *MSM* Middle scalene muscle, *ASM* Anterior scalene muscle, *SCM* Sternocleidomastoid. Image credit: Antoun Nader, MD.

Between the clavicle and the first rib, the brachial plexus lies anterior and lateral to the subclavian artery. The supraclavicular block is performed by injection of local anesthetic around the brachial plexus lateral to the artery at this level and will result in a blockade of the brachial plexus branches that innervate the upper extremity [3].

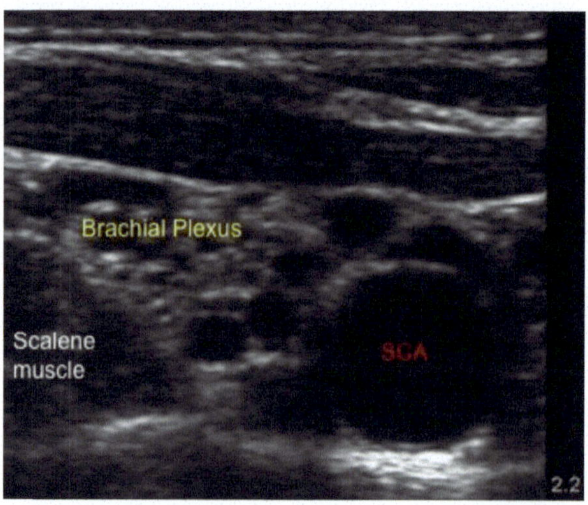

SCA Subclavian artery. Image credit: Antoun Nader, MD.

In the third part of the axilla, the cords of brachial plexus surround the axillary artery: the lateral cord is situated lateral to the artery, the medial cord is situated medial to the artery, and the posterior cord is situated posterior to the artery. The infraclavicular block is performed by injection of local anesthetic at this level and will result in blockade of the terminal branches of the brachial plexus innervating the upper extremity below the elbow [4].

Techniques Different techniques can be used to localize the brachial plexus and surrounding structures. The interscalene muscles and interscalene groove can be easily identified by surface anatomy palpation. The paresthesia technique for blocking the brachial plexus above the clavicle relies on introducing a needle between the scalene muscles and electing a paresthesia in the targeted area. The nerve stimulation guidance technique relies on eliciting a motor response in the targeted myotome. Recently, ultrasound guidance has gained popularity. The ultrasound wave reflections allow identification of the scalene muscles, interscalene groove, the brachial plexus, and other surrounding vascular structures such as the vertebral artery and the thyrocervical trunk.

Blockade the brachial plexus in the axilla, the axillary block, relies on depositing local anesthetic around the axillary artery. The artery can be easily palpable by hand, and local anesthetic can be deposited posterior and anterior to the artery using a trans-arterial technique. Using nerve stimulator, an elicited motor response in a muscle innervated by the radial and median nerve is sought and local anesthetic is injected around these nerves. Using ultrasound guidance, the axillary artery and vein, the brachial plexus, and the conjoint tendons of the latissimus dorsi and teres major are identified. Injection of local anesthetic medial to the conjoint tendon around the artery will result in blockade of the brachial plexus below the elbow [5]. Distal to the axilla, the individual median, ulnar, and radial nerves can be identified using ultrasound guidance and blocked separately.

Indication Interscalene brachial plexus block is mostly done for shoulder surgery. Brachial plexus block between the clavicle and first rib is performed for surgery below the shoulder. Axillary block is performed for surgery below the elbow.

Medication Intermediate (ropivacaine) or long-acting (bupivacaine) local anesthetic in concentration of 0.5% are injected for surgical anesthesia after bony surgery. Lower concentrations are used for analgesia. Short-acting (mepivacaine) or intermediate-acting (ropivacaine) local anesthetic are used for soft tissue surgery.

8.2 Lower Extremity Blocks

Anatomy The lumbar plexus is formed by the anterior divisions of the first (L1), second (L2), third (L3), and part of the fourth lumbar (L4) nerve roots with contribution from the lower twelfth thoracic (T12) nerve. It gives branches to the femoral nerve, the lateral femoral cutaneous nerve, obturator nerve, the ilioinguinal, iliohypogastric, and genitofemoral nerves. Below the inguinal ligament, the femoral nerve (L2–3–4) is located lateral to the femoral artery and vein below the fascia iliaca of the psoas muscle. The femoral nerve gives rise to an anteromedial division and posterolateral division. The anteromedial division innervates the sartorius muscle and contributes to the skin innervation of the medial thigh. The posterolateral division innervates the quadriceps muscle and is a major contributor to the knee joint innervation. The femoral nerve branches to the vastus medialis muscle, the saphenous nerve, and the infrapatellar branches of the femoral nerve accompany the superficial femoral artery to the adductor canal. The saphenous nerve exits the adductor canal and continues distally to innervate the medial aspect of the lower extremity below the knee. The lateral femoral cutaneous nerve (L2–3) separates from the plexus on the anterior surface of the psoas muscle and continues below the inguinal ligament to innervate the lateral thigh. The obturator nerve innervates the adductor muscles. In the groin, it divides into a posterior branch that runs between the adductor magnus and brevis and to an anterior branch that runs between the adductor longus and brevis. The obturator nerve contributes to the skin innervation of the medial thigh and gives articular branches to the knee [6].

The sacral plexus is derived from branches of the lower part of the fourth lumbar nerve (L4), the fifth lumbar nerve (L5), the first sacral (S1), part of the second sacral (S2), and part of the third sacral (S3) nerve. It gives branches to the sciatic nerve which runs along the posterior part of the thigh. The sciatic nerve is formed by two separate divisions: the tibial and common peroneal. These two divisions are engulfed by a common perineural sheet. They separate in the popliteal fossa into two distinct components. The tibial nerve follows the popliteal artery to the leg and continues as the posterior tibial nerve. The common peroneal nerve runs around the head of the fibula and gives branches to the superficial and deep peroneal nerve [6]. The posterior femoral cutaneous nerve originates from the first (S1), second (S2), and third sacral (S3) nerve roots. It separates from the sciatic nerve in the gluteal area and innervates the posterior thigh, posterior leg, and perineum. The pudendal nerve originates from the second (S2), third (S3), and fourth sacral (S4) nerves. It crosses from the greater sciatic notch to the lesser sciatic notch over the ischial spine where it can be easily identified in close proximity to the pudendal artery.

Techniques The lumbar plexus can be blocked anterior to the transverse process of the corresponding lumbar vertebra most commonly done at the fourth lumbar level using the transverse process of the corresponding vertebra as bony landmark. The needle is then advanced anterior to the process to obtain loss of resistance or to elicit a quadriceps response using a nerve stimulator [7].

The femoral nerve is commonly blocked at the inguinal crease where it is most superficial. When using a nerve stimulating technique, a quadriceps contraction (patella dance) is sought. With ultrasound guidance, the femoral artery, fascia lata, fascia iliaca, and femoral nerve are identified. The nerve lies lateral to the femoral artery and deep to the fascia iliaca [6]. An injection below the fascia iliaca, closer to the lateral component of the femoral nerve, will provide analgesia to the quadriceps muscle and the anteromedial part of the knee joint. The saphenous nerve may be blocked at the level of the midthigh, deep to the sartorius muscle, in the adductor canal [8].

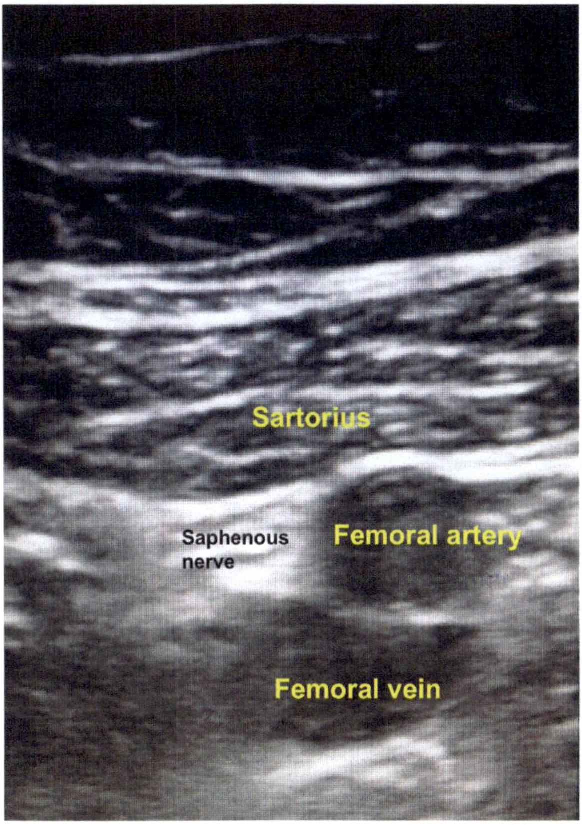

Image credit: Ryan Zaglama, MD.

The branches of obturator nerve are commonly blocked in the facial planes between the adductor muscles. The lateral femoral cutaneous nerve is blocked medial to the anterior superior iliac spine and anterior to the sartorius muscle.

The sciatic nerve can be blocked at any point along its course from the sacral foramina to the distal leg. The most common location is at the level of the gluteal crease. At this point, the sciatic nerve is fairly superficial covered only by the inferior part of the gluteal muscle [9]. It lays lateral to the biceps femoris and medial to the femur, which are easily identifiable. Another common location for sciatic nerve blockade is at the popliteal fossa, posterior to the popliteal vessels. The sciatic nerve typically bifurcates into the tibial and common peroneal nerves 5–10 cm cephalad of the level of the popliteal fossa. When using a nerve stimulator, the most commonly sought response is foot inversion. When using ultrasound guidance, a circumferential spread of local anesthetic is sought.

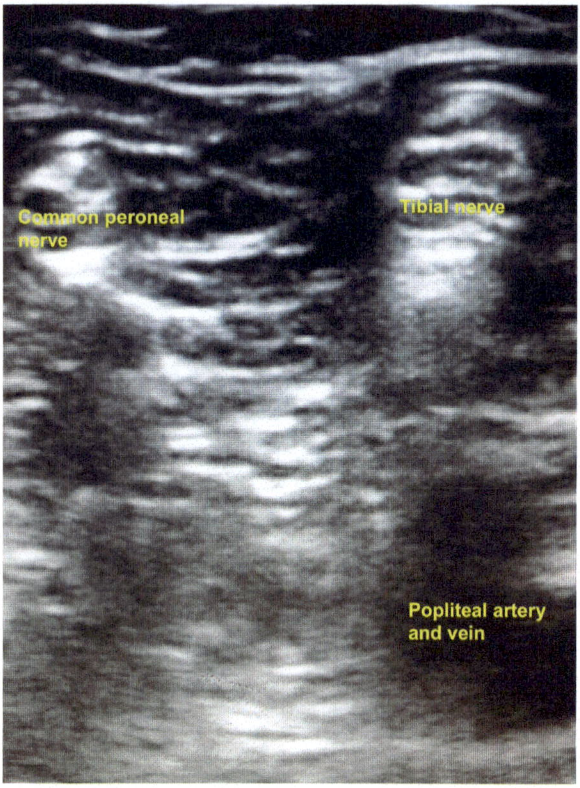

Image credit: Ryan Zaglama, MD.

Indication Femoral nerve block is performed for knee surgery and surgery of the distal femur and anterior thigh. Sciatic nerve block is performed for ankle and foot surgery and occasionally for knee surgery. Posterior femoral cutaneous and lateral femoral cutaneous blocks which block cutaneous innervation of the posterior and lateral thigh, respectively, are performed for some surgeries above the knee.

Medication Intermediate (ropivacaine) or long-acting (bupivacaine) local anesthetic with a concentration of 0.5% are injected for surgical anesthesia after bony surgery. Lower concentrations are used for analgesia.

8.3 Truncal Blocks

Anatomy The anterior abdominal wall is innervated by spinal nerve roots from the sixth thoracic (T6) to the first lumbar (L1) vertebra. In the lateral abdominal wall, the nerves run in a fascial plane between the internal oblique muscle and the transverse abdominis muscle [10]. The ilioinguinal nerve and the iliohypogastric nerve are accompanied by a corresponding identifiable artery. The intercostal nerves run below the ribs in a fascial plane between the internal intercostal and innermost intercostal muscles in close proximity to the intercostal artery below the corresponding rib. More proximally, the intercostal nerves are located in the paravertebral space medial to the pleural, lateral to the vertebral foramen, and anterior to the transverse process. The medial pectoral nerve runs on the deep surface of pectoralis minor. The lateral pectoral nerve travels between the pectoralis major and minor. Both nerves, in addition to the intercostal nerves, innervate the anterior chest wall.

Techniques Blockade of the anterior abdominal wall muscles was initially described in the triangle of the Petit at the lateral abdominal wall just above the iliac spine using loss of resistance technique. Using ultrasound guidance, the transversus abdominis plane (TAP) block involves identifying the external oblique muscle, the internal oblique muscle, the transversus muscle, and the peritoneum. Local anesthetic is deposited between the internal oblique muscle and the transversus muscle. A modification of the technique, the rectus sheath block, involves injection of local anesthetic in the anterior subcostal area between the rectus muscle and the transversus muscle. Another modification of the technique, the quadratus lumborum block, involves injection of local anesthetic more proximally in proximity of the quadratus lumborum muscle. Blockade of the ilioinguinal and iliohypogastric nerves involves identifying the ilioinguinal artery between the internal oblique muscle and transversus muscle and injecting local anesthetic around the artery [10].

Blockade of the nerves supplying the anterior chest wall muscles involves injecting local anesthetic in the intercostal plane between the internal intercostal and innermost intercostal to block the intercostal nerves and injecting local anesthetic between the pectoralis major and minor and between the pectoralis minor and serratus muscle to block the lateral and medial pectoral nerves [11].

Indications These facial plane nerve blocks are performed for surgery on the anterior abdomen and for surgery on the anterior chest wall, such as mastectomy.

8.4 Common Superficial Nerve Blocks

Superficial nerve blocks are commonly used to diagnose and treat peripheral neuralgias, joint pain and as a supplement for regional analgesia. These mostly sensory nerves are commonly blocked using ultrasound guidance. The superficial cervical plexus originates from the second to the fourth cervical nerves. The superficial cervical plexus can be identified between the middle scalene muscle and the sternocleidomastoid muscle where it can be easily blocked as a supplement for surgeries involving the neck [1]. The phrenic nerve can be identified anterior to the anterior scalene muscle and deep to the sternocleidomastoid muscle. This nerve can be blocked to treat persistent hiccups. The suprascapular nerve can be easily identified in the suprascapular notch below the suprascapular ligament and adjacent to the suprascapular artery. This nerve block can be used to diagnose and treat acute and chronic shoulder pain [12]. The ilioinguinal nerve and artery can be easily identified in the area between the anterior superior iliac spine and the umbilicus. The nerve and accompanying artery are easily identified between the internal oblique and the transversus muscle [10]. The nerve can be blocked as diagnostic and therapeutic tools for ilioinguinal neuralgia as well as for post-operative analgesia after inguinal hernia repair.

The lateral femoral cutaneous nerve can be blocked as a diagnostic and therapeutic modality for meralgia paresthetica. The saphenous and infrapatellar nerve can be blocked distal to the adductor canal for saphenous neuralgias and for medial knee pain. Peripheral nerve blocks are commonly performed for foot and ankle surgery. The posterior tibial nerve can be blocked posterior to the tibial artery and the medial malleolus [13]. The deep peroneal nerve can be blocked lateral to the deep peroneal artery at the level of the ankle. The sural and saphenous nerves can be easily blocked close to their corresponding veins, the small and great saphenous veins, respectively.

8.5 Head and Neck Blocks

8.5.1 Cervical Sympathetic Chain Block

The cervical sympathetic chain lies in the prevertebral fascia anterior to the longus colli muscle and posterior to the carotid artery and longus capitis muscle. It includes three cervical ganglia: the upper, the middle, and the lower ganglia. The lower ganglion is commonly fused with the first thoracic ganglia to form the stellate ganglion. Blockade of these ganglia can interrupt the sympathetic outflow to the head and neck. When combined with the stellate ganglion block, the sympathetic innervation of the upper extremity can be blocked. Interruption of the sympathetic outflow can be used as a diagnostic and therapeutic modality to treat sympathetic mediated pain. Blockade of these ganglia requires careful understating of the neck anatomy.

Technique Cervical sympathetic chain block is mostly performed at the level of the sixth cervical transverse process. At this level, the sympathetic chain is anterior to the vertebral artery and longus colli muscle, medial to the brachial plexus, posterior to the carotid artery and the thyroid gland, and lateral to the esophagus. In addition, at this level, the vertebral artery is localized within the anterior tubercle (Chassaignac's tubercle). Ultrasound guidance can provide an excellent tool to identify these structures [14].

Indication Cervical sympathetic chain block is performed for a variety of conditions involving head and neck and upper extremity pain. These include complex regional pain syndromes of the upper extremity and sympathetic mediated vascular insufficiency conditions.

8.5.2 Occipital Nerve Block

The occipital nerve can be blocked at the level of the nuchal line in close proximity to the occipital artery. More frequently, the nerve is blocked at the level of the second cervical vertebra. At this level, the nerve lies in a fascial plan superior to the obliquus capitis inferior muscle and deep to the trapezius and spinalis muscle. Blockade of the nerve at this level (C2) provides analgesia in the distribution of the greater and lesser occipital nerve. As with the cervical sympathetic chain block, ultrasound guidance can prove to be a great imaging tool to identify soft tissue structures surrounding the nerve as well as to identify the vertebral and occipital artery. Blockade of this nerve can be used as a diagnostic and therapeutic modality to treat occipital neuralgia.

Technique The bifid spinous process of C2 and the transverse process of C1 are identified. The obliquus capitis muscle extending between the spinous process of C2 and transverse process of C1 is identified. The fascial plane between the obliquus capitis inferior and semispinalis muscle is identified [15]. The occipital nerve is identified in is this plane and local anesthetic or steroid is injected at this level.

Indication Occipital nerve block is performed mostly for occipital neuralgia and other painful conditions involving the posterior scalp such as posterior craniotomy.

8.5.3 Trigeminal Nerve Block

The nucleus of the trigeminal nerve is located in the brainstem at the level of the pons. The trigeminal nerve ganglion (Gasserian ganglion) is located in the Meckel's cave, an indentation in the middle cranial fossa. The ganglion gives three divisions. The first division exits the cranium throughout the supraorbital fossa and provides innervation to the forehead, eyelid and cornea, and frontal sinus. The second division exits the cranium through the foramen rotundum and innervates the lower eyelid, nose, cheek and upper jaw, nasal mucosa, upper teeth, and maxillary sinus. The third division exits through the foramen ovale and innervates the mandible, lower tip, and lower teeth. The sphenopalatine ganglion which is a major parasympathetic ganglion of the head lies in close proximity and is closely associated with the maxillary branch of the trigeminal nerve.

Techniques Many techniques have been described to block the Gasserian ganglion and its branches. A commonly used technique involves using ultrasound guidance to identify the lateral pterygoid muscle and maxillary artery. This upper part of this muscle originates from infratemporal surface of the sphenoid bone and inserts onto the capsule of the temporomandibular joint. The maxillary artery can be easily identified deep to the muscle. Injection deep to the lateral pterygoid muscle will result in blockade of the branches of the trigeminal nerve and of the sphenopalatine ganglion. In addition, the injectate can flow retrograde to block the Gasserian ganglion.

Indication This injection can be used to treat trigeminal neuralgia and atypical facial pain [16].

8.6 Thoracic and Lumbar Sympathetic Chain Blocks

8.6.1 Celiac Plexus Block

The celiac plexus provides innervation to the small bowel, large bowel proximal to the transverse colon, liver, gallbladder and biliary tract, kidney, and pancreas. Blockade of the autonomic innervation to these organs can be performed by either blocking the greater (T5–9), lesser (T10–11), and least (T12) splanchnic nerves or by blocking the celiac plexus anterior to the aorta around the celiac artery.

Technique Many techniques have been described to block the splanchnic nerves or the celiac plexus. The posterior retrocrural approach involves blocking the splanchnic nerve at the level of the twelfth thoracic vertebra posterior to the crura of the diaphragm. This approach is commonly done using fluoroscopic or CAT scan guidance. A diagnostic block is initially performed using local anesthetic and is followed by a neurolytic block. The posterior transcrural approach is performed by crossing the crura of the diaphragm at the T12 level and deposing local anesthetic lateral or anterior to the aorta around the celiac plexus. A trans-aortic approach has been described. It involves passing the needle through the aorta to deposit the drugs anterior to the artery around the celiac plexus. An anterior approach can be performed going the stomach using CAT scan guidance or ultrasound guidance. It involves identifying the aorta and celiac artery and deposing local anesthetic anterior to the aorta.

Indication The celiac plexus block is used to treat malignant visceral pain originating from the small bowel, large bowel proximal to transverse colon, biliary tract, and pancreas [17, 18].

The hypogastric plexus provides innervation to the pelvic organs. It is located anterior to the vertebral disc located between L5 and S1. A hypogastric block is performed using fluoroscopic or CAT scan guidance.

Technique A needle is advanced to the space anterior to the L5–S1 disc. After needle tip position confirmation, local anesthetic or a neurolytic agent is deposited.

Indication Hypogastric plexus block can be used to diagnose and treat pelvic pain.

8.6.2 The Lumbar Sympathetic Chain

The lumbar sympathetic chain is located anterior to the vertebral body of the second, third, and fourth vertebral body. The sympathetic outflow to the lower extremity can be interrupted by blocking the sympathetic chain at these levels. The block is usually performed using fluoroscopic or CAT scan guidance. A diagnostic block is initially performed followed by a neurolytic block [18].

Technique A needle is advanced to reach the anterolateral part of the vertebral body at the L2, L3, L4 level, anterior to the origin of the psoas muscle on the affected side. After needle tip position confirmation, a local anesthetic or neurolytic agent is deposited.

Indication Lumbar sympathetic block is performed for sympathetic mediated pain of the lower extremity, such as CRPS or vascular insufficiency of the lower extremity.

The ganglion impar is the most distal part of the sympathetic chain. It is located anterior to the sacrococcygeal junction and to the coccyx. This ganglion provides nociceptive and sympathetic innervation to perineum. Ganglion impar block is usually performed using fluoroscopic guidance. A small amount of local anesthetic is deposited anterior to the sacrococcygeal junction [18].

References

1. Neal JM, Gerancher J, Hebl JR, Ilfeld BM, Mccartney CJ, Franco CD, et al. Upper extremity regional anesthesia. Reg Anesth Pain Med. 2009;34(2):134–70.
2. Winnie AP, Ramamurthy S, Durrani Z. Interscalene cervical plexus block: a single injection technic. Anesth Analg. 1975;54:370–5.
3. Chan VW, Perlas A, Rawson R, Odukoya O. Ultrasound-guided supraclavicular brachial plexus block. Anesth Analg. 2003;97:1514–7.
4. Salazar CH, Espinosa W. Infraclavicular brachial plexus block: variation in approach and results in 360 cases. Reg Anesth Pain Med. 1999;24:411–6.
5. Liu FC, Liou JT, Tsai YF, Li AH, Day YY, Hui YL, et al. Efficacy of ultrasound-guided axillary brachial plexus block: a comparative study with nerve stimulator-guided method. Chang Gung Med J. 2005;28:396–402.
6. Enneking F, Chan V, Greger J, Hadzic A, Lang S, Horlocker T. Lower-extremity peripheral nerve blockade: essentials of our current understanding. Reg Anesth Pain Med. 2005;30(1):4–35.
7. Capdevila P, Macaire C, Dadure O, Choquet P, Biboulet Y, Ryckwaert F. D'Athis. Continuous psoas compartment block for postoperative analgesia after total hip arthroplasty: new landmarks, technical guidelines and clinical evaluation. Anesth Analg. 2002;94:1606–13.
8. Bouaziz H, Henhamou D, Narchi P. A new approach for saphenous nerve block (letter). Reg Anesth. 1996;21:490.
9. di Benedetto P, Casati A, Bertini L, Fanelli G. Posterior subgluteal approach to block the sciatic nerve: description of the technique and initial clinical experiences. Eur J Anaesthesiol. 2002;19:682–6.
10. Chin KJ, Mcdonnell JG, Carvalho B, Sharkey A, Pawa A, Gadsden J. Essentials of our current understanding: abdominal wall blocks. Reg Anesth Pain Med. 2017;42(2):133–83.
11. Blanco R. The 'pecs block': a novel technique for providing analgesia after breast surgery. Anaesthesia. 2011;66(9):847–8.
12. Bansal V, Shastri U, Canlas C, Gadsden JC. Diaphragm-sparing nerve blocks for shoulder surgery. Reg Anesth Pain Med. 2017;42(4):544–5.
13. Redborg KE, Antonakakis JG, Beach ML, Chinn CD, Sites BD. Ultrasound improves the success rate of a tibial nerve block at the ankle. Reg Anesth Pain Med. 2009;34(3):256–60.
14. Stellate ganglion (cervical sympathetic trunk) block. Regional anaesthesia, stimulation, and ultrasound techniques. 2014. p. 245–52.

15. Greher M, Moriggl B, Curatolo M, Kirchmair L, Eichenberger U. Sonographic visualization and ultrasound-guided blockade of the greater occipital nerve: a comparison of two selective techniques confirmed by anatomical dissection. Br J Anaesth. 2010;104:637–42.
16. Nader A, Kendall MC, De Oliveria GS, Chen JQ, Vanderby B, Rosenow JM, et al. Ultrasound-guided trigeminal nerve block via the pterygopalatine fossa: an effective treatment for trigeminal neuralgia and atypical facial pain. Pain Physician. 2013;16(5):E537–45.
17. Jankovic D, Shankar H. Celiac plexus block. Regional nerve blocks in anesthesia and pain therapy. Basel: Springer; 2015. p. 673–84.
18. Gunduz OH, Coskun OK. Ganglion blocks as a treatment of pain: current perspectives. J Pain Res. 2017;10:2815–26.

Chapter 9
Other Methods: Minimally Invasive Techniques in Pain Clinic

Koki Shimoji and Tatsuhiko Kano

9.1 Introduction

There are several methods for treating chronic pain in conjunction with nerve blocks. Regarding the methods of treating chronic pain, Swedish Council on Health Technology Assessment advocates as follows: The research on treating chronic pain unequivocally demonstrates a strong negative correlation between pain and quality of life, i.e., pain reduction improves quality of life. Living with chronic pain requires a new orientation in life and the opportunity to talk about the experience. Patients with chronic pain are eager to retain their sense of dignity. This assessment is very important for treating chronic pain patients. After the precise assessment, following treatments with single or combined may be effective.

9.2 Methods in Conjunction with Nerve Blocks

9.2.1 Multimodal Rehabilitation

The long-term impact of broad-based, coordinated rehabilitation programs, referred to as multimodal rehabilitation (usually a combination of psychological interventions and physical activity, physical exercise, or physical therapy) show that pain decreases more, a greater number of people return to work, and sick leaves are shorter than with passive control and/or limited, separate interventions.

K. Shimoji (✉)
Niigata University Graduate School of Medicine, Niigata, Japan

Pain Control Institute, Tokyo, Japan
e-mail: koki-shimoji@nifty.com

T. Kano
Kurume University Medical School, Kurume, Japan

K. Shimoji et al. (eds.), *Chronic Pain Management in General and Hospital Practice*, https://doi.org/10.1007/978-981-15-2933-7_9

9.2.2 Cognitive Behavioral Therapy

Cognitive behavioral therapy provides better social and physical function, as well as 25% greater ability to cope, in chronic pain patients than other behavioral therapies, medications, and physical therapy that have been studied and to no treatment at all (moderately strong scientific evidence).

9.2.3 *Analgesic Drugs* (See Chap. 5)

Drugs, oral, rectal, percutaneous or intravenous route, should be minimal and effective to avoid side effects. These side effects should be carefully monitored. *Paracetamol* (*acetaminophen*) somewhat alleviates the pain of mild to moderate osteoarthritis. Paracetamol is more effective in combination with tramadol or another weak opioid than as monotherapy. *COX-2 inhibitors* and other nonsteroidal anti-inflammatory drugs (NSAIDs) reduce the pain of osteoarthritis and arthritis by at least 30%. Combining them with tramadol or another weak opioid can increase their effectiveness. All COX-2 inhibitors and other NSAIDs increase the risk of cardiovascular events. It should be reminded that COX-2 inhibitors can be a cost-effective option for chronic pain patients with an elevated risk of gastrointestinal bleeding. *Amitriptyline* reduces the pain of peripheral and central neuropathic pain due to herpes zoster, diabetes, and stroke patients by more than 20%. Tricyclic antidepressants moderately alleviate fibromyalgia pain. *Carbamazepine* is effective (NNT 1.4–2.8) in trigeminal neuralgia. *Gabapentin* (*Neurontin*) reduces neuropathic pain (NNT 3.8 for at least 50%) in diabetes and in patients with post-herpetic (NNT 3.2) pain. *Tramadol* is more effective than placebo for nociceptive pain—approximately 20% of tramadol patients, as opposed to 40% of placebo patients, stop taking their medication due to insufficient relief. Tramadol alleviates neuropathic pain (NNT 4.3 for at least 50% pain relief). Tramadol is as effective as weak opioids for musculoskeletal pain. Tramadol causes adverse effects to the same extent as weak and strong opioids. *Capsaicin* reduces (NNT 8 for at least 50%) neuropathic pain and osteoarthritis pain in small joint pain. The research results are contradictory when it comes to the effectiveness of *glucosamine* in relieving osteoarthritis pain. *Weak opioids* reduce mild to moderate osteoarthritis and low back pain. They are just as effective as NSAIDs for moderate pain. *Strong opioids* alleviate neuropathic, diabetic, or herpetic pain. Strong opioids reduce severe osteoarthritis pain by approximately 24%. Both weak and strong opioids, however, cause unpleasant adverse effects such as constipation, fatigue, dizziness, nausea, and vomiting in more than half of the patients.

9.2.4 Instrumental Interventions

Brain, spinal cord, or peripheral nerve stimulation reduces the frequency of angina attacks by approximately 50% and improves quality of life, both short-term and long-term, even in patients with severe angina pectoris or the ischemic symptoms of peripheral arterial disease. *Acupuncture* may alleviate chronic low back pain more effectively than placebo.

Radiofrequency denervation can provide short-term relief of chronic neck and back pain but may pose a risk of minor or serious complications.

9.2.5 Physical Intervention

Physical exercise, relaxation, biofeedback, massage, manipulation, physical therapy, and orthosis. All these methods may alleviate chronic pain 20–30% more effectively than a treatment that does not involve physical activity. Treatment strategies that include physical activity may be more cost-effective in alleviating chronic low back pain than standard primary care that does not involve specific measures.

9.3 Brain Stimulation

Although there are arguments that brain stimulation itself is invasive, it may depend upon the techniques, skills of operators, diseases. The techniques of brain stimulation may provide the chronic pain patients one of the minimally invasive methods to overcome the distress if properly used. First employed by Croft in 1952 [1], brain stimulation represents one of the earliest uses to treat chronic pain that is refractory to medical therapy.

Motor cortex stimulation (MCS) and deep brain stimulation (DBS) have been shown to be effective for treating several neuropathic and refractory pain states that are not responsive or amenable to other therapies.

MCS has shown particularly promising for the treatment of trigeminal neuropathic pain and central pain syndromes such as thalamic pain syndrome. DBS may be employed for several nociceptive and neuropathic pain states, including cluster headaches, chronic low back pain, failed back surgery syndrome, peripheral neuropathic pain, and facial deafferentation pain [2].

Transcranial stimulation techniques might be more promising for out-patient treatments in pain clinic in terms of non-invasiveness.

9.3.1 Motor Cortex Stimulation (MCS)

Chronic stimulation of the precentral cortex for the treatment of pain was first reported by Tsubokawa and his colleagues in 1991 [3]. Interestingly, stimulation of the motor cortex gave better results than stimulation of the sensory cortex, the latter of which caused some patients' pain to worsen. Many reports have followed describing the use of MCS for intractable pain syndromes including post-stroke pain, phantom limb pain, spinal cord injury pain, post-herpetic neuralgia, and neuropathic pain of the limbs or face [3]. Most of studies involving MCS focus on its use in post-stroke and trigeminal neuropathic pain, for which other treatments failed to control [4–6].

MCS has shown particularly promising in the treatment of trigeminal neuropathic pain and central pain syndromes such as thalamic pain syndrome.

Approximately two-thirds of patients with post-stroke pain and trigeminal neuropathic pain respond well to MCS [6, 7].

9.3.1.1 Methods

Prior to the surgical procedure, an MRI or a functional MRI (fMRI) is performed to precisely localize the site of the motor cortex that is stimulated to treat a pain region [6–11]. A small craniotomy is performed for electrode placement under local or general anesthesia [7, 8]. Image-guided neuronavigation is used to precisely identify the motor cortex intraoperatively [7–9]. Then a linear incision, approximately 10 cm long, is made, followed by a circular craniotomy approximately 5 cm in diameter [9].

Electrophysiologic monitoring is recommended by several authors to demonstrate the efficacy of electrode placement. The central sulcus may be identified by recording brain surface electrical activity using an epidural grid electrode. A waveform I appears approximately 20 msec after stimulation, and its waveform reverses from negative to positive at the central sulcus (an effect known as the N20/P20 waveform phase reversal) [12, 13]. In response to stimulation of the cortex both somatosensory-evoked potentials and electromyogram (EMG) could be monitored for precise location of the electrodes at the area of the motor cortex that corresponds to the pain region.

After surgery, the electrode cable is externalized for trial stimulation, and a trial stimulation is performed usually lasting 3–7 days. During MCS, patients feel a degree of pain reduction without experience of stimulation-induced sensory phenomenon in contrast to spinal cord stimulation which induces muscle trembling feeling.

There are considerable variations in the stimulation parameters among the investigators. Stimulus intensities and frequencies are tested by asking patients' feeling during this period. If patients obtain sufficient pain relief, the electrodes are connected to an implanted pulse generator, which are usually placed subcutaneously over the pectoralis muscle, in the operating room.

9.3.1.2 Efficacy

A review of the literature showed that 76% of patients with neuropathic facial pain achieved more than 50% pain relief with MCS [7, 8, 11]. Post-stroke pain responds nearly as well, with approximately two-thirds of patients obtaining good to excellent relief [4, 6].

MCS appears to be a relatively safe and effective neuromodulation technique for appropriately selected patients [14].

9.3.1.3 Complications

Seizure induction has been reported following MCS programming and during chronic MCS [5, 9–11], which does not develop to seizure.

Serious complications include intracranial bleeding, infection, and permanent neurological deficits in few patients [4, 7, 9, 11].

9.3.2 Deep Brain Stimulation (DBS)

Heath [15] in 1954 first reported successful pain relief with stimulation of the septal region nuclei in patients with psychiatric disease. Mazars et al. [16] and Hosobuchi et al. [17] in 1973 and Adams et al. [18] in 1974 reported the first experience of using chronic stimulation of the sensory thalamic nuclei to treat neuropathic pain. Richardson and Akil [19, 20] and Hosobuchi and coworkers [21–24] reported pain relief in patients undergoing chronic stimulation of the periaqueductal gray (PAG) and the periventricular gray (PVG) at the level of the posterior third ventricle. This result has been subsequently confirmed by several investigations [25–34].

9.3.2.1 Methods

DBS electrodes are implanted using stereotactic guidance (Fig. 9.1), and most surgeons use frame-based stereotaxic apparatus for electrode implantation. After the frame is applied, patients undergo high-resolution stereotactic MRI. In many cases, surgery is performed under local anesthesia supplemented as needed by intravenous sedation.

A parasagittal frontal burr hole is created through a small incision. Intraoperative electrical stimulation is required to define the exact target for stimulation, which is only approximated by the stereotactic MRI. Thus, the stereotactic coordinates represent only starting points for localization of the physiological targets. Microelectrode recording and microstimulation can define the process of localization [35, 36]. Microelectrode recording can help locate targets based on their electrophysiologic activity [37]. Once the physiologic targets have been defined with stimulation, permanent electrodes are introduced to those sites, and the leads are externalized through a separate stab wound in the scalp for trial stimulation.

CT scan or MRI is obtained to confirm electrode placement and to assess possible intracerebral hemorrhage. After postoperative recovery and resolution of any peri-electrode edema, test stimulation is initiated to evaluate the patient's pain relief [37–39].

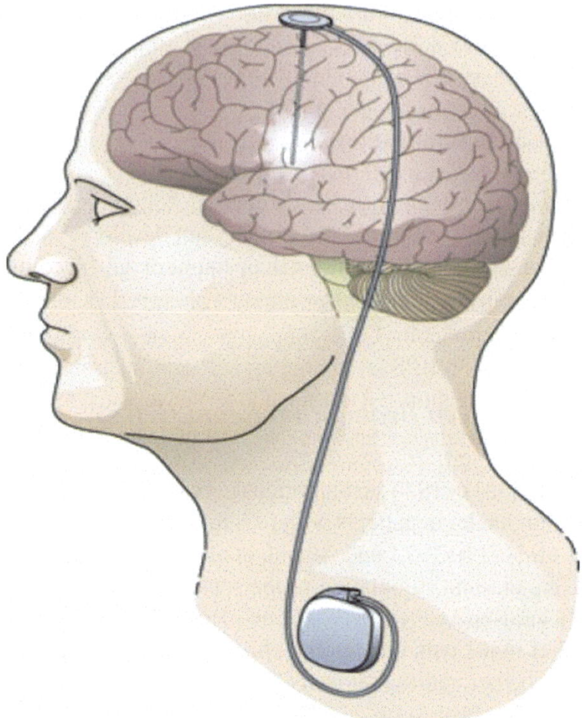

Fig. 9.1 Deep brain stimulation (Permission granted to use NINDS illustration of Deep Brain Stimulation, Girolami, Paul (NIH/NINDS))

All possible stimulation combinations can be tested during a trial stimulation period that generally lasts 5–9 days. If satisfactory pain relief is obtained, the patient is returned to the operating room and the electrodes are connected to an implantable pulse generator [40].

9.3.2.2 Efficacy

Approximately 40% of patients with neuropathic pain had success at long-term follow-up, ranging from 19% to 79%. Long-term efficacy of DBS.

The effects of DBS are varied depending on the authors and sites of stimulation (PAG/PVG and/or VPM thalamic stimulation). It may be important to note the clarification of patient selection and target criteria.

It has been observed that stimulation efficacy was correlated with the stimulation target. Thus, PAG/PVG stimulation may produce good to excellent results in approximately 80% of patients, and the addition of sensory thalamic or internal capsule stimulation may increase the success rate. Nociceptive pain may respond better to DBS than neuropathic pain. Cephalalgias also have promising results, with cluster headaches carrying the best success rates [41–43].

Further, randomized, blinded, and controlled clinical trials are desirable to evaluate the efficacy of DBS in patients who are refractory to other therapies [43, 44], and also comparison with surgical methods should be made [45–47].

9.3.2.3 Complications

Intracranial hemorrhage is the most significant complication of DBS. It can occur at the time of the insertion or removal of the electrode. The reported incidence of hemorrhage ranges between 1.9% and 4.1%. Using contemporary coaxial DBS electrodes, there has been a significant decrease in the incidence of intracranial hemorrhage [29–31, 33, 34, 38, 39].

Permanent neurological deficits have been reported in 2.0–3.4% of the patients. The deficits most commonly resulted from intracranial hemorrhage [38, 39].

Mortality is rare from DBS, ranging from 0 to 1.6%, resulting from complications of intracranial hemorrhage [48].

The incidence of infectious complications from DBS ranges from 3.3 to 13.3%. These complications included meningitis, encephalitis, and infection of the scalp or IPG site [38]. Most of cases required wound debridement and removal of all hardware in addition to systemic antibiotics for successful resolution of the infection.

Transient headaches were observed in halves of cases, most of which were believed to be a direct result of the intracranial operation and resolved by the time of patient discharge from the hospital [38]. PAG/PVG stimulation can cause other transient side effects, including diplopia, nausea, vertical gaze palsies, blurred vision, nystagmus, and persistent oscillopsia [49].

9.3.3 MCS Vs DBS

There are little data providing a direct comparison between these two techniques [2]. Katayama et al. reported no difference between MCS and thalamic DBS for phantom limb pain [5]. The same group reported the effects of spinal cord stimulation (SCS), thalamic DBS, and MCS in 45 patients with post-stroke pain. Satisfactory pain control was obtained more frequently as the stimulation site was moved to higher levels (7% by SCS, 25% by DBS, and 48% by MCS) [6].

Long-term pain relief with DBS has been widely documented in a number of patients. Recent data moderately supports the use of DBS for refractory pain associated with cephalgia and failed back surgery syndrome and suggests that the therapy may have a value for treating post-stroke pain, central pain syndromes, and peripheral deafferentation pain [50, 51].

DBS has had its best success in treating cluster headaches [52, 53] and nociceptive syndromes such as chronic low back pain [54], while thalamic pain syndrome, postherpetic neuralgia, and pain due to spinal cord injury are not well treated with DBS.

MCS may be an appropriate treatment for neuropathic facial pain, post-stroke pain, or chronic pain conditions that do not respond to other types of neurostimulation. However, there may be occasions in which MCS is indicated without being preceded by such neurostimulation, as is the case in patients with complete deafferentation conditions. There is no compelling evidence that MCS is less effective than DBS for treating chronic pain.

While many case series have been published on the use of MCS or DBS for pain, no randomized, controlled trials exist to confirm the effectiveness. MCS is probably better suited because of its minimum invasiveness than DBS.

9.3.4 Non-invasive Brain Stimulation: Transcranial Electric or Magnetic Stimulation

Clinical application of transcranial direct-current stimulation (tDCS) or transcutaneous brain stimulation (electroanesthesia) (EA) was developed in 1969 at our laboratory for general anesthesia during major surgery [55, 56]. Our clinical trial was succeeded even in major surgical procedures such as open heart surgery, and more than fifty cases were reported with some remaining tasks. The tasks included pain during the start of electrical stimulation and hypertension throughout the procedures. The former was combatted with the use of ultrashort acting intravenous anesthetics, the latter was controlled by hypotensive drugs. During the procedures of EA, we frequently noticed its more analgesic effect than hypnotic effect.

Relief of chronic pain by direct electrical stimulation of the motor cortex has recently sparked development of non-invasive technologies: transcranial direct-current stimulation (tDCS) and transcranial magnetic stimulation (TMS) [57].

The effects of tDCS have been studied in the patients with stroke or other central pain [58–61] for improving activities of daily living (ADL) and with visceral pain [58].

Repetitive transcranial magnetic stimulation (rTMS) can induce long-lasting, potentially therapeutic brain plasticity [58]. Although adverse effects of rTMS are minimal, primarily headaches and rarely single provoked seizures have been reported [58].

Transcranial magnetic stimulation devices are developed for depression and migraine and for various indications elsewhere. Although multiple studies report that high-frequency rTMS of the motor cortex reduces neuropathic pain, their quality remains to be justified for routine clinical use [59, 60].

Chronic central neuropathic pain (CCNP) is a debilitating condition that affects populations such as stroke survivors, amputees, spinal cord injury patients, and patients with multiple sclerosis, with prevalence rates between 30% and 80%. This condition can be caused by a lesion or disease affecting the somatosensory system. CCNP is notoriously drug resistant, and few effective CCNP treatment or management strategies exist. The emergence of non-invasive brain stimulation technique may provide a novel avenue for managing chronic central neuropathic pain [61]. The recent study suggests that the technique also provides activation of function in the motor and somatosensory area [62] (Fig. 9.2).

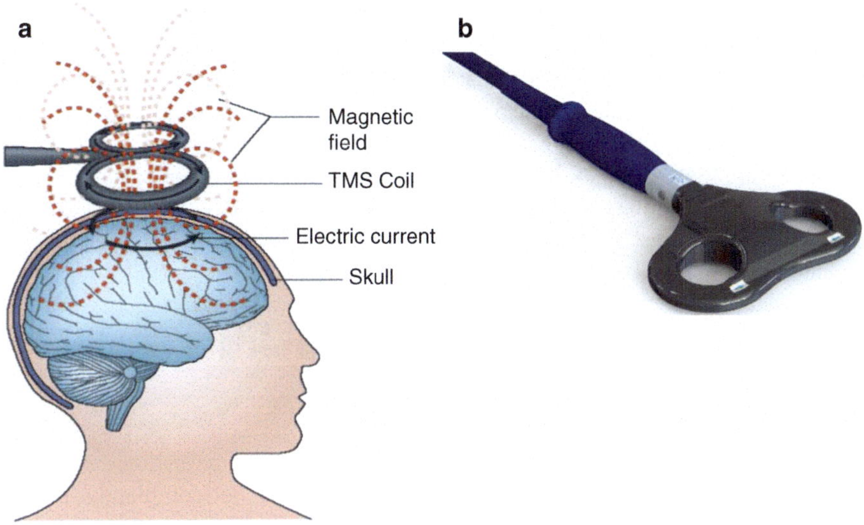

Fig. 9.2 (**a**) Schematic presentation of transcranial magnetic stimulation. (**b**) A magnetic apparatus for magnetic stimulation, manufactured by Magstim Co., Ltd. (Ridding MC & Rothwell JC, Nature Reviews Neuroscience, 2007)

9.4 Spinal Cord Stimulation (SCS)

Spinal cord stimulation (SCS) or dorsal column stimulation (DCS) is a type of technique that is used to send electrical signals to selected areas of the dorsal spinal cord for the treatment of certain pain conditions which hardly respond to the analgesics or other measures [63, 64].

SCS has also been applied for various kinds of chronic pain such as failed back surgery syndrome (FBSS), complex regional pain syndrome, pain caused by nerve damage, and even intractable angina [65],

9.4.1 Historical Background

Electrotherapy of pain by neurostimulation including SCS is based on the gate control theory proposed by Melzack and Wall in 1965 [66]. This theory proposed that small nerves carrying painful peripheral stimuli and large nerves carrying touch and vibratory sensation both terminate in the dorsal horn (the gate) of spinal cord [66]. It was hypothesized that input to the latter could be manipulated to "close the gate" to the former.

As an application of the gate control theory, Shealy et al. [67] implanted the first spinal cord stimulation device directly on the dorsal column for the treatment of chronic pain. In 1971, Shimoji and his colleagues [68] first reported clinical application of electroanesthesia, and also the analgesic properties of epidural spinal cord stimulation by the epidural catheter electrodes, based on the techniques of continuous epidural block and also first recorded human spinal cord potentials epidurally with the same technique [63, 64]. Since then this epidural stimulation technique has undergone numerous technical and clinical developments. The developments include the implantation of the epidural electrodes, these materials, and subcutaneous simulator [65].

9.4.2 Mechanism of Action

The neurophysiologic mechanisms of action of SCS are not completely understood but may involve masking effect on pain sensation by altering the pain processing of the central nervous system [65, 66, 69, 70]. The mechanisms of analgesia by SCS in neuropathic pain and ischemic pain states of limb may be different [71, 72]. Experimental evidence shows that SCS alters the local neurochemistry in dorsal horn, suppressing the hyperexcitability of the neurons in neuropathic pain states, such as increased levels of GABA and serotonin release. Thus, suppression of levels of some excitatory transmitters, including glutamate and aspartate, may be induced by SCS. In the case of ischemic pain, analgesia seems to derive from restoration of the oxygen demand/supply by suppression of sympathetic activities [73].

9.4.3 Methods

The direct implantation of the plate electrodes on the dorsal surface of the cord attempted by Shealy et al. caused severe complications such as arachnoiditis, subdural hemorrhage.

It was demonstrated that SCS from the epidural space using the epidural catheter electrodes did not cause any complications [69, 73, 74]. The catheter electrodes were inserted into the posterior epidural space percutaneously and remained for several days just as used in the continuous epidural block (Fig. 9.3). The methods have been advanced with epidural implantation of the electrodes and also subcutaneous implantation of the electric stimulator [63, 73, 75] (Figs. 9.4 and 9.5).

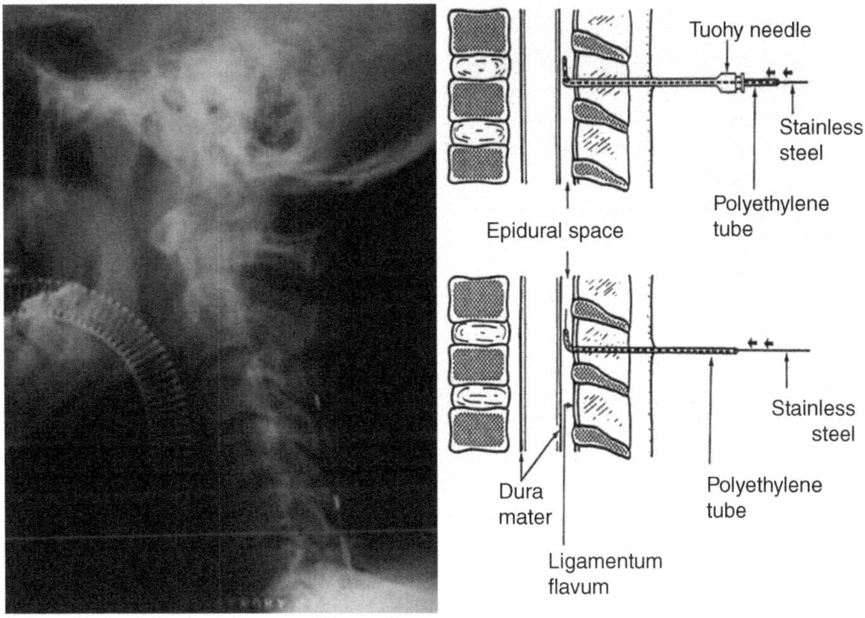

Fig. 9.3 Left: lateral view of X-ray in a patient with cerebral palsy, in whom the two stimulation catheter electrodes were inserted into the epidural space at C3 and C5 levels under general anesthesia, since the procedures of epidural electrode placement was difficult due to severe involuntary muscle movement. The patient, 47-year-old female, complained of neck and arm pain caused by muscle rigidity and involuntary movements (unpublished data). Right: schematic presentation of placement of an epidural catheter electrode into the posterior epidural space, based on the method of continuous epidural anesthesia

9.4.4 Application

The most common use of SCS is neuropathic pain, failed back surgery syndrome (FBSS), peripheral or myocardial ischemic pain [63, 65, 71–79], and chronic pain syndromes which do not respond to other pain treatments.

Usually, a temporary implant, called a trial, to determine the best stimulation pattern for several days is tested with external pulse generator. When pain control was achieved, a permanent system, with leads and a pulse generator, may be placed.

SCS must be carefully carried out in people who have coagulation related disorders, or are on anticoagulant therapy [63]. Contraindications may include local and systemic infection, pacemaker implants, or those people in whom imaging studies show anatomical anomalies or epidural adhesion that make placement difficult [63, 69, 77], or those with psychological problems [63].

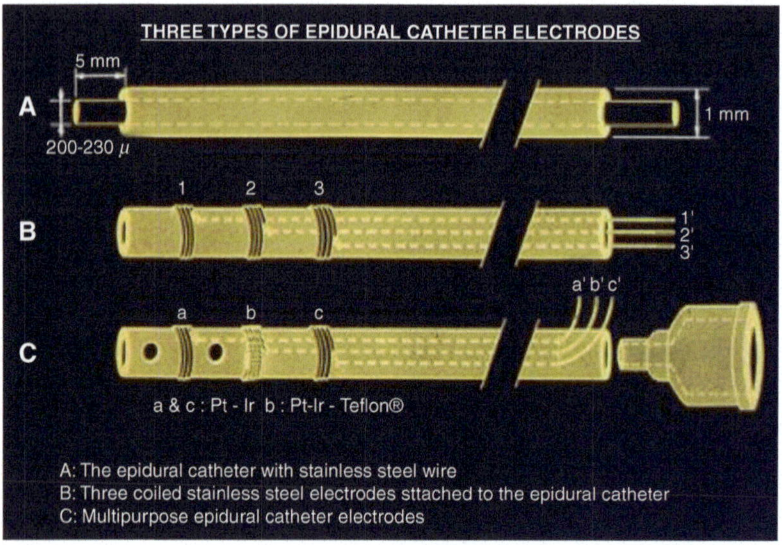

Fig. 9.4 Three kinds of epidural catheter electrodes. Catheter electrode A can be used to record the spinal cord potentials, and also to stimulate spinal cord epidurally. Electrodes B and C were also developed for multiple uses. (A) stainless steel was advanced through an epidural catheter, which was used routinely for the continuous epidural anesthesia or block, 5 mm beyond the tip of the catheter when the catheter was placed properly in the posterior epidural space. (B) an epidural catheter with attached three coiled stainless steel electrodes which are commercially available (Unique Medical, Inc. and Inter Medical, Inc.). (C) an epidural catheter with two side orifices, attached to three platinum wire electrodes developed in our laboratory for multipurpose uses, i.e., for electrical stimulation, recordings of electrical activities of the spinal cord, local blood flow, and tissue oxygen pressure. The catheter also could be used for injecting local anesthetics

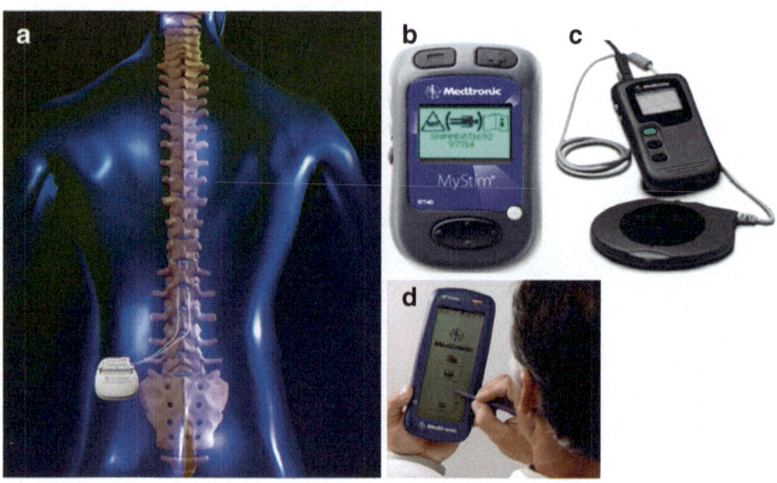

Fig. 9.5 (**a**) Schematic presentation of the epidurally implanted electrodes and subcutaneous stimulator. (**b**) The modulator for the patient. (**c**) The modulator for the pain therapist. (**d**) The therapist checking the implanted stimulator (By courtesy of Medtronic)

9.4.5 *Adverse Effects and Complications*

Complications with SCS from the epidural space range from simple easily correctable problems to devastating paralysis. The common complications include lead migration, lead breakage, infection, rotation of the pulse generator, subcutaneous or epidural hematomas, cerebrospinal fluid (CSF) leak, post-dural puncture headache, discomfort at pulse generator site, seroma, and transient paraplegia [63] Almost all these complications are due to undue manipulations.

Some patients may complain of the tingling sensation unpleasant [63, 73, 74]. This complication can be released by reprogramming of pulse frequency and/or voltage [73]. The lead migration may require resetting the lead placement [73, 74].

9.4.6 *Non-invasive SCS*

Recently, even non-invasive electrical or magnetic stimulation from the skin surface of the scalp and the back has been shown to affect brain and spinal cord functions, respectively [80]. There is increasing evidence that it can also induce prolonged functional neuroplastic changes [80, 81]. When delivered repetitively, magnetic stimulation could also modulate spinal cord functions and thus lead to pain relief [80]. More researches, however, remain to be undertaken to show clinical benefits of these non-invasive maneuvers [80].

9.4.7 *Minimally Invasive and Simple Method of SCP*

Minimally invasive, simple, and cost-effective method of SCP may be the use of the technique of continuous epidural block [64]. The commercially available epidural catheter, 20~50 cm long, containing a stainless steel inside, is introduced into the dorsal part of the spinal epidural space at the appropriate spinal segment, the stainless steel is further advanced beyond the catheter tip approximately 5 mm [63, 64].

The catheter with steel inside is sutured and fixed to the skin surface by the adhesive tape. The other part of the steel is connected to the electric simulator.

This method, based on the continuous epidural block, can be carried out in the out-patient clinic, is simple and inexpensive. The method can be applied even in the patient's home using water-protective adhesive tape if needed [73, 74].

9.5 Percutaneous Electric Nerve Stimulation (PENS) or Transcutaneous Electric Nerve Stimulation (TENS)

Percutaneous electric nerve stimulation (PENS) by a needle electrode or transcutaneous electrical nerve stimulation (TENS) by a surface electrode may provide a safe and simple alternative to narcotics and anti-inflammatory analgesics utilized in chronic pain.

Treatment of chronic pain with TENS demonstrated significant pain reduction. The application of TENS may lead to less pain medication usage and should be incorporated into the treatment strategy for chronic pain.

This technique has been used for the treatment of chronic pain for many decades. Even a permanent implantation of the electrodes to a peripheral nerve has been tried [82–84].

For patients in whom maximal medical therapy has failed, the peripheral nerve stimulation (PNS) (TENS or PENS) might be a potential alternative. Since these techniques have been described for several decades, clinicians have preferred to use these relative to other modes of neuromodulation such as spinal cord stimulation (SCS) and brain stimulation. Like other methods of neuromodulation, the mechanisms of action of PNS are not completely understood but are believed to function by activating a gating mechanism of pain transmission when stimulating low-threshold kinesthetic and discriminative touch large-diameter afferent fibers (alpha to beta fibers), subsequently inhibiting nociceptive transmission along a multitude of pain pathways, resulting in diminished pain perception [85].

Peripheral nerve stimulation has proven benefit even in an assembly of neuropathic pain conditions [82] as well as other intractable pain states. Both PNS and peripheral nerve field stimulation (PNfS) have been shown to be effective treatment modalities for conditions associated with truncal pain, intractable abdominal pain, and fibromyalgia. Peripheral nerve stimulation has also been successfully applied toward the treatment of a variety of chronic headache etiologies, including occipital neuralgia, transformed migraine, chronic refractory migraines, craniofacial neuropathic pain, cervical headaches, chronic cluster headaches [86], and chronic refractory headaches [87, 88].

Advantages of PNS versus stimulation motor cortex or deep brain stimulation (MCS or DBS) and spinal cord stimulation (SCS) are less invasive lead placement, greater target accessibility through minimally invasive techniques, lower morbidity, and potentially lower costs. Although peripheral nerve stimulators are still considered experimental in many situations, numerous patients have experienced a significant amount of pain relief, increased functionality, and improved quality of life [87].

9.5.1 Methods

Technology has advanced to the point where PNS electrodes and leads can feasibly be implanted at the time of trialing without the cost of expensive implanted pulse generators [88].

For the relatively smaller proportion of patients with isolated peripheral neuropathic pain, compared with the overall chronic pain population, PNS might be beneficial because of its lower economic priority than SCS. PNS remains predominantly a simple and relatively inexpensive method to identify favorable candidates for peripheral neuromodulation. This method takes advantage of the routine nerve block procedure used to inject a local anesthetic or corticosteroids, recasting it as an access technique for peripheral nerve neuromodulation. In this fashion, patients can undergo a stimulation trial while helping physicians with clinical decision making and identifying favorable candidates for subsequent permanent peripheral nerve stimulator implantation surgery [82].

Even in facial neuropathic pain, the infraorbital and supraorbital nerve stimulations afforded good pain relief.

A week-long trial of stimulation is preferable as same as that in case of SCS.

Standardizing the trial duration and perhaps extending the period of stimulation beyond 1 h may improve selection specificity.

Stimulus frequency and intensity are usually 10–100 Hz and 10~500 mV, respectively. Even low-frequency stimulation 1–5 Hz is sometimes used as in the case of spinal cord stimulation.

Peripheral nerve stimulation is a well-established yet underutilized method for treating chronic pain [82, 84]. Patient identification is of prime importance for subsequent permanent peripheral stimulator implantation if needed.

Several types of peripheral nerve stimulators have been developed [88], thus providing various kinds of waveforms have been studied (Fig. 9.6) [89], including 1/f pulses [90].

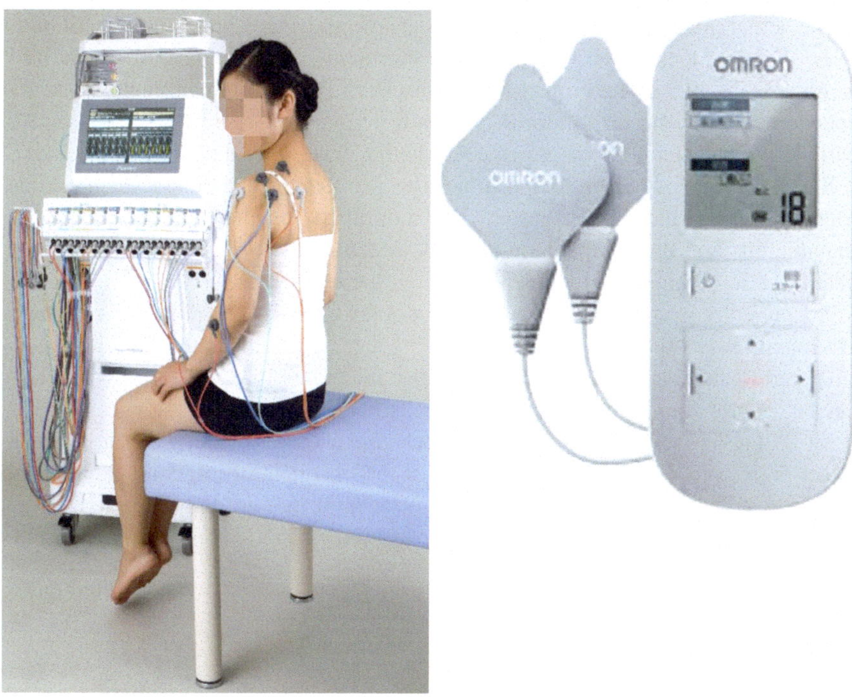

Fig. 9.6 The two examples of electric peripheral nerve stimulators. Left: A large peripheral nerve stimulator for medical use, which can deliver various kinds of pulse-waves with 1/f fluctuations, responding to the evaluation by the patients (By courtesy of Nihon Medix, Ltd.) Right: A handy and simple simulator commercially available (By courtesy of Omron, Ltd)

9.6 Acupuncture

Acupuncture is believed to be devised before 2500 BC in China and widely introduced in the late twentieth century in many other areas of the world. Acupuncture consists of the insertion of one or several small metal needles into the skin and underlying tissues at meridian points on the body.

Acupuncture grew out of ancient Chinese philosophy's dualistic cosmic theory of the yin and the yang. The theory says as follows: The yin, the female principle, passive and dark and is represented by the earth; the yang, the male principle, is active and light and is represented by the heavens. The forces of yin and yang act in the human body as they do throughout the natural universe as a whole. Disease or physical disharmony is caused by an imbalance or undue preponderance of these two forces in the body. The goal of Chinese medicine is to bring the yin and the yang back into balance with each other, thus restoring the person to health. An imbalance of yin and yang results in an obstruction of the life force, or qi(気)[1], in the body. Qi flows through 12 meridians, or pathways, in the body, each in turn associated with a major visceral organ (liver, kidney, etc.) and with a functional body system. Acupuncture is designed to affect the distribution of yin and yang in these channels so that the qi will be enabled to flow freely and harmoniously [91].

The actual practice of acupuncture consists of inserting needles into any of hundreds of points located over the 12 basic meridians and over several specialized meridians (Fig. 9.7). The typical needle insertion is 3–10 mm in depth; in some procedures it may be up to almost 250 mm or more. A needle may be twisted, twirled, or connected to a low-voltage alternating current for the duration of its use.

Briefly, the mechanism responsible for acupuncture-mediated analgesia is believed to activate opioid-based pain inhibition, mediated by endogenous cannabinoids and the sympathetic nervous system, and non-opioid pain-relieving system via serotonin and norepinephrine from the brain stem.

Acupuncture is commonly used for pain control but doubts about its effectiveness remain [91, 92]. It may be associated with a greater immediate pain relief effect compared to sham acupuncture and analgesic injections [93], and its effectiveness may be different among the conditions, diseases, or techniques [94].

Most of reviews were positive for low back pain and osteoarthritis. For myofascial trigger point pain, a positive trend exists. For the treatment of migraine, rheumatoid arthritis, and tension headache, the effects of acupuncture are largely negative. For dysmenorrhea and temporomandibular joint pain, the evidence is contradictory [92–96].

9.6.1 Definition of Trigger Points

The term "trigger point" is said to be defined by Dr. Travell [97] in 1942, known as President John F. Kennedy's personal physician, to describe a clinical finding with

---

[1] Acupuncture in the narrower sense of using metal needles to treat illnesses by stimulating specific points along circulation channels (meridians) in accordance with theories related to the circulation of qi [91, 92].

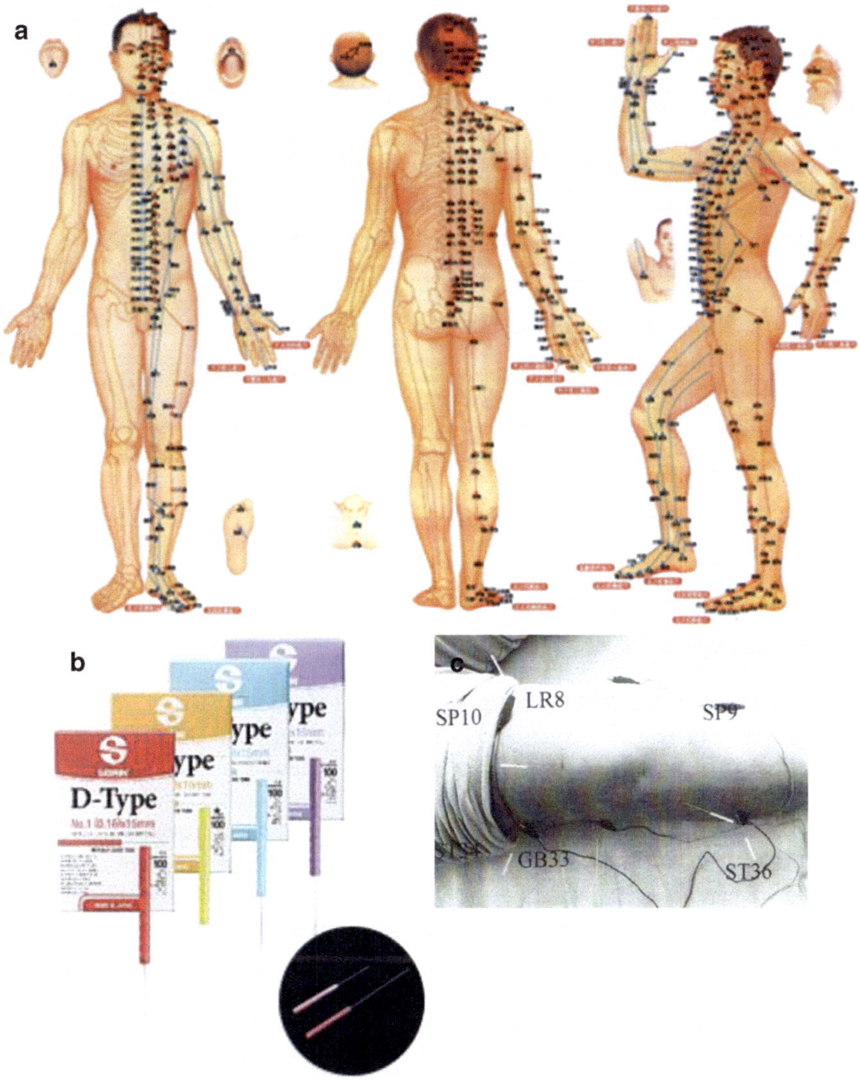

Fig. 9.7 (**a**) Acupuncture points, drawing from a Chinese manuscript (Adopted from Kesihatan/Health in Web). (**b**) The disposable acupuncture needles commercially available. (**c**) Needling and electrical stimulation procedure for a patient with degenerative knee arthritis, pointing to the meridians (Takahashi H: Chapter IV, Stimulation produced analgesia by acupuncture. In Shimoji K (Ed). All about Stimulation Produced Analgesia, Shinko Igaku Shuppan, Tokyo, 2010, pp. 55–64, in Japanese)

the following characteristics: (1) Pain related to a discrete, irritable point in skeletal muscle or fascia, not caused by acute local trauma, inflammation, degeneration, neoplasm, or infection. (2) The painful point can be felt as a nodule or band in the muscle, and a twitch response can be elicited on stimulation of the trigger point. (3) Palpation of the trigger point reproduces the patient's complaint of pain, and the pain radiates in a distribution typical of the specific muscle harboring the trigger point. (4) The pain cannot be explained by findings on neurological examination [98].

While this explanation provides an excellent theoretical construct for how myofascial trigger points (TrPs) form and ultimately lead to pain, it does not necessarily imply that trigger points are the primary target for acupuncture procedures. Presently, there is a lack of robust, empirical evidence validating the clinical diagnostic criteria for TrPs [97] proposed by Travell and other investigators [97–99]. In a systematic review, "tenderness" is the only criteria found to be moderately reliable for trigger point identification and only in the upper trapezius [99].

9.6.2 Mechanism of Analgesia

The following mechanisms have been hypothesized for development of acupuncture analgesia:

1. Activation of hypothalamic system: The acupuncture has been shown to activate centrally the hypothalamic–pituitary–adrenal axis and activate peripherally the corticotropin releasing hormone pro-opiomelanocortin (the precursor of β-endorphin) corticosteroid axis to inhibit COX-2, reducing inflammatory cytokines [100].
2. To reverse hyperalgesia: Acupuncture has been demonstrated to reverse protein kinase C (PKC)-mediated peripheral hyperalgesia by normalizing nociceptive channels, including transient receptor potential vanilloid (TRPV), acid-sensing ion channel (ASIC), tetrodotoxin (TTX), and purinergic (P2X/Y) [101].
3. Stimulation of immune cells: Acupuncture also stimulates immune cells, fibroblasts, and keratinocytes to release calcitonin gene-related peptide (CGRP) and substance-P, altering the stimulation of TTX receptors to reverse hyperalgesia [102].
4. The effect on mast cells: The number of mast cells (MCs) located at acupoints, including ST36, SP6, GB34, LI4, LI11, and PC6, has been shown to be 50% higher than non-acupoint locations. Several studies have linked the physical stimulation of needles with the activation of stretch-sensitive chloride channels on MC, resulting in degranulation [103–106].
5. To promote tissue healing: Acupuncture needling has been shown to decrease cytokines responsible for inflammation via activation of toll-like receptors on fibroblasts [106, 107].
6. The effect on CGRP and SP:

   Evidence from the acupuncture literature suggests that electric dry needling (EDN) results in a significant increase in peripheral calcitonin gene regulated peptide (CGRP) and substance-P (SP) [108, 109].
7. Angiogenesis: A recent study demonstrated that acupuncture dry needling can promote tendon healing via angiogenesis and fibroblast migration via CGRP release from sensory nerve endings and mechanical stimulation of collagen fibers, respectively [108, 110–112].
8. Aß and Aδ fiber stimulation

   While Aδ and C fibers open the pain gait, Aβ stimulation attempts to keep it closed. In the case of chronic pain, the gait is continually left open.

Multiple systematic reviews have demonstrated the increased Aβ fiber activation with acupuncture [85]. Like Aβ fibers, many systematic reviews have reported Aδ stimulation with acupuncture [113].

9. Activation of descending inhibitory systems: Acupuncture needling has also been shown to activate the descending pain modulatory system, which is mediated by a synergic relationship between opioids and non-opioids, including serotonin and norepinephrine [96, 114, 115].
10. Effects on volume transmission: Volume transmission (VT) is a widespread mode of intercellular communication that occurs in the extracellular fluid (ECF) and in the cerebrospinal fluid (CSF) of the brain with volume transmission signals moving from source to target cells via energy gradients leading to diffusion and convection [116]. Short and long distance VT may take place in meridian channels via diffusion and flow in the interstitial fluid. Acupuncture can produce VT signals by releasing transmitters and modulators from nerve terminals and mast cells [116].

9.6.3 Diseases or Conditions Treated by Acupuncture

Acupuncture successfully treats conditions ranging from musculoskeletal problems such as back pain, neck pain, to nausea, migraine headache, anxiety, depression, insomnia, and infertility [92, 93, 96]. Further, acupuncture has been reported to be effective for pain or hyperesthesia related to the following diseases, symptoms, or conditions: allergic rhinitis, biliary colic, depression, dysentery, acute bacillary, primary dysmenorrhea, epigastralgia, peptic ulcer, gastritis, gastrospasm, facial pain, headache, essential hypertension, primary hypotension, induction of labor, knee pain, leukopenia, low back pain, correction of fetus malposition, morning sickness, nausea and vomiting, neck pain, dental pain, temporomandibular dysfunction, periarthritis of shoulder, postoperative pain, renal colic, rheumatoid arthritis, sciatica, sprain, stroke, Alzheimer's disease, obesity, tennis elbow, etc. [117, 118].

9.7 Vagal Nerve Stimulation (VNS)

Recent human and animal studies provide growing evidence that vagal nerve stimulation (VNS) has analgesic effects besides therapeutic efficacy in the treatment of refractory epilepsy and depression. Analgesia is believed to be mediated by vagal afferents that inhibit spinal nociceptive reflexes and transmission and have strong anti-inflammatory properties [119]. VNS has been applied for various chronic pain syndromes, including fibromyalgia, pelvic pain [120], and headaches [63, 121] and even Alzheimer's disease.

Non-invasive VNS (nVNS), which stimulates the carotid vagus nerve with the use of a personal handheld device, also demonstrated efficacy for acute migraine or cluster headache attacks. Long-term use of nVNS seems to exert even a prophylactic effect for both chronic migraine and chronic cluster headache. In animal studies, nVNS modulated multiple pain pathways and lessen cortical spreading depression [121].

9.7.1 *Mechanism*

Vagus nerve (the tenth cranial nerve) arises from the medulla and carries both afferent and efferent fibers. The afferent vagal fibers connect to the nucleus of the solitary tract which in turn projects to other locations in the central nervous system.

The proposed mechanism of action of VNS is alteration of epinephrine release by projections of solitary tract to locus coeruleus in the medulla, and elevation of gamma aminobutyric acid (GABA) levels in the brain stem.

VNS also drives activation of neuromodulatory nuclei that are associated with plasticity, including the cholinergic basal forebrain besides the noradrenergic locus coeruleus. Repeatedly pairing brief bursts of VNS has been shown to drive sensory or motor events producing event-specific plasticity in neural circuits [122].

9.7.2 *Procedure*

In conventional vagus nerve stimulation, a device is surgically implanted under the skin on the chest, and a wire is threaded under the skin connecting the device to the left vagus nerve. The right vagus nerve is not commonly used because it carries fibers that supply nerves to the heart. Even an implantable device that stimulates the right vagus nerve is also studied for the treatment of heart failure [122, 123] (Fig. 9.8).

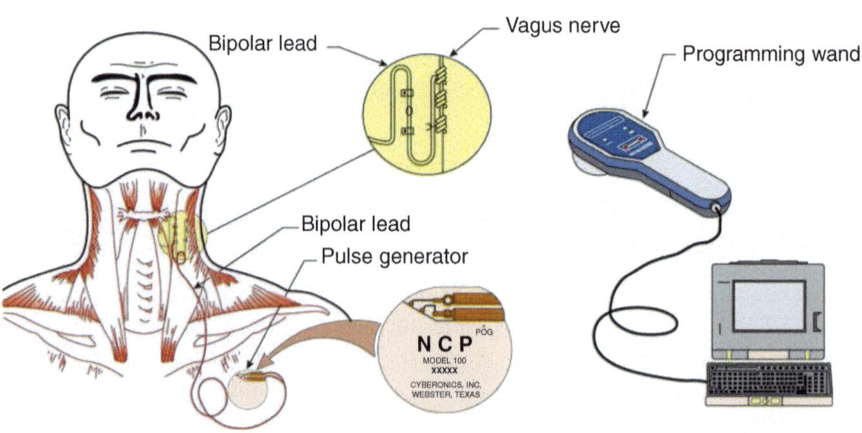

Fig. 9.8 Placement of vagus nerve stimulation device. As illustrated in the insert (upper right box), the distal end of the lead is wrapped around the nerve. The most proximal electrode is helical and helps to anchor the lead to the vagus nerve. The ECG sensing vector triggers the generator which in turn can stimulate the negative electrode (Open access: Vagus Nerve Stimulation Therapy, Website Neupsy Key)

9.7.3 Application

The VNS is originally an approach mainly used in cases of intractable epilepsy resistant to all other therapies. Its benefits have also been shown in severe cases of depression resistant to typical treatment [123].

Long-term use of nVNS seems to exert even a prophylactic effect for both chronic migraine and chronic cluster headache. In animal studies, nVNS has been shown to modulate multiple pain pathways and even lessen cortical spreading depression. Progression in nVNS clinical efficacy over time suggests an underlying disease-modifying neuromodulation [121]. Non-invasive VNS appears to be as effective as the invasive counterpart for many indications. With an enormous potential therapeutic gain and a high safety profile, further development and application of nVNS is promising.

Multiple studies have also documented significant improvements in quality of life after VNS therapy in individuals with neurodevelopmental disorders [124]. Moreover, recent findings indicate that VNS significantly enhances the benefits of rehabilitative training in animal models and patients, leading to greater recovery in a variety of neurological diseases, including chronic pain syndromes.

VNS paired with behavioral therapy may represent a potential new approach to enhance rehabilitation that could significantly improve even the outcomes of individuals with neurodevelopmental disorders.

9.7.4 Adverse Effects

The most frequently encountered side effects include coughing, chest pain, sense of compression of the chest, and coarsening of voice, all of which will diminish in time. None of these side effects is epileptic or in similar nature. The side effects may be related to the dysfunction of the vagus nerve, but removal of the device will rarely be necessary. VNS will create no cognitive or systemic adverse effects. Perioperative complications of VNS are mostly related with cardiac dysrhythmias.

Recent studies have shown that the changes in the cardiac rhythm and fluctuations on the blood pressure change with the on/off periods of the stimulation phases [125]. Such findings can be improved significantly only by elongating the off period and adjusting the electrode placements. Another rare complication is the infection at the implantation site. The most frequent acute complications of VNS implantation include temporary excessive salivation, mild coughs, paralysis of the vocal cord, lower facial weakness, rarely bradycardia, and very rarely, asystole, all of which are reversible [125].

9.8 Percutaneous Disc Coagulation Therapy (PDCT)

The results of open surgical discectomy for contained disc herniation have been poor. Consequently, several less invasive techniques have been developed including percutaneous lumbar laser disc decompression.

The percutaneous access to the disc was first used in the 1950s to biopsy the disc with needles. The minimally invasive access to the disc using endoscopic techniques was developed in the 1970s, cited by Singh et al. [126].

Disc herniation causing lumbar pain and disability is one of the most common spinal diseases. Lumbar open discectomy has been the most frequently used methods for treating lumbar disc herniation that requires spinal surgery. However, the surgery needs an incision dissection of muscles and ligaments which may cause undesirable results to lumbar spine post-operatively. Percutaneous techniques are rapidly replacing traditional open surgery in operations requiring discectomy, decompression, and fusion [126–128].

Technical advances in the use of intradiscal therapies led to the development of intradiscal electrothermal annuloplasty (IDET), DISC nucleoplasty along with laser-assisted, endoscopic, and nucleotome disc decompressions [129–132].

The most advanced theory of PDCT is that PDCT can deliver stable thermal damage to the center of nucleus pulposus and annulus part as well with ball shaped plasma light, and several similar methods have been tried [133] (Fig. 9.9).

9.8.1 The Techniques

A patient is basically prepared in prone or lateral position just the same as in spinal or epidural block. Under C-arm guide, a sufficient area is sterilized to be draped with a disposable sterile swab. Entry point is started at 8–10 cm away from lateral in spinous process. Stabbing point is determined under C-arm guide with local anesthesia. There are several modified methods tested.

After administering local anesthesia, insert a small guide probe into to disc under the C-arm guidance. Over the probe, a slightly larger tube is inserted down to the annulus. One to two millimeter diameter nucleotome probe or coagulation needle is then inserted through the tube and into the disc (Fig. 9.9). In case of coagulation 40–60 centigrade heat is applied for 30~60 min dependent on the case. In case of the suction method, the nucleotome probe is used to remove small pieces of the nucleus and suction some nucleus out of the disc [126]. The procedure takes about 30~45 min. Patients can be discharged from the hospital within a day.

These PDCT methods are considered as a very effective minimally invasive surgery capable of obtaining a satisfactory outcome in patients with the lumbar disc herniation. However, further long-term clinical evaluations are still awaited [134].

Further, Disc-FX®, minimally invasive spine system, was developed to efficiently access the damaged disc without injury to surrounding disc anatomy. This system may be helpful in selected patients with symptomatic degenerative disc disease providing favorable outcomes lasting up to 2 years or more [135].

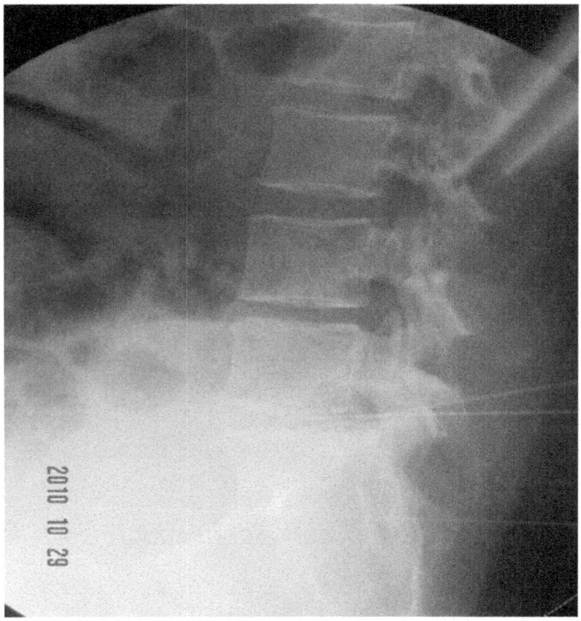

Fig. 9.9 X-ray image of the spine showing the two coagulation needles were inserted (unpublished data)

9.9 MRI-Guided Focused Ultrasound Surgery

MRI-guided focused ultrasound (MRgFUS) surgery is a minimally invasive thermal ablation method that uses magnetic resonance imaging (MRI) for target definition, treatment planning, and closed-loop control of energy deposition. Integrating FUS and MRI as a therapy delivery system allows us to localize, target, and monitor in real time, and thus to ablate targeted tissue without damaging normal structures [136]. This precision makes MRgFUS an attractive alternative to surgical resection or radiation therapy of benign and/or malignant tumors, leading to pain relief. As it is already used for the treatment of uterine fibroids, MRgFUS is in ongoing clinical trials for the treatment of breast, liver, prostate, and brain cancer and for the palliation of pain in bone metastasis in several countries [136]. In addition to thermal ablation, focused ultrasound (FUS), with or without the use of microbubbles, can temporarily change vascular or cell membrane permeability and release or activate various compounds for targeted drug delivery or gene therapy [136]. Thus, MRgFUS may provide a new therapeutic approach to pain management associated with varieties of diseases, including motor system diseases [137–139].

9.9.1 Neurosurgical Application

MRgFUS is an emerging technique that uses acoustic energy to treat minimally invasively intracranial disorders. At high frequencies, it can be used to raise tissue temperatures and ablate discrete brain targets with sub-millimeter accuracy. This application is currently under investigation for a broad range of clinical applications, including brain tumors, movement disorders, and psychiatric conditions. At low frequencies, MRI-guided focused ultrasound can be used to modulate neuronal activity and in conjunction with injected microbubbles, can open the blood–brain barrier to enhance the delivery of therapeutic compounds. The last decade has shown dramatic advances in the science of MRgFUS, helping elucidate both its mechanisms and potential in pre-clinical models, and its translational promise across myriad clinical applications, even including Parkinson's disease [137–139].

9.9.2 Uterine Fibroids Application

MRgFUS is a minimally invasive technique for the treatment of uterine fibroids.

The role of MRgFUS in the treatment of fibroids has been evolving since its introduction by Hindley J et al. in 2004 [140]. Several new devices and techniques including location-specific treatment, volumetric therapy, and vessel-targeted therapy have been introduced over the last few years. Several case series report uncomplicated pregnancy following MRgFUS; however, results of the ongoing studies will further elucidate the utility of MRgFUS in patients planning future fertility. A systematic review of the literature was completed and studies that reported quality of life at baseline and after 6 months were included in a meta-analysis [141].

Thus, MRgFUS represents a minimally invasive treatment for uterine fibroids that is able to improve the quality of life including abdominal uneasiness or pain and fibroid size with durability. There are several rare, but important side effects and complications related to MRI-guided HIFU treatment which include: pain, inflammation of subcutaneous fatty tissue and muscles of the abdominal wall, skin burns, deep vein thrombosis, paresthesia of the leg due to the nerve irritation or damage, bowel perforation (extremely rare) [142].

It is possible that MRgFUS could be the treatment of choice for patients desiring future fertility; however, further investigation is needed [141].

9.9.3 Application to Metastatic Cancer

Magnetic resonance-guided focused ultrasound (MRgFUS) may be an alternative local therapy for patients with painful bone metastasis for whom standard conventional radiation therapy is not successful.

Recent findings [143–145] suggest that MRgFUS provides a similar treatment response rate but faster pain relief compared with conventional radiation therapy and has the potential to serve as the first-line treatment for painful bone metastasis in selected patients.

References

1. Croft PG. The effect of electrical stimulation of the brain on the perception of pain. J Ment Sci. 1952;98:421–6.
2. Honey CM, Tronnier VM, Honey CR. Deep brain stimulation versus motor cortex stimulation for neuropathic pain: a minireview of the literature and proposal for future research. Comput Struct Biotechnol J. 2016;14:234–7.
3. Tsubokawa T, Katayama Y, Yamamoto T, Hirayama T, Koyama S. Chronic motor cortex stimulation for the treatment of central pain. Acta Neurochir Suppl (Wien). 1991;52:137–9.
4. Katayama Y, Fukaya C, Yamamoto T. Poststroke pain control by chronic motor cortex stimulation: neurological characteristics predicting a favorable response. J Neurosurg. 1998;89:585–91.
5. Katayama Y, Yamamoto T, Kobayashi K, et al. Motor cortex stimulation for phantom limb pain: comprehensive therapy with spinal cord and thalamic stimulation. Stereotact Funct Neurosurg. 2001;77:159–62.
6. Katayama Y, Yamamoto T, Kobayashi K, et al. Motor cortex stimulation for post-stroke pain: comparison of spinal cord and thalamic stimulation. Stereotact Funct Neurosurg. 2001;77:183–6.
7. Monsalve GA. Motor cortex stimulation for facial chronic neuropathic pain: a review of the literature. Surg Neurol Int. 2012;3(Suppl. 4):S290–311.
8. Fontaine D, Hamani C, Lozano A. Efficacy and safety of motor cortex stimulation for chronic neuropathic pain: critical review of the literature. J Neurosurg. 2009;110:251–6.
9. Lefaucheur JP, Drouot X, Cunin P. Motor cortex stimulation for the treatment of refractory peripheral neuropathic pain. Brain. 2009;132(Pt 6):1463–71.
10. Nguyen JP, Velasco F, Brugières P. Treatment of chronic neuropathic pain by motor cortex stimulation: results of a bicentric controlled crossover trial. Brain Stimul. 2008;1:89–96.
11. Velasco F, Argüelles C, Carrillo-ruiz JD. Efficacy of motor cortex stimulation in the treatment of neuropathic pain: a randomized double-blind trial. J Neurosurg. 2008;108:698–706.
12. Velasco F, Carrillo-Ruiz JD, Castro G, et al. Motor cortex electrical stimulation applied to patients with complex regional pain syndrome. Pain. 2009;147:91–8.
13. Cedzich C, Taniguchi M, Schäfer S, Schramm J. Somatosensory evoked potential phase reversal and direct motor cortex stimulation during surgery in and around the central region. Neurosurgery. 1996;38:962–70.
14. Kurt E, Henssen DJHA, Steegers M, Staal M, Beese U, et al. Motor cortex stimulation in patients suffering from chronic neuropathic pain: summary of an expert meeting and premeeting questionnaire, combined with a literature review. World Neurosurg. 2017;108: 254–63.
15. Heath R. Studies in schizophrenia: a multidisciplinary approach to mind brain relationships. Cambridge: Harvard University Press; 1954.
16. Mazars G, Merienne L, Cioloca C. Thalamic stimulation for intermittent analgesia: preliminary notes [in French]. Rev Neurol. 1973;128:273–9.
17. Hosobuchi Y, Adams JE, Rutkin B. Chronic thalamic stimulation for the control of facial anesthesia dolorosa. Arch Neurol. 1973;29:158–61.
18. Adams JE, Hosobuchi Y, Fields HL. Stimulation of the internal capsule for relief of chronic pain. J Neurosurg. 1974;41:740–4.

19. Richardson DE, Akil H. Pain reduction by electrical brain stimulation in man, part I: acute administration in periaqueductal and periventricular sites. J Neurosurg. 1977;47:178–83.
20. Richardson DE, Akil H. Pain reduction by electrical stimulation, part II: chronic self-administration in the periventricular gray matter. J Neurosurg. 1977;47:184–94.
21. Hosobuchi Y, Adams JE, Linchitz R. Pain relief by electrical stimulation of the central gray matter in humans and its reversal by naloxone. Science. 1977;197:183–6.
22. Hosobuchi Y, Adams JE, Bloom FE, Guilleum R. Stimulation of human periaqueductal grey for pain relief increases immunoreactive B-endorphin in ventricular fluid. Science. 1979;203:279–81.
23. Hosobuchi Y, Lamb S, Bascim D. Tryptophan loading may reverse tolerance to opiate analgesics in humans: a preliminary report. Pain. 1980;9:161–9.
24. Hosobuchi Y, Rossier J, Bloom FE. Oral loading with L-tryptophan may augment the simultaneous release of ACTH and beta-endorphin that accompanies periaqueductal stimulation in humans. Adv Biochem Psychopharmacol. 1980;22:563–70.
25. Akil H, Richardson DE, Hughes J, Barchas JD. Enkephalin-like material elevated in ventricular cerebrospinal fluid of pain patients after analgesic focal stimulation. Science. 1978;201:463–5.
26. Richardson DE, Akil H. Long term results of periventricular gray-self stimulation. Neurosurgery. 1977;1:199–202.
27. Amano K, Kitamura H, Kawamura H, et al. Alterations of immunoreactive beta-endorphin in the third ventricular fluid in response to electrical stimulation of the human periaqueductal gray matter. Appl Neurophysiol. 1980;43:150–8.
28. Gybels J. Electrical stimulation of the brain for pain control in humans [in German]. Verhandl Deutsch Gesellsch Inn Med. 1980;86:1553–9.
29. Ray CD, Bruton CV. Deep brain stimulation for severe, chronic pain. Acta Neurochir. 1980;3:289–93.
30. Dieckmann GJ, Witzmann A. Initial and long-term results of deep brain stimulation for chronic intractable pain. Appl Neurophysiol. 1982;45:167–72.
31. Plotkin R. Results in 60 cases of deep brain stimulation for chronic intractable pain. Appl Neurophysiol. 1982;45:173–8.
32. Richardson DE. Analgesia produced by stimulation of various sites in the human beta-endorphin system. Appl Neurophysiol. 1982;45:116–22.
33. Hosobuchi Y. Subcortical electrical stimulation for control of intractable pain in humans. J Neurosurg. 1986;64:543–53.
34. Levy RM, Lamb S, Adams JE. Treatment of chronic pain by deep brain stimulation: long term follow-up and review of the literature. Neurosurgery. 1987;21:885–93.
35. Hosobuchi Y. Intracerebral stimulation for the relief of chronic pain. In: Youmans JR, editor. Neurological surgery. Philadelphia: WB Saunders; 1990. p. 4128–43.
36. Kumar K, Toth C, Nath RK. Deep brain stimulation for intractable pain: a 15-year experience. Neurosurgery. 1997;40:736–46.
37. Rinaldi PC, Young RF, Albe-Fessard D, Chodakiewitz J. Spontaneous neuronal hyperactivity in the medial and intralaminar thalamic nuclei of patients with deafferentation pain. J Neurosurg. 1991;74:415–21.
38. Kumar K, Wyant GM, Nath R. Deep brain stimulation for control of intractable pain in humans, present and future: a ten-year follow-up. Neurosurgery. 1990;26:774–82.
39. Hosobuchi Y. Dorsal periaqueductal gray matter stimulation in humans. Pacing Clin Electrophysiol. 1987;10:213–6.
40. Mazars GJ, Merienne L, Cioloca C. Comparative study of electrical stimulation of posterior thalamic nuclei, periaqueductal gray and other midline mesencephalic structures in man. In: Bonica JJ, editor. Advances in pain research and therapy, vol. 3. New York: Raven Press; 1979. p. 541–6.
41. Falowski SM. Deep brain stimulation for chronic pain. Curr Pain Headache Rep. 2015;19:27.

42. Farrand S, Evans AH, Mangelsdorf S, et al. Deep brain stimulation for severe treatment-resistant obsessive-compulsive disorder: an open-label case series. Aust N Z J Psychiatry. 2018;52(7):699–708.
43. Sugiyama K, Nozaki T, Asakawa T, et al. The present indication and future of deep brain stimulation. Neurol Med Chir (Tokyo). 2015;55:416–21.
44. Boccard SG, Pereira EA, Aziz TZ. Deep brain stimulation for chronic pain. J Clin Neurosci. 2015;22:1537–43.
45. Hassan S, Lagrata S, Levy A, et al. Microvascular decompression or neuromodulation in patients with SUNCT and trigeminal neurovascular conflict? Cephalalgia. 2018;38(2):393–8.
46. Lempka SF, Malone DA Jr, Hu B, et al. Randomized clinical trial of deep brain stimulation for poststroke pain. Ann Neurol. 2017;81:653–63.
47. Boccard SGJ, Prangnell SJ, Pycroft L, et al. Long-term results of deep brain stimulation of the anterior cingulate cortex for neuropathic pain. World Neurosurg. 2017;106:625–37.
48. Sweet W. Intracerebral electrical stimulation for the relief of chronic pain. In: Youmans JR, editor. Neurological surgery. Philadelphia: WB Saunders; 1982. p. 3739–48.
49. Akram H, Miller S, Lagrata S, et al. Ventral tegmental area deep brain stimulation for refractory chronic cluster headache. Neurology. 2016;86(18):1676–82.
50. Bittar RG, Kar-Purkayastha I, Owen SL, Bear R, Green A, Wang S, Aziz T. Deep brain stimulation for pain relief: a meta-analysis. J Clin Neurosci. 2005;12:515–9.
51. Green AL, Owen SL, Davies P, Moir L, Aziz TZ. Deep brain stimulation for neuropathic cephalalgia. Cephalalgia. 2006;26:561–7.
52. Schoenen J, Di Clemente L, Vandenheede M, et al. Hypothalamic stimulation in chronic cluster headache: a pilot study of efficacy and mode of action. Brain. 2005;128:940–7.
53. Franzini A, Ferroli P, Leone M, et al. Hypothalamic deep brain stimulation for the treatment of chronic cluster headaches: a series report. Neuromodulation. 2004;7:1–8.
54. Mogilner AY, Rezaih AR. Brain stimulation: current clinical indications and future prospects. Suppl Clin Neurophysiol. 2004;57:721–32.
55. Shimoji K, Asai A, Toei M, et al. Clinical application of electroanesthesia. 1. Method. Masui. 1969;18:1479–85.
56. Shimoji K, Higashi H, Terasaki H, et al. Physiologic changes associated with clinical electroanesthesia. Anesth Analg. 1971;50:490–7.
57. Thibaut A, Russo C, Hurtado-Puerto AM, et al. Effects of transcranial direct current stimulation, transcranial pulsed current stimulation, and their combination on brain oscillations in patients with chronic visceral pain: a pilot crossover randomized controlled study. Front Neurol. 2017;8:576.
58. Klein MM, Treister R, Raij T. Transcranial magnetic stimulation of the brain: guidelines for pain treatment research. Pain. 2015;156:1601–14.
59. Elsner B, Kugler J, Pohl M, Mehrholz JD. Transcranial direct current stimulation (tDCS) for improving activities of daily living, and physical and cognitive functioning, in people after stroke. Cochrane Database Syst Rev. 2016;(3):CD009645.
60. O'Connell NE, Wand BM, Marston L, et al. Non-invasive brain stimulation techniques for chronic pain. Cochrane Database Syst Rev. 2014;(4):CD008208.
61. Chen ML, Yao L, Boger J, Mercer K, Thompson B, Jiang N. Non-invasive brain stimulation interventions for management of chronic central neuropathic pain: a scoping review protocol. BMJ Open. 2017;7:e016002.
62. Galhardoni R, Correia GS, Araujo H, et al. Repetitive transcranial magnetic stimulation in chronic pain: a review of the literature. Arch Phys Med Rehabil. 2015;96(4 Suppl):S156–72.
63. Shimoji K. Stimulation produced analgesia. Tokyo: Shinko Pub. Co; 2010.
64. Shimoji K, Higashi H, Kano T, Asai S, Morioka T. Electrical management of intractable pain. Masui (Jap J Anesth). 1971;20:444–7.
65. Wong SS, Chan CW, Cheung CW. Spinal cord stimulation for chronic non-cancer pain: a review of current evidence and practice. Hong Kong Med J. 2017;23:517–23.
66. Melzack R, Wall PD. Pain mechanism: anew theory. Science. 1965;150:971–9.

67. Shealy CN, Mortimer JT, Reswick JB. Electrical inhibition of pain by stimulation of the dorsal columns: preliminary clinical report. Anesth Analg. 1967;46:489–91.
68. Shimoji K, Higashi H, Terasaki H, Morioka T. Clinical electroanesthesia with several methods of current application. Anesth Analg. 1971;50:409–16.
69. Shimoji K, Kitamura H, Ikezono E, et al. Spinal hypalgesia and analgesia by low-frequency electrical stimulation in the epidural space. Anesthesiology. 1974;41:91–4.
70. Vallejo R, Bradley K, Kapural L. Spinal cord stimulation in chronic pain: mode of action. Spine (Phila Pa 1976). 2017;42(Suppl 14):S53–60.
71. Peppucci E, Di Bonaventura R, Esposito V, et al. Update on mechanism and therapeutic implications of spinal cord stimulation and cerebral hemodynamics: a narrative review. Acta Neurochir Suppl. 2017;124:27–36.
72. Deer TR, Mekhail N, Provenzano D. The appropriate use of neurostimulation of the spinal cord and peripheral nervous system for the treatment of chronic pain and ischemic diseases: the neuromodulation appropriateness consensus committee. Neuromodulation. 2014;17:515–50.
73. Shimoji K. Analgesia by spiral cord stimulation. Masui. 1994;43(Suppl):S67–76.
74. Shimoji K, Hokari T, Kano T, et al. Management of intractable pain with percutaneous epidural spinal cord stimulation: differences in pain-relieving effects among diseases and sites of pain. Anesth Analg. 1993;77(1):110–6.
75. Howard-Quijano K, Takamiya T, Dale EA, et al. Spinal cord stimulation reduces ventricular arrhythmias during acute ischemia by attenuation of regional myocardial excitability. Am J Physiol Heart Circ Physiol. 2017;313:H421–31.
76. Shimoji K, Matsuki M, Shimizu H, et al. Low-frequency, weak extradural stimulation in the management of intractable pain. Br J Anaesth. 1977;49:1081–6.
77. Kin K, Agari T, Yasuhara T. The factors affecting the difficulty of percutaneous cylindrical electrode placement for spinal cord stimulation. World Neurosurg. 2018;113: e391–8.
78. Kumar K, Hunter G, Demeria D. Spinal cord stimulation in treatment of chronic benign pain: challenges in the treatment planning and present status, a 22-year experience. Neurosurgery. 2006;58:481–96.
79. Kinfe TM, Pintea B, Vatter H. Is spinal cord stimulation useful and safe for the treatment of chronic pain of ischemic origin? A review. Clin J Pain. 2016;32:7–13.
80. Rossini PM, Burke D, Chen R, et al. Non-invasive electrical and magnetic stimulation of the brain, spinal cord, roots and peripheral nerves: basic principles and procedures for routine clinical and research application. An updated report from an I.F.C.N. Committee. Clin Neurophysiol. 2015;126:1071–107.
81. Phillips AA, Squair JW, Sayenko DG, et al. An autonomic neuroprosthesis: non-invasive electrical spinal cord stimulation restores autonomic cardiovascular function in individuals with spinal cord injury. J Neurotrauma. 2018;35(3):446–51.
82. Reddy CG, Flouty OE, Holland MT, et al. Novel technique for trialing peripheral nerve stimulation: ultrasonography-guided StimuCath trial. Neurosurg Focus. 2017;42:E5.
83. Aló KM, Abramova MV, Richter EO. Percutaneous peripheral nerve stimulation. Prog Neurol Surg. 2011;24:41–57.
84. Dworkin RH, O'Connor AB, Backonja M, et al. Pharmacologic management of neuropathic pain: evidence-based recommendations. Pain. 2007;132:237–51.
85. Melzack R, Wall PD. Pain mechanisms: a new theory. Science. 1965;150:971–9.
86. Meng DW, Zhang JG, Zheng Z, et al. Chronic bilateral sphenopalatine ganglion stimulation for intractable bilateral chronic cluster headache: a case report. Pain Physician. 2016;19:E637–42.
87. Mobbs RJ, Nair S, Blum P. Peripheral nerve stimulation for the treatment of chronic pain. J Clin Neurosci. 2007;14:216–23.
88. Kano T. Electroanesthesia. In: Shimoji K, editor. Stimulation produced analgesia. Tokyo: Shinko Pub. Co; 2003.

89. Shimoji K, Takahashi N, Nishio Y, et al. Pain relief by transcutaneous nerve stimulation with bidirectional modulated sine waves in patients with chronic back pain: a randomized, double-blind, sham-controlled study. Neuromodulation. 2007;10:42–51.
90. Takakura K, Sano K, Kosugi Y, Ikebe J. Pain control by transcutaneous electrical nerve stimulating using irregular pulse of 1/f fluctuation [proceedings]. Appl Neurophysiol. 1979;42:314–5.
91. Chen YL, Zhao C, Zhang L, et al. Toward evidence-based Chinese medicine: Status quo, opportunities and challenges. Chin J Integr Med. 2018;24(3):163–70.
92. Emst E, Lee MS, Choi TY. Acupuncture: does it alleviate pain and are there serious risks? A review of reviews. Pain. 2011;152:755–64.
93. Xiang A, Cheng K, Shen X, et al. The immediate analgesic effect of acupuncture for pain: a systematic review and meta-analysis. Evid Based Complement Alternat Med. 2017;2017:3837194.
94. Armour M, Dahlen HG, Zhu X, et al. The role of treatment timing and mode of stimulation in the treatment of primary dysmenorrhea with acupuncture: an exploratory randomised controlled trial. PLoS One. 2017;12:e0180177.
95. Tejada MA, Montilla-García A, Cronin SJ, et al. Sigma-1 receptors control immune-driven peripheral opioid analgesia during inflammation in mice. Proc Natl Acad Sci U S A. 2017;114:8396–401.
96. Zhao ZQ. Neural mechanism underlying acupuncture analgesia. Prog Neurobiol. 2008;85:355–75.
97. Travell W, Travell JG. Technic for reduction and ambulatory treatment of sacroiliac displacement. Arch Phys Ther. 1942;23:222–32.
98. Travell JG, Simons DG. Myofascial pain and dysfunction: the trigger point manual: the lower extremities, vol. 2. Baltimore: Williams & Wilkins; 1992.
99. Dunning J, Butts R, Mourad F, et al. Dry needling: a literature review with implications for clinical practice guidelines. Phys Ther Rev. 2014;19:252–65.
100. Wang X, Zhang B, Zhang L, Liu S. Electroacupuncture suppresses morphine reward-seeking behavior: lateral hypothalamic orexin neurons implicated. Neurosci Lett. 2017;661: 84–9.
101. Yen LT, Hsu YC, Lin JG, Hsieh CL, Lin YW. Role of ASIC3, Nav1.7 and Nav1.8 in electroacupuncture-induced analgesia in a mouse model of fibromyalgia pain. Acupunct Med. 2018;36(2):110–6.
102. Chen L, Xu A, Yin N, Zhao M, et al. Enhancement of immune cytokines and splenic CD4+ T cells by electroacupuncture at ST36 acupoint of SD rats. PLoS One. 2017;12: e0175568.
103. Chen B, Li MY, Guo Y, et al. Mast cell-derived exosomes at the stimulated acupoints activating the neuro-immune regulation. Chin J Integr Med. 2017;23:878–80.
104. Yao W, Yang H, Yin N, Ding G. Mast cell-nerve cell interaction at acupoint: modeling mechanotransduction pathway induced by acupuncture. Int J Biol Sci. 2014;10:511–9.
105. Wu ML, Xu DS, Bai WZ, Cui JJ, Shu HM, et al. Local cutaneous nerve terminal and mast cell responses to manual acupuncture in acupoint LI4 area of the rats. J Chem Neuroanat. 2015;68:14–21.
106. Wang L, Sikora J, Hu L, Shen X, Grygorczyk R, et al. ATP release from mast cells by physical stimulation: a putative early step in activation of acupuncture points. Evid Based Complement Alternat Med. 2013;2013:350949.
107. Su TF, Zhao YQ, Zhang LH, Peng M, Wu CH, et al. Electroacupuncture reduces the expression of proinflammatory cytokines in inflamed skin tissues through activation of cannabinoid CB2 receptors. Eur J Pain. 2012;16:624–35.
108. Zijlstra FJ, van den Berg-de Lange I, Huygen FJ, Klein J. Anti-inflammatory actions of acupuncture. Mediat Inflamm. 2003;12:59–69.
109. Zhu LX, Zhao FY, Cui RL. Effect of acupuncture on release of substance P. Ann N Y Acad Sci. 1991;632:488–9.

110. Fung PC. Probing the mystery of Chinese medicine meridian channels with special emphasis on the connective tissue interstitial fluid system, mechanotransduction, cells durotaxis and mast cell degranulation. Chin Med. 2009;4:10.
111. MacPherson H, Hammerschlag R, Coeytaux RR, et al. Unanticipated insights into biomedicine from the study of acupuncture. J Altern Complement Med. 2016;22:101–7.
112. Zhang R, Lao L, Ren K, Berman BM. Mechanisms of acupuncture-electroacupuncture on persistent pain. Anesthesiology. 2014;120:482–503.
113. Bardoni R, Takazawa T, Tong CK, Choudhury P, Scherrer G, et al. Pre- and postsynaptic inhibitory control in the spinal cord dorsal horn. Ann N Y Acad Sci. 2013;1279:90–6.
114. Yonehara N. Influence of serotonin receptor antagonists on substance P and serotonin release evoked by tooth pulp stimulation with electro-acupuncture in the trigeminal nucleus caudalis of the rabbit. Neurosci Res. 2001;40:45–51.
115. Mi W, Wang S, You Z, et al. Nortriptyline enhances morphine-conditioned place preference in neuropathic rats: role of the central noradrenergic system. Anesth Analg. 2017;125:1032–41.
116. Fuxe K, Borroto-Escuela DO, Romero-Fernandez W. Volume transmission and its different forms in the central nervous system. Chin J Integr Med. 2013;19:323–9.
117. Beaussier M, Sciard D, Sautet A. New modalities of pain treatment after outpatient orthopaedic surgery. Orthop Traumatol Surg Res. 2016;102(1 Suppl):S121–4.
118. Lau CH, Wu X, Chung VC, et al. Acupuncture and related therapies for symptom management in palliative cancer care: systematic review and meta-analysis. Medicine (Baltimore). 2016;95:e2901.
119. Chakravarthy K, Chaudhry H, Williams K, Christo PJ. Review of the uses of vagal nerve stimulation in chronic pain management. Curr Pain Headache Rep. 2015;19:54.
120. Napadow V, Edwards RR, Cahalan CM, et al. Evoked pain analgesia in chronic pelvic pain patients using respiratory-gated auricular vagal afferent nerve stimulation. Pain Med. 2012;13:777–89.
121. Yuan H, Silberstein SD. Vagus nerve stimulation and headache. Headache. 2017;57(Suppl 1):29–33.
122. Hays SA. Enhancing rehabilitative therapies with vagus nerve stimulation. Neurotherapeutics. 2016;13:382–94.
123. Verrier RL, Nearing BD, Olin B, Boon P, Schachter SC. Baseline elevation and reduction in cardiac electrical instability assessed by quantitative T-wave alternans in patients with drug-resistant epilepsy treated with vagus nerve stimulation in the AspireSR E-36 trial. Epilepsy Behav. 2016;62:85–9.
124. Engineer CT, Hays SA, Kilgard MP. Vagus nerve stimulation as a potential adjuvant to behavioral therapy for autism and other neurodevelopmental disorders. J Neurodev Disord. 2017;9:20.
125. Ekmekçi H, Hülagu Kaptan H. Vagus nerve stimulation. Open Access Maced J Med Sci. 2017;5:391–4.
126. Singh V, Manchikanti L, Calodney AK, et al. Percutaneous lumbar laser disc decompression: an update of current evidence. Pain Physician. 2013;16(2 Suppl):SE229–60.
127. Park CW, Lee JY, Choi WJ. Percutaneous disc coagulation therapy (PDCT) comparing with automated percutaneous lumbar discectomy (APLD) in patients of herniated lumbar disc disease: preliminary report. Korean J Spine. 2012;9:159–64.
128. Kim SH, Kim SC, Cho KH. Clinical outcomes of percutaneous plasma disc coagulation therapy for lumbar herniated disc diseases. J Korean Neurosurg Soc. 2012;51:8–13.
129. Bonaldi G. Automated percutaneous lumbar discectomy: technique, indications and clinical follow-up in over 1000 patients. Neuroradiology. 2003;45:735–43.
130. Botsford JA. Radiological considerations: patient selection for percutaneous laser disc decompression. J Clin Laser Med Surg. 1994;12:255–9.
131. Bressler HB, Keyes WJ, Rochon PA, Badley E. The prevalence of low back pain in the elderly. A systemic review of the literature. Spine. 1999;24:1813–9.

132. Cassidy JD, Carroll LJ, Cote P. The Saskatchewan health and back pain survey: the prevalence of low back pain and related disability in Saskatchewan adults. Spine. 1998;23:1860–7.
133. Choy DS. Percutaneous laser disc decompression (PLDD): twelve years' experience with 752 procedures in 518 patients. J Clin Laser Med Surg. 1998;16:325–31.
134. Abrishamkar S, Kouchakzadeh M. Mirhosseini a et al: comparison of open surgical discectomy versus plasma-laser nucleoplasty in patients with single lumbar disc herniation. J Res Med Sci. 2015;20:1133–7.
135. Kumar N, Zaw AS, Kumar N, et al. Annulo-nucleoplasty using disc-fx in the management of degenerative lumbar disc pathology: how long can the effect last? Global Spine J. 2018;8:365–73.
136. Jolesz FA. MRI-guided focused ultrasound surgery. Annu Rev Med. 2009;60:417–30.
137. Martínez-Fernández R, Rodríguez-Rojas R, Del Álamo M, et al. Focused ultrasound subthalamotomy in patients with asymmetric Parkinson's disease: a pilot study. Lancet Neurol. 2018;17:54–63.
138. Meng Y, Suppiah S, Mithani K, Solomon B, Schwartz ML, Lipsman N. Current and emerging brain applications of MR-guided focused ultrasound. J Ther Ultrasound. 2017;5:26.
139. Zaaroor M, Sinai A, Goldsher D. Magnetic resonance-guided focused ultrasound thalamotomy for tremor: a report of 30 Parkinson's disease and essential tremor cases. J Neurosurg. 2018;128:202–10.
140. Hindley J, Gedroyc WM, Regan L, et al. MRI guidance of focused ultrasound therapy of uterine fibroids: early results. AJR Am J Roentgenol. 2004;183:1713–9.
141. Clark NA, Mumford SL, Segars JH. Reproductive impact of MRI-guided focused ultrasound surgery for fibroids: a systematic review of the evidence. Curr Opin Obstet Gynecol. 2014;26:151–61.
142. Łoziński T, Filipowska J, Gurynowicz G, Gabriel I, Czekierdowski A. Non-invasive therapeutic use of high-intensity focused ultrasound (HIFU) with 3 tesla magnetic resonance imaging in women with symptomatic uterine fibroids. Ginekol Pol. 2017;88:497–503.
143. Lee HL, Kuo CC, Tsai JT, et al. Magnetic resonance-guided focused ultrasound versus conventional radiation therapy for painful bone metastasis: a matched-pair study. J Bone Joint Surg Am. 2017;99:1572–8.
144. Joo B, Park MS, Lee SH, et al. Pain palliation in patients with bone metastases using magnetic resonance-guided focused ultrasound with conformal bone system: a preliminary report. Yonsei Med J. 2015;56:503–9.
145. Barile A, Arrigoni F, Zugaro L, et al. Minimally invasive treatments of painful bone lesions: state of the art. Med Oncol. 2017;34:53.

Chapter 10
Pain Measurements

Koki Shimoji and Sumihisa Aida

10.1 Introduction

Can we measure pain intensity? As pain is a personal and subjective experience, it is influenced by various factors such as his or her own personal history, local culture, social situation, education, and psychological states of the patient.

Approaches to the measurement of pain have been approached by (1) verbal or numeric self-rating scales, (2) behavioral observation scales, and (3) physiologic variables, etc. The complex nature of the experience of pain, however, suggests that measurements from these variables may not always show high validity.

Patients' self-reports may provide the most valid measure of the pain experience at a usual outpatient clinical setting as compared with behavioral measurements including vital signs. In terms of pain dimension, unidimensional and multidimensional measurements are advocated. For instance, the visual analog scale (VAS), a unidimensional measurement, and the McGill Pain Questionnaire (MPQ), a multidimensional measurement, may be the most frequently used self-rating instruments for the measurement of pain in clinical settings.

The MPQ is designed to assess the multidimensional nature of pain experience and has been demonstrated to be a reliable, valid, and consistent measurement tool [1]. However, MPQ is somewhat time-consuming and not always easy to use at a very busy outpatient clinic. A short-form MPQ is developed for use when the time to obtain information from patients is limited [1], but still hard to use in a busy clinical setting.

K. Shimoji (✉)
Niigata University Graduate School of Medicine, Niigata, Japan

Pain Control Institute, Tokyo, Japan
e-mail: koki-shimoji@nifty.com

S. Aida
Department of Anesthesiology, International University of Health and Welfare Hospital, Otawara, Japan

K. Shimoji et al. (eds.), *Chronic Pain Management in General and Hospital Practice*, https://doi.org/10.1007/978-981-15-2933-7_10

When selecting a pain assessment tool, consideration should be given to the patient's age, physical, emotional, and cognitive status, and personal preferences. The pain tool selected should be used on a regular basis to assess pain and to monitor the effects of interventions. It should not, however, be used as the sole measure of pain as advocated by the Agency for Healthcare Research and Quality (AHRQ) and other investigators. Pain assessment tools should be quantitative, qualitative, and should also measure psychological factors reflected on distress or specific pain behaviors such as grimacing, muscle tension, protective movements, and even breathing. At present, there are no ideal scales to assess pain multidimensionally by a single number.

Further, although there have been reported various pain scales, there is no one-to- one relationship between the amount or type of pathophysiology and pain intensity. Particularly, the chronic pain experience is shaped by a myriad of biomedical, psychosocial, and behavioral factors. Assessing each of these three domains through a comprehensive evaluation of the person with chronic pain is essential for treatment decisions and to facilitate optimal treatments [2].

Behavioral approaches to the measurement of pain may also provide valuable data. Descriptor differential scale (DDS) was also developed using sophisticated psychophysical techniques and was designed to measure separately the sensory and unpleasantness dimensions of pain [3]. Although DDS has also been shown to be a valid and reliable measurement of pain with ratio-scaling properties applying psychophysical principles, it has not been used frequently in a clinical setting, seemingly because of time-consuming. Further development and refinement of pain measurement techniques will lead to increasingly accurate tools with greater predictive powers.

10.2 Unidimensional Measures

10.2.1 Visual Analog Scale (VAS)

The VAS is a unidimensional measure of pain intensity [1], which has been widely used in almost all adult patients [1].

The VAS is a continuous scale comprised of a horizontal (HVAS) or vertical (VVAS) line, usually 10 cm (100 mm) in length, anchored by 2 verbal descriptors, one for each symptom extreme [4, 5].

The scale is most commonly determined by "no pain" (score of 0) and "worst imaginable pain" (score of 100 [100-mm scale]) for pain intensity [6].

Respondents or patients are asked to report "current pain intensity" or "pain intensity in the last 24 hours" and asked to place a line perpendicular to the VAS line at the point that represents their pain intensity [4, 7, 8] (Fig. 10.1).

The VAS is available in the public domain at no cost, and its graphic formats may be obtained from Drs Scott & Huskisson or online: http://www.amda.com/tools/library/whitepapers/hospiceinltc/appendix-a.pdf.

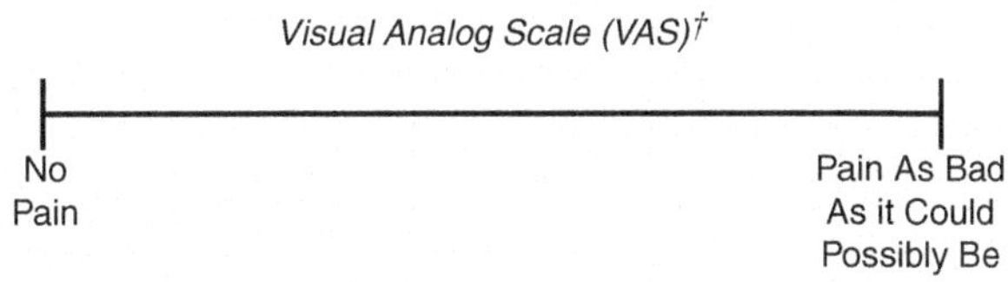

Fig. 10.1 The visual analog scale. The left end point (0) corresponds to "no pain" and the right end point (100) is defined as "pain as intense as it can be." †A 10-cm baseline is recommended for VAS scales. (Source: Adopted from Public domain)

Using a ruler, the score is determined by measuring the distance (mm) on the 10-cm line between the "no pain" (0 mm) and the patient's mark. The VAS is measured on a paper, and thus cannot be administered verbally or by phone.

The VAS was originally developed in the field of psychology to measure well-being [9]. Hayes and Patterson [10] was the first to use the VAS scales for determining the worker's mood.

Woodforde and Merskey [11] first reported the use of the VAS pain scale with the descriptor extremes "no pain at all" and "my pain is as bad as it could possibly be" in patients with a variety of pain.

Older patients with cognitive impairment may have difficulty understanding or completing the scale [12–14], and may need supervision during completion [15]. The patients with motor diseases may also have difficulty to complete the VAS.

The VAS has been shown to be highly correlated with a verbal descriptive scale and numerical rating scale [16, 17].

The VAS has demonstrated to be sensitive to changes in pain assessed hourly for a maximum of 4 h and weekly for up to 4 weeks following analgesic therapy in patients with chronic inflammatory or degenerative joint pain [8]. Minimal clinically significant change has been estimated as 1.1 points on the VAS scale in patients with rheumatoid arthritis [18], while a minimum clinically important difference of 1.37 cm has been determined in patients with rotator cuff disease evaluated after 6 weeks of non-operative treatment [19].

Older patients, however, may have difficulty completing the VAS due to cognitive or motor impairments. Thus, scoring in the VAS is more complicated than that in the numeric rating scale (NRS) as described below, and it cannot be administered by telephone [20].

10.2.2 Numeric Rating Scale (NRS)

The NRS is a numeric version of the visual analog scale (VAS). The respondent selects a number from the whole number (from 0 to 10) that best reflects the intensity of the respondent's pain [21]. The common format is a horizontal bar or line, similar to the VAS [12, 13, 16, 21]. A 11-point numeric scale with 0 representing "no pain" and 10 representing "worst pain imaginable." Respondents are asked to report pain intensity "in the last 24 h" or average pain intensity [22].

The NRS can be administered verbally, by telephone or graphically [13]. The number that the respondent indicates on the scale to rate their pain intensity is recorded, ranging from 0 to10.

High reliability between the tests has been observed in both literate and illiterate patients with rheumatoid arthritis before and after medical consultation [23]. The NRS was shown to be highly correlated to the VAS in patients with various chronic pain conditions [23].

Like the VAS, however, the NRS is inadequate in capturing the complexity and idiosyncratic nature of the pain experience or improvements due to symptom fluctuations in the patients with chronic back pain and/or symptomatic hip and knee osteoarthritis (OA) [24, 25].

Analyses of the relationships between changes in NRS scores and patient reports of overall improvement, measured using a standard 7-point patient global impression of change, demonstrated a reduction of two points, or 30%, on the NRS scores were found to be clinically important in clinical trials of pregabalin for diabetic neuropathy, postherpetic neuralgia, chronic low back pain, fibromyalgia, and osteoarthritis [26]. Similar results were found in low back pain patients when changes in NRS scores were compared to patient improvements in pain after physical therapy, using a 15-point Global Rating of Change scale [27, 28].

The NRS is a valid and reliable scale to measure pain intensity. Advantages of this measure over the VAS are its ability to be provided verbally (or by telephone) or in writing, and also its simplicity of scoring. However, similar to the VAS, the NRS evaluates only one component of the pain experience, pain intensity, and therefore does not express the complexity and idiosyncratic nature of pain or symptom fluctuations.

As compared with VAS and verbal rating scale (VRS), NRSs are applicable for unidimensional assessment of pain intensity in most settings [29] (Fig. 10.2).

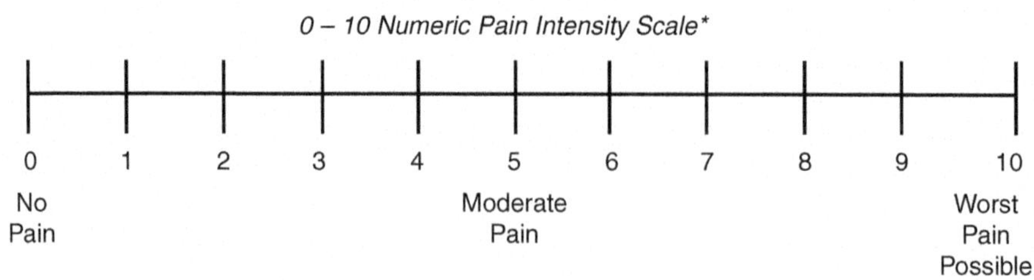

Fig. 10.2 The numeric rating scale. Indicated for adults and children (>9 years old) in all patient care settings in which patients are able to use numbers to rate the intensity of their pain. The NRS consists of a straight horizontal line numbered at equal intervals from 0 to 10 with anchor words of "no pain," "moderate pain," and "worst pain." (Source: Adapted from Acute Pain Management Guideline Panel 1992; AHCPR 1994, Adopted from Public domain)

10.2.3 Verbal Rating Scale

The verbal rating scale (VRS) is simple, and classifies pain as no pain, mild, moderate, or severe. Some studies indicate that older adults prefer to characterize their pain using the VRS. The description can be translated to a number for charting and works particularly well if everyone on the unit uses the same scale (Table 10.1, Fig. 10.3). For simplicity patients prefer the verbal rating scale, but it lacks sensitivity and the data it produces can be misunderstood [17]. Pearson correlation coefficient and p value were demonstrated to show excellent correlation between the VRS and VAS although VRS showed a tendency to be higher than VAS [30].

Another study indicated that two-thirds of the individual subjects had significant correlations between the VRS and VAS with a mean of 0.68. The one-third of the subjects who did not have significant correlations also had significantly less variability in their ratings than did subjects with significant correlations [31].

The use of the VRS was the most successful with cognitively impaired group, completed by most respondents with moderately impaired, and by some of even those with severe cognitive impairment [32].

The VRS might also be reliable for assessment of pain after surgery. However, the validity of intermittent questioning about possible change in pain intensity may not be valid [33].

It was shown that although the relatively high Spearman correlations between original VAS and VRS were found, the low ordinal association and low probability of agreement between discrete VAS and VRS [34]. Thus, VAS and VRS should not be used interchangeably in the clinical setting or for increased statistical power in pain research.

Table 10.1 Verbal rating scale expressed in number

Verbal rating scale	
Description	Points assigned
No pain	0
Mild pain	2
Moderate	5
Severe	10

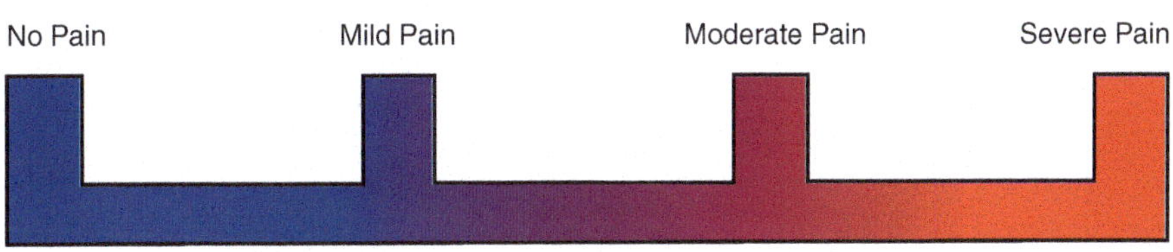

Fig. 10.3 Verbal rating scale in table and color (adopted from public domain)

10.2.4 Verbal Descriptor Scale: Pain Thermometer (Modified Method of VRS)

The Pain Thermometer (PT), a modified vertical VDS (or called VRS) alongside a graphic thermometer, has also been validated as a measure for pain in older adults [35] (Fig. 10.4).

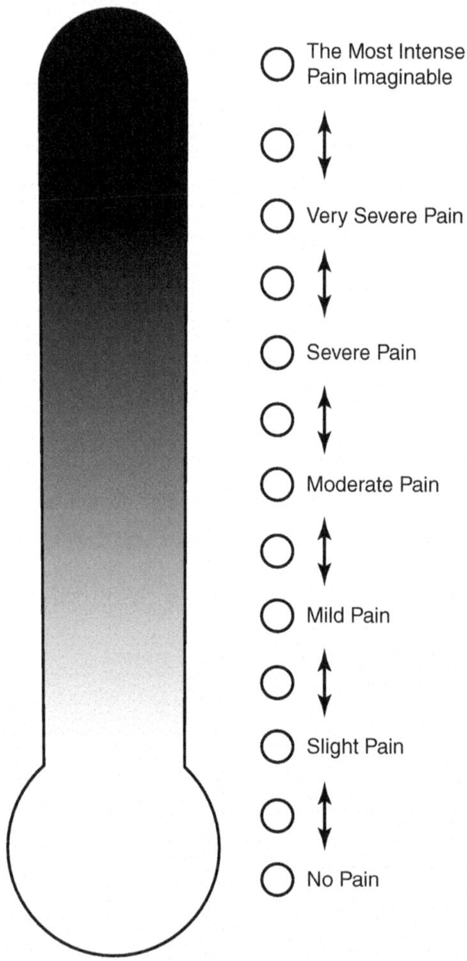

Fig. 10.4 Iowa pain thermometer (printed with permission from Dr. Keela Herr, The University of Iowa)

10.2.5 The Faces Pain Scale (FPS) and Revised Scales

The Faces Pain Scale (FPS) [36] is a self-report measure used also to assess the intensity of children's pain, showing them the pictures of faces, which express no pain to severe pain. Three studies were carried out to revise the original scale and validate the adapted version. In the first phase, the FPS was revised from its original seven faces to six, while maintaining its desirable psychometric properties, in order to make it compatible in scoring with other self-rating and observational scales which use a common metric (0–5 or 0–10). Using a computer-animated version of the FPS developed by Champion and colleagues (Sydney Animated Facial Expressions Scale) [37], psychophysical methods were applied to identify four faces representing equal intervals between the scale values representing least pain and most pain.

In the second phase, children used the new six-face Faces Pain Scale-Revised (FPS-R) to rate the intensity of pain from ear piercing. Its validity is supported by a strong positive correlation ($r = 0.93$, $N = 76$) with a visual analog scale (VAS) measure in children aged 5–12 years [37].

In the third phase, a clinical sample of pediatric inpatients aged 4–12 years used the FPS-R and a VAS or the colored analog scale (CAS) to rate pain during hospitalization for surgical and non-surgical painful conditions. The validity of the FPS-R was further supported by strong positive correlations with the VAS [38].

The FPS-R is shown to be appropriate for use in assessment of the intensity of children's acute pain from age 4 or 5 onward. It has the advantage of being suitable for use with the most widely used metric for scoring (0–10) and related closely to a linear interval scale [37].

Children's ability to describe pain increases with age and experience, and changes throughout their developmental stages. Therefore, the self-report of pain by numeric scales, pictorial scales, or verbal scales should be used appropriately depending on age [39].

There are a large number of self-report measures of pediatric pain intensity; and there is some agreement that professionals in the clinical and research practice should assess pain intensity using the Pieces of Hurt Tool, the Faces Pain Scale, or Visual Analog Scales because these measures have shown to have sound psychometric properties and clinical utility [40].

No single observational measure is broadly recommended for pain assessment across all contexts [38].

In children, three main methods are currently used to measure pain intensity: (1) self-reporting, (2) behavioral measures, (3) physiologic measures.

Nonverbal behaviors such as facial expression, limb movement, grasping, holding, and crying are considered more reliable and objective measures of pain than self-reports [39].

Most 2-year-old children can report the incidence and location of pain, but do not have the adequate cognitive skills to describe its severity. Three-year-old children can start to differentiate the severity of pain and are able to use a three-level pain intensity scale with simple terms like "no pain," "a little pain," or "a lot." [39]. By the age of 4 years, most children are able to use 4- to 5-item pain discrimination scales. Their ability to recognize the influence of pain appears around the age of 5 years, when they are able to rate the intensity of pain. Facial expression scales are most commonly used with this age group to obtain self-reports of pain. These scales require children to point to the face that represents how they feel or the amount of pain they are experiencing.

In school-aged children, healthcare professionals usually depend on self-reports of pain. Although children at this age understand pain, their use of language to report it is different from adults.

Adolescents tend to minimize or even deny pain, so it is important to provide them with privacy and choice. They may or may not choose to have parents or friends present during an examination. To assess pain, specifically chronic pain, the Adolescent Pediatric Pain Tool (APPT) or the McGill Pain Questionnaire may be helpful [39].

10.3 Multidimensional Measures

10.3.1 McGill Pain Questionnaire (MPQ)

Its purpose is to measure the different qualities of the subjective pain experience [41]. Three classes of words (total of 78) that describe the sensory, affective, and evaluative aspects of pain, and a 5-point pain intensity scale (present pain intensity [PPI]).

There are 20 subclasses, each containing two to six words, and one pain intensity scale consisting of one item. Pain Rating Index (PRI) contains four subscales (sensory, affective, evaluative, and a miscellaneous category) (Table 10.2).

The questionnaire was developed for use in adult populations with a variety of chronic pain problems.

The respondent is given the questionnaire with the words grouped into 20 subclasses. An interviewer then instructs respondents to choose one word from each subclass if a word within that class fits their present pain. If no word fits, then no word should be chosen from that subclass. The interviewer defines any words that the respondent does not understand.

Thus, the interviewer must be able to define each word. Time to administer/complete is 5–15 min. Equipment needed are pencil and paper.

Table 10.2 McGill Pain Questionnaires (reproduced with permission from Dr. Merzack R)

McGill-Metzack Pain Questionnaire

Patient's Name ______ Date ______ Time ______ am/pm
Analgesic(S) ______ Dosage ______ Time Given ______ am/pm
______ Dosage ______ Time Given ______ am/pm

Analgesic Time Difference (hours): +4 +1 +2 +3

PRI: S ______ (1-10) A ______ (11-15) E ______ (16) M(S) ______ (17-19) M(AE) ______ (20) M(T) ______ (17-20) PRT(T) ______ (1-20)

1 FLICKERING, QUIVERING, PULSING, THROBBING, BEATING, POUNDING	11 TRING, EXHAUSTING
2 JUMBING, FLASHING, SHOOTING	12 SICKENING, SUFFOCATING
3 PRICKING, BORING, DRILLING, STABBING, LANCINATING	13 FEARFUL, FRIGHTFUL, TERRIFYING
4 SHARP, CUTTING, LACERATING	14 PUNISHING, GRUELING, CRUEL, VICIOUS, KILLING
5 PINCHING, PRESSING, GNAWING, CRAMPING, CRUSHING	15 WRETCHED, BLINDING
6 TUGGING, PULLING, WRENCHING	16 ANNOYING, TROUBLESOME, MISERABLE, INTENSE, UNBEARABLE
7 HOT, BURNING, SCALDING, SEARING	17 SPREADING, RADIATING, PENETRATING, PIERCING
8 TINGLING, ITCHY, SMARTING, STINGING	18 TIGHT, NUMB, DRAWING, SQUEEZING, TEARING
9 DULL, SORE, HURTING, ACHING, HEAVY	19 COOL, COLD, FREEZING
10 TENDER, TAUT, RASPING, SPLITTING	20 NAGGING, NAUSEATING, AGONIZING, DREADFUL, TORTURING
	PPI: 0 No pain, 1 MILD, 2 DISCOMFORTING, 3 DISTREASSING, 4 HORRIBLE, 5 EXCRUCIATING

PPI ______ COMMENTS:

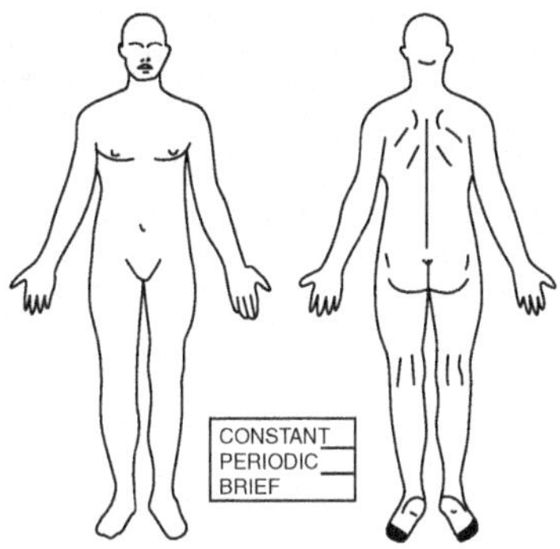

CONSTANT ___
PERIODIC ___
BRIEF ___

ACCOMPANYING SYMPTOMS:	SLEEP:	FOOD INTAKE:
NAUSEA	GOOD	GOOD
HEADACHE	FITFUL	SOME
DIZZINESS	CAN'T SLEEP	LITTLE
DROWSINESS	COMMENTS:	NONE
CONSTIPATION		COMMENTS:
DIARRHEA		
COMMENTS:	ACTIVITY: GOOD, SOME, LITTLE, NONE	COMMENTS:

Key:
PPI = present pain intensity
PRI = pain rating index
S = sensory components of pain
A = affective, or emotional, components of pain
E = evaluative terms
M = miscellaneous terms

Combinations of words can be identified: M(S) and M(AE) and the entire number totaled: PRI(T). (Copyright 1970. Ronald Melzack)

The MPQ is available at no cost from the author, and also available online at http://www.qolid.org by paying a membership fee.

Each word within the PRI has an assigned value based on its placement within the subclass. The PPI is a 5-point scale. Scores on the PRI can range from 0 to 20 words chosen (number of words chosen [NWC]), 0–78 for the total score based on rank value. Scores on the PPI can range from 0 to 5.

The PRI is interpreted both in terms of quantity of pain as evidenced by the number of words used and the rank values of the words, as well as the quality of pain as evidenced by the particular words that are selected. A meta-analysis [42] concluded that normative scores across painful conditions range from 24% to 50% of the maximum scores.

The MPQ is scored by hand by first counting the number of words used to obtain a total word score (number of words chosen). Then the rank values of the words chosen are summed to give a total PRI score and scores on each of the four subscales. The PPI is scored by noting the number-word combination chosen by the respondent. The time to score is within 2 min.

Retest over 3–7 days showed that respondents tended to choose the same words in the PRI and report the same PPI level.

Validity is indicated by respondents' tendency to use all 20 subclasses of pain words. It was found that arthritis patients used similar sets of words to describe their pain and that a substantial affective dimension underlies their responses [43].

Early work by Melzack [41] indicated that the MPQ was sensitive to change as a result of biofeedback or hypnotic training. Language versions other than English may not match exactly the words on the original English version. Therefore, one must be cautious about comparing populations across language and cultural groups. The MPQ requires a fairly sophisticated vocabulary and may not be appropriate for low literacy respondents. Research on both adults and children indicates that there may be sex and ethnic differences in the selection of pain descriptors [44].

The McGill Pain Questionnaire asks patients to describe subjective psychological feelings of pain. More than 70 pain descriptors such as pulsing, shooting, stabbing, burning, grueling, radiating, and agonizing are grouped together to convey a patient's pain response.

The questionnaire combines questions about the nature and frequency of pain with a body-map diagram to pinpoint its location. It uses word lists separated into four classes (sensory, affective, evaluative, and miscellaneous) to assess the total pain experience. Patients rate their pain words and the administrator allocates a numerical score, called the "Pain Rating Index" [45]. Scores vary from 0 to 78, with the higher score indicating greater pain.

10.3.2 Short-Form McGill Pain Questionnaire (SF-MPQ)

The SF-MPQ is a multidimensional measure of perceived pain in adults with chronic pain [43, 45]. The SF-MPQ is comprised of 15 words (11 sensory and 4 affective) from the original MPQ [45].

The Pain Rating Index is comprised of two subscales: (1) sensory subscale with 11 words or items and (2) affective subscale with four words or items, which are rated on an intensity scale as 0 = none, 1 = mild, 2 = moderate, or 3 = severe. The SF-MPQ also includes one item for present pain intensity and one item for a 10-cm visual analog scale (VAS) for average pain. It is valuable to discriminate among different pain syndromes [46] and evaluate the responsiveness of different symptoms to treatment [47–49].

Thus, each selected word is scored from 0 (none) to 3 (severe) for the Pain Rating Index. The total Pain Rating Index score is obtained by summing the item scores (range 0–45). Scores on the Present Pain Intensity range from 0 to 5 and on the VAS from 0 to 10.

Some difficulties in completing the scale have been reported and attributed to unfamiliar descriptors and unclear written instructions. However, experience in completing the SF-MPQ and verbal instructions improved completion in patients with osteoarthritis (OA), low back pain and also, in patients with several other diseases in different cultures.

For internal consistency, using the SF-MPQ in rheumatoid arthritis (RA) and fibromyalgia patients, Cronbach's alphas were estimated at 0.73–0.89 (acceptable to good number) but ranged from 0.45 to 0.73 for 1-month and 3-month intervals. Among rheumatic patients, test–retest reliability was 0.79–0.93 at intervals of 1–3 days, and high intraclass correlations were demonstrated for the total, sensory, affective, and average pain scores (5-day period): 0.96, 0.95, 0.88, and 0.89, respectively, in an OA population [50].

Although designed for descriptive purposes, the SF-MPQ has been found to be sensitive to the effects of pain therapies in a variety of population settings [51–53].

The SF-MPQ is easier to use and takes less time to administer and complete than the original longer form. The word choices are not as complex, and the intensity ranking of mild, moderate, and severe is better understood by patients [45]. However, sufficient experience is required to adequately complete the SF-MPQ. Therefore, new users require supervision during completion [50].

The short form was further revised for use in neuropathic and non-neuropathic pain conditions (SF-MPQ-2) [54]. The SF-MPQ-2 includes seven additional symptoms relevant to neuropathic pain, for a total of 22 items with 0–10 numerical response options.

The SF-MPQ-2 has demonstrated excellent reliability and validity in a sample of patients with chronic neuropathic, non-neuropathic pain [55], and acute low back pain [54]. The SF-MPQ-2 has also been found to be valid in respondents with different cultures [56–60]. Further psychometric testing of this revised measure remains awaited, which may play a useful role with respect to identifying neuropathic versus nociceptive pain.

10.3.3 Brief Pain Inventory (BPI)

The Brief Pain Inventory (BPI) was developed by the Pain Research Group of the WHO Collaborating Centre for Symptom Evaluation in Cancer Care [61].

The ability to resume activity, maintain a positive affect or mood, and sleep are relevant functions for patients. The BPI uses a numeric rating scale to assess difficulties with walking, general activity, mood, and sleep.

The Brief Pain Inventory–Short Form (BPI-sf) is a 9-item self-administered questionnaire used to evaluate the severity of a patient's pain and the impact of this pain on the patient's daily functioning. The patient is asked to rate their worst, least, average, and current pain intensity, list current treatments and their perceived effectiveness, and rate the degree that pain interferes with general activity, mood, walking ability, normal work, relations with other persons, sleep, and enjoyment of life on a 10-point scale [62].

The BPI-sf is a modification of the Brief Pain Inventory (Long Form), which includes additional questions on demographics (date of birth, marital status, education, employment), pain history, aggravating and easing factors, treatment and medication, pain quality, and response to treatment. The brevity of the BPI-sf makes it suitable for settings in which pain is assessed on a daily basis (e.g., in a randomized control trial), whereas the long-form may be more appropriate as a baseline measure.

The questionnaire exists within the biopsychosocial model of pain, as it addresses sensory, emotional, and functional aspects of the pain experience [62]. Thus, the tool is responsive to changes in pain associated with both pharmacological, physical, and psychological interventions [63].

Originally intended for use in epidemiological studies and clinical trials involving patients with cancer-related pain, the BPI-sf is now widely used in a range of chronic cancer-related and non-malignant pain conditions, including HIV/AIDS, phantom limb pain, critical limb ischemia, neuropathy, low back pain, and osteoarthritis. The tool has also been used to assess individuals experiencing nonmalignant or acute pain and has been translated into numerous languages [64]. The questionnaire can be completed via self-report or interview. The short form version takes 5 min for the patient to complete.

The psychometric properties of the tool have been analyzed in a range of populations with cancer and non-cancer related pain. Acceptable reliability has been reported in studies of patients with advanced cancer pain [65, 66], osteoarthritis pain [67, 68], postoperative pain [69], chronic pain in neuropathic and nociceptive pain patients [70].

A number of studies have utilized a confirmatory factor approach (CFA) to determine the construct validity of the BPI. A three-factor representation (pain intensity, activity interference, and affective interference) was compared with a two-factor (pain intensity, activity interference) and one-factor (pain intensity) approach. Both two- and three-factor representations in the HIV/AIDS and cancer populations were supported by Atkinson and colleagues [71]. Other reports showed that a two-factor model had greater validity for patients with non-cancer pain, including arthritis, back/neck pain, injury-/trauma-related pain, neuropathic pain, and fibromyalgia-related pain [64, 72].

The BPI has also been utilized for the influence of non-cancer pain on quality of life measures [73, 74] (Table 10.3).

10.3.4 Simple Combination Method (VAS + ADL)

Combined evaluation of pain by VAS or NRS and pain relief score of activities of daily life (ADL) by observers (PRSO) have been also advocated [76].

In 56 patients with severe chronic pain, pain relief was evaluated by observation of changes in activities of daily life (ADL), drug intake, and patients' mood. The

Table 10.3 Brief pain inventory—short form (permission from Cleeland [75], AACR)

Date: ______________ **Study ID:** ______________

Hospital: ______________

Brief Pain Inventory (Short Form)

1. **Throughout our lives, most of us have had pain from time to time (such as minor headaches, sprains, and toothaches). Have you had pain other than these everyday kinds of pain today?**

   ☐ Yes ☐ No

2. **On the diagram, shade in the areas where you feel pain. Put an X on the area that hurts the most.**

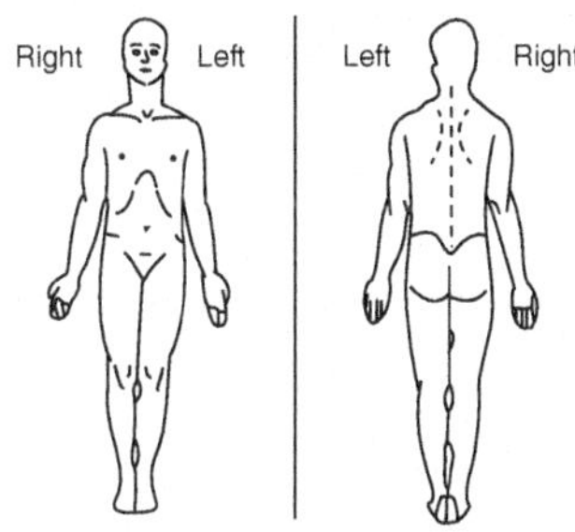

3. **Please rate your pain by marking the box beside the number that best describes your pain at its <u>worst</u> in the last 24 hours.**

   ☐ 0 ☐ 1 ☐ 2 ☐ 3 ☐ 4 ☐ 5 ☐ 6 ☐ 7 ☐ 8 ☐ 9 ☐ 10

   No Pain — Pain As Bad As You Can Imagine

4. **Please rate your pain by marking the box beside the number that best describes your pain at its <u>least</u> in the last 24 hours.**

   ☐ 0 ☐ 1 ☐ 2 ☐ 3 ☐ 4 ☐ 5 ☐ 6 ☐ 7 ☐ 8 ☐ 9 ☐ 10

   No Pain — Pain As Bad As You Can Imagine

5. **Please rate your pain by marking the box beside the number that best describes your pain on the <u>average.</u>**

   ☐ 0 ☐ 1 ☐ 2 ☐ 3 ☐ 4 ☐ 5 ☐ 6 ☐ 7 ☐ 8 ☐ 9 ☐ 10

   No Pain — Pain As Bad As You Can Imagine

6. **Please rate your pain by marking the box beside the number that tells how much pain you have <u>right now.</u>**

   ☐ 0 ☐ 1 ☐ 2 ☐ 3 ☐ 4 ☐ 5 ☐ 6 ☐ 7 ☐ 8 ☐ 9 ☐ 10

   No Pain — Pain As Bad As You Can Imagine

Page 1 of 2

degree of pain relief was scored on the basis of these evaluations by a pain clinic physician, a nurse, and a member of the patient's family. The resulting score was termed "pain relief score by observers" (PRSO). Subjective pain relief was evaluated by the visual analog scale (VAS). Although a significant correlation was demonstrated between the mean VAS and PRSO values, there was some dissociation between the two values in patients with underlying personal problems such as compensation lawsuits or job loss. The results suggest that an objective evaluation of pain relief is possible by PRSO alone without subjective assessment, and that PRSO can be used for patients with various types of pain. This simple combined assessment of pain relief by the VAS and PRSO methods may be useful to detect the influence of personal background factors in patients with chronic pain.

10.3.5 Chronic Pain Grade Scale (CPGS)

The CPGS is a multidimensional measure that assesses two dimensions of overall chronic pain severity: pain intensity and pain-related disability. It is suitable for use in all chronic pain conditions, including chronic musculoskeletal (MSK) and low back pain [77].

Subscale scores for pain intensity and disability are combined to calculate a chronic pain grade that enables classification of chronic pain patients into five hierarchical categories: grades 0 (no pain) to IV (high disability-severely limiting).

The CPGS is comprised of seven items. All items are scored on a 11-point Likert scale, with responses ranging from 0 to 10. Recall period for items is in the past 3–6 months.

The CPGS has been used in epidemiologic studies and clinical trials to evaluate and compare pain severity across groups and in response to treatment effects, and in clinical practice to improve the prognostic judgments of physicians [78].

The scale is available in the original reference [77] as well as directly from the author. The CPGS is an interview administered questionnaire that can also be self-completed by respondents (Table 10.4).

Scores are calculated for three subscales: (1) the characteristic pain intensity score, which ranges from 0 to 100, is calculated as the mean intensity ratings for reported current, worst, and average pain; (2) the disability score, which ranges from 0 to 100, is calculated as the mean rating for difficulty performing daily, social, and work activities; (3) the disability points score, which ranges from 0 to 3, is derived from a combination of ranked categories of number of disability days and disability score.

The four subscale scores (characteristic pain intensity, disability score, and the disability points score) are used to classify subjects into one of the 5 pain severity grades: grade 0 for no pain, grade I for low disability-low intensity, grade II for low disability-high intensity, grade III for high disability-moderately limiting, and grade IV for high disability-severely limiting.

The CPGS is easy to administer and time to complete the CPGS may not exceed 10 min.

The CPGS has originally been adapted into England [79] and an Italian version has been developed to evaluate severity in chronic pain patients [80].

Interviews were conducted with primary care patients with back pain, headache, and temporo-mandibular disorder [77]. The development of the graded classifica-

Table 10.4 Chronic pain grade scale

Appendix A

Graded Chronic Pain Scale

1. On how many days in the last six months have had [ANATOMICAL SITE] pain?

PAIN DAYS

___ ___ ___

IF PAIN NOT PRESENT IN THE PRIOR SIX MONTHS, SKIP THE REMAINING QUESTIONS

2. How would you rate your *[ANATOMICAL SITE]* pain on a 0 to 10 scale at the present time, that is right now, where 0 is “no pain” and 10 is “pain as bad as could be”?

NO PAIN										PAIN AS BAD COULD BE
0	1	2	3	4	5	6	7	8	9	10

3. In the past six months (or three months), how intense was your worst pain rated on a 0 to 10 scale where 0 is “no pain” and 10 is “pain as bad as could be”?

NO PAIN										PAIN AS BAD COULD BE
0	1	2	3	4	5	6	7	8	9	10

4. In the past six months (or three months), on the average, how intense was your pain rated on a 0 to 10 scale where 0 is “no pain” and 10 is “pain as bad as could be”? [That is, your usal pain at times you were experiencing pain].

NO PAIN										PAIN AS BAD COULD BE
0	1	2	3	4	5	6	7	8	9	10

5. About how many days in the last six months (or three months) have you been kept from your usal activities (work, school or housework) becase of *[ANATOMICAL SITE]* pain?

DISABILTY DAYS

___ ___ ___

6. In the past six months (or three months), how much has *[ANATOMICAL SITE]* pain interfered with your daily activities rated on a 0 to 10 scale where 0 is “no interference” and 10 is “unable to carry on any activities”?

NO INTERFERENCE										UNABLE TO CARRY ON ANY ACTIVITIES
0	1	2	3	4	5	6	7	8	9	10

7. In the past six months (or three months), how much has *[ANATOMICAL SITE]* pain interfered with your ablity to take part in recreational,social and family activities where 0 is “no interference” and 10 is “unable to carry on any activities”?

NO INTERFERENCE										UNABLE TO CARRY ON ANY ACTIVITIES
0	1	2	3	4	5	6	7	8	9	10

8. In the past six months (or three months), how much has *[ANATOMICAL SITE]* pain interfered with your ablity to work (including house work) where 0 is “no interference” and 10 is “unable to carry on any activities”?

NO INTERFERENCE										UNABLE TO CARRY ON ANY ACTIVITIES
0	1	2	3	4	5	6	7	8	9	10

tion drew on concepts by Turk and Rudy of chronic pain severity [81, 82]. Two of the items used in the disability score were adapted from their Multidimensional Pain Inventory [83]. The Guttman scaling[1] [84] method was used to develop the graded classification of chronic pain.

---

[1] Guttman scaling is a method of scale construction developed by Louis Guttman in 1944. Widely used in the measurement of attitudes and public opinion, the goal of Guttman scaling is to establish unidimensional measurement instruments. A typical Guttman scale includes a series of items or statements tapping progressively higher levels of a single attribute.

The CPGS is easy to understand and complete based on a high response rate (76.3%) to a postal survey sent to general practice patients in the UK [79]. Among musculoskeletal (MSK) chronic pain patients, missing values were only noted in <3% of each of the questions in an Italian version of the CPGS [85].

For internal consistency, the internal consistency was shown to be within acceptable (Cronbach's alpha, 0.74) among patients with chronic back pain [77]. In an Italian version of CPGS, the internal consistency was noted to be good (Cronbach's alpha ranged from 0.81 to 0.89) for subscales and global scores in patients with chronic MSK pain [80]. Test–retest reliability was found to be high after a 2-week interval (weighted 0.81) in patients with low back pain [86].

Comparisons of CPGS scores with the Short Form 36 Health Survey (SF-36) indicate that a higher chronic pain grade using the CPGS is associated with poorer physical, psychological, social, and general health as measured by the SF-36 ($P < 0.001$) [87] and worse scores on the SF-36 bodily pain scale [80]. Spearman's correlation coefficients for the CPGS scores and the various dimensions of SF-36 were highest for the pain dimension and lowest for the mental health dimension [79].

The CPGS is a valid and reliable tool that is useful for the evaluation of chronic musculoskeletal (MSK) pain. It allows for grading of the global severity of chronic pain and therefore analysis of the qualitative changes in chronic pain over time. The CPGS assesses not only aspects of the pain itself, but also the impact of the pain on daily, social, and work activities, which may be a significant advantage over many other pain questionnaires. A limitation of the CPGS relative to the other scales is the complexity of scoring.

10.3.6 The West Haven-Yale Multidimensional Pain Inventory (WHYMPI)

The West Haven-Yale Multidimensional Pain Inventory (WHYMPI) was developed by Kerns RD et al. [83] in order to fill a widely recognized void in the assessment of clinical pain. Assets of the inventory are its brevity and clarity, its foundation in contemporary psychological theory, its multidimensional focus, and its strong psychometric properties. Three parts of the inventory, comprised of 12 scales, examine the impact of pain on the patients' lives, the responses of others to the patients' communications of pain, and the extent to which patients participate in common daily activities. The instrument is recommended for use in conjunction with behavioral and psychophysiological assessment strategies in the evaluation of chronic pain patients in clinical settings.

Reliability tests in the Swedish version of the WHYMPI showed Cronbach's alpha ranging from 0.68 to 0.93 (internal consistency: from questionable to excellent) [88]. The Turkish version of WHYMPI was shown to be reliable and valid for the measurement of pain in patients with cancer [89], while the reliability and validity of its German version were shown to be variable in chronic pain patients [90].

The further findings additionally supported the value of the WHYMPI for multiple theoretical perspectives such as the stress appraisal and attentional models in research and clinical applications [91] but not for the early clinical course of recurrent and persistent low back pain in chiropractic patients [92].

10.3.7 Short Form 36 Bodily Pain Scale (SF-36 BPS)

The SF-36 BPS is one of the eight subscales of the Medical Outcomes Study SF-36 questionnaire, a generic measure of health status designed for use in population surveys vitality, physical functioning, bodily pain, general health perceptions, physical role functioning, emotional role functioning, social role functioning, mental health [93, 94].

In 1996, version 2.0 of the SF-36 (SF-36v2) was introduced to correct deficiencies identified in the original version, SF-36v1; the 2-item SF-36 BPS subscale assesses bodily pain as a dimension of health status [95]. The SF-36 BPS assesses bodily pain intensity and interference of pain with normal activities.

Intensity of bodily pain is evaluated using a 6-point rating scale of "none" to "very severe." The extent to which pain has interfered with work is evaluated on a 5-point rating scale from "not at all" to "extremely." The SF-36 BPS is available in both standard (4 week) and acute (1 week) recall versions [93]. The SF-36 and its subscales, including the BPS, have been used in epidemiologic studies to compare health status across populations and within population subgroups, such as in estimating the relative burden of different diseases, and differentiating the health benefits of different treatments [95].

The SF-36 and its various versions have been developed by the Rand Corporation and John E. Ware (SF-36 Health Survey, The Health Institute, New England Medical Center Hospitals, Box 345, 750 Washington Street, Boston, MA, 02111). The Medical Outcomes Trust, Health Assessment Lab, and Quality Metric Incorporated are copyright holders of all SF-36 and SF-12 surveys. All SF-36 survey instruments, scoring manuals, and licenses for use are available from QualityMetric at www.qualitymetric.com. Different charges are levied for academic and commercial use.

The SF-36 BPS is suitable for self-administration, computerized administration, or administration by a trained interviewer in person or by telephone. Telephone voice recognition interactive systems and online administrations are currently being evaluated [96]. Responses for each of the 2 SF-36 BPS items are recoded into final item values. The raw scale score is computed as a simple algebraic sum of the recoded item values. The raw scale score is then transformed to a 0–100 scale. Norm-based scores may be calculated for SF-36v2 by including population normative data in the scoring algorithms. The BPS score is only calculated if both items are completed.

SF-36v1 BPS scores range from 0 to 100. A higher score indicates lack of bodily pain. SF-36v2 uses norm-based scoring, where 50 is the "average" for the population. Therefore, scores above or below 50 can be considered above or below, respectively, the population average health status for bodily pain, and scores can be interpreted based on deviance from the mean.

SF-36 has been translated and adapted for use in more than 50 countries as part of the International Quality of Life Assessment (IQOLA) Project.

Information about translations is available from the IQOLA Program of the Health Assessment Lab in Boston, Massachusetts (http://www.iqola.org).

SF-36 is generally easy to administer and complete [97]. Although the SF-BPS is designed to measure the health status of populations, it has been shown to be responsive to improvements in pain.

The SF-36 BPS is a valid and reliable generic questionnaire designed to evaluate bodily pain as a dimension of overall health status and has been widely used internationally and in diverse populations. Its advantages include simplicity of administration and usefulness in making comparisons across populations for research purposes.

10.3.8 Measure of Intermittent and Constant Osteoarthritis Pain (ICOAP)

The ICOAP measure is a multidimensional osteoarthritis (OA)-specific measure designed to comprehensively evaluate the pain experience in people with hip or knee OA, including pain intensity, frequency, and impact on mood, sleep, and quality of life, independent of the effect of pain on physical function [24]. It is intended for use alongside a measure of physical disability.

The ICOAP is a 11-item scale evaluating two pain domains: a 5-item scale evaluates constant pain and a 6-item scale evaluates intermittent pain or "pain that comes and goes." Two supplementary questions can be used to assess predictability of intermittent pain when present. Both a hip and knee joint version of the ICOAP are available [24, 98].

Eleven items in two domains with two supplementary items are provided on intermittent pain predictability.

All items are constructed as rating scales with five levels of response. For items asking about intensity, response options are "not at all," "mildly," "moderately," "severely," and "extremely." For items about frequency, response options are "never," "rarely," "sometimes," "often," and "very often" [24]. For the supplementary items asking about predictability of pain, the response options are "never," "rarely," "sometimes," "often," and "very often" [98].

The ICOAP and ICOAP Users Guide can be obtained free of charge from the OARSI web site, www.oarsi.org.

Method of administration. The measure can be interviewer-administered in person or by telephone. Respondents should complete both subscales (ICOAP User's Guide).

Scoring. Each ICOAP item is scored from 0 to 4. A score is separately produced for each subscale by summing the items' subscale scores and then normalizing each score from 0 (no pain) to 100 (extreme pain). A total ICOAP score can be calculated by summing the two subscale scores, and normalizing from 0 (no pain) to 100 (extreme pain). Rules have been created to deal with missing data (ICOAP User's Guide). No scoring guidelines are available for the two supplementary items.

The ICOAP has been shown to be easy to understand and complete; subjects felt positive about the inclusion of the two distinct pain domains (constant pain and pain that comes and goes) [99].

Regarding content validity, Cronbach's alpha was 0.93 for 100 individuals with hip and knee OA [24]. Test–retest reliability in 76 individuals with hip and knee OA, age more than 40 years, demonstrated an intraclass correlation coefficient of 0.85 (95% confidence interval 0.76–0.91) [100].

10.4 Behavioral Measures of Pain in Critically Ill Patients

The behavioral measures of pain look at behavioral features and responses such as facial expressions, body postures, vocalizations, and movements and are useful for assessing pain where communication is difficult. This can also include the assessment of (1) behavioral responses, (2) sleep patterns, (3) activity levels, and (4) appetite.

10.4.1 Behavioral Pain Scale (BPS)

The Behavioral Pain Scale (BPS) and Critical-Care Pain Observation Tool (CPOT) are behavioral pain assessment tools for uncommunicative and sedated intensive care unit (ICU) patients [101].

The BPS was developed for use with critically ill patients in the ICU. It evaluates and scores three categories of behavior on a 1–4 scale: (1) facial expression: 1 for relaxed to 4 for grimacing, (2) upper-limb movement: 1 for no movement to 4 for permanently retracted, (3) ventilator compliance: 1 for tolerating ventilator to 4 for unable to control ventilation (Agency for Health Care Research and Quality, USA).

A cumulative score above three may indicate pain is present; the score can be used to evaluate intervention but cannot be interpreted to mean pain intensity. The patient must be able to respond in all categories of behavior—for example, the BPS should not be used in a patient who is receiving a neuromuscular blocking agent.

The implementation of the BPS can be recommended in intensive care units and may improve the management of pain among sedated patients by providing a systematic and consistent approach to pain assessment to guide interventions. The CPOT may also prove useful in assessing pain among sedated patients, but first

Table 10.5 Behavioral Pain Scale

Item	Description	Score
Facial expression	Relaxed	1
	Partially tightened (e.g., brow lowering)	2
	Fully tightened (e.g., eyelid closing)	3
	Grimacing	4
Upper limbs	No movement	1
	Partially bent	2
	Fully bent with finger flexion	3
	Permanently retracted	4
Compliance with mechanical ventilation	Tolerating movement	1
	Coughing but tolerating ventilation most of the time	2
	Fighting ventilator	3
	Unable to control ventilation	4

Reproduced with permission from Payen et al. [103]

requires further validation. Also, further research is needed into the effects of pain assessment tools on pain management practices and patient outcomes [101, 102] (Table 10.5).

10.4.2 Critical-Care Pain Observation Tool (CPOT)

The CPOT (Table 10.4) was developed on the basis of retrospective chart reviews to determine common pain notations and findings with focus groups of ICU clinicians [104–106].

This instrument is designed for use in both intubated and nonintubated critical care patients. Four domains—facial expressions, movements, muscle tension, and ventilator compliance—are scored from 0 to 2; total scores range from 0 (no pain) to 8 (most pain). The CPOT contains evidence-based descriptors that are operationally defined for each domain, and the content validity index of all indicators was 0.88–1.0, according to an analysis of the results of a questionnaire provided to physicians and critical care nurses.

The CPOT was originally developed in French and was tested in a convenience sample of 105 cardiac surgery patients [104].

After completion of the assessment by two observers, the patient was asked to indicate the presence or absence of pain by nodding the head yes or no. Patients who had delirium (as indicated by the Confusion Assessment Method for the Intensive Care Unit) were excluded from the study. Interrater reliability was moderate to high (weighted κ coefficient = 0.52–0.88) when tested between the same two data collectors.

Physical motion is known to increase heart rate and blood pressure to compensate for increased oxygen demand, making this method of establishing validity problematic. However, when patients' self-reported pain values were compared with the observer derived CPOT scores, the positive predictive value of the CPOT was high (85.7%). All of the nurse respondents reported that the CPOT directives were clear and that the tool was easy to use.

The first report of the internal consistency of the CPOT (56%–100% agreement) [107] had a high internal consistency (Cronbach α, 0.71) and good discriminate validity (mean scale scores = 0.27 at rest to 0.56 after noxious stimulation) and a low interrater reliability (Pearson correlation coefficient, 0.63; $P < 0.001$). However, this poor reliability could be due to the limited amount of training the assessors received before data collection. Repeated measures study showed that interrater reliability of the CPOT was excellent ($\kappa = 0.79$), and discriminate validity was good; mean scores were 0.27 (SD, 0.64) at rest and 1.93 (SD, 1.41) during the procedure [108].

10.5 Pain Assessment in Cognitively Impaired Patients

The assessment of pain in patients with cognitive impairment is a significant challenge. Cognitively impaired patients tend to voice fewer pain complaints but may become agitated or manifest unusual or sudden changes in behavior when they are in pain. Caregivers may have difficulty knowing when cognitively impaired patients are in pain and when they are experiencing pain relief. This may make the patient vulnerable to both under-treatment and over-treatment.

10.5.1 Pain Assessment in Advanced Dementia Scale (PAINAD)

The Pain Assessment in Advanced Dementia Scale (PAINAD) can be used when severe dementia is present. This tool involves the assessment of breathing, negative vocalization, facial expression, body language, and consolability (Table 10.6).

Table 10.6 Pain Assessment in Advanced Dementia (PAINAD)

	0	1	2	Score[a]
Breathing	Normal	• Occasional labored breathing • Short period of hyperventilation	• Noisy labored breathing • Long period of hyperventilation • Cheyne–Stokes respirations	
Negative vocalization	None	• Occasional moan/groan • Low level speech with a negative or disapproving quality	• Repeated, troubled calling out • Loud moaning or groaning • Crying	
Facial expression	Smiling or inexpressive	• Sad • Frightened • Frown	Facial grimacing	
Body language	Relaxed	• Tense • Distressed • Pacing • Fidgeting	• Rigid • Fists clenched • Knees pulled up • Pulling/pushing away • Striking out	
Consolability	No need to console	Distracted or reassured by voice or touch	Unable to console, distract, or reassure	
Total				

Reproduced with permission from Warden et al. [109], Elsevier
PAINAD scoring: 1–3 = mild; 4–6 = moderate; 7–10 = severe
[a]Some institutions have developed policies in which a PAINAD score of four or greater must be addressed in the nursing care plan. Source: Public domain

10.5.2 Pain Assessment in Seniors with Limited Ability to Communicate

The Pain Assessment Checklist for Seniors with Limited Ability to Communicate (PACSLAC) evaluates 60 behaviors such as facial expressions, activities, and mood [110]. A checkmark is made next to any behavior the patient exhibits. The total number of behaviors may be scored but cannot be equated with a pain intensity score. It is unknown if a high score represents more pain than a low score. In other words, a patient who scores ten out of 60 behaviors does not necessarily have less pain than a patient who scores 20. However, in an individual patient, a change in the total pain score may suggest more or less pain.

The PACSLAC Checklist is used to screen for pain in older adults who have dementia or other cognitive impairment with a limited ability to communicate and should be used by a professional nurse.

It should be used at the following time points: (1) at the initial intake/admission to services, (2) for an older adult with behavioral symptoms suggestive of pain, assess at least every 8 h, (3) at any time a change in pain status is reported, (4) in 1 h following a pain intervention to assess effectiveness, (5) for older adults residing in long term health care settings, and assessments should be completed at each quarterly review.

The PACSLAC Checklist should be complete, based on observations of the older adult during activity or movement (such as transferring out of bed or walking) after a day-long shift of observation. Presence or absence of each behavior is determined on the checklist. The total score after each use should be compared with the previous score received.

An increased score suggests that an increase in pain is likely. On the other hand, a lower score suggests that pain has decreased. All scores are documented and recorded in a location that is readily accessible by other health care providers.

The PACSLAC is a screening tool and not a definitive indicator of pain. Behavior observation scores should be considered alongside knowledge of existing painful conditions and reports from someone who knows the older adult (like a family member or nursing assistant) and their pain behaviors [111].

This analysis may inform a more rigorous theoretical underpinning and (re) development of pain and discomfort tools and the comparative analysis of this checklist with other similar tools calls for empirical testing of a broad item pool for sensitivity and specificity in detecting and discriminating pain from other sources of discomfort [112].

In the patients with dementia and expected death, a low symptom burden was observed with validated instruments, also in dehydrated patients. A good death is possible but might be enhanced if the symptom burden is regularly assessed with validated instruments. The use of observation tools may have influenced the physicians to make treatment decisions [113, 114].

References

1. Katz J, Melzack R. Measurement of pain. Surg Clin North Am. 1999;79:231–52.
2. Dansie EJ, Turk DC. Assessment of patients with chronic pain. Br J Anaesth. 2013;111:19–25.
3. Gracely RH, Kwilosz DM. The descriptor differential scale: applying psychophysical principles to clinical pain assessment. Pain. 1988;35:279–88.
4. Huskisson EC. Measurement of pain. Lancet. 1974;2:1127–31.
5. Huskisson EC, Wojtulewski JA, Berry H, et al. Treatment of rheumatoid arthritis with fenoprofen: comparison with aspirin. Br Med J. 1974;1:176–80.
6. Burckhardt CS, Jones KD. Adult measures of pain: the McGill pain questionnaire (MPQ), rheumatoid arthritis pain scale (RAPS), short-form McGill pain questionnaire (SF-MPQ), verbal descriptive scale (VDS), visual analog scale (VAS), and West Haven-Yale multidisciplinary pain inventory (WHYMPI). Arthritis Rheum. 2003;49:S96–104.
7. Scott J, Huskisson EC. Vertical or horizontal visual analogue scales. Ann Rheum Dis. 1979;38:560.
8. Joyce CR, Zutshi DW, Hrubes VF, Mason RM. Comparison of fixed interval and visual analogue scales for rating chronic pain. Eur J Clin Pharmacol. 1975;8:415–20.

9. Aitken RC. Measurement of feelings using visual analogue scales. Proc R Soc Med. 1969;62:989–93.
10. Hayes MHS, Patterson DG. Experimental development of the graphic rating method. Psychol Bull. 1921;18:98–9.
11. Woodforde JM, Merskey H. Some relationships between subjective measures of pain. J Psychosom Res. 1972;16:173–8.
12. Jensen MP, McFarland CA. Increasing the reliability and validity of pain intensity measurement in chronic pain patients. Pain. 1993;55:195–203.
13. Jensen MP, Karoly P, Braver S. The measurement of clinical pain intensity: a comparison of six methods. Pain. 1986;27:117–26.
14. Kremer E, Atkinson JH, Ignelzi RJ. Measurement of pain: patient preference does not confound pain measurement. Pain. 1981;10:241–8.
15. Scott J, Huskisson EC. Graphic representation of pain. Pain. 1976;2:175–84.
16. Downie WW, Leatham PA, Rhind VM, et al. Studies with pain rating scales. Ann Rheum Dis. 1978;37:378–81.
17. Williamson A, Hoggart B. Pain: a review of three commonly used pain rating scales. J Clin Nurs. 2005;14:798–804.
18. Wolfe F, Michaud K. Assessment of pain in rheumatoid arthritis: minimal clinically significant difference, predictors, and the effect of anti-tumor necrosis factor therapy. J Rheumatol. 2007;34:1674–83.
19. Tashjian RZ, Deloach J, Porucznik CA, Powell AP. Minimal clinically important differences (MCID) and patient acceptable symptomatic state (PASS) for visual analog scales (VAS) measuring pain in patients treated for rotator cuff disease. J Shoulder Elb Surg. 2009;18:927–32.
20. Bourdel N, Alves J, Pickering G, et al. Systematic review of endometriosis pain assessment: how to choose a scale? Hum Reprod Update. 2015;21:136–52.
21. Rodriguez CS. Pain measurement in the elderly: a review. Pain Manag Nurs. 2001;2:38–46.
22. Dworkin RH, Turk DC, Farrar JT, et al. Core outcome measures for chronic pain clinical trials: IMMPACT recommendations. Pain. 2005;113:9–19.
23. Ferraz MB, Quaresma MR, Aquino LR, et al. Reliability of pain scales in the assessment of literate and illiterate patients with rheumatoid arthritis. J Rheumatol. 1990;17:1022–4.
24. Hawker GA, Davis AM, French MR, Cibere J, Jordan JM, March L, et al. Development and preliminary psychometric testing of a new OA pain measure: an OARSI/OMERACT initiative. Osteoarthr Cartil. 2008;16:409–14.
25. Hush JM, Refshauge KM, Sullivan G, et al. Do numerical rating scales and the Roland-Morris disability questionnaire capture changes that are meaningful to patients with persistent back pain? Clin Rehabil. 2010;24:648–57.
26. Farrar JT, Young JP Jr, LaMoreaux L, Werth JL, Poole RM. Clinical importance of changes in chronic pain intensity measured on an 11-point numerical pain rating scale. Pain. 2001;94:149–58.
27. Childs JD, Piva SR, Fritz JM. Responsiveness of the numeric pain rating scale in patients with low back pain. Spine. 2005;30:1331–4.
28. Morrisette DC, Cholewicki J, Logan S, Seif G, McGowan S. A randomized clinical trial comparing extensible and inextensible lumbosacral orthoses and standard care alone in the management of lower back pain. Spine. 2014;39:1733–42.
29. Hjermstad MJ, Fayers PM, Haugen DF, et al. Studies comparing numerical rating scales, verbal rating scales, and visual analogue scales for assessment of pain intensity in adults: a systematic literature review. J Pain Symptom Manag. 2011;41:1073–93.
30. Holdgate A, Asha S, Craig J, Thompson J. Comparison of a verbal numeric rating scale with the visual analogue scale for the measurement of acute pain. Emerg Med (Fremantle). 2003;15:441–6.
31. Linton SJ, Götestam KG. A clinical comparison of two pain scales: correlation, remembering chronic pain, and a measure of compliance. Pain. 1983;17:57–65.

32. Closs SJ, Dowding D, Allcock N, et al. Towards improved decision support in the assessment and management of pain for people with dementia in hospital: a systematic meta-review and observational study. Southampton: NIHR Journals Library; 2016.
33. Bech RD, Lauritsen J, Ovesen O, Overgaard S. The verbal rating scale is reliable for assessment of postoperative pain in hip fracture patients. Pain Res Treat. 2015;2015:676212.
34. Kliger M, Stahl S, Haddad M, et al. Measuring the intensity of chronic pain: are the visual analogue scale and the verbal rating scale interchangeable? Pain Pract. 2015;15:538–47.
35. Herr K, Spratt KF, Garand L, Li L. Evaluation of the Iowa pain thermometer and other selected pain intensity scales in younger and older adult cohorts using controlled clinical pain: a preliminary study. Pain Med. 2007;8:585–600.
36. Bieri D, Reeve RA, Champion GD, Addicoat L, Ziegler JB. The faces pain scale for the self-assessment of the severity of pain experienced by children: development, initial validation, and preliminary investigation for ratio scale properties. Pain. 1990;41:139–50.
37. Hicks CL, von Baeyer CL, Spafford PA, van Korlaar I, Goodenough B. The faces pain scale-revised: toward a common metric in pediatric pain measurement. Pain. 2001;93:173–83.
38. von Baeyer CL, Spagrud LJ. Systematic review of observational (behavioral) measures of pain for children and adolescents aged 3 to 18 years. Pain. 2007;127:140–50.
39. Srouji R, Ratnapalan S, Schneeweiss S. Pain in children: assessment and nonpharmacological management. Int J Pediatr. 2010;2010:474838.
40. Huguet A, Stinson JN, McGrath PJ. Measurement of self-reported pain intensity in children and adolescents. J Psychosom Res. 2010;68:329–36.
41. Melzack R. The McGill pain questionnaire: major properties and scoring methods. Pain. 1975;1:277–99.
42. Wilkie DJ, Savedra MC, Holzemer WL, Tesler MD, Paul SM. Use of the McGill pain questionnaire to measure pain: a meta-analysis. Nurs Res. 1990;39:36–41.
43. Burckhardt CS. The use of the McGill pain questionnaire in assessing arthritis pain. Pain. 1984;19:305–14.
44. Seymour RA, Charlton JE, Phillips ME. An evaluation of dental pain using visual analogue scales and the Mcgill pain questionnaire. J Oral Maxillofac Surg. 1983;41:643–8.
45. Melzack R. The short-form McGill pain questionnaire. Pain. 1987;30:191–7.
46. Rasmussen PV, Sindrup SH, Jensen TS, Bach FW. Symptoms and signs in patients with suspected neuropathic pain. Pain. 2004;110:461–9.
47. Gilron I, Bailey JM, Tu D, Holden RR, Weaver DF, Houlden RL. Morphine, gabapentin, or their combination for neuropathic pain. N Engl J Med. 2005;352:1324–34.
48. Aradillas E, Schwartzman RJ, Grothusen JR, Goebel A, Alexander GM. Plasma exchange therapy in patients with complex regional pain syndrome. Pain Physician. 2015;18:383–94.
49. Goldberg H, Firtch W, Tyburski M, Pressman A, Ackerson L, Hamilton L, Smith W, Carver R, Maratukulam A, Won LA, Carragee E, Avins AL. Oral steroids for acute radiculopathy due to a herniated lumbar disk: a randomized clinical trial. JAMA. 2015;313:1915–23.
50. Grafton KV, Foster NE, Wright CC. Test-retest reliability of the short-form McGill pain questionnaire: assessment of intraclass correlation coefficients and limits of agreement in patients with osteoarthritis. Clin J Pain. 2005;21:73–82.
51. Birch S, Jamison RN. Controlled trial of Japanese acupuncture for chronic myofascial neck pain: assessment of specific and nonspecific effects of treatment. Clin J Pain. 1998;14: 248–55.
52. Ruoff GE, Rosenthal N, Jordan D, Karim R, Kamin M. Tramadol/ acetaminophen combination tablets for the treatment of chronic lower back pain: a multicenter, randomized, double-blind, placebo-controlled outpatient study. Clin Ther. 2003;25:1123–41.
53. Pison L, Peeters P, Blaauw Y, Vernooy K, Kumar N, Philippens S, Crijns HJ, Vlaeyen J, Schoenen J, Timmermans C. Headache during cryoballoon ablation for atrial fibrillation. Europace. 2015;17:898–901.

54. Dworkin RH, Turk DC, Trudeau J, et al. Validation of the short-form McGill pain Questionnaire-2 (SF-MPQ-2) in acute low back pain. J Pain. 2015;16:357–66.
55. Lovejoy TI, Turk DC, Morasco BJ. Evaluation of the psychometric properties of the revised short-form McGill pain questionnaire. J Pain. 2012;13:1250–7.
56. Gauthier LR, Young A, Dworkin RH, Rodin G, Zimmermann C, Warr D, Librach SL, Moore M, Shepherd FA, Pillai Riddell R, Macpherson A, Melzack R, Gagliese L. Validation of the short-form McGill pain questionnaire-2 in younger and older people with cancer pain. J Pain. 2014;15:756–70.
57. Adelmanesh F, Jalali A, Attarian H, Farahani B, Ketabchi SM, Arvantaj A, Raissi GR. Reliability, validity, and sensitivity measures of expanded and revised version of the short-form McGill pain questionnaire (SF-MPQ-2) in Iranian patients with neuropathic and non-neuropathic pain. Pain Med. 2012;13:1631–6.
58. Maruo T, Nakae A, Maeda L, Shi K, Takahashi K, Morris S, Hosomi K, Kanatani H, Matsuzaki T, Saitoh Y. Validity, reliability, and assessment sensitivity of the Japanese version of the short-form McGill pain questionnaire 2 in Japanese patients with neuropathic and non-neuropathic pain. Pain Med. 2014;15:1930–7.
59. Choi SA, Son C, Lee JH, Cho S. Confirmatory factor analysis of the Korean version of the short-form McGill pain questionnaire with chronic pain patients: a comparison of alternative models. Health Qual Life Outcomes. 2015;13:15.
60. Kachooei AR, Ebrahimzadeh MH, Erfani-Sayyar R, Salehi M, Salimi E, Razi S. Short form-McGill pain questionnaire-2 (SF-MPQ-2): a cross-cultural adaptation and validation study of the Persian version in patients with knee osteoarthritis. Arch Bone Jt Surg. 2015;3:45–50.
61. Cleeland CS, Ryan KM. Pain assessment: global use of the brief pain inventory. Ann Acad Med Singap. 1994;23:129–38.
62. Mendoza T, Mayne T, Rublee D, Cleeland C. Reliability and validity of a modified brief pain inventory short form in patients with osteoarthritis. Eur J Pain. 2006;10:353–61.
63. Hwang SS, Chang VT, Kasimis B. Dynamic cancer pain management outcomes: the relationship between pain severity, pain relief, functional interference, satisfaction and global quality of life over time. J Pain Symptom Manage. 2002;23:190–200.
64. Tan G, Jensen MP, Thornby JI, Shanti BF. Validation of the brief pain inventory for chronic nonmalignant pain. J Pain. 2004;5:133–7.
65. Pelayo-Alvarez M, Perez-Hoyos S, Agra-Varela Y. Reliability and concurrent validity of the palliative outcome scale, the Rotterdam symptom checklist, and the brief pain inventory. J Palliat Med. 2013;16:867–74.
66. Kumar SP. Utilization of brief pain inventory as an assessment tool for pain in patients with cancer: a focused review. Indian J Palliat Care. 2011;17:108–15.
67. Kapstad H, Rokne B, Stavem K. Psychometric properties of the brief pain inventory among patients with osteoarthritis undergoing total hip replacement surgery. Health Qual Life Outcomes. 2010;8:1–8.
68. Williams VS, Smith MY, Fehnel SE. The validity and utility of the BPI interference measures for evaluating the impact of osteoarthritic pain. J Pain Symptom Manag. 2006;31:48–57.
69. Lavand'homme PM, Grosu I, France MN, Thienpont E. Pain trajectories identify patients at risk of persistent pain after knee arthroplasty: an observational study. Clin Orthop Relat Res. 2014;472:1409–15.
70. Erdemoglu AK, Koc R. Brief pain inventory score identifying and discriminating neuropathic and nociceptive pain. Acta Neurol Scand. 2013;128:351–8.
71. Atkinson TM, Rosenfeld BD, Sit L, et al. Using confirmatory factor analysis to evaluate construct validity of the brief pain inventory (BPI). J Pain Symptom Manag. 2011;41:558–65.
72. Lapane KL, Quilliam BJ, Benson C, Chow W, Kim M. One, two, or three? Constructs of the brief pain inventory among patients with non-cancer pain in the outpatient setting. J Pain Symptom Manag. 2014;47:325–33.

73. Lapane KL, Quilliam BJ, Benson C, Chow W, Kim MS. Impact of noncancer pain on health-related quality of life. Pain Pract. 2015;15:333–42.
74. Tyler EJ, Jensen MP, Engel JM, Schwartz L. The reliability and validity of pain interference measures in persons with cerebral palsy. Arch Phys Med Rehabil. 2002;83:236–9.
75. Cleeland CS. The measurement of pain from metastatic bone disease: capturing the patient's experience. Clin Cancer Res. 2006;12(20):6236s.
76. Aida S, Tomita M, Lee C, Fukuda S, Shimoji K. Simple pain relief score by observers (PRSO) for assessing chronic pain. J Anesth. 1997;11:100–4.
77. Von Korff M, Ormel J, Keefe FJ, Dworkin SF. Grading the severity of chronic pain. Pain. 1992;50:133–49.
78. Elliott AM, Smith BH, Penny KI, Smith WC, Chambers WA. The epidemiology of chronic pain in the community. Lancet. 1999;354:1248–52.
79. Smith BH, Penny KI, Purves AM, Munro C, Wilson B, Grimshaw J, et al. The chronic pain grade questionnaire: validation and reliability in postal research. Pain. 1997;71:141–7.
80. Salaffi FF, Stancati AF, Grassi W. Reliability and validity of the Italian version of the chronic pain grade questionnaire in patients with musculoskeletal disorders. Clin Rheumatol. 2006;25:619–31.
81. Turk DC, Rudy TE. Towards a comprehensive assessment of chronic pain patients. Behav Res Ther. 1987;25:237–49.
82. Turk DC, Rudy TE. Toward an empirically derived taxonomy of chronic pain patients: integration of psychological assessment data. J Consult Clin Psychol. 1988;56:233–8.
83. Kerns RD, Turk DC, Rudy TE. The west haven-Yale multidimensional pain inventory (WHYMPI). Pain. 1985;23:345–56.
84. Guttman LA. A basis for scaling qualitative data. Am Sociol Rev. 1944;91:139–50.
85. Krebs EE, Bair MJ, Damush TM, Tu W, Wu J, Kroenke K. Comparative responsiveness of pain outcome measures among primary care patients with musculoskeletal pain. Med Care. 2010;48:1007–14.
86. Dunn KM, Jordan K, Croft PR. Does questionnaire structure influence response in postal surveys? J Clin Epidemiol. 2003;56:10–6.
87. Penny KI, Purves AM, Smith BH, Chambers WA, Smith WC. Relationship between the chronic pain grade and measures of physical, social and psychological well-being. Pain. 1999;79:275–9.
88. Jakobsson U. Psychometric testing of the brief screening version of multidimensional pain inventory (Swedish version). Scand J Caring Sci. 2009;23:171–9.
89. Cetin AA, Bektas H, Ozdogan M. The West Haven Yale multidimensional pain inventory: reliability and validity of the Turkish version in individuals with cancer. Eur J Oncol Nurs. 2016;20:1–9.
90. Flor H, Rudy TE, Birbaumer N, Streit B, Schugens MM. The applicability of the West Haven-Yale multidimensional pain inventory in German-speaking countries. Data on the reliability and validity of the MPI-D. Schmerz. 1990;4:82–7.
91. Chatkoff DK, Leonard MT, Maier KJ. Pain catastrophizing differs between and within West Haven-Yale multidimensional pain inventory (MPI) pain adjustment classifications: theoretical and clinical implications from preliminary data. Clin J Pain. 2015;31:349–54.
92. Eklund A, Bergström G, Bodin L, Axén I. Do psychological and behavioral factors classified by the West Haven-Yale multidimensional pain inventory (Swedish version) predict the early clinical course of low back pain in patients receiving chiropractic care? BMC Musculoskelet Disord. 2016;17:75.
93. Ware JE Jr, Sherbourne CD. The MOS 36-item short-form health survey (SF-36). I. Conceptual framework and item selection. Med Care. 1992;30:473–83.
94. McHorney CA, Ware JE, Raczek AE. The MOS 36-item short-form health survey (SF-36) II: psychometric and clinical tests of validity in measuring physical and mental health constructs. Med Care. 1993;31:247–63.

95. Ware JE, Gandek B. Overview of the SF-36 health survey and the international quality of life assessment (IQOLA) project. J Clin Epidemiol. 1998;51:903–12.
96. Hawker GA, Mian S, Kendzerska T, French M. Measures of adult pain: visual analog scale for pain (VAS pain), numeric rating scale for pain (NRS pain), McGill pain questionnaire (MPQ), short-form McGill pain questionnaire (SF-MPQ), chronic pain grade scale (CPGS), short form-36 bodily pain scale (SF-36 BPS), and measure of intermittent and constant osteoarthritis pain (ICOAP). Arthritis Care Res (Hoboken). 2011;63(Suppl 11):S240–52.
97. Quintana JM, Escobar A, Bilbao A, Arostegui I, Lafuente I, Vidaurreta I. Responsiveness and clinically important differences for the WOMAC and SF-36 after hip joint replacement. Osteoarthr Cartil. 2005;13:1076–83.
98. Hawker GA, French MR, Elkayam JG, Davis AM. Unpredictability of intermittent knee OA pain: impact on pain, function, and mood [abstract]. Arthritis Rheum. 2010;62(Suppl 10):S284–5.
99. Maillefert JF, Kloppenburg M, Fernandes L, Punzi L, Gunther KP, Martin Mola E, et al. Multi-language translation and cross-cultural adaptation of the OARSI/OMERACT measure of intermittent and constant osteoarthritis pain (ICOAP). Osteoarthr Cartil. 2009;17:1293–6.
100. Bombardier C, Melfi C, Paul J, Green R, Hawker GA, Wright J, et al. Comparison of a generic and a disease-specific measure of pain and physical function after knee replacement surgery. Med Care. 1995;33:AS131–44.
101. Bouajram RH, Sebat CM, Love D, Louie EL, Wilson MD, Duby JJ. Comparison of self-reported and behavioral pain assessment tools in critically ill patients. J Intensive Care Med. 2018; https://doi.org/10.1177/0885066618757450.
102. Cade CH. Clinical tools for the assessment of pain in sedated critically ill adults. Nurs Crit Care. 2008;13:288–97.
103. Payen JF, Bru O, Bosson JL, et al. Assessing pain in critically ill sedated patients by using a behavioral pain scale. Crit Care Med. 2001;29:2258–63.
104. Gélinas C, Fillion L, Puntillo KA, Viens C, Fortier M. Validation of the critical-care pain observation tool in adult patients. Am J Crit Care. 2006;15:420–7.
105. Gélinas C, Fillion L, Puntillo K. Item selection and content validity of the critical-care pain observation tool for non-verbal adults. J Adv Nurs. 2008;65:203–16.
106. Herr K, Coyne PJ, Ely E, Gélinas C, Manworren RC. APMN 2019 position statement: pain assessment in the patient unable to self-report. Pain Manag Nurs. 2019;20(5):402–3.
107. Wibbenmeyer L, et al. Evaluation of the usefulness of two established pain assessment tools in a burn population. J Burn Care Res. 2011;32:52–60.
108. Vázquez M, et al. Pain assessment in turning procedures for patients with invasive mechanical ventilation. Nurs Crit Care. 2011;16:178–85.
109. Warden V, Hurley AC, Volicer L. Development and psychometric evaluation of the pain assessment in advanced dementia (PAINAD) scale. J Am Med Dir Assoc. 2003;4:9–15.
110. Fuchs-Lacelle S, Hadjistavropoulos T. Development and preliminary validation of the pain assessment checklist for seniors with limited ability to communicate (PACSLAC). Pain Manag Nurs. 2004;5:37–49.
111. van Dalen-Kok AH, et al. Pain assessment in impaired cognition (PAIC): content validity of the Dutch version of a new and universal tool to measure pain in dementia. Clin Interv Aging. 2018;13:25–34.
112. van der Steen JT, et al. Tools to assess pain or lack of comfort in dementia: a content analysis. J Pain Symptom Manage. 2015;50:659–75.e3.
113. Klapwijk MS, et al. Symptoms and treatment when death is expected in dementia patients in long-term care facilities. BMC Geriatr. 2014;14:99.
114. van der Maaden T, et al. Improving comfort in people with dementia and pneumonia: a cluster randomized trial. BMC Med. 2016;14:116.

Part II
Pain Management Techniques

Chapter 11
Back Pain

Pierluigi di Vadi

11.1 Introduction

Back pain is a common condition affecting most people at least once in their life. It is the commonest musculoskeletal reason for consulting medical doctors and has a huge social impact with a high number of days lost from work. Episodes of simple back pain are often difficult to interpret, and consequently it is not simple to provide the appropriate management.

A careful history and clinical examination are essential first steps of clinical practice. Still, an unambiguous pathology can only be found in a minority of patients affected by back pain; but patients expect a diagnosis.

Frequently, patients can be reassured about the absence of serious or underlying malignant conditions, but it may be a challenge to provide them with an appropriate specific diagnosis. A large percentage of individuals with back pain worry about the consequence of it and the repercussion that their disability has on their quality of daily life and particularly on their jobs. Quite often there is only little relationship between coincidental local pathology and the perceived pain and disability. In fact, episodes of back pain may occur without any predictable sign of onset. It is an interesting observation that people in less developed countries suffer from back pain but not necessarily consequent disability [1], possibly because they expect to have back pain as part of their life [1], contrary to what often happens in advanced countries.

Back pain is not a disease but a syndrome. There is no objective measurement for it. There are several different subjective tools to assess its severity. They vary from simple linear scales (visual analogue scale, numerical pain scale, verbal pain intensity, etc.) to more complicated questionnaires (McGill pain questionnaire and its short form, Pain Outcomes Questionnaire-Short Form, The DN4 Questionnaire,

P. di Vadi (✉)
Department of Anaesthetics and Pain Management, University Hospital Lewisham, London, UK
e-mail: pdv@doctors.org.uk

K. Shimoji et al. (eds.), *Chronic Pain Management in General and Hospital Practice*, https://doi.org/10.1007/978-981-15-2933-7_11

etc.). All of them require a patient's ability to appropriately describe their problem and are based on their personal experience, culture, beliefs, age, and psychosocial underlying factors. Consequently, any subjective measurement varies substantially between individuals. Back pain is indeed a bio-psycho-social problem.

Many epidemiological studies have been conducted on back pain worldwide. A literature-based review conducted in Europe showed a general population prevalence of back pain varying between 5.9% and 11.1% [2]. These data are confirmed by a more recent study in low- and middle-income countries, showing that the prevalence of back pain is widespread irrespectively of general wealth [3]. Approximately, 60–70% of persons surveyed report at least one episode of back pain at some point in their life. The "Duprin Pain Report" [5] found back pain being the second most common syndrome after headache in the USA. The prevalence of back pain increases with age reaching 77.3% and 81.7%, respectively, in man and women above 70 years of age [6]. This is a problem on the increase with the average life expectance becoming longer. The prevalence rate for children and adolescents is lower than that seen in adults but is rising [4, 7].

Back pain is the leading cause of activity limitation and absence from work throughout much of the world, imposing a high economic burden on individuals, families, communities, industry, and governments [7, 8]. Several studies have been performed in Europe to evaluate the social and economic impact of low back pain. In the UK, back pain has been identified as the most common cause of disability in young adults, with more than 100 million workdays lost per year [9]. In Sweden, a survey suggested that back pain accounted for a progressive increase of the number of workdays lost, from seven million in 1980 to 28 million by 1987 [9]. In the USA, an estimated 149 million workdays are lost every year because of back pain [10], with total cost estimated to be between US$ 100 and 200 billion a year [11, 12]. Back pain is indeed a worrying economic burden worldwide.

Back muscles as well as other components of the back play important roles in the initial development and the consequent establishment of long-standing chronic back pain.

1. The intervertebral disk is a hydrodynamic elastic structure interposed between each vertebra. It comprises mucopolysaccharide gel containing annular collagen fibres and an enclosed central nucleus. The disk undergoes compression, rotation, and shear; these combined stresses are responsible for tear or disruption of the annular fibres, which can be one of the starting points of the back pain syndrome. The disk is no longer able to absorb the continuous stress of daily life activity partially or totally. Differences between age, weight, activity, rest, and external condition such as dampness and cold are relevant to this process. (Fig. 11.1). Secondary innervation of the disc following degeneration may be important for the development of discogenic pain.
2. The appropriate alignment of each vertebra is also of fundamental importance. When vertebrae are not aligned properly as it happens in spondylolisthesis (grade I, II, III, IV) the overall stress over the intervertebral disk, the apophyseal joints, and the neighbouring tissues could become unsustainable, causing again back pain (Fig. 11.2).

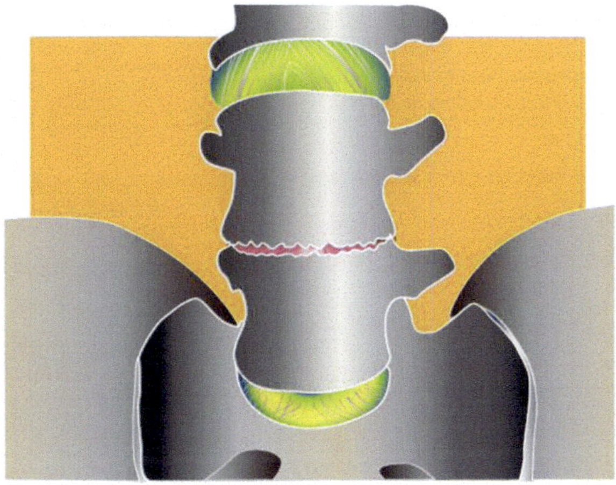

Fig. 11.1 Intervertebral disc totally worn out at L4/L5, causing natural vertebral fusion

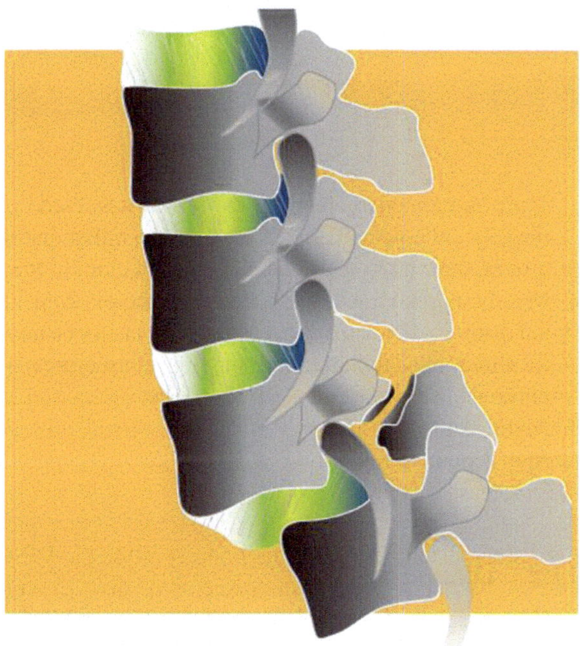

Fig. 11.2 Example of spondylolisthesis causing a non-alignment of the vertebrae with consequent abnormal stress over the invertebral discs and neighbour tissues

3. Apophyseal joints (facet joints) are hinge-like joints that allow flexion, extension, and torsion of the spine. These joints also interlock the vertebra to make the spine more stable. These joints are in almost constant motion and quite commonly with time wear out or become degenerated. When apophyseal joints become worn or torn, the cartilage may become thinner or even disappear completely with consequent damage to the bone of the joint underneath, producing overgrowth of bone

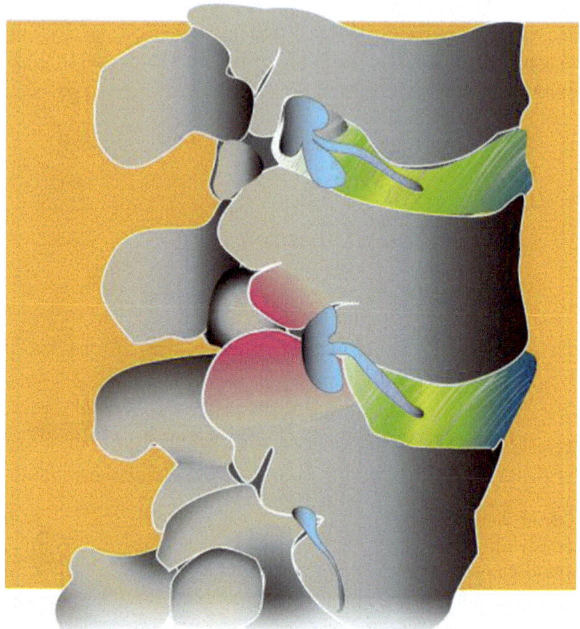

Fig. 11.3 Degenerated apophyseal joints causing impingement of the nerve root and/or spinal stenosis

spurs and an enlargement of the joints, which can pinch the nerve root running directly underneath (Fig. 11.3). Chronic inflammation of the sacroiliac joint can also be the cause for the development of chronic low back pain.

4. Vertebral crush fracture as a consequence of physical accident or systemic medical pathologies (osteoporosis, myeloma, metastasis) produce a bio-mechanic localised change, affecting the local structures, resulting in usually severe chronic back pain (Fig. 11.4).
5. Myofascial pain
6. Spinal stenosis

11.2 Diagnosis

At the beginning of making a diagnosis it is essential to rule out red and yellow flags, conditions that could masquerade as chronic back pain [13]. Red flag conditions need to be attended to in their own right immediately. Yellow flags should be seen to as far as possible as part of the back pain treatment.

Red Flags are

1. Thoracic pain
2. Fever and unexplained weight loss
3. History of malignant disease

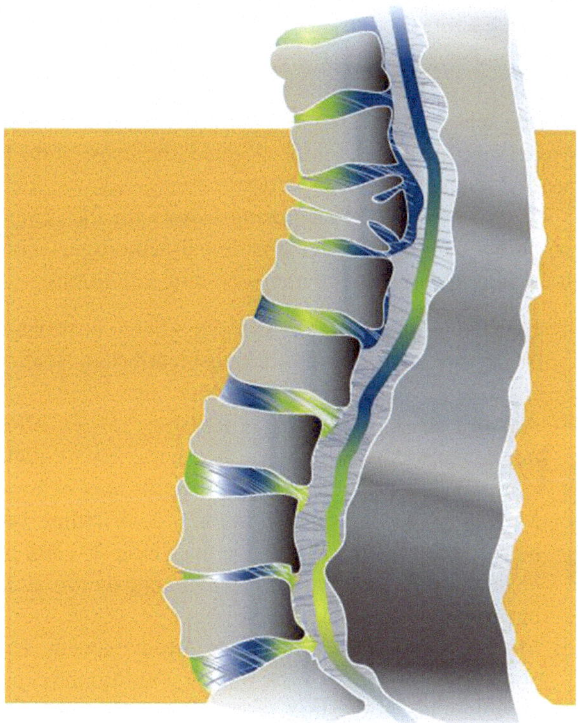

Fig. 11.4 Example of vertebral crush fracture producing an abnormal bio-mechanical pressure over the neighbour tissues

4. Ill health or presence of other medical illness
5. Progressive neurological deficit
6. Disturbed gait, saddle anaesthesia

Yellow Flags are psychosocial factors shown to be indicative of long-term chronicity and disability

1. A negative attitude that back pain is harmful or potentially severely disabling
2. Fear avoidance behaviour and reduced activity levels
3. An expectation that passive, rather than active, treatment will be beneficial
4. A tendency to depressive, low morale, and social withdrawal
5. Social or financial problems

Diagnosis is the foundation of the management of back pain. It is based on clinical assessment and is supplemented by radiological and other tests. It is essential to start with taking a detailed history of the symptoms and related issues from the beginning. This is followed by a careful clinical examination of the tender areas and assessment of the dermatomes involved.

A full neurological examination of the lower limbs is mandatory. Based on the data collected, different investigation needs to be arranged. The gold standard is a simple X-ray of the spine, which provides information of the vertebral condition (wedge fracture, spondylolysis, scoliosis, osteoarthritic changes of the apophyseal joints) and of the intervertebral space. In case the intervertebral space is reduced in size and is associated with referred pain and or signs of nerve irritation (numbness, tingling sensation, etc. into a specific dermatome), a MRI scan should be performed to assess the level of the spine affected, the shape of the discs and the entity, size and location of any bulge or prolapse.

There are several predisposing factors for the development of back pain. They can be divided into pre-existing spinal pathologies, concomitant medical and psychological features, social and economic conditions.

(a) Disc dehydration with or without a bulge or prolapse, spondylolisthesis, ankylosing spondylitis, vertebral osteoarthritis, scoliosis, vertebral osteoporotic fracture are all contributing factors.
(b) Anxiety, depression, stress and distress, anger. All of them often produce back muscle spasm, usually associated with lack of quality sleep. Additionally, as a consequence individual pain thresholds may be lowered.
(c) Manual work is often a substantial contributing factor. Lifting (particularly if heavy) and twisting, long standing, long driving, prolonged sitting, all have a negative impact and are important contributors to the onset and establishment of prolonged back pain.
(d) Miscellaneous causes such as recurrent exposure to dampness and bad weather conditions have their own impact. Additionally, psychosocial factors such as monotonous work, little control over its own job, job dissatisfaction, and domestic problems also contribute to the back pain syndrome.
(e) Central sensitization, particularly when the nerve roots are compromised or encroached on by a prolapsed disc, hypertrophy of the apophyseal joints and/or the ligamentum flavum, even if affected only mildly.
(f) Age also plays a role with the inevitable general aspects of degeneration, independently of the patient's ability to control his or her weight and physical activity.

Chronic back pain often develops on basis of a combination of some predisposing factors.

11.3 Management

In the absence of red flags and having addressed yellow flags as far as possible, the initial management of back pain is conservative with the emphasis to remain active as far as reasonably possible. In detail, conservative management depends on the severity and the characteristics of the presenting condition.

Acute episodes of back pain are usually relieved by initial short periods of rest, medication such as non-steroidal anti-inflammatory drugs (NSAIDs) and, if needed, simple analgesics such as paracetamol [14] with or without mild opioids (codeine,

Table 11.1 Initial pharmacological treatment of acute back pain episodes

NSAIDs	NSAIDs	NSAIDs	NSAIDs
	Paracetamol	Paracetamol	Paracetamol
		Codeine, etc.	
			Buprenorphine, etc.

Table 11.2 Advised radiological investigations in recurrent episodes of back pain

Spine X-Ray	Spine X-Ray	Spine X-Ray
	Spine CT scan	Spine MRI scan

dihydrocodeine, etc.) Table 11.1. The use of paracetamol on its own has recently been questioned by a Cochrane review [15] which came to the conclusion that its use in acute and probably chronic back pain its efficacy will not go beyond its placebo effect.

It is important to gently mobilise the tender muscle area quite soon to avoid the consequence of localised muscle stiffness, which would increase the length and severity of the acute back pain episode and prolong the period of disability.

The management of recurrent episodes of back pain becomes more complicated, particularly if they become frequent. First, it is important to re-evaluate the severity of the condition by repeating a simple neurological examination of the lower limbs to find out if there is a degree of impingement of the main lumbar nerve roots, with shooting pain in a dermatomal distribution with or without the association of other symptoms such as numbness, pins and needles, or tingling sensation, accompanied by altered sensitivity and possibly motor weakness. It is also important to deeply palpate the back muscle area close to the spine to localise possible tenderness. If there are clinical signs of any nerve root involvement, a MRI scan should be performed (or a CT scan if an MRI is contraindicated) (Table 11.2).

If there is a history of osteoarthritis or osteoporosis, then an X-ray of the spinal column should probably be preferred as first diagnostic investigation. It is essential to have a clear understanding of the underlying spinal condition, of the daily activity of the patient, his/her job characteristics, and the individual psychosocial features, if any (Table 11.2).

Chronic back pain has repercussions on patients' daily life by interfering with the quality of life often facilitating the development of depression and anxiety symptoms [16].

The use of the so-called alternative techniques such as acupuncture, percutaneous neuromodulation, trans-cutaneous-nerve-stimulator (TENS) is still in place, although the evidence of beneficial effects, as appears in the literature, is quite limited [17–20]. A major issue is that in particular acupuncture may need to be administered quite frequently, which can be difficult where budgetary considerations are important.

Physical therapy has always played an important role in the treatment of back pain, but it is very much based on the willingness of the patient to pursue it fully. "Back School" consists of a therapeutic programme given to groups of people that

Table 11.3 Non-pharmacological techniques used in chronic back pain

TENS, acupuncture	Physiotherapy	Back school

Table 11.4 Multi-disciplinary techniques employed in complex chronic back pain

CBT	PMP	Mindfulness

Table 11.5 Adjuvant analgesics in chronic back pain

TCA	Anticonvulsants	SNRI
Amitriptyline, etc.	Gabapentin, pregabalin, etc.	Duloxetine, etc.

includes both education and exercise. It is, however, uncertain if "Back School" is effective in relieving chronic low back pain (Table 11.3). In a systematic review, the results showed no difference or only a trivial effect in favour of it [20]. Although the quality of the evidence was mostly low, there are myriad potential variants on the "Back School approach" regarding the employment of different exercises and educational methods [20].

Cognitive and behavioural techniques (CBT) and Pain Management Programmes (PMP) have been implemented for complex chronic back pain [21–23]. More recently, the mindfulness approach has become more popular [24, 25].

Analgesics should be used in back pain but with caution. NSAIDs appear to be slightly more effective than paracetamol (Cochrane review [15]). Their use should be restricted to not more than 1–2 weeks avoiding them where they are contraindicated (Asthma, COPD, severe heart conditions, renal failure, and anticoagulant treatment). Combinations of mild opioids (codeine/dihydrocodeine of different strength) with paracetamol are widely used in primary care with long-term limited results.

The use of adjuvant analgesics such as gabapentin, pregabalin, and amitriptyline mostly in chronic back pain is also widely used in the UK primary care (Table 11.4); however, the current evidence on the use of such compounds is limited with risks of adverse effects without any demonstrated effectiveness [26].

Atkinson et al. [27] could find no difference in pain relief in patients with mechanical low back pain without a neuropathic component when pregabalin was compared with placebo. Even among the cohorts of individual subjects, there were no outlying results who could have been averaged out in the statistical process. Pregabalin may be possibly more effective in back pain patients with a neuropathic component, e.g., nerve root compromise (Table 11.5).

The use of strong opiates and opioids in chronic back pain is very controversial. In the past particularly over the 1980s and the 1990s, when the use of these substances did increase substantially in the management of chronic pain in general and of non-malignant back pain specifically. Today, there is general consensus among physicians to limit the use of opiates in non-malignant chronic pain. This is the consequence of increasing cases of documented dependency and lethal side effects, the development of opiate induced hyperalgesia and other of severe long-standing side effects [28–32]. Table 11.6.

Table 11.6 Strong opioids in chronic back pain

Strong opiates
Morphine, oxycodone, fentanyl, etc.

Table 11.7 Analgesics with dual mechanism of action used in chronic back pain

Dual action analgesics
Tramadol, Tapentadol

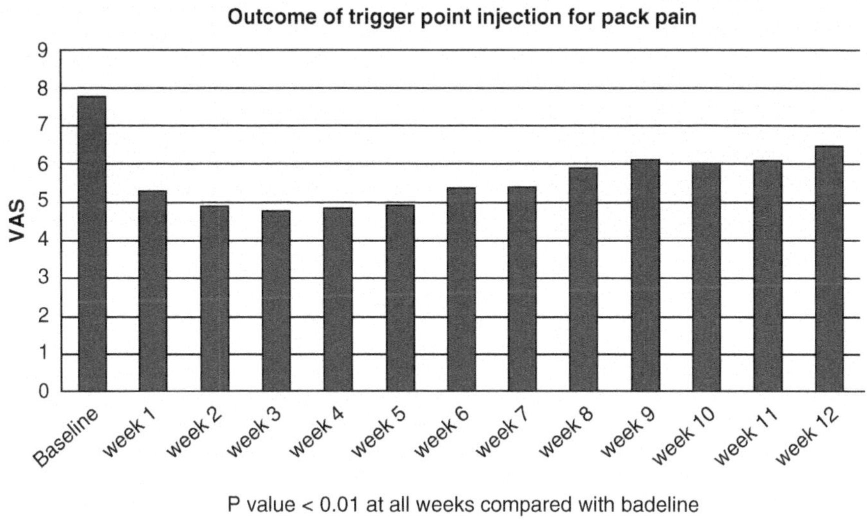

Fig. 11.5 Pain relieving effects of trigger point injections expressed with visual analogue scale (VAS) over 12 weeks

Medication with dual action (opioid receptors and serotoninergic agonist effect) have also been used quite widely with Tramadol in particular. The more recent "dual action agonist drug" Tapentadol appears to have a better profile and effectiveness [33–35] Table 11.7.

In some patients, conventional treatment does not provide sufficient pain relief or improvement in quality of life. Interventional strategies (spinal injections) will then have a role in the management of back pain. A course of trigger point injections (TPI) at 8–10 weeks interval provides an average benefit limited in time, with the symptoms coming back after 6–8 weeks as an average [36]. In general, the course would assure beneficial effects for 6 months approximately. The other advantage of such simple technique is that they are very safe. The active medication injected is usually methylprednisolone [34] (Fig. 11.5); however, other cortisone-based medications are also widely used.

In some cases, dry needling of hardened portions of muscle may be as effective as steroid injections (see chapter covering procedures).

A course of lumbar epidural injections (LEI) or lumbar root injections (LRI) under fluoroscopic guidance may be performed [37–39] (Figs. 11.6 and 11.7), if the back pain is associated with lumbar radiculopathy over a specific dermatome as diagnosed by neurological examination of the lower limbs and MRI evidence of a disc bulge.

Lumbar Nerve Root Injection

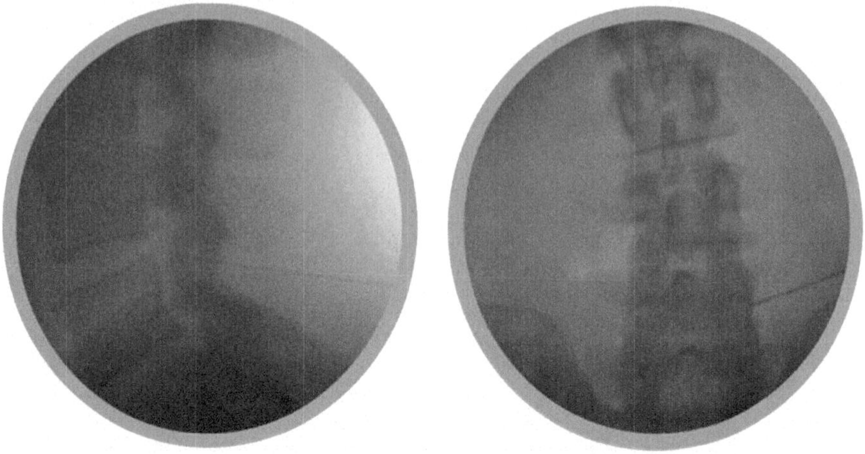

Fig. 11.6 Needle position in LRI as seen in antero-posterior and lateral view

Fig. 11.7 Contrast medium spread after a lumbar epidural injection as seen in lateral view

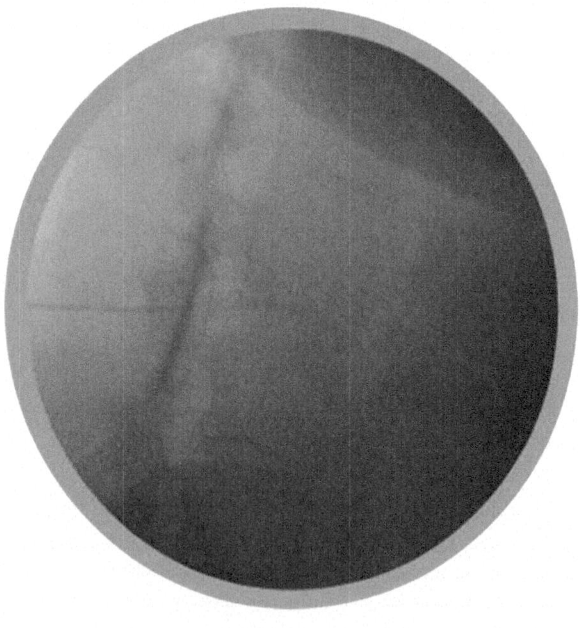

Inflamed facet joints may be the source of back pain. Unfortunately, there are no reliable clinical indicators for facet joint pain. In the past, facet joint injections were performed for diagnostic purposes. This procedure is no longer supported by Nice [40]. Radiofrequency denervation of the medial branch in experienced hands has still a place in the treatment of back pain [40–43].

There are also clear indications for more advanced procedures like spinal cord stimulation [44, 45], peripheral, neuromodulation [46] or treatment of discogenic pain.

11.4 Case Report 1

Patient FD, male of 50 years of age was referred to the Pain Clinic. He was complaining of constant chronic low back pain, without any radiculopathy in the lower limbs. He was an active person, riding the bicycle daily. His BMI was 21.6. The patient was mainly complaining of severe stiffness in the early morning and of a dull ache across the lower back, becoming more severe in the late afternoon and evening. He used to take NSAIDs but developed an allergic reaction and stopped. He was not keen on taking mild opiates because of side effects, particularly constipation and drowsiness. He had gone to visit his GP on several occasions, received different analgesics, including the adjuvant analgesics with no results. He attended physiotherapy but again did not find it useful.

The neurological examination of the lower limbs did not reveal any abnormality in terms of peripheral sensitivity, motor power and stretch reflexes. However, when taking his personal history, he mentioned to have been a regular rugby player from the age of 15–35 and to have suffered several unspecified back injuries. An MRI scan of the thoraco-lumbar spine showed the presence of an old crush fracture at the level of T12 and total dehydration of the L5 disc with the L5 vertebra laying directly on the top of the sacrum.

The cause of his back pain became clear. He was continuing to have a physically demanding life style. He was feeling good in himself and enjoyed riding his professional bicycle on a daily base. I had a long conversation with him, explained in detail the results of the MRI scan and the neurological examination and the implication of them. Then, I suggested the most appropriate management strategy in my opinion.

The management of his back pain was based on the following advice:

1. Change professional bicycle to a smoother amateur bicycle provided with soft suspensions and saddle.
2. To go swimming 3–4 times weekly
3. To start yoga exercises
4. To use a transcutaneous nerve stimulator (TENS) to be applied to the tender area of the back, first in the morning and few additional times during the day for periods of 2 h approximately at each time.

The patient agreed with the plan and implemented the advised management strategy. His back pain is not an issue anymore and he was discharged from the Pain Clinic back to his general practitioner. Basically, the patient needed a detailed explanation of his condition and a tailored pain management strategy.

11.5 Case Report 2

Patient MMC, female of 57 years of age, was referred to the Pain Clinic by her General Practitioner (GP). She had a history of Crohn's disease for which several abdominal surgical interventions were necessary over the years. Three years before being referred to the Pain Clinic she underwent an open cholecystectomy and 8 months after the surgery she had developed severe pain, particularly related to physical activities, in the upper right abdominal quadrant, radiating to the lower thoracic and upper lumbar back. The GP and the Surgeon had fully investigated the patient, but nothing pathological was found.

A neurological examination of the affected area did not show any peripheral abnormality with normal sensitivity of the entire painful area and of the surgical scar. The most probable diagnosis was of phantom visceral pain following the removal of the entire painful gall bladder. The patient had been previously prescribed different medications for neuropathic pain, but she had decided to stop them due to the limited effectiveness combined with unpleasant side effects, mostly characterised by drowsiness.

A clear explanation of the peripheral and central mechanism of developing phantom visceral pain was given to the patient. The analogy with peripheral limb pain following an amputation was a helpful model for the patient to understand her condition.

The patient needed to know why she did not get any similar problem following several abdominal surgeries to treat the Crohn's disease when, on the contrary, she had developed this specific localised pain after the cholecystectomy. She was prepared to cope with the pain after the explanation to her symptoms. Consequently, patient MMC was satisfied and discharged from the Pain Clinic.

11.6 Case Report 3

Patient CM, male of 73 years of age was referred to the Pain Clinic for long-standing mechanical low back and right sided lumbar radiculopathy. He had been suffering from low back pain for several years and more recently had developed a severe right lumbar radiculopathy in the L4/L5 and L5/S1 distribution. An MRI scan performed soon after his referral revealed the presence of diffuse dehydration of the lumbar discs, particularly evident at L4 and L5 levels with bulges at these levels causing narrowing of the exit foramina more pronounced over the right side, associated with facet joint hypertrophy and producing compression of the nerve roots. Prior to his referral to the Pain Clinic, he had tried different pain management strategies without achieving tangible benefits but, on the other end, in some cases causing severe side effects. A long list of "opioids based" analgesics combined with "adjuvant" analgesics was trailed. The major issue was that as soon the dose of medications was increased to higher levels side effects would appear.

Apart from suffering from Parkinson Disease and essential hypertension, however, patient AM was in general good health.

A course of right lumbar root injections (LRI) with methylprednisolone, under fluoroscopic guidance was planned. Patient AM received three consecutive LRI at 8 weeks interval. The treatment was extremely effective reducing the pain from severe to very mild. The improvement remained substantial at 6 months follow up. The conservative treatment consisted on the use of clonazepam 0.5 mg and quinine sulphate 300 mg at night, and pregabalin 75 mg twice daily.

Patient AM is currently attending the outpatient's consultation clinic for review at 6 monthly intervals.

References

1. Anderson RT. An orthopaedic ethnography in rural Nepal. Med Anthropol. 1984;8:46–59.
2. Juniper M, Le TK, Mladis D. The epidemiology, economic burden, and pharmacological treatment of chronic low back pain in France, Germany, Italy, Spain, and the UK: a literature-based review. Expert Opin Pharmacother. 2009;10(16):2581–92.
3. Stubbs B, Korangi A, Thompson T, Veronese N, Carvalho AF, Solomon M, Miesha J, Schofield P, Cresco T, Wilson N, Namport D. The epidemiology of back pain and its relationship with depression, psychosis, anxiety, sleep disturbances, and stress sensitivity: data from 43 low and middle-income countries. Gen Hosp Psychiatry. 2016;43:63–70.
4. Balague F, Troussier B, Salminen JJ. Non-specific low back pain in children and adolescents: risk factors. Eur Spine J. 1999;8:429–38.
5. Taylor H, Curran NM. The Duprin pain report. New York: Louis Harris and Associates; 1985. p. 1–233.
6. Makris UE, Frenkel L, Han L, Leo-Summers L, Gill TM. Epidemiology of restricting back pain in community living older persons. J Am Geriatr Soc. 2011;59(4):610–4.
7. Taimela S, Kujala UM, Salminen JJ, Viljanen T. The prevalence of low back pain among children and adolescents: a nationwide, cohort-based questionnaire survey in Finland. Spine. 1997;22:1132–6.
8. Andersson GBJ. The epidemiology of spinal disorders. In: Frymoyer JW, editor. The adult spine: principles and practice. Philadelphia: Lippincott-Raven; 1997. p. 93–141.
9. Croft P, et al. The prevalence and characteristics of chronic widespread pain in the general population. J Rheumatol. 1993;20:710–3.
10. Guo HR, Tanaka S, Halperin WE, Cameron LL. Back pain prevalence in US industry and estimates of lost workdays. Am J Public Health. 1999;89(7):1029–35.
11. Katz JN. Lumbar disc disorders and low-back pain: socioeconomic factors and consequences. J Bone Joint Surg Am. 2006;88(suppl 2):21–4.
12. Rubin DI. Epidemiology and risk factors for spine pain. Neurol Clin. 2007;25(2):353–71.
13. Samanta J, Kendall J, Samanta A. Chronic low back pain. BMJ. 2003;326:535–542.G.
14. Ostojic P, Radunovic G, Lazovic M, Tomanovic-Vujadinovic S. Ibuprofen plus paracetamol versus ibuprofen in acute low back pain: a randomized open label multicenter clinical study. Acta Reumatol Port. 2017;42(1):18–25.
15. Saragiotto BT, Machado GC, Ferreira ML, Pinheiro MB, Abdel Shaheed C, Maher CG. Paracetamol for low back pain. Cochrane Database Syst Rev. 2016, 2016;(6):CD012230.
16. Fernandez M, Colodro-Conde L, Hartvigsen J, Ferreira ML, Refshauge KM, Pinheiro MB, Ordonana JR, Ferreira PH. Chronic low back pain and the risk of depression or anxiety symptoms: insights from a longitudinal twin study. Spine J. 2017;17(7):905–12.

17. Khadilkar A, Odebiyi DO, Brosseau L, Wells GA. Transcutaneous electrical nerve stimulation (TENS) versus placebo for chronic low-back pain. Cochrane Database Syst Rev. 2008;(4):CD003008.
18. Johnson MI, Jones G. Transcutaneous electrical nerve stimulation: current status of evidence. Pain Manag. 2017;7(1):1–4.
19. Trigkilidas D. Acupuncture therapy for chronic lower back pain: a systematic review. Ann R Coll Surg Engl. 2010;92(7):595–8. https://doi.org/10.1308/003588410X12699663904196.
20. Wise J. NICE recommends exercise and not acupuncture for low back pain. BMJ. 2016;352:i1765. https://doi.org/10.1136/bmj.i1765.
21. Andersen LN, Juul-Kristensen B, Sørensen TL, Herborg LG, Roessler KK, Søgaard K. Longer term follow-up on effects of tailored physical activity or chronic pain self-management programme on return-to-work: a randomized controlled trial. J Rehabil Med. 2016;48(10):887–92. https://doi.org/10.2340/16501977-2159.
22. Gregg CD, Hoffman CW, Hall H, McIntosh G, Robertson PA. Outcomes of an interdisciplinary rehabilitation programme for the management of chronic low back pain. J Prim Health Care. 2011;3(3):222–7.
23. van Hooff ML, van der Merwe JD, O'Dowd J, Pavlov PW, Spruit M, de Kleuver M, van Limbeek J. Daily functioning and self-management in patients with chronic low back pain after an intensive cognitive behavioral programme for pain management. Eur Spine J. 2010;19(9):1517–26. https://doi.org/10.1007/s00586-010-1435-5.
24. Cherkin DC, Sherman KJ, Balderson BH, Cook AJ, Anderson ML, Hawkes RJ, Hansen KE, Turner JA. Effect of mindfulness-based stress reduction vs cognitive behavioral therapy or usual care on back pain and functional limitations in adults with chronic low back pain: a randomized clinical trial. JAMA. 2016;315(12):1240–9. https://doi.org/10.1001/jama.2016.2323.
25. Bawa FL, Mercer SW, Atherton RJ, Clague F, Keen A, Scott NW, Bond CM. Does mindfulness improve outcomes in patients with chronic pain? Systematic review and meta-analysis. Br J Gen Pract. 2015;65(635):e387–400. https://doi.org/10.3399/bjgp15X685297.
26. Shanthanna H, Gilron I, Rajarathinam M, AlAmri R, Kamath S, Thabane L, Devereaux PJ, Bhandari M. Benefits and safety of gabapentinoids in chronic low back pain: a systematic review and meta-analysis of randomized controlled trials. PLoS Med. 2017;14(8):e1002369. https://doi.org/10.1371/journal.pmed.1002369.
27. Atkinson JH, Slater MA, Caparelli EV, et al. A randomized controlled trial of gabapentin for chronic low back pain with and without a radiating component. Pain. 2016;157:1499–503.
28. Bohnert AS, Valenstein M, Bair MJ, Ganoczy D, McCarthy JF, Ilgen MA, Blow FC. Association between opioid prescribing patterns and opioid overdose-related deaths. JAMA. 2011;305(13):1315–21. https://doi.org/10.1001/jama.2011.370.
29. Darnall BD, Stacey BR, Chou R. Medical and psychological risks and consequences of long-term opioid therapy in women. Pain Med. 2012;13(9):1181–211. https://doi.org/10.1111/j.1526-4637.2012.01467.x.
30. Phillips JK, Ford MA, Bonnie RJ. Pain management and the opioid epidemic: balancing societal and individual benefits and risks of prescription opioid use. Washington, DC: National Academies Press; 2017.
31. Miller M, Barber CW, Leatherman S, Fonda J, Hermos JA, Cho K, Gagnon DR. Prescription opioid duration of action and the risk of unintentional overdose among patients receiving opioid therapy. JAMA Intern Med. 2015;175(4):608–15. https://doi.org/10.1001/jamainternmed.2014.8071.
32. Edlund MJ, Martin BC, Devries A, Fan MY, Braden JB, Sullivan MD. Trends in use of opioids for chronic noncancer pain among individuals with mental health and substance use disorders: the TROUP study. Clin J Pain. 2010;26(1):1–8. https://doi.org/10.1097/AJP.0b013e3181b99f35.
33. Sánchez Del Águila MJ, Schenk M, Kern KU, Drost T, Steigerwald I. Practical considerations for the use of tapentadol prolonged release for the management of severe chronic pain. Clin Ther. 2015;37(1):94–113. https://doi.org/10.1016/j.clinthera.2014.07.005.

34. Hofmann JF, Lal A, Steffens M, Boettger R. Patient-relevant outcomes and health-related quality of life in patients with chronic, severe, noncancer pain treated with tapentadol prolonged release-using criteria of health technology assessment. J Opioid Manag. 2016;12(5):323–31. https://doi.org/10.5055/jom.2016.0349.
35. Afilalo M, Morlion B. Efficacy of tapentadol ER for managing moderate to severe chronic pain. Pain Physician. 2013;16(1):27–40.
36. Ayob F, Liu M, di Vadi P. Myofascial Trigger point injection for chronic lower back pain (Poster). European Acute and Chronic Joint Pain Symposium, Dubrovnik, 2016.
37. Sencan S, Ozcan-Eksi EE, Cil H, Tay B, Berven S, Burch S, Deviren V, Demir-Deviren S. The effect of transforaminal epidural steroid injections in patients with spondylolisthesis. J Back Musculoskelet Rehabil. 2017;30(4):841–6. https://doi.org/10.3233/BMR-160543.
38. Taskaynatan MA, Tezel K, Yavuz F, Tan AK. The effectiveness of transforaminal epidural steroid injection in patients with radicular low back pain due to lumbar disc herniation two years after treatment. J Back Musculoskelet Rehabil. 2015;28(3):447–51. https://doi.org/10.3233/BMR-140539.
39. Altun I, Yuksel KZ. Impact of position on efficacy of caudal epidural injection for low back pain and radicular leg pain due to central spinal stenosis and lumbar disc hernia. J Korean Neurosurg Soc. 2017;60(2):205–10. https://doi.org/10.3340/jkns.2016.0405.007.
40. Al-Najjim M, Shah R, Rahuma M, Gabbar OA. Lumbar facet joint injection in treating low back pain: radiofrequency denervation versus SHAM procedure. Systematic review. J Orthop. 2017;15(1):1–8. https://doi.org/10.1016/j.jor.2017.10.001.
41. Leggett LE, Soril LJ, Lorenzetti DL, Noseworthy T, Steadman R, Tiwana S, Clement F. Radiofrequency ablation for chronic low back pain: a systematic review of randomized controlled trials. Pain Res Manag. 2014;19(5):e146–53.
42. Falco FJ, Manchikanti L, Datta S, Sehgal N, Geffert S, Onyewu O, Singh V, Bryce DA, Benyamin RM, Simopoulos TT, Vallejo R, Gupta S, Ward SP, Hirsch JA. An update of the effectiveness of therapeutic lumbar facet joint interventions. Pain Physician. 2012;15(6):E909–53.
43. Van Zundert J, Vanelderen P, Kessels A, van Kleef M. Radiofrequency treatment of facet-related pain: evidence and controversies. Curr Pain Headache Rep. 2012;16(1):19–25. https://doi.org/10.1007/s11916-011-0237-8.
44. Deckers K, De Smedt K, Mitchell B, Vivian D, Russo M, Georgius P, Green M, Vieceli J, Eldabe S, Gulve A, van Buyten JP, Smet I, Mehta V, Ramaswamy S, Baranidharan G, Sullivan R, Gassin R, Rathmell J, Gilligan C. New therapy for refractory chronic mechanical low back pain-restorative neurostimulation to activate the lumbar multifidus: one year results of a prospective multicenter clinical trial. Neuromodulation. 2018;21(1):48–55.
45. Grider JS, Manchikanti L, Carayannopoulos A, Sharma ML, Balog CC, Harned ME, Grami V, Justiz R, Nouri KH, Hayek SM, Vallejo R, Christo PJ. Effectiveness of spinal cord stimulation in chronic spinal pain: a systematic review. Pain Physician. 2016;19(1):E33–54.
46. Verrills P, Russo M. Peripheral nerve stimulation for back pain. Prog Neurol Surg. 2015;29:127–38.

Chapter 12
Postherpetic Neuralgia

Christine El-Yahchouchi and Antoun Nader

12.1 Causes

Postherpetic neuralgia is a common neuropathic pain syndrome, caused by a viral infection specifically the varicella zoster virus. A primary exposure to varicella zoster virus during childhood can cause chickenpox; however, herpes zoster is a reactivation of the dormant virus in the dorsal root or cranial nerve that typically occurs later in life or when the immune system is compromised [3, 5].

Around 90–95% of people in North America show seropositivity to the varicella zoster virus and are considered at risk to develop herpes zoster and postherpetic neuralgia [3, 6].

HZ infection is characterized by a vesicular rash in a dermatomal fashion accompanied with a neuropathic pain that can even begin as a prodromal few days before the appearance of the typical rash. Typically the rash begins as maculopapular lesions that progress to vesicles that finally crust and heal within 2–4 weeks [1]. Scarring and changes in skin pigmentation is not uncommon.

The definition of postherpetic neuralgia varies in the literature. Some suggested that if the pain persists beyond 3 months after the acute rash it qualifies for postherpetic neuralgia. Rarely PHN onset can be months or even years after the initial rash has resolved [7]. The incidence of postherpetic neuralgia varies between 9% and 34%, depending on the definition [8] therefore it is classified as third most common cause of neuropathic pain following chronic radicular pain and diabetic neuropathy.

C. El-Yahchouchi (✉)
Department of Anesthesiology, American University of Beirut Medical Center, Beirut, Lebanon
e-mail: ce18@aub.edu.lb

A. Nader
Feinberg School of Medicine, Northwestern University Feinberg School of Medicine, Chicago, IL, USA
e-mail: ANader@nm.org

K. Shimoji et al. (eds.), *Chronic Pain Management in General and Hospital Practice*, https://doi.org/10.1007/978-981-15-2933-7_12

The cause of the pain is thought to be related to the inflammation caused by the reactivation of the virus which will lead to demyelination and axonal degeneration and fibrosis as demonstrated by early studies. This will lead to overexpression of channels and receptors such as sodium channels, TPRV1, and adrenoreceptors on damaged neurons sensitizing pain specific fibers that can elicit continuous pain even with the absence of stimulus.

12.2 Diagnosis

Diagnosis of PHN is a clinical diagnosis based on recognizing the signs and identifying the risk factors. Age, immunosuppression, autoimmune disease, and gender are described as potential risks factors to develop this syndrome. Under the age of 60, female gender was a risk factor [9]. Intensity and duration of pain during the acute phase of the rash, the involvement of the ophthalmic branch of the trigeminal nerve was also described as risk factor in some reviews [10].

Pain may start before, during, or after the acute vesicular rash, it is typically localized, dermatomal, and does not cross the midline. The patients usually report itching, burning, or throbbing quality of pain, consistent with any other neuropathic pain that might be aggravated by light touch. However, the history of HZ provides evidence for a diagnosis of PHN. In some cases diagnosing HZ is difficult and the rash can be mistaken for a different diagnosis, in these cases, detection of viral DNA by polymerase chain reaction using fluid from the lesions is the most sensitive and specific test. In addition, direct fluorescent antibody staining, [11] immunoperoxidase staining, histopathology, and Tzanck smear can also be useful.

Pain may be the sole presentation in some cases (zoster sine herpete) where rash does not appear at all making the diagnosis more difficult.

In addition to the pain, cognitive impairment, sleep disturbance as well as psychological implications are often associated with this syndrome and treating the pain alone is not always enough.

Physical examination can complete the diagnosis, examining areas of previous AHZ may show evidence of cutaneous scarring [12]. Due to the central and peripheral sensitization discussed above, hyperalgesia and allodynia are common. However, decreased sensation or numbness can also be experienced by the patient.

HZ is highly contagious when the rash appears and until the lesions crust [13].

It is well known that the most common locations of HZ are fifth cranial nerves (with its ophthalmicus branch being most commonly affected) and intercostal nerves. Reports of uncommon localization of herpes zoster include the ulnar nerve [14] and the C6 nerve root. Interestingly, Jason et al. reported a female patient who presented 6 months post ACDF with recurrent C6 radiculopathy consisting with restenosis, shortly after, the appearance of the pathognomonic rash along C6 distribution confirmed the diagnosis of HZ. Patient was diagnosed later on with postherpetic neuralgia and persistent pain even after 2 years from the appearance of the rash.

12.3 Treatments

12.3.1 Prevention

The VZV and HZ vaccines that are traditionally used are live attenuated vaccines therefore limiting its use in immunocompromised patients. Multiple studies showed decrease efficacy with age, despite the uncertainty about its effectiveness and duration of action, the advisory committee on immunization practices recommended in 2014 that the VZ vaccines should be given for adults aged >60 years.

An experimental recombinant vaccine HZ/su that contains a non-live VZ glycoprotein with a subunit antigen AS01B was recently developed.

During a recent clinical trial, zoster efficacy study in adult 50 years of age or older (ZOE 50) subjects received HZ/su vaccine or placebo and were followed over a period of 3.2 years, results were promising showing 96% efficacy against HZ. A similar ongoing study ZOE-70 is currently ongoing including subjects over 70 years of age. Accordingly, the FDA recently approved Shingrix; HZ/su vaccine for the prevention of shingles in patients over 50 years of age, following that, the ACIP revised the previous recommendations and voted for the use of Shingrix over the traditional live attenuated Zostavax vaccine.

12.3.2 Treatment

The mainstay treatment of postherpetic neuralgia is primarily a prevention from HZ virus which is the direct cause of this syndrome. Multiple treatment modalities are currently described and used for the treatment of acute pain from HZ virus such as antiviral drugs, topical creams, membrane stabilizers, corticosteroids, Interleukins as well as epidural injections with or without steroids. Unfortunately, none of these treatments demonstrated evidence in the prevention or treatment of PHN. Oral antiviral agents may reduce the duration of postherpetic neuralgia if taken during acute herpes zoster specially if started within 72 h of the skin lesions [2, 15].

The available antiviral agents can be divided into two classes: the first are nucleoside analogues that rely on viral phosphorylation to be activated such as acyclovir, famciclovir, and valacyclovir. The second is independent from viral phosphorylation such as foscarnet, vidarabine, and cidofovir. Famciclovir was shown to be superior to valacyclovir in reducing acute zoster symptoms [16].

The treatment recommendations are based on general consensus of societies, the most recent recommendations are those of the IASP in 2015. As with any complex syndrome, multimodal and multidisciplinary approach is a must.

Approved medications for neuropathic pain should be the first-line therapy such as Gabapentinoid, TCA, and SNRIs. Gabapentinoid being the only approved agent for this condition SNRIs were never described in patients with PHN and therefore lack evidence. Combination of these drugs is an alternative option to monotherapy, especially if the patient does not tolerate increasing the dose of one agent.

Second line therapy include Lidocaine patches (5%), capsaicin patches (8%) applied to the painful area for 60 min, and tramadol. Tramadol should be used carefully when combined with antidepressant medication especially those with serotonin activity due to its interaction potential. For elderly patients who could not tolerate the side effects of the first-line treatments, lidocaine patches can be a first-line option due to its high safety profile. Finally opioids and botulinum toxin A are recommended as third line therapy by IASP. Opioids have demonstrated efficacy, however, due to safety concerns they are viewed as third line therapy [4].

12.3.3 Interventional Therapies

Due to the low quality of the available evidence no general consensus on the role of interventional therapies such as spinal cord stimulation, deep brain stimulation, intrathecal medication delivery, cryoablation/pulsed radiofrequency of intercostal nerves. Moreover the IASP recommended against sympathetic blocks or intrathecal injections for PHN treatment.

12.3.4 Spinal Cord Stimulation

Some suggested that it may be helpful in cases where there is partial and not complete deafferentation from postherpetic neuralgia. Temporary stimulation during acute pain might decrease pain and prevent postherpetic pain [1].

Spinal cord stimulation provided long-term pain relief in 47.1% of reported patients with PHN [17], making SCS and peripheral nerve stimulation a promising therapy that requires further investigations to prove its efficacy.

12.3.5 Deep Brain Stimulation

Deep brain stimulation of the contralateral periventricular gray area and ventral posterior lateral thalamic nucleus was reported to be effective in treating postherpetic pain [18]. Several studies have also shown efficacy of high frequency repetitive transcranial magnetic stimulation of the primary motor cortex, in treating chronic pain syndrome [19].

The incorporation of these techniques in the treatment of postherpetic neuralgia algorithm remains controversial and restricted to patients with intractable pain who failed more conservative management.

12.3.6 *Intrathecal and Epidural Injections*

Spinal intrathecal injections of corticosteroids were reported to be effective in one randomized, controlled trial; however, another trial failed to replicate these positive results [3]. A meta-analysis showed that epidural steroids can reduce the pain during the acute zoster pain, however, failed to prevent postherpetic neuralgia [20].

References

1. Koshy E, Mengting L, Kumar H, Jianbo W. Epidemiology, treatment and prevention of herpes zoster: a comprehensive review. Indian J Dermatol Venereol Leprol. 2018;84(3):251–62. https://doi.org/10.4103/ijdvl.IJDVL_1021_16.
2. Jalali MH, Ansarin H, Soltani-Arabshahi R. Broad-band ultraviolet B phototherapy in zoster patients may reduce the incidence and severity of postherpetic neuralgia. Photodermatol Photoimmunol Photomed. 2006;22(5):232–7.
3. Johnson RW, Rice AS. Clinical practice. Postherpetic neuralgia. N Engl J Med. 2014;371(16):1526–33. https://doi.org/10.1056/NEJMcp1403062.
4. Hadley GR, Gayle JA, Ripoll J, Jones MR, Argoff CE, Kaye RJ, Kaye AD, Hadley GR. Postherpetic neuralgia a review. Curr Pain Headache Rep. 2016;20(3):17. https://doi.org/10.1007/s11916-016-0548-x.
5. Hope-Simpson RE. Postherpetic neuralgia. J R Coll Gen Pract. 1975;25(157):571–5.
6. Johnson RW. Herpes zoster and postherpetic neuralgia. Expert Rev Vaccines. 2010;9(3 Suppl):21–6. https://doi.org/10.1586/erv.10.30.
7. Feller L, Khammissa RAG, Fourie J, Bouckaert M, Lemmer J. Postherpetic neuralgia and trigeminal neuralgia. Pain Res Treat. 2017;2017:1681765. https://doi.org/10.1155/2017/1681765.
8. van Wijck AJ, Opstelten W, Moons KG, van Essen GA, Stolker RJ, Kalkman C, et al. The PINE study of epidural steroids and local anaesthetics to prevent postherpetic neuralgia: a randomised controlled trial. Lancet. 2006;367(9506):219–24.
9. Forbes HJ, Bhaskaran K, Thomas SL, Smeeth L, Clayton T, Mansfield K, et al. Quantification of risk factors for postherpetic neuralgia in herpes zoster patients: a cohort study. Neurology. 2016;87(1):94–102. https://doi.org/10.1212/WNL.0000000000002808.
10. Jung BF, Johnson RW, Griffin DR, Dworkin RH. Risk factors for postherpetic neuralgia in patients with herpes zoster. Neurology. 2004;62(9):1545–51.
11. O'Connor KM, Paauw DS. Herpes zoster. Med Clin North Am. 2013;97(4):503–22, ix. https://doi.org/10.1016/j.mcna.2013.02.002.
12. Chen N, Li Q, Yang J, Zhou M, Zhou D, He L. Antiviral treatment for preventing postherpetic neuralgia. Cochrane Database Syst Rev. 2014;(2):CD006866. https://doi.org/10.1002/14651858.CD006866.pub3.
13. Seward J, Jumaan A. VSV: persistence in the population. In: Human herpesviruses: biology, therapy, and immunoprophylaxis. Cambridge: Cambridge University Press; 2007.
14. Cukic V. The uncommon localization of herpes zoster. Med Arch. 2016;70(1):72–5. https://doi.org/10.5455/medarh.2016.70.72-75.
15. Watson CP. Herpes zoster and postherpetic neuralgia. CMAJ. 2010;182(16):1713–4. https://doi.org/10.1503/cmaj.101409.
16. Ono F, Yasumoto S, Furumura M, Hamada T, Ishii N, et al. Comparison between famciclovir and valacyclovir for acute pain in adult Japanese immunocompetent patients with herpes zoster. J Dermatol. 2012;39(11):902–8. https://doi.org/10.1111/j.1346-8138.2012.01584.x.

17. Kurklinsky S, Palmer SC, Arroliga MJ, Ghazi SM. Neuromodulation in postherpetic neuralgia: case reports and review of the literature. Pain Med. 2017;19:1237. https://doi.org/10.1093/pm/pnx175.
18. Green AL, Nandi D, Armstrong G, Carter H, Aziz T. Post-herpetic trigeminal neuralgia treated with deep brain stimulation. J Clin Neurosci. 2003;10(4):512–4.
19. Ma SM, Ni JX, Li XY, Yang LQ, Guo YN, Tang YZ. High-frequency repetitive transcranial magnetic stimulation reduces pain in postherpetic neuralgia. Pain Med. 2015;16(11):2162–70. https://doi.org/10.1111/pme.12832.
20. Chen N, Yang M, He L, Zhang D, Zhou M, Zhu C. Corticosteroids for preventing postherpetic neuralgia. Cochrane Database Syst Rev. 2010;(12):CD005582. https://doi.org/10.1002/14651858.CD005582.pub3.

Chapter 13
Neuropathic Pain: Complex Regional Pain Syndrome (CRPS)

Mansoor M. Aman, Ammar Mahmoud, and Taruna Waghray-Penmetcha

13.1 Introduction

Chronic pain affects 100 million Americans [1] and is broadly subcategorized as neuropathic, nociceptive (somatic and visceral), and sympathetically mediated. Epidemiologic studies on complex regional pain syndrome are scarce. A regional report from Mayo Clinic retrospectively examined their records between years 1989 and 1999 for the incidence and prevalence of CRPS I in a population of 106,470. The incidence was 5.46 per 100,000 person-years at risk and a period prevalence of 20.57 per 100,000. The diagnosis favored a female:male distribution at 4:1 with a median age of onset of 46 years. Fracture was found to be the most common trigger (46%), and diagnostic work-up included a triple-phase bone scan and autonomic testing in the majority of patients (>80%) [2]. A review of data from 1996 to 2005 reported a higher incidence of 26.2 per 100,000 with a 3:1 distribution [3].

The cumulative economic burden of various chronic pain conditions is estimated at $635 billion [4]. While the prevalence of complex regional pain syndrome (CRPS) only accounts for 1.2% of this patient population [5], it is associated with significant morbidity and financial implications due to difficulty in diagnosis, multiple treatment algorithms, as well as chronic medication costs. Reaching a correct diagnosis is often challenging and patients can often be misdiagnosed with generalized pain

M. M. Aman
Division of Pain Medicine, Department of Anesthesiology, Harvard Medical School/Brigham and Women's Hospital, Boston, MA, USA

A. Mahmoud
Division of Pain Medicine, Department of Anesthesiology, Cleveland Clinic Foundation, Cleveland, OH, USA

T. Waghray-Penmetcha (✉)
Division of Pain Medicine, Department of Anesthesiology, John H. Stroger Jr. Hospital of Cook County, Chicago, IL, USA
e-mail: tpenmetcha@cookcountyhhs.org

K. Shimoji et al. (eds.), *Chronic Pain Management in General and Hospital Practice*, https://doi.org/10.1007/978-981-15-2933-7_13

disorder, fibromyalgia, and various other pain disorders for years. It has been demonstrated that in the 3 years leading up to a formal diagnosis of CRPS, the cost of medical care is approximately $15,000. The median cost after CRPS diagnosis over an eight-year span is over $55,000 including inpatient, outpatient, and prescription costs [6]. This does not include work hours lost, co-morbid conditions and their treatment, and cost associated with interventional/surgical therapies such as neuromodulation. A diagnosis of CRPS carries not only physical pain, but also psychological, social, and financial implications that must be taken into consideration. In this chapter, we aim to provide an in-depth review of the history of CRPS, its pathophysiology, diagnostic criteria, and various available and emerging treatment modalities.

13.2 A Historical Perspective

Complex regional pain syndrome (CRPS) is a debilitating, often progressive pain disorder that can affect the limbs, trunks, or can have a full body presentation. In understanding this once elusive disease, it is important to consider its historical significance. While there are many physicians who played an instrumental role in our understanding of pain today, we will briefly discuss contributions by a select few.

The early clinical manifestations of neuropathic pain can be traced back to the sixteenth century anatomist and the father of modern surgery Ambroise Paré—physician to French King Charles IX of Valois. The King underwent multiple phlebotomy treatments for smallpox, which led to chronic burning pain. Centuries later, a British surgeon named Denmark first described post traumatic neuropathic pain in a wounded soldier in 1812. Years later, the early works by Neurologist Silas Weir Mitchell who cared for wounded soldiers during the American civil war led to what we now understand as "causalgia," derived from the Greek words for heat and pain. In the 1900s, following the introduction of X-ray, Paul Sudek described atrophy that could persist beyond the stages of acute injury leading to chronic pain. The mechanisms of disease were further explored by Rene Leriche who hypothesized that the sympathetic nervous system was also contributing to this pervasive pain state and went on to perform the first periarterial sympathectomy for arm pain. James Evans was also a strong proponent of the sympathetically mediated mechanisms of this disease. He later coined the term reflex sympathetic dystrophy (RSD). Also in the 1940s while Evans emphasized the sympathetic mechanism, Froise proposed arterial vasospasm as the likely starting point of chronic pain following tissue injury. John Bonica, an anesthesiologist, by training would go on to form the International Association for the Study of Pain (IASP) and help classify the disease by stages. He described three distinct stages: Acute (Stage 1), Dystrophic (stage 2), and Atrophic (stage 3)—now obsolete and only mentioned for historical significance. He also emphasized that the dystrophic changes were secondary to pain, and not always localized to the distribution of nerves or roots [7, 8]. The names RSD and causalgia were subsequently changed to complex regional pain syndrome type-I and type-II, respectively.

13.3 Taxonomy

The International Association for the Study of Pain initially defined RSD as "continuous pain in a portion of an extremity after trauma which may include fracture but does not involve a major nerve." A known nerve injury was necessary to make a diagnosis of causalgia [9]. As ongoing research revealed etiologies apart from sympathetic over activity, in 1994 the terminology was again modified. Regional sympathetic dystrophy was renamed complex regional pain syndrome (CRPS I), and causalgia replaced with CRPS II. The current IASP definition of CRPS I is a "syndrome that usually develops after an initiating noxious event, not limited to the distribution of a single peripheral nerve and is apparently disproportionate to the inciting event." The definition of CRPS II includes a painful condition associated with a peripheral nerve injury [10].

13.4 Pathophysiology

The pathophysiology of both CRPS Type I and Type II has perplexed scientist for decades. Proposed theories suggest alterations in autonomic, peripheral, and central nervous systems. Other mechanisms likely to play a significant role include ischemia reperfusion injury, micro vascular spasm, inflammatory, genetic, and autoimmune changes. It is critical to understand the various pathologic alterations in order to both manage, and develop future treatment modalities (Fig. 13.1).

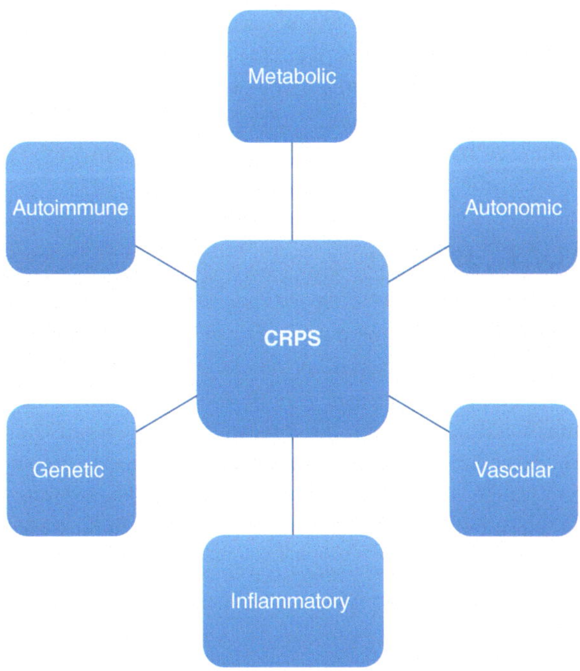

Fig. 13.1 The multi-compartment model describing the pathophysiology of CRPS

13.4.1 Metabolic and Autonomic

Early theories suggested excessive bony metabolism that persisted beyond the stage of initial injury to be the primary etiology [11]. This mechanism was studied by radiographic changes in patients with chronic pain following injury but failed to explain the various other constellation of symptoms. The works of James Evans proposed an autonomic basis for the rubor, pallor, sweating, and/or atrophy present in his patients [12]. He suggested that excessive nociceptive afferent signals from the peripheral nervous system enter the central nervous system (CNS) post-traumatic injury. In the CNS, these nociceptive afferents converge with and stimulate fibers of the autonomic system. This internunical pool was responsible for post-ganglionic efferent output that subsequently induced arterial capillary spasm causing ischemic pain. An increase in capillary filtration pressure would explain the edema and swelling. Clinically, the pain would subside following sympathetic blockade in a large proportion of patients, presumably due to a decrease in this efferent limb. This proved to be both diagnostic and therapeutic and would be the foundation of research for generations thereafter [13, 14].

13.4.2 Sympathetically Mediated and Sympathetically Independent CRPS

With years of experience in diagnosis and management, the underlying mechanisms of CRPS were also called into question. Clinically, some patients experience dramatic improvement in symptoms following chemical sympathectomy while others experience little to no relief. This gave rise to proponents of sympathetically maintained [15], and sympathetically independent CRPS [16]. While other groups argued that early stages of disease actually demonstrate a decrease in sympathetic tone as evidenced by a warm, erythematous, edematous limb [17, 18].

13.4.3 Vascular

Around the same time period, Froise proposed another theory to explain the symptoms of CRPS—arterial spasms being the primary cause of pain [19]. This traumatic arterial vasospasm was thought to occur in the small arterioles, leading to nutritional deprivation of the tissue and degenerative changes of the affected limb. The large vessels are unaffected ensuring adequate tissue perfusion and limiting the occurrence of limb threatening ischemia. The edema was thought to occur from disruption of the microvasculature resulting in increased capillary permeability and extravasation of plasma. Both of these mechanisms supported an underlying ischemia, and treatment with sympathetic blockade to increase flow. The primary difference being, Evans reported alternations in sympathetic tone being the driving force to the clinical changes, while Froise regarded the ischemia to be the dominant factor.

13.4.4 Inflammatory

In 1993, a large prospective study of RSD failed to demonstrate significant autonomic involvement [20]. The authors suggested that symptoms were resultant of an exaggerated inflammatory response, possibly owing to oxygen radicals. The disease was renamed the following year to CRPS. Higher levels of local inflammatory markers such as interleukin (IL)-6 and tumor necrosis factor (TNF)-alpha have been shown in a CRPS extremity when compared to an uninvolved extremity [21]. Skin biopsy immunoassay in early stages of CRPS has shown keratinocyte activation resulting in epidermal thickening and upregulation of TNF-alpha, IL-6, and tryptase. This suggests increased mast cell activity in patients with early CRPS. In contrast, chronic cases of CRPS had reduced keratinocyte activity that led to epidermal thinning and no increase in mast cell numbers [22]. Mast cells are generated in the bone marrow and secrete various molecules such as histamine, nitric oxide, and heparin. Treatment agents for prevention of division and killing mast cells (Imatinib), and prevention of release from mast cells (antihistamines, glucocorticoids) have been explored as possible targets for treatment [23].

The concept of neurogenic inflammation is also thought to play a role wherein microglia and astrocytes respond to an injury, but can also lead to hypersensitivity and chronic pain. It is proposed that blood borne macrophages and monocytes can penetrate the central nervous system and differentiate into microglia and contribute to pain. A study examined the plasma cytokines of CRPS patients compared to match controlled and found elevated levels of CD14 (+) CD16 (+) monocyte/macrophage subgroup and significantly lower anti-inflammatory cytokine IL-1 [24]. Subsequently, there has been data to suggest the role of immunomodulating medications such as bisphosphonates, glucocorticoids, immunoglobulins, and TNF-alpha antagonist agents [25].

The upregulation of the pro-inflammatory cytokines is thought to be responsible for peripheral sensitization and increased nociception. This constant, intense peripheral noxious input from nerve injury or tissue damage increases the excitability of nociceptive neurons of the spinal cord—a phenomenon known as central sensitization [26]. Associated with central sensitization is the windup phenomenon, wherein the repeated stimulation of the dorsal root afferents including nociceptive C fibers increases the number of action potentials generated [27].

13.4.5 Genetic

It has been long proposed that certain populations may have a genetic predisposition to developing CRPS [28]. With the Human Genome Project it is possible to map specific loci and identify patterns in genetic susceptibility. Studies reported human leukocyte antigen (HLA)—DR13, HLA-DR2, and HLA-DQ1—may play a significant role for select phenotypes [29]. The idea that trivial trauma may lead to significant disability in certain patients while others heal appropriately is explained by genetic factors conferring susceptibility. Two distinct genetic loci at D6S1014∗36 and D6S1014∗37 alleles were found in significantly higher frequency only in CRPS with multifocal or generalized tonic dystonia [30]. Interesting, HLA-DQ8 was found to be associated with CRPS despite phenotypic variance (with and without dystonia) [31].

13.4.6 Autoimmune

Whether autoantibodies are directly linked to the pathogenesis of CRPS or simply a phenomenon not directly related to its development is unknown. Active agnostic type autoantibodies directed at β2 adrenergic receptor and/or the muscarinic-2 receptor peptide were found in the serum samples of CRPS patients [32]. While this suggests an autoimmune component present in select patients, further study is required to discern causality versus coincidence. When screening for autoimmune disease, one of the most common tests performed is the antinuclear antibodies (ANA). Serum assay of 82 CRPS (as defined by Harden–Bruehl criteria) demonstrated a positive ANA at much higher rates when compared to healthy general population, 33% vs. 4%. There was no correlation between the presence of ANA in cold versus warm CRPS [33].

13.5 Diagnosis and Clinical Presentation

The diagnostic criteria for CRPS have evolved drastically over the years. An international consensus meeting was held in Budapest, Hungary to help standardize diagnosis and improve specificity from prior IASP diagnostic criteria [34, 35]. Unlike many other disease processes, the diagnosis of CRPS is made clinically and does not warrant confirmatory testing. The Budapest criteria have a sensitivity of 0.99 and a specificity of 0.68 [36].

CRPS most commonly develops after trauma, surgery, or prolonged immobilization of an affected limb, but has been reported to occur spontaneously. CRPS type I does not have a definable nerve injury, whereas in type II, a nerve injury is present. To meet these diagnostic criteria, the patient must have continuing pain that is out of

Table 13.1 Budapest criteria for diagnosis of CRPS

Symptom (patient reports at least one symptom in three or more categories)	Sign (evidence of at least one sign in two or more categories)
Sensory: Hyperesthesia and/or allodynia	Sensory: Hyperalgesia (to pinprick) and/or allodynia (to light touch and/or temperature sensation and/or deep somatic pressure and/or joint movement)
Vasomotor: Temperature asymmetry and/or skin color changes	Vasomotor: Temperature asymmetry (>1 °C) and/or skin color changes
Sudomotor/edema: Edema and/or sweating changes	Sudomotor/EDEMA: Edema and/or sweating changes
Motor/trophic: Decreased range of motion and/or motor dysfunction (weakness, tremor, dystonia) and/or trophic changes (hair, nail, skin)	Motor/trophic: Decreased range of motion and/or motor dysfunction (weakness, tremor, dystonia) and/or trophic changes (hair, nail, skin)

Adapted from original publication by Harden et al. [35]

Table 13.2 CRPS severity score

Symptoms	Signs
Allodynia	Hyperalgesia
Bilateral temperature asymmetry	Allodynia
Skin color changes	Temperature asymmetry
Edema	Skin color changes
Sweating asymmetry	Edema
Trophic/dystrophic changes (hair, skin or nails)	Sweating asymmetry
Motor changes (weakness, tremor or dystonia)	Trophic/dystrophic changes
Decreased range of motion	Motor changes
	Decreased range of motion

proportion to its inciting injury, no other diagnosis explaining injury, at least one sign in two categories, and at least one symptom in three categories (Table 13.1). Signs and symptoms usually affect one limb and may include disturbances in sensation, motor function, edema, altered hair and nail growth, and autonomic disturbances.

While this dichotomous criterion is essential in making an initial diagnosis, it does not allow for longitudinal monitoring of clinical progression or improvement. The CRPS Severity Score (CSS) is a validated [37, 38] measure that looks at the presence or absence of 17 signs and symptoms of CRPS. The range of scores is from 0 to 17, one point for each sign/symptom. The higher scores were associated with greater pain intensity, functional disability, and greater variance in bilateral temperature asymmetry (Table 13.2). It is important to note that a patient with long-standing CRPS may fall outside of the diagnostic criteria but still have significant pain and functional impairment. While anxiety and psychological factors may play a role in the global assessment of pain, a recent study reported that these factors do not concern patients. Above all else, patients reported needing physicians to address not only their CRPS related pain, but also their generalized pain, movement difficulties, and reliance on medication to consider themselves recovered [39].

13.6 Management

13.6.1 Prevention of CRPS

A variety of pharmacological agents including free radical scavengers (vitamin C), corticosteroids, and calcitonin have been studied for primary prevention of CRPS following an injury or surgery. Clinically, there are multiple limitations surrounding the utility of these therapies in the perioperative and post-traumatic periods. These limitations include difficulty in identifying patients who are at increased risk, appropriate duration and dose of the selected therapy, and lack of randomized controlled trials supporting the use of such agents. In effort to limit progression of existing CRPS, patients undergoing surgery should undergo a pre-operative evaluation to discuss recommendations on the timing of surgery, perioperative pain management options, and anesthetic technique.

13.6.1.1 Vitamin C

Vitamin C is a potent water-soluble antioxidant with promising results in the prevention of CRPS following both traumatic injury and orthopedic surgery. Of the available preventative therapies, vitamin C has been the most studied and verified. The American Academy of Orthopedic Surgeons (AAOS) currently recommends 500 mg of vitamin C every day for 50 days after distal radius fracture to prevent occurrence of CRPS [40]. Evidence supporting this practice includes a recent meta-analysis of four randomized control trials (three in upper extremity distal radius fractures and one in lower extremity following foot and ankle surgery) concluding that a vitamin C daily dose of more than 500 mg for 45–50 days post-trauma or surgery may help reduce the occurrence of CRPS [41]. Included in this meta-analysis, a multicenter dose-response study explored the role of various dosing regimens (200 mg, 500 mg, and 1500 mg/day) and concluded that 200 mg daily dosing is no more effective than placebo, while 500 mg and 1500 mg daily dosing resulted in significantly lower ratios of CRPS [42].

13.6.2 Treatment Options

13.6.2.1 Physical Therapy and Occupational Therapy

Physical and occupation therapy are considered the cornerstone for treatment of patients with CRPS. Physiotherapy can be used to treat mild cases of CRPS; however, it is commonly combined with medical management for greater efficacy. Prior to physiotherapy referral, patient centered goals surrounding pain intensity reduction and functional restoration should be discussed. Additionally, referral to a therapist familiar with the different phases and clinical features of CRPS is key to ensure patient compliance and treatment success. There are multiple physical therapy interventions that are beneficial in patients with CRPS. These interventions include desensitization therapy, mirror box therapy, gradual weight-bearing exercises, transcutaneous electrical nerve stimulation (TENS), isotonic stretching, and aerobic conditioning. Finally, therapy should be tailored to a patient specific treatment algorithm with a goal towards vocational and functional rehabilitation.

13.6.2.2 Desensitization Therapy

Desensitization can be effective in treating the hypersensitivity and allodynia associated with CRPS. It commonly involves progressive stimuli (textures/fabrics, vibration, heat, and cold) to the affected areas. Additionally, tactile discrimination can decrease pain and increase tactile acuity when patients are required to discriminate between type and location of tactile stimulus (two-point discrimination) [43].

13.6.2.3 Mirror Box Therapy

Mirror box therapy (MBT) is a simple and noninvasive technique that can be utilized in the treatment of patients with CRPS. The patient is positioned to view the unaffected limb in the mirror, while the painful limb is hidden. Mirror reflection permits the patient to visualize and rehearse movement of the affected limb. The goal of MBT is to restore cortical processing thereby resulting in pain reduction and functional restoration of the affected limb. Interestingly, MBT has been regarded as a "time sensitive" treatment modality. Patients with recent (8 weeks or less) onset of CRPS experienced significant pain reduction, while patient with intermediate onset (>1 year) reported reduced stiffness [44].

13.6.2.4 Pharmacotherapy

Appropriate medication selection and management in patients with CRPS can be challenging. Prior to starting any medication regimen it is pivotal for the clinician to be familiar with current evidence-based medicine recommendations and published randomized controlled trials. Referral and consultation with a pain management specialist with expertise in the multiple treatment regimens for CRPS should be utilized.

There are multiple medication classes that can be employed in the treatment of patients with CRPS. Common categories of medications used include anti-inflammatory, antidepressants, anticonvulsants, antihypertensive, bisphosphonates, NMDA receptor antagonist, and opioids. Additionally, emerging drug therapies including botulinum toxin type A, topical compound formulations, free radical scavengers, and intravenous immunoglobulin are being studied and may suggest novel treatment modalities in the future.

Appropriate agent selection will help manage the presenting symptoms of CRPS and allow patients to successfully start and advance in their rehabilitation programs. Given that multiple physiological systems are affected in patients with CRPS, it is unlikely that a single medication class will effectively manage the different presenting symptoms. To overcome this, a combination of multiple medications from different classes should be employed. Combination therapy is regarded superior than long-term opioid therapy. Finally, modification of any current treatment regimen should occur on a case-by-case basis and patients should be counseled regarding the adverse effects and associated costs to ensure compliance.

13.6.2.5 Anticonvulsants

There are multiple anticonvulsant medications that could be used in the management of CRPS. It is important to recognize that these medications have different mechanisms and can be combined for synergistic and additive effects. Of the available antiepileptic medications only a few have been studied in patients with CRPS. Commonly used anticonvulsants in treatment of CRPS include gabapentin, pregabalin, lamotrigine, and carbamazepine.

13.6.2.6 Gabapentin

Gabapentin is commonly regarded as a first line treatment option for patients with neuropathic pain. It exerts its effect at the $\alpha_2\delta$ subunit of voltage gated calcium channels. Familiarity with its administration and associated side effects has led to its use in the management of patients with CRPS. To date, there is one double-blind randomized controlled trial exploring the role of gabapentin in patients with CRPS. Gabapentin has been shown to have a mild effect on pain reduction but significant reduction in sensory deficits (hyperalgesia and allodynia) in the affected limb [45].

13.6.2.7 Tricyclic Antidepressants (TCA)

Tricyclic antidepressants are commonly utilized in the management of neuropathic pain. TCA's are highly efficacious with a number needed to treat (NNT) of 2.6 [46]. The mechanism of pain relief is complex and involves a variety of mechanisms including inhibition of presynaptic reuptake of serotonin and norepinephrine [46] and sodium channel blockade [47, 48]. In patients with CRPS suffering from painful mono/polyneuropathies, clomipramine demonstrated greater efficacy and pain improvement when compared to acetylsalicylic acid [49]. Despite the lack of clinical trials exploring the role of TCA's in patients with CRPS, they are still commonly used to address the neuropathic component of pain in patients with CRPS.

13.6.2.8 Corticosteroids

The anti-inflammatory effects of corticosteroids are complex. In addition to the molecular effect of steroids, a stimulatory effect on the endogenous opioid system has been demonstrated in patients with CRPS [50]. The mechanism of pain relief in patients with CRPS is unclear and the data is divided. Clinically, corticosteroid therapy should be reserved for acute flares and breakthrough pain management due to their prohibitive side effect profile with long-term use. In a randomized placebo-controlled trial, (RCT) prednisone therapy for 12 weeks resulted in more than 75% clinical improvement in patients with CRPS when compared to placebo [51]. In post-stroke CRPS patients the use of corticosteroid therapy (methylprednisolone 32 mg/day for 2 weeks, followed by a tapered dose over 2 weeks) resulted in improved symptoms in 86% of patients [52].

However, there are multiple RCTs that have shown no benefit of corticosteroid therapy in patients with CRPS. The addition of corticosteroid (Prednisone 5 mg/day) to an established rehabilitation regimen did not result in any improvement in swelling, discoloration, and functional status. Another group evaluated the utility of Bier block with Lidocaine and Methylprednisolone and found no significant difference in pain score, range of motion, and edema acutely or at 1.5 months follow up [53].

13.6.2.9 Nonsteroidal Anti-Inflammatory Drugs (NSAIDs)

NSAIDs exert their analgesic effect through inhibition of prostaglandin synthesis, namely cyclo-oxygenase enzymes (COX-1 and COX-2). COX-2 is induced in inflammatory cells, making it the likely site of action or pain relief. A recent randomized, double-blinded placebo-controlled trial exploring the role of Parecoxib in CRPS did not demonstrate any difference in pain intensity or edema [54]. Unfortunately, high quality studies exploring the role COX-2 inhibition in patients with CRPS are lacking. A comparison of NSAID's to corticosteroids exploring its efficacy in patients with CRPS has been studied. Prednisone therapy resulted in significant improvement in signs of CRPS following stroke when compared to piroxicam [55].

13.6.2.10 Bisphosphonates

Bisphosphonates have been used in the management of metabolic bone diseases and osteoporosis due to their potent antiresorptive effects. Evidence of increased tracer uptake on triple-phase bone scintigraphy in patients with early CRPS [56] has led to interest in exploring their utility during the early phases of CRPS. This increased tracer uptake suggests a local drug concentration effect that is likely responsible for their observed clinical effect [57]. In patients with long standing CRPS, decreased tracer uptake on triple-phase bone scintigraphy may be responsible for their less pronounced clinical effects.

The mechanism of pain relief through which bisphosphonates exert their effect in patients with CRPS is complex. In addition to their anti-osteoclastic activity, their therapeutic effect lies in their ability to modulate various inflammatory mediators that are upregulated in CRPS [58]. There are a total of five randomized control trials that have been published documenting the efficacy of alendronate [59, 60], clodronate [61], pamidronate [62], and neridronate [63] in improving pain score, functional status, and edema. Of particular interest, the largest RCT involved Neridronate (four 100-mg infusions over 10 days for a total of 40 days) in patients with early stage CRPS (less than 4 months onset). Neridronate therapy demonstrated a 50% or greater VAS pain reduction in 73% of patients (vs. 33% in control group) with significantly greater improvement in physical functioning, allodynia, hyperalgesia, and edema. Neridronate therapy was highly effective with an estimated NNT of 2.4. Most remarkable observation was that 100% of neridronate treated patients did not demonstrate any clinical signs or symptoms of CRPS at 1 year follow up [63].

13.6.2.11 Alpha-Adrenergic Agents

Alpha-adrenergic antagonists exert their effect on the sympathetic nervous system. Their ability to block alpha 1 and alpha 2 receptors can be utilized to attenuate sympathetically mediated pain in patients with CRPS. Upregulation of alpha 1-adrenoceptors in dermal nerves and epidermal cells has been demonstrated in patients with CRPS and may augment pain and neuroinflammatory disturbances [64]. Antagonism of these receptors can decrease peripheral sensitization, while inhibition of alpha-1 adrenergic mediated vasoconstriction will increase peripheral tissue perfusion.

Phenoxybenzamine (Intravenous regional blockade and oral dosing) has been shown to be effective in patients with CRPS [65, 66]. In contrast to previous studies with a high target dose range (up to 120 mg/day) [67], therapeutic benefits have been demonstrated at 10 mg/day dosing [66]. Careful titration should be exercised to avoid common side effects associated with alpha blockade (orthostatic hypotension, dizziness, and sexual dysfunction). With the same rationale, selective alpha-1 antagonists (terazosin and prazosin) may be utilized in the management of CRPS. Despite the lack of high-level evidence to support their efficacy, they are often utilized for their cost-effectiveness and better-tolerated side effect profile when compared to phenoxybenzamine.

13.6.2.12 NMDA Antagonists

Windup and central sensitization appear to be involved in the induction and maintenance of CRPS/neuropathic pain [68, 69]. Over excitation of the N-methyl-D-Aspartate (NMDA) receptor plays a major role in the development of central sensitization and plasticity. Intense or prolonged painful stimulus causes release of glutamate from peripheral nociceptive afferents in the dorsal horn of the spinal cord. The glutamate stimulates NMDA receptors on second-order neurons that produce windup and central sensitization. Therefore, NMDA receptor antagonists have been used to block the cellular mechanisms supporting windup and central sensitization [68]. Ketamine is one of the potent NMDA-blocking drugs currently available for clinical use. It can be administered topically or intravenously. Pain relief and complete remission is reported in resistant patients, in few placebo-controlled studies [70–73]. Retrospective analysis of subanesthetic ketamine infusion (0.1 mg/kg/h to 0.5 mg/kg/h) has shown some benefit in management of pain in CRPS [74]. A randomized double-blind placebo-controlled trial showed that IV ketamine (0.35 mg/kg/h, not to exceed 25 mg/h over a 4-h period daily for 10 days, resulted in statistically significant ($P < 0.05$) reductions in many pain parameters. Side effects including nausea, vomiting, headaches, and hallucinations are reported with ketamine use [71].

13.6.2.13 Opioids

There is much debate surrounding the clinical utility of opioid analgesics in patients with CRPS. Concerns surrounding their efficacy, adverse effects, tolerance, and abuse potential make them a less desirable treatment option. There is a vacancy of evidence exploring their efficacy in patients with CRPS. One randomized control trial evaluating controlled-release morphine (90 mg/day) did not show a difference in pain reduction when compared to placebo [75]. Despite the lack of evidence supporting their use, opioid analgesics are commonly used to attenuate the neuropathic component of CRPS. Cochrane review exploring the utility of opioids in neuropathic pain syndromes demonstrated efficacy with short and intermediate therapy [76]. A theoretical benefit may exist with methadone, tramadol, and tapentadol owing to their respective NMDA and SNRI effects. Individualized therapy should be practiced and opioid therapy should be limited to pain relief during acute pain crises. The use of long-term opioid therapy results in opioid induced hyperalgesia a troubling superimposition on existing sensory disturbances in CRPS.

13.6.3 Interventional Therapies

13.6.3.1 Sympathetic Blocks

Given the longstanding belief that CRPS has a predominantly autonomic mediated pathogenesis: chemical, lytic, radiofrequency induced neurotomy and surgical sympathectomies have been performed for decades in effort to interrupt aberrant afferent signals. Unfortunately, there is limited high quality evidence to support this. As alluded to earlier, the response to sympatholytic blocks (SB) is variable. This highlights the existence of different variants within CRPS—the sympathetically mediated and independent. Clinically, it is difficult to discern the difference in such variances and the delineation is made depending on the response to SB. Upper extremity sympathectomy can be achieved with stellate ganglion block (SGB) and thoracic (T2) sympathetic block (TSB). Lower extremity sympathectomy can be achieved by lumbar sympathetic block (LSB). These procedures may be performed with fluoroscopic, ultrasound, or computed tomography guidance. Surgical sympathectomy via transection of the sympathetic chain, and radiofrequency lesioning has been performed with limited benefit in refractory CRPS [77, 78].

In a study attempting to establish predictors for SB success (both stellate and lumbar) a 31% moderate success rate was reported. Moderate improvement was defined by pain relief of greater than 50% for at least 6 h and good response was defined as at least 50% for 2–7 days. The authors concluded that no sign or symptom predicted good success, and that the presence of allodynia or hypoesthesia is a negative predictor for block success. Their transient complication rate following injection was 84% including increased pain, headache, dysphagia, nausea, blurred vision, and groin pain [79]. A double-blinded placebo-controlled cross over trial designed to assess the diagnostic and therapeutic value of LSB revealed that local anesthetics provided a longer duration of pain relief (90 h) when compared to saline (20 h). However, this study had a small sample size, and the practical application of this is questionable [80]. The first double-blinded, randomized, and controlled study evaluating the utility of TSB yielded encouraging results. While the average pain intensity did not differ between the treatment and control group at 1 month, at 12 months the TSB treatment group had lower visual analog pain scores than the control (3.47 ± 3.5 vs. 5.86 ± 2.9; $P = 0.046$). Furthermore, the Hospital Anxiety and Depression scores were lower in the TSB group when compared to the control at 1 and 12-month intervals [81]. Even if a sympathetic block is considered to be successful, it is important to appreciate that the duration of this success may be limited. Low quality evidence such as retrospective analyses and case reports has shown some benefit with repeat sympathetic blocks. Systemic reviews continue to demonstrate that the evidence is scarce and relatively underpowered (small sample size). Therefore, no conclusions can be drawn from the existing literature [82, 83]. The limited data in support of sympathetic blockade is retrospective, case series, or pilot studies [84]. In conclusion, in patients with refractory CRPS having failed conservative therapy it is sensible to proceed with a sympathetic block. If the block provides 50% pain reduction, it may be repeated with local anesthetic or radiofrequency lesioning. If symptoms persist, the patient should be evaluated by psychology and assessed for spinal cord stimulation [85].

13.6.4 Neuromodulation

13.6.4.1 Spinal Cord Stimulation

Alternation of spinal cord nerve activity via application of a targeted electrical or chemical stimulus is commonly referred to as neuromodulation. The fundamental principle stems from the Gate Theory of Pain [86] described by Melzack in 1965. In an overly simplistic overview, the stimulation of large A-Beta fibers leads to the activation of inhibitory interneurons, and subsequent inhibition of second-order nociceptive neurons in the dorsal horn of the spinal cord. This paresthesia sensation interrupts or supersedes the painful stimuli carried by the A delta and C fibers. Shortly thereafter, in 1967 Shealy placed the first dorsal column stimulator in patients suffering from cancer pain [87]. The technology has since evolved at an exponential rate and has been studied in a variety of pain disorders including CRPS. In patients who have failed the plethora of conservative measures including physical therapy, medical management, and sympathetic blockade, spinal cord stimulation (SCS) should be considered [85]. With the available devices, traditional (paresthesia based) or paresthesia free stimulation can be programmed and individualized to each patient. The procedure is most commonly performed in two steps—a trial and permanent implant. A percutaneous trial procedure is first performed wherein epidural leads with conducting electrodes are placed, and connected to an external pulse generator. The patient is advised to return to usual activity for a number of days to test if the stimulation adequately covers and helps alleviate their usual pain. Various metrics may be used to document trial success; these include reduction in pain score, reduction in pain medication, and improvement in functional status. If the trial is successful, the leads are removed and a permanent procedure scheduled at a future date. The implant procedure is performed in a similar fashion and involves placement of epidural leads and connection to an implantable pulse generator that is placed in a subcutaneous pocket most often in the flank or buttock. A clinical trial of 54 patients randomized in a 2:1 to receive SCS plus physical therapy or physical therapy alone showed favorable outcomes for the SCS plus therapy group. The SCS plus physical therapy group had a mean reduction of 2.4 cm in pain intensity at 6 months compared to 0.2 cm in the physical therapy alone group. The SCS group had a larger proportion of patients reporting significant improvement in pain (39% vs 6%), while there was no clinically important improvement in functional status. The implant group had an improved health related quality of life, and the complication rate was 25%, with one patient warranting explant [88]. While SCS is an advantageous therapy for the treatment of CRPS related pain, patient selection remains paramount. A 11-year prospective case series report suggested that at least a 50% reduction in pain following a trial procedure is needed for long-term success with implant, with an efficacy of 63% in their implanted patients [89]. In a recent literate review of SCS in CRPS patients, it was demonstrated that SCS remains an efficacious treatment modality with high-level evidence (1B+) for perceived pain relief, pain score, and quality of life. The evidence for functional improvement, CRPS signs, analgesic sparing effects, psychological health, and sleep hygiene is less clear [90].

13.6.4.2 Dorsal Root Ganglion Stimulation

Primary sensory neurons (PSN) are large cells that span from the peripheral receptors to the dorsal horns of the spinal cord. The dorsal root ganglion (DRG) is the site where the soma (cell body) of the PSN resides hence playing a critical role in the transmission of stimuli. Hogan described that "approximately 15,000 neurons are housed per DRG at segmental levels where major plexuses innervate the limbs" [91]. Unlike peripheral nerve fascicles that are surrounded by perineurium, the DRG lacks a capsular membrane, making it more highly permeable [92]. This lack of a membrane is advantageous when using epidural medications to interrupt nociceptive stimuli. As certain disease processes (neuropathic, zoster, radiculopathy, and causalgia) follow a dermatomal pattern, the selected DRG are attractive targets for treatment [91]. In 2013, a study in rat models demonstrated that direct stimulation of the DRG by electrical fields reduces neuronal excitability and could be a new target for pain relief [93]. This target was quickly adapted as potential site for neuromodulation and a small prospective study showed promise [94, 95]. It was also suggested that DRG stimulation is less susceptible to positional changes when compared with traditional stimulation of the dorsal columns [96]. The ACCURATE trial was a large multicenter randomized comparative effectiveness trial in 152 patients with CRPS or causalgia of the lower extremities receiving either DRG stimulation or conventional dorsal column SCS. The DRG group had higher pain relief as defined by ≥50% improvement (81.2% vs. 55.7%) at 3 months. The DRG group also demonstrated less postural variation in stimulation intensity, reduced stimulation to non-painful areas suggested enhanced targeted therapy, and increased quality of life [97]. At the present time, Class A randomized control trial evidence supports the use of DRG for CRPS and other pain syndromes [98]. Once again, the detailed description of surgical technique is beyond the scope of this chapter. The methodology of implant is similar to SCS using a percutaneous approach accessing the epidural space. The technique requires more advanced skills as strain relief loops are made in the epidural space. The leads may be connected to an external pulse generator during the trial phase, and an implantable pulse generator surgically placed if the trial proves to be successful. We recommend reading the various guidelines on patient selection, safety, coagulation management, and prevention of neurologic injury published by the Neuromodulation Appropriateness Consensus Committee [99–101].

13.6.5 Future Directives

Hyperbaric oxygen therapy: The anti-nociceptive effect of hyperbaric oxygen therapy (HBOT) is via neural nitric oxide-dependent release of the endogenous opioid, dynorphin, which subsequently activates k- and μ-opioid receptors [102]. In animal models, HBOT was shown to be effective at reducing edema and improving range of motion in the acute phase.

Botulinum toxin-A (BTX-A): Provides relief of neuropathic pain, and may therefore demonstrate efficacy in managing CRPS. In clinical practice, there is still limited information to guide the choice, formulation, and dose of the toxin, which are mainly based on the experience of the clinician.

Plasma exchange: The autoimmune etiology of CRPS explains the use of plasma exchange therapy, used in other autoimmune disorders. Large, randomized placebo-controlled plasma exchange trials are needed to validate and expand on the findings.

13.7 Case Report

A 40-year-old male with no significant past medical history, presented with a 2-month history of left foot injury. He developed CRPS with foot pain, swelling, and allodynia. Patient was unable to bear weight on the affected foot and was using crutches to ambulate. Extensive work-up revealed no other etiology for his pain. No fracture or evidence of nerve injury was present. Pain was minimally controlled with gabapentin, ibuprofen, tramadol, and physical therapy. Lumbar sympathetic block was done with pain relief lasting for a week. Block was repeated with a similar response. SCS was discussed as an option to provide long-term benefit. Patient underwent a successful SCS trial and subsequent implant with significant improvement in pain and functionality.

13.8 Summary

The complex pathophysiology, multifactorial nature of this condition, and varied clinical presentations make it challenging for physicians to diagnose and treat CRPS effectively. A multidisciplinary approach with input from pain physicians, neurologists, psychologists, and PM&R physicians is vital not only for optimal pain management but also for functional and psychological recovery.

References

1. Nahin RL. Estimates of pain prevalence and severity in adults: United States, 2012. J Pain. 2015;16(8):769–80.
2. Sandroni P, Benrud-Larson LM, McClelland RL, Low PA. Complex regional pain syndrome type I: incidence and prevalence in Olmsted county, a population-based study. Pain. 2003;103(1–2):199–207.
3. de Mos M, de Bruijn AG, Huygen FJ, Dieleman JP, Stricker BH, Sturkenboom MC. The incidence of complex regional pain syndrome: a population-based study. Pain. 2007;129(1–2):12–20.
4. Gaskin DJ, Richard P, Institute of Medicine (US) Committee on Advancing Pain Research, Care, and Education. The economic costs of pain in the United States. In: Relieving pain in America: a blueprint for transforming prevention, care, education, and research. Washington, DC: National Academies Press; 2011. Appendix C Available from: https://www.ncbi.nlm.nih.gov/books/NBK92521.
5. Murphy KR, Han JL, Yang S, Hussaini SM, Elsamadicy AA, Parente B, et al. Prevalence of specific types of pain diagnoses in a sample of United States adults. Pain Physician. 2017;20(2):E257–e68.
6. Elsamadicy AA, Yang S, Sergesketter AR, Ashraf B, Charalambous L, Kemeny H, et al. Prevalence and cost analysis of complex regional pain syndrome (CRPS): a role for neuromodulation. Neuromodulation. 2018;21:423.
7. Iolascon G, de Sire A, Moretti A, Gimigliano F. Complex regional pain syndrome (CRPS) type I: historical perspective and critical issues. Clin Cases Miner Bone Metab. 2015;12(Suppl 1):4–10.
8. Coderre TJ. Complex regional pain syndrome – type I: what's in a name? J Pain. 2011;12(1):2–12.
9. Classification of chronic pain. Descriptions of chronic pain syndromes and definitions of pain terms. Prepared by the International Association for the Study of Pain, Subcommittee on Taxonomy. Pain Suppl. 1986;3:S1–226.
10. Merskey H, Bogduk N. Classification of chronic pain: descriptions of chronic pain syndromes and definition of pain terms. Seattle, WA: IASP Press; 1994.
11. Sudeck P. Über die akute entzündliche Knochenatrophie. Arch Klin Chir. 1900;62:147–56.
12. Evans JA. Reflex sympathetic dystrophy. Surg Gynecol Obstet. 1946;82:36–43.
13. Evans JA. Sympathectomy for reflex sympathetic dystrophy; report of twenty-nine cases. J Am Med Assoc. 1946;132(11):620–3.
14. Evans JA. Reflex sympathetic dystrophy; report on 57 cases. Ann Intern Med. 1947;26(3):417–26.
15. Roberts WJ. A hypothesis on the physiological basis for causalgia and related pains. Pain. 1986;24(3):297–311.
16. Frost SA, Raja SN, Campbell JN, Meyer RA, Khan AA. Does hyperalgesia to cooling stimuli characterize patients with sympathetically maintained pain (reflex sympathetic dystrophy)? In: Dubner R, Gebhart GF, Bond MR, editors. Proceedings of the 5th world congress on pain, pain research and clinical management, vol. 3. Amsterdam: Elsevier; 1988. p. 151–6.
17. Schurmann M, Gradl G, Zaspel J, Kayser M, Lohr P, Andress HJ. Peripheral sympathetic function as a predictor of complex regional pain syndrome type I (CRPS I) in patients with radial fracture. Auton Neurosci. 2000;86(1–2):127–34.
18. Wasner G, Heckmann K, Maier C, Baron R. Vascular abnormalities in acute reflex sympathetic dystrophy (CRPS I): complete inhibition of sympathetic nerve activity with recovery. Arch Neurol. 1999;56(5):613–20.
19. Foisie PS. Traumatic arterial vasospasm. N Engl J Med. 1947;237(9):295–302.
20. Veldman PH, Reynen HM, Arntz IE, Goris RJ. Signs and symptoms of reflex sympathetic dystrophy: prospective study of 829 patients. Lancet. 1993;342(8878):1012–6.

21. Huygen FJ, De Bruijn AG, De Bruin MT, Groeneweg JG, Klein J, Zijlstra FJ. Evidence for local inflammation in complex regional pain syndrome type 1. Mediat Inflamm. 2002;11(1):47–51.
22. Birklein F, Drummond PD, Li W, Schlereth T, Albrecht N, Finch PM, et al. Activation of cutaneous immune responses in complex regional pain syndrome. J Pain. 2014;15(5):485–95.
23. Dirckx M, Groeneweg G, van Daele PL, Stronks DL, Huygen FJ. Mast cells: a new target in the treatment of complex regional pain syndrome? Pain Pract. 2013;13(8):599–603.
24. Ritz BW, Alexander GM, Nogusa S, Perreault MJ, Peterlin BL, Grothusen JR, et al. Elevated blood levels of inflammatory monocytes (CD14+ CD16+) in patients with complex regional pain syndrome. Clin Exp Immunol. 2011;164(1):108–17.
25. Dirckx M, Stronks DL, Groeneweg G, Huygen FJ. Effect of immunomodulating medications in complex regional pain syndrome: a systematic review. Clin J Pain. 2012;28(4):355–63.
26. Bruehl S. An update on the pathophysiology of complex regional pain syndrome. Anesthesiology. 2010;113(3):713–25.
27. Baranauskas G, Nistri A. Sensitization of pain pathways in the spinal cord: cellular mechanisms. Prog Neurobiol. 1998;54(3):349–65.
28. Mailis A, Wade J. Profile of Caucasian women with possible genetic predisposition to reflex sympathetic dystrophy: a pilot study. Clin J Pain. 1994;10(3):210–7.
29. Kemler MA, van de Vusse AC, van den Berg-Loonen EM, Barendse GA, van Kleef M, Weber WE. HLA-DQ1 associated with reflex sympathetic dystrophy. Neurology. 1999;53(6):1350–1.
30. van de Beek WJ, Roep BO, van der Slik AR, Giphart MJ, van Hilten BJ. Susceptibility loci for complex regional pain syndrome. Pain. 2003;103(1–2):93–7.
31. van Rooijen DE, Roelen DL, Verduijn W, Haasnoot GW, Huygen FJ, Perez RS, et al. Genetic HLA associations in complex regional pain syndrome with and without dystonia. J Pain. 2012;13(8):784–9.
32. Kohr D, Singh P, Tschernatsch M, Kaps M, Pouokam E, Diener M, et al. Autoimmunity against the beta2 adrenergic receptor and muscarinic-2 receptor in complex regional pain syndrome. Pain. 2011;152(12):2690–700.
33. Dirckx M, Schreurs MWJ, de Mos M, Stronks DL, Huygen FJPM. The prevalence of autoantibodies in complex regional pain syndrome type I. Mediat Inflamm. 2015;2015:718201.
34. Bruehl S, Harden RN, Galer BS, Saltz S, Bertram M, Backonja M, et al. External validation of IASP diagnostic criteria for complex regional pain syndrome and proposed research diagnostic criteria. International Association for the Study of Pain. Pain. 1999;81(1–2):147–54.
35. Harden RN, Bruehl S, Stanton-Hicks M, Wilson PR. Proposed new diagnostic criteria for complex regional pain syndrome. Pain Med. 2007;8(4):326–31.
36. Harden RN, Bruehl S, Perez RSGM, Birklein F, Marinus J, Maihofner C, et al. Validation of proposed diagnostic criteria (the "Budapest Criteria") for complex regional pain syndrome. Pain. 2010;150(2):268–74.
37. Harden RN, Maihofner C, Abousaad E, Vatine JJ, Kirsling A, Perez R, et al. A prospective, multisite, international validation of the complex regional pain syndrome severity score. Pain. 2017;158(8):1430–6.
38. Harden RN, Bruehl S, Perez RS, Birklein F, Marinus J, Maihofner C, et al. Development of a severity score for CRPS. Pain. 2010;151(3):870–6.
39. Llewellyn A, McCabe CS, Hibberd Y, White P, Davies L, Marinus J, et al. Are you better? A multi-centre study of patient-defined recovery from complex regional pain syndrome. Eur J Pain. 2018;22:551.
40. Lichtman DM, Bindra RR, Boyer MI, Putnam MD, Ring D, Slutsky DJ, et al. Treatment of distal radius fractures. J Am Acad Orthop Surg. 2010;18(3):180–9.
41. Shibuya N, Humphers JM, Agarwal MR, Jupiter DC. Efficacy and safety of high-dose vitamin C on complex regional pain syndrome in extremity trauma and surgery—systematic review and meta-analysis. J Foot Ankle Surg. 2013;52(1):62–6.

42. Zollinger PE, Tuinebreijer WE, Breederveld RS, Kreis RW. Can vitamin C prevent complex regional pain syndrome in patients with wrist fractures? A randomized, controlled, multicenter dose-response study. J Bone Joint Surg Am. 2007;89(7):1424–31.
43. Moseley GL, Zalucki NM, Wiech K. Tactile discrimination, but not tactile stimulation alone, reduces chronic limb pain. Pain. 2008;137(3):600–8.
44. McCabe CS, Haigh RC, Ring EF, Halligan PW, Wall PD, Blake DR. A controlled pilot study of the utility of mirror visual feedback in the treatment of complex regional pain syndrome (type 1). Rheumatology. 2003;42(1):97–101.
45. van de Vusse AC, Stomp-van den Berg SG, Kessels AH, Weber WE. Randomised controlled trial of gabapentin in complex regional pain syndrome type 1 [ISRCTN84121379]. BMC Neurol. 2004;4:13.
46. Sindrup SH, Jensen TS. Pharmacologic treatment of pain in polyneuropathy. Neurology. 2000;55(7):915–20.
47. Wang GK, Russell C, Wang SY. State-dependent block of voltage-gated Na+ channels by amitriptyline via the local anesthetic receptor and its implication for neuropathic pain. Pain. 2004;110(1–2):166–74.
48. Woolf CJ, Max MB. Mechanism-based pain diagnosis: issues for analgesic drug development. Anesthesiology. 2001;95(1):241–9.
49. Langohr HD, Stohr M, Petruch F. An open and double-blind cross-over study on the efficacy of clomipramine (Anafranil) in patients with painful mono- and polyneuropathies. Eur Neurol. 1982;21(5):309–17.
50. Figuerola Mde L, Levin G, Bertotti A, Ferreiro J, Barontini M. Normal sympathetic nervous system response in reflex sympathetic dystrophy. Funct Neurol. 2002;17(2):77–81.
51. Christensen K, Jensen EM, Noer I. The reflex dystrophy syndrome response to treatment with systemic corticosteroids. Acta Chir Scand. 1982;148(8):653–5.
52. Braus DF, Krauss JK, Strobel J. The shoulder-hand syndrome after stroke: a prospective clinical trial. Ann Neurol. 1994;36(5):728–33.
53. Taskaynatan MA, Ozgul A, Tan AK, Dincer K, Kalyon TA. Bier block with methylprednisolone and lidocaine in CRPS type I: a randomized, double-blinded, placebo-controlled study. Reg Anesth Pain Med. 2004;29(5):408–12.
54. Breuer AJ, Mainka T, Hansel N, Maier C, Krumova EK. Short-term treatment with parecoxib for complex regional pain syndrome: a randomized, placebo-controlled double-blind trial. Pain Physician. 2014;17(2):127–37.
55. Kalita J, Vajpayee A, Misra UK. Comparison of prednisolone with piroxicam in complex regional pain syndrome following stroke: a randomized controlled trial. QJM. 2006;99(2):89–95.
56. Lee GW, Weeks PM. The role of bone scintigraphy in diagnosing reflex sympathetic dystrophy. J Hand Surg Am. 1995;20(3):458–63.
57. Varenna M. Bisphosphonates beyond their anti-osteoclastic properties. Rheumatology. 2014;53(6):965–7.
58. Varenna M, Adami S, Sinigaglia L. Bisphosphonates in complex regional pain syndrome type I: how do they work? Clin Exp Rheumatol. 2014;32(4):451–4.
59. Adami S, Fossaluzza V, Gatti D, Fracassi E, Braga V. Bisphosphonate therapy of reflex sympathetic dystrophy syndrome. Ann Rheum Dis. 1997;56(3):201–4.
60. Manicourt DH, Brasseur JP, Boutsen Y, Depreseux G, Devogelaer JP. Role of alendronate in therapy for posttraumatic complex regional pain syndrome type I of the lower extremity. Arthritis Rheum. 2004;50(11):3690–7.
61. Varenna M, Zucchi F, Ghiringhelli D, Binelli L, Bevilacqua M, Bettica P, et al. Intravenous clodronate in the treatment of reflex sympathetic dystrophy syndrome. A randomized, double blind, placebo controlled study. J Rheumatol. 2000;27(6):1477–83.
62. Robinson JN, Sandom J, Chapman PT. Efficacy of pamidronate in complex regional pain syndrome type I. Pain Med. 2004;5(3):276–80.

63. Varenna M, Adami S, Rossini M, Gatti D, Idolazzi L, Zucchi F, et al. Treatment of complex regional pain syndrome type I with neridronate: a randomized, double-blind, placebo-controlled study. Rheumatology. 2013;52(3):534–42.
64. Finch PM, Drummond ES, Dawson LF, Phillips JK, Drummond PD. Up-regulation of cutaneous alpha-1-adrenoceptors in complex regional pain syndrome type I. Pain Med. 2014;15(11):1945–56.
65. Malik VK, Inchiosa MA Jr, Mustafa K, Sanapati MR, Pimentel MC Jr, Frost EA. Intravenous regional phenoxybenzamine in the treatment of reflex sympathetic dystrophy. Anesthesiology. 1998;88(3):823–7.
66. Inchiosa MA Jr, Kizelshteyn G. Treatment of complex regional pain syndrome type I with oral phenoxybenzamine: rationale and case reports. Pain Pract. 2008;8(2):125–32.
67. Muizelaar JP, Kleyer M, Hertogs IA, DeLange DC. Complex regional pain syndrome (reflex sympathetic dystrophy and causalgia): management with the calcium channel blocker nifedipine and/or the alpha-sympathetic blocker phenoxybenzamine in 59 patients. Clin Neurol Neurosurg. 1997;99(1):26–30.
68. Carpenter KJ, Dickenson AH. NMDA receptors and pain—hopes for novel analgesics. Reg Anesth Pain Med. 1999;24(6):506–8.
69. Bennett GJ. Update on the neurophysiology of pain transmission and modulation: focus on the NMDA-receptor. J Pain Symptom Manag. 2000;19(1 Suppl):S2–6.
70. Kiefer RT, Rohr P, Ploppa A, Dieterich HJ, Grothusen J, Koffler S, et al. Efficacy of ketamine in anesthetic dosage for the treatment of refractory complex regional pain syndrome: an open-label phase II study. Pain Med. 2008;9(8):1173–201.
71. Schwartzman RJ, Alexander GM, Grothusen JR, Paylor T, Reichenberger E, Perreault M. Outpatient intravenous ketamine for the treatment of complex regional pain syndrome: a double-blind placebo controlled study. Pain. 2009;147(1–3):107–15.
72. Sigtermans MJ, van Hilten JJ, Bauer MC, Arbous MS, Marinus J, Sarton EY, et al. Ketamine produces effective and long-term pain relief in patients with complex regional pain syndrome type 1. Pain. 2009;145(3):304–11.
73. Finch PM, Knudsen L, Drummond PD. Reduction of allodynia in patients with complex regional pain syndrome: a double-blind placebo-controlled trial of topical ketamine. Pain. 2009;146(1–2):18–25.
74. Correll GE, Maleki J, Gracely EJ, Muir JJ, Harbut RE. Subanesthetic ketamine infusion therapy: a retrospective analysis of a novel therapeutic approach to complex regional pain syndrome. Pain Med. 2004;5(3):263–75.
75. Harke H, Gretenkort P, Ladleif HU, Rahman S, Harke O. The response of neuropathic pain and pain in complex regional pain syndrome I to carbamazepine and sustained-release morphine in patients pretreated with spinal cord stimulation: a double-blinded randomized study. Anesth Analg. 2001;92(2):488–95.
76. McNicol ED, Midbari A, Eisenberg E. Opioids for neuropathic pain. Cochrane Database Syst Rev. 2013;(8):Cd006146.
77. Forouzanfar T, van Kleef M, Weber WE. Radiofrequency lesions of the stellate ganglion in chronic pain syndromes: retrospective analysis of clinical efficacy in 86 patients. Clin J Pain. 2000;16(2):164–8.
78. Straube S, Derry S, Moore RA, Cole P. Cervico-thoracic or lumbar sympathectomy for neuropathic pain and complex regional pain syndrome. Cochrane Database Syst Rev. 2013;(9):Cd002918.
79. van Eijs F, Geurts J, van Kleef M, Faber CG, Perez RS, Kessels AG, et al. Predictors of pain relieving response to sympathetic blockade in complex regional pain syndrome type 1. Anesthesiology. 2012;116(1):113–21.
80. Price DD, Long S, Wilsey B, Rafii A. Analysis of peak magnitude and duration of analgesia produced by local anesthetics injected into sympathetic ganglia of complex regional pain syndrome patients. Clin J Pain. 1998;14(3):216–26.

81. Rocha Rde O, Teixeira MJ, Yeng LT, Cantara MG, Faria VG, Liggieri V, et al. Thoracic sympathetic block for the treatment of complex regional pain syndrome type I: a double-blind randomized controlled study. Pain. 2014;155(11):2274–81.
82. Cepeda MS, Carr DB, Lau J. Local anesthetic sympathetic blockade for complex regional pain syndrome. Cochrane Database Syst Rev. 2005;(4):Cd004598.
83. O'Connell NE, Wand BM, Gibson W, Carr DB, Birklein F, Stanton TR. Local anaesthetic sympathetic blockade for complex regional pain syndrome. Cochrane Database Syst Rev. 2016;7:Cd004598.
84. Wei K, Feldmann RE Jr, Brascher AK, Benrath J. Ultrasound-guided stellate ganglion blocks combined with pharmacological and occupational therapy in complex regional pain syndrome (CRPS): a pilot case series ad interim. Pain Med. 2014;15(12):2120–7.
85. van Eijs F, Stanton-Hicks M, Van Zundert J, Faber CG, Lubenow TR, Mekhail N, et al. Evidence-based interventional pain medicine according to clinical diagnoses. 16. Complex regional pain syndrome. Pain Pract. 2011;11(1):70–87.
86. Melzack R, Wall PD. Pain mechanisms: a new theory. Science. 1965;150(3699):971–9.
87. Shealy CN, Mortimer JT, Reswick JB. Electrical inhibition of pain by stimulation of the dorsal columns: preliminary clinical report. Anesth Analg. 1967;46(4):489–91.
88. Kemler MA, Barendse GA, van Kleef M, de Vet HC, Rijks CP, Furnee CA, et al. Spinal cord stimulation in patients with chronic reflex sympathetic dystrophy. N Engl J Med. 2000;343(9):618–24.
89. Geurts JW, Smits H, Kemler MA, Brunner F, Kessels AG, van Kleef M. Spinal cord stimulation for complex regional pain syndrome type I: a prospective cohort study with long-term follow-up. Neuromodulation. 2013;16(6):523–9; discussion 9.
90. Visnjevac O, Costandi S, Patel BA, Azer G, Agarwal P, Bolash R, et al. A comprehensive outcome-specific review of the use of spinal cord stimulation for complex regional pain syndrome. Pain Pract. 2017;17(4):533–45.
91. Hogan Q. Labat lecture: the primary sensory neuron: where it is, what it does, and why it matters. Reg Anesth Pain Med. 2010;35(3):306–11.
92. Abram SE, Yi J, Fuchs A, Hogan QH. Permeability of injured and intact peripheral nerves and dorsal root ganglia. Anesthesiology. 2006;105(1):146–53.
93. Koopmeiners AS, Mueller S, Kramer J, Hogan QH. Effect of electrical field stimulation on dorsal root ganglion neuronal function. Neuromodulation. 2013;16(4):304–11; discussion 10-1.
94. Deer TR, Grigsby E, Weiner RL, Wilcosky B, Kramer JM. A prospective study of dorsal root ganglion stimulation for the relief of chronic pain. Neuromodulation. 2013;16(1):67–71; discussion 2.
95. Liem L, Russo M, Huygen FJ, Van Buyten JP, Smet I, Verrills P, et al. One-year outcomes of spinal cord stimulation of the dorsal root ganglion in the treatment of chronic neuropathic pain. Neuromodulation. 2015;18(1):41–8; discussion 8-9.
96. Kramer J, Liem L, Russo M, Smet I, Van Buyten JP, Huygen F. Lack of body positional effects on paresthesias when stimulating the dorsal root ganglion (DRG) in the treatment of chronic pain. Neuromodulation. 2015;18(1):50–7; discussion 7.
97. Deer TR, Levy RM, Kramer J, Poree L, Amirdelfan K, Grigsby E, et al. Dorsal root ganglion stimulation yielded higher treatment success rate for complex regional pain syndrome and causalgia at 3 and 12 months: a randomized comparative trial. Pain. 2017;158(4):669–81.
98. Harrison C, Epton S, Bojanic S, Green AL, FitzGerald JJ. The efficacy and safety of dorsal root ganglion stimulation as a treatment for neuropathic pain: a literature review. Neuromodulation. 2018;21:225.
99. Deer TR, Mekhail N, Provenzano D, Pope J, Krames E, Leong M, et al. The appropriate use of neurostimulation of the spinal cord and peripheral nervous system for the treatment of chronic pain and ischemic diseases: the Neuromodulation Appropriateness Consensus Committee. Neuromodulation. 2014;17(6):515–50; discussion 50.

100. Deer TR, Narouze S, Provenzano DA, Pope JE, Falowski SM, Russo MA, et al. The Neurostimulation Appropriateness Consensus Committee (NACC): recommendations on bleeding and coagulation management in neurostimulation devices. Neuromodulation. 2017;20(1):51–62.
101. Deer TR, Lamer TJ, Pope JE, Falowski SM, Provenzano DA, Slavin K, et al. The Neurostimulation Appropriateness Consensus Committee (NACC) safety guidelines for the reduction of severe neurological injury. Neuromodulation. 2017;20(1):15–30.
102. Zelinski LM, Ohgami Y, Chung E, Shirachi DY, Quock RM. A prolonged nitric oxide-dependent, opioid-mediated antinociceptive effect of hyperbaric oxygen in mice. J Pain. 2009;10(2):167–72.

Chapter 14
Neuropathic Pain Syndrome: Diabetic and Other Neuropathies

Atsushi Sawada and Michiaki Yamakage

14.1 Cause of Pain

The symptoms associated with painful diabetic neuropathy include pain, paresthesia, allodynia, impairment of vibration sense, reduced thermal sensation, and loss of pinprick sensation [1]. Long-term exposure to hyperglycemia can damage peripheral nerves and cause painful diabetic neuropathy. Furthermore, it is assumed that combinations of other risk factors might also be able to induce even more nerve damage. The major risk factors of painful diabetic neuropathy consist of diabetes duration, hyperglycemia, and age. Additional risk factors include prediabetes, height, hypertension, obesity, metabolic syndrome, oxidative stress, low vitamin D, generic factors, inflammation, and low physical activity [2].

14.1.1 Diabetes Duration

Duration of diabetes has been reported to be significantly correlated with the occurrence of DPN [3]. However, maintaining long-term near-normoglycemia after a diagnosis of type 1 diabetes is associated with a complete prevention of painful DPN. A study of patients with type 1 diabetes who were followed for 24 years reported that 64% of poorly controlled patients developed confirmed clinical DPN, while DPN did not occur in any of the strictly controlled patients [4].

A. Sawada (✉) · M. Yamakage
Department of Anesthesiology, Sapporo Medical University School of Medicine, Sapporo, Japan

K. Shimoji et al. (eds.), *Chronic Pain Management in General and Hospital Practice*, https://doi.org/10.1007/978-981-15-2933-7_14

14.1.2 Hyperglycemia

Hyperglycemia increases the risk of DPN. Furthermore, it has also been reported that every 1% increment in the HbA1c corresponds to a risk of approximately a 10–15% higher frequency of DPN [5]. Results of a meta-analysis of randomized controlled trials suggested that optimized glycemic control produced clinical benefits in some patients, with the development of DPN prevented in patients with type 1 diabetes. However, the effect was not clearly evident in patients with type 2 diabetes [6–8]. These findings potentially indicate that there might be a pathophysiological difference for DPN between the two types of diabetes.

14.1.3 Age

Several studies have confirmed the association of DPN with age. The results of these studies demonstrated that age was an independent risk factor of DPN and could directly increase the risk of neuropathy [3, 5, 9].

14.2 Pain Management

Treatments designed to manage painful DPN have targeted the various pathogenetic mechanisms of DPN [1]. Due to a growing understanding of the association between metabolic syndrome and DPN, pain management therapies for DPN have placed more emphasis on pathophysiological aberrations, such as obesity, dyslipidemia, and hypertension [7, 8]. Concomitant treatments, such as glycemic control, lifestyle intervention, lipid lowering therapies, and angiotensin-converting enzyme (ACE) inhibitors, in patients with diabetes mellitus have also positively impacted DPN.

14.2.1 Glycemic Control

Optimal glycemic control is the primary treatment approach recommended for managing diabetic symptoms and preventing further peripheral nerve damage. The results of the Diabetes Control and Complications Trial clearly demonstrated that glycemic control prevented DPN in patients with type 1 diabetes [10]. Although a meta-analysis of 7 randomized trials confirmed that intensive glycemic control prevented DPN in patients with type 1 diabetes, DPN was not prevented in patients with type 2 diabetes [7, 8]. However, the role of glycemic control in the prevention of DPN has been controversial in patients with type 2 diabetes, as there were significant limitations for the meta-analyses with regard to the targeted glucose levels, therapeutic strategies, trial design, and neuropathy end-points, such as foot exam and vibration perception.

14.2.2 Lifestyle Intervention

Lifestyle intervention, including diet and exercise, promoted cutaneous nerve fiber regeneration and slowed the progression of DPN in patients with diabetes. Although 1 year of exercise has been shown to be a useful preventative therapy [11], long-term aerobic exercise has additionally been shown to prevent the development of DPN [12]. Furthermore, it has also been demonstrated that both diet and exercise induce small-fiber regeneration [11].

14.2.3 Lipid Lowering Therapies

It has been consistently found that plasma lipids are associated with the progression of DPN [13]. The European Diabetes Prospective Complications study examined patients with type 1 diabetes and reported that total cholesterol, LDL cholesterol, and triglycerides levels were significantly associated with the progression of DPN [14]. Furthermore, the Fremantle Diabetes Study examined the use of lipid lowering therapies aimed at reducing TG levels and confirmed that these therapies did decrease the progress of DPN [15].

14.2.4 ACE Inhibitors

The development of nephropathy and retinopathy is closely associated with the progression of DPN in the patients with diabetes. The ACE inhibitor, trandolapril, improved DPN in patients with diabetes after 12 months of treatment [16]. In hypertensive type 2 diabetic patients, the ACE inhibitor, delapril, safely ameliorated the development and progression of DPN [17].

14.3 Other Signs and Symptoms Related to Pain

DPN development is known to be heterogeneous, based on the symptoms, risk covariates, pathologic alterations, and underlying mechanisms. In accordance with the evidence available in 2010, the Toronto Consensus Panel classified DPN into the two major subgroups, typical and atypical DPN [18]. The symptoms of the typical diabetic polyneuropathy were defined as "a chronic, symmetrical, length-dependent sensorimotor polyneuropathy due to metabolic and microvessel alterations as a result of chronic hyperglycemia and cardiovascular risk covariates" [19]. Typical DPN development has been reported to be associated with a background of prolonged exposure to hyperglycemia, associated metabolic syndrome, and cardiovascular risk factors [20]. The development of nephropathy, retinopathy, and neuropathy is closely associated due to the similar pathological alterations [16]. Atypical DPN has not been researched and characterized as well as typical DPN. However, atypical diabetic neuropathy differs from typical DPN due to several variations in the onset, course, manifestations, and putative mechanisms [19]. The onset of symptoms may be acute, subacute, or chronic in patients with atypical DPN [18]. In addition, the other signs and symptoms associated with painful DPN include sensorimotor polyneuropathy, cardiovascular autonomic neuropathy, and gastrointestinal autonomic neuropathy [18].

14.3.1 Diabetic Sensorimotor Polyneuropathy

The use of nerve conduction testing has been proposed as a reliable indicator of the occurrence of typical DPN for epidemiologic surveys. In addition, several studies have also emphasized the importance of the proficiency of the medical personnel in performing the clinical neurological assessments [21]. Currently, atypical DPN has yet to be characterized and researched as well as typical DPN.

14.3.2 Cardiovascular Autonomic Neuropathy

Cardiovascular autonomic neuropathy (CAN) is defined as the dysfunction of the autonomic control of the cardiovascular system. Clinical predictors of CAN include hyperglycemia, presence of DPN, nephropathy, retinopathy, hypertension, obesity, smoking, and dyslipidemia [22]. CAN is closely correlated with mortality and morbidity such as myocardial ischemia, stroke, and diabetic nephropathy progression [23]. The assessment of CAN is also clinically useful for classifying cardiovascular risks as indicators so that they can then be used for more intensive pharmacotherapeutic and lifestyle management of comorbid conditions [18]. Cardiovascular reflex tests, which are the gold standard for assessing CAN, have good sensitivity, specificity, and reproducibility. Relatively simple tests that are widely used to assess CAN include heart rate variability to deep breathing, a Valsalva maneuver, and blood pressure changes in response to posture [24]. The optimal period for CAN assessment may be at the time of the type 2 diabetes diagnosis and at 5 years after diagnosis of type 1 diabetes in patients with risks of CAN due to long-term hyperglycemia, cardiovascular risks, DPN, and angiopathic diabetic complications [18].

14.3.3 Gastrointestinal Autonomic Neuropathy

Gastrointestinal secretions are modulated by interactions between the autonomic and enteric nervous system. Gastrointestinal symptoms associated with considerable morbidity frequently occur among patients with diabetes mellitus [25]. However, it can be difficult to evaluate gastrointestinal autonomic function in humans. Therefore, the diagnosis of gastrointestinal autonomic neuropathy is frequently based on exclusion. Gastrointestinal symptoms are common in patients with poor glycemic control or with psychological factors associated with disordered gastric motor function induced by diabetes [26]. Delayed gastric emptying was present in approximately 50% of patients with type 2 diabetes and may be correlated with regurgitation, dysphagia, and esophageal strictures. For the management of impaired gastric emptying, it has been recommended that erythromycin, metoclopramide, and high-fiber diets be used [27]. Recent evidence indicates that gastroparesis, delayed gastric emptying, or esophageal dysmotility in patients with diabetes mellitus should be clinically managed by using proton pump inhibitors [28]. Lower gastrointestinal symptoms, such as diarrhea and constipation, are present in 20–25% of patients with diabetes [29]. For the management of diarrhea, it has been recommended that loperamide, clonidine, and electrolyte balance be used. Constipation is commonly managed with diet and exercise. In severe cases, the use of laxatives may be considered [29].

14.4 Diagnosis

DPN is diagnosed by board certified neurologists using a standardized evaluation to identify symptoms, signs, and nerve abnormality [30]. Although DPN is defined as, "the presence of symptoms and/or signs of peripheral nerve dysfunction in people with diabetes after the exclusion of other causes" [31], the diagnosis should only be made after a careful clinical examination. In 2010, the Toronto Consensus Panels on DPN provided definitions of typical and atypical DPN and the associated diagnostic criteria [32]. DPN is classified into at least two major subgroups that include generalized symmetric polyneuropathies, and focal and multifocal neuropathies [33]. Generalized symmetric polyneuropathies contain acute sensory neuropathy, chronic sensorimotor diabetic polyneuropathy, and autonomic neuropathy. Early diagnosis of DPN is important in order to prevent irreversible nerve damages [34]. Examination of responses to pinpricks, temperature, and vibration perception threshold, 10-g monofilament pressure sensation at the distal halluces, and ankle reflexes are useful for diagnosing patients with diabetes mellitus for DPN. A 10-g monofilament is also helpful for detecting DPN in order to prevent ulcer risks. A small decrease in the duration of a vibratory stimulus sensation is also an early indicator of DPN [34]. By using combinations of more than one of these tests, DPN can be detected with more than 87% sensitivity [32]. Electrophysiological studies can be extremely helpful when trying to distinguish focal and multifocal neuropathies from other neuropathies caused by cerebral infarcts and spinal stenosis in patients with diabetes mellitus [35]. Other causes of polyneuropathy, such as alcohol use, deficiency of vitamin B12, obstructive vessel diseases, vasculitis, infections, and cancer should also be assessed [36].

14.5 General Treatments (Medical, Surgical, and Others) and Prognosis

Pregabalin and duloxetine are the only two drugs that have been approved by the U.S. Food and Drug Administration (FDA) for the treatment of DPN. However, the guidelines issued by the American Academy of Neurology (AAN) encourage clinicians to use a broader range of drugs after careful consideration of the patient's age, quality-of-life, physical function, and comorbidities, including the adverse effects associated with these other medications [37]. Several organizations, professional societies, and expert panels including the AAN have produced guidelines for the treatment of neuropathic pain. In general, these guidelines have recommended considering the use of anticonvulsants including the calcium channel alpha-2-delta ligand, tricyclic antidepressants, and serotonin norepinephrine reuptake inhibitors as first-line agents, followed by the use of opioids and topical treatments [38].

14.5.1 Anticonvulsants

Anticonvulsants have a long history of use in treating neuropathic pain. Carbamazepine is one of the traditional anticonvulsants, which acts by inhibiting voltage-gated sodium channels and reduces neuronal excitability in the central and peripheral nervous systems. In early studies, carbamazepine was reported to successfully be able to control neuropathic pain [34]. Results of a meta-analysis showed that carbamazepine was just as effective as other agents in the treatment of DPN [39]. However, carbamazepine is associated with side effects that include dizziness, ataxia, sedation, confusion, myelosuppression, and osteoporosis in the elderly. Pregabalin and gabapentin are the ligands of the alpha-2-delta subunit of calcium channels, which decrease central sensitization by reducing calcium influx [40]. The newer calcium channel alpha-2-delta ligand class anticonvulsants (pregabalin) have been shown to be an efficacious and safe treatment for the pain of DPN [41], and currently are the only medication given a level A recommendation by the AAN guidelines for the treatment of painful DPN [42]. Gabapentin has been given a level B recommendation. However, a recent analysis showed that gabapentin provided the best pain relief as compared to six other antidepressants and anticonvulsants used to treat painful DPN [43]. Even so, both of these medications are associated with the side effects that include somnolence, dizziness, weight gain, headache, dry mouth, and peripheral edema.

14.5.2 Tricyclic Antidepressants

Tricyclic antidepressants are commonly used for the treatment of DPN, with the effect occurring via a pathway that differs from that of the antidepressant effect. Tricyclic antidepressants have a wide range of effects, including inhibition of serotonin and noradrenaline reuptake from synaptic junctions and acting as antagonists on N-methyl-D-aspartate, histamine, muscarinic, and alpha-adrenergic receptors [44]. The precise mechanism by which they ameliorate neuropathic pain remains unknown. Amitriptyline has also been used as an effective first-line medication for painful DPN with its use primarily based on cost considerations [45]. Despite its potential benefit, amitriptyline is less frequently used because of the higher incidence and severity of the adverse anticholinergic and cardiac effects [38]. However, imipramine and desipramine have a lower side effect burden than amitriptyline.

14.5.3 Serotonin Norepinephrine Reuptake Inhibitors (SNRIs)

SNRIs, such as duloxetine and venlafaxine, are selective inhibitors of serotonin and norepinephrine that act by regulating the descending inhibitory pathway to alleviate pain [46]. Duloxetine was a first-line medication approved by the FDA in 2004 for the treatment of painful DPN [42]. Although the safety profile of duloxetine is superior to amitriptyline, the common adverse side effect of duloxetine is nausea. Furthermore, it has been reported that 14–20% of patients treated with a daily 60 g dose of duloxetine suffered from somnolence and constipation [47]. Though not approved by the FDA, another SNRI, venlafaxine, has been found to be efficacious for the treatment of painful DPN [48]. The most common adverse effect associated with venlafaxine is gastrointestinal disturbance. However, the AAN guidelines concluded that there was not sufficient data to recommend the use of duloxetine and venlafaxine for the treatment of DPN [42].

14.5.4 Opioid Analgesia

Opioids ameliorate pain by acting on spinal and supraspinal mechanisms via opioid receptors. Tramadol, which is primarily a μ receptor agonist and a weak inhibitor of norepinephrine and serotonin reuptake, has been shown to provide significant pain relief of polyneuropathies [49]. The adverse effects of tramadol include nausea, constipation, sedation, and headache. In addition, tramadol has a lower potential for abuse than other opioids. Extended-release tapentadol, which combines an opioid agonist and a norepinephrine antagonist, received approval from the FDA for the treatment of neuropathic pain, although it has not been specifically used for painful DPN [50]. Opioid therapy should be reserved for patients, who are non-responder to first-line medications, as prolonged use of opioids can lead to tolerance, dependence, and abuse. Therefore, the risk–benefit ratio of opioid therapy for patients with DPN remains unclear. In several studies, a combination therapy of opioids and other medications has been reported to improve efficacy without increasing adverse effects. Furthermore, a combination therapy of long-acting morphine sulfate plus gabapentin has been confirmed to be superior to either drug alone [51]. Moreover, the combination therapy of tramadol plus acetaminophen also improved pain relief as compared to gabapentin alone [52].

14.5.5 Topical Treatments

A previous meta-analysis has demonstrated that capsaicin, which is a transient receptor potential vanilloid type 1 agonist, was an effective treatment for DPN [53]. Subsequently, however, it was reported that capsaicin therapy should not be recommended as a treatment of DPN, as it is associated with epidermal denervation and has a potential risk of foot ulceration [54]. In contrast, 5% lidocaine plasters, which block sodium channels, have been shown to improve pain scores and the quality of life in patients with DPN [55]. Therefore, the AAN has recommended the use of lidocaine patch therapy for the treatment of DPN, as a level C recommendation.

14.6 Case Reports

Uluduz et al. have reported on the use of intravenous immunoglobulin (IVIG) therapy to treat asymmetrical, simultaneous multiple cranial nerve palsies, which were mild signs of peripheral neuropathies, in a 55-year-old woman with uncontrolled type 2 diabetic mellitus for 12 years [56]. Her symptoms included right peripheral facial paralysis, ptosis, and restricted left eye movements with spared pupils. Laboratory investigations revealed high lipid profiles and glucose levels. Although she was put on aggressive insulin treatment with a dose of 58 units/day, there were no changes in her glucose level. IVIG treatment was started on the 15th day of her hospitalization with a dose of 0.4 g/kg/day and continued for 5 days. IVIG treatment decreased her blood glucose level on the first day. All of her cranial nerve palsies improved during the first month and there has been no recurrence observed during the following 8 months. Immunotherapy has been previously reported to be effective for treating diabetic polyneuropathies, including radiculoplexopathy [57]. Although the mechanisms of IVIG in autoimmune disorders remain uncertain, the IVIG treatment in this patient did reduce the high glucose level on the first day, with her clinical symptoms disappearing by the end of the first month. This case report suggested that IVIG may have a potential clinical role in some patients with diabetic polyneuropathies.

14.7 Recent Topics

Spinal cord stimulation (SCS) has been clinically used to treat neuropathic pain [58]. Slangen et al. reported that SCS provided pain relief in painful DPN during a multicenter randomized clinical trial [59]. In this trial, they randomly allocated 36 patients with severe lower limb pain into a group that was given a combination of the best medical treatment (BMT) plus SCS (SCS group, $n = 22$) and a group that only received BMT (BMT group, $n = 14$). Study results showed that the SCS group exhibited a relatively improved treatment success (59% for the SCS group vs. 7% for the BMT group; $P < 0.01$), and better pain relief during both the daytime and nighttime (41% and 36% in the SCS group vs. 0% and 7% in the BMT group; $P < 0.05$). Thus, these results show that SCS provides positive effects for both painful DPN and neuropathic pain.

14.8 Summary

DPN is the most common complication of diabetes, with the management of DPN clinically important due to its association with morbidity and mortality. Although the management and treatment of painful DPN remains difficult, the recent development of specific clinical examinations and diagnostic criteria has made it possible to detect DPN at an earlier stage and thus, provide aggressive intervention. The management of DPN should include patient education, lifestyle modification including smoking cessation, exercise, and healthy diet. However, since limitations still exist for the present treatments of painful DPN, further research into the best treatments for DPN will need to be undertaken.

References

1. Javed S, Petropoulos IN, Tavakoli M, Malik RA. Clinical and diagnostic features of small fiber damage in diabetic polyneuropathy. Handb Clin Neurol. 2014;126:275–90.
2. Papanas N, Ziegler D. Risk factors and comorbidities in diabetic neuropathy: an update 2015. Rev Diabet Stud. 2015;12:48–62.
3. Tesfaye S, Stevens LK, Stephenson JM, Fuller JH, Plater M, Ionescu-Tirgoviste C, Nuber A, Pozza G, Ward JD. Prevalence of diabetic peripheral neuropathy and its relation to glycemic control and potential risk factors: the EURODIAB IDDM Complications Study. Diabetologia. 1996;39:1377–84.
4. Ziegler D, Behler M, Schroers-Teuber M, Rodenn M. Near-normoglycemia and development of neuropathy: a 24-year prospective study from diagnosis of type 1 diabetes. BMJ Open. 2015;5:e006559. https://doi.org/10.1136/bmjopen-2014-006559.
5. Adler AI, Boyko EJ, Ahroni JH, Stensel V, Forsberg RC, Smith DG. Risk factors for diabetic peripheral sensory neuropathy. Results of the Seattle Prospective Diabetic Foot Study. Diabetes Care. 1997;20:1162–7.

6. Boussageon R, Bejan-Angoulvant T, Saadatian-Elahi M, Lafont S, Bergeonneau C, Kassai B, Erpeldinger S, Wright JM, Gueyffier F, Cornu C. Effect of intensive glucose lowering treatment on all cause mortality, cardiovascular death, and microvascular events in type 2 diabetes: meta-analysis of randomized controlled trials. BMJ. 2011;343:d4169. https://doi.org/10.1136/bmj.d4169.
7. Callaghan BC, Cheng HT, Stables CL, Smith AL, Feldman EL. Diabetic neuropathy: clinical manifestations and current treatments. Lancet Neurol. 2012;11:521–34.
8. Callaghan BC, Little AA, Feldman EL, Hughes RA. Enhanced glucose control for preventing and treating diabetic neuropathy. Cochrane Database Syst Rev. 2012;(6):CD007543. https://doi.org/10.1002/14651858.CD007543.pub2.
9. Franklin GM, Shetterly SM, Cohen JA, Baxter J, Hamman RF. Risk factors for distal symmetric neuropathy in NIDDM. The San Luis Valley Diabetes Study. Diabetes Care. 1994;17:1172–7.
10. Diabetes Control and Complications Trial Research Group, Nathan DM, Genuth S, Lachin J, Cleary P, Crofford O, Davix M, Rand L, Siebert C. The effect of intensive treatment of diabetes on the development and progression of long-term complications in insulin-dependent diabetes mellitus. N Engl J Med. 1993;329:977–86.
11. Smith AG, Russell J, Feldman EL, Goldstein J, Peltier A, Smith S, Hamwi J, Pollari D, Bixby B, Bixny B, Howard J, Singleton JR. Lifestyle intervention for prediabetic neuropathy. Diabetes Care. 2006;29:1294–9.
12. Balducci S, Lacobellis G, Parisi L, Di Biase N, Calandriello E, Leonetti F, Fallucca F. Exercise training can modify the natural history of diabetic peripheral neuropathy. J Diabetes Complicat. 2006;20:216–23.
13. Perez-Matos MC, Morales-Alvarez MC, Mendivil CO. Lipids: a suitable therapeutic target in diabetic neuropathy? J Diabetes Res. 2017;2017:6943851. https://doi.org/10.1155/2017/694385.
14. Tesfaye S, Chaturvedi N, Eaton SE, Ward JD, Manes C, Ionescu-Trigoviste C, Witte DR, Fuller JH. EURODIAB Prospective Complications Study Group. Vascular risk factors and diabetic neuropathy. 2005;352:341–50.
15. Davis TM, Yeap BB, Davis WA, Bruce DG. Lipid-lowering therapy and peripheral sensory neuropathy in type 2 diabetes: the Fremantle Diabetes Study. Diabetologia. 2008;51: 562–6.
16. Malik RA, Williamson S, Abbott C, Carrington AL, Igbal J, Schady W, Boulton AJ. Effect of angiotensin-converting-enzyme (ACE) inhibitor trandolapril on human diabetic neuropathy: randomized double-blind controlled trial. Lancet. 1998;352:1978–81.
17. Ruggenenti P, Lauria G, Fassi A, Ileva AP, Rota S, Chiurchiu C, Barlovic DP, Sqhirlanzoni A, Lombardi R, Penza P, Cavaletti G, Piatti ML, Frigeni B, Filipponi M, Rubis N, Noris G, Motterlini N, Enelordache B, Gaspari F, Perna A, Zaletel J, Bossi A, Dodesini AR, Trevisan R, Remuzzi G, DEMAND Study Investigators. Effects of manidipine and delapril in hypertensive patients with type 2 diabetes mellitus: the delapril and manidipine for nephroprotection in diabetes (DEMAND) randomized clinical trial. Hypertension. 2011;58:776–83.
18. Tesfaye S, Boulton AJ, Dyck PJ, Freeman R, Horowitz M, Kempler P, Lauria G, Malik RA, Spallone V, Vinik A, Bernardi L, Valensi P, Toronto Diabetic Neuropathy Expert Group. Diabetic neuropathies: update on definitions, diagnostic criteria, estimation of severity, and treatments. Diabetes Care. 2010;33:2285–93.
19. Javed S, Alam U, Malik RA. Treating diabetic neuropathy: present strategies and emerging solutions. Rev Diabet Stud. 2015;12:63–83.
20. Dyck PJ, Davies JL, Wilson DM, Service FJ, Melton LJ 3rd, O'Brien PC. Risk factors for severity of diabetic polyneuropathy: intensive longitudinal assessment of the Rochester Diabetic Neuropathy Study cohort. Diabetes Care. 1999;22:1479–86.
21. Dyck PJ, Overland CJ, Low PA, Litchy WJ, Davies JL, Dyck PJ, O'Brien PC, CI vs. NPhys Trial Investigators, Albers JW, Andersen H, Bolton CF, England JD, Klein CJ, Llewelyn JG, Mauermann ML, Russell JW, Singer W, Smith AG, Tesfaye S, Vella A. Signs and symptoms versus nerve conduction studies to diagnose diabetic sensorimotor polyneuropathy: CI vs. NPhys trial. Muscle Nerve. 2010;42:157–64.

22. Valensi P, Paries J, Attali JR, French Group for Research and Study of Diabetic Neuropathy. Cardiac autonomic neuropathy in diabetic patients: influence of diabetes duration, obesity, and microangiopathic complications—the French multicenter study. Metabolism. 2003;52:815–20.
23. Vinik AI, Ziegler D. Diabetic cardiovascular autonomic neuropathy. Circulation. 2007;115:387–97.
24. Freeman R. Assessment of cardiovascular autonomic function. Clin Neurophysiol. 2006;117:716–30.
25. Gatopoulou A, Papanas N, Maltezos E. Diabetic gastrointestinal autonomic neuropathy: current status and new achievements for everyday clinical practice. Eur J Intern Med. 2012;23:499–505.
26. Jones KL, Russo A, Stevens JE, Wishart JM, Berry MK, Horowitz M. Predictors of delayed gastric emptying in diabetes. Diabetes Care. 2001;24:1264–9.
27. Ma J, Rayner CK, Jones KL, Horowitz M. Diabetic gastroparesis: diagnosis and management. Drugs. 2009;69:971–86.
28. Rayner CK, Horowitz M. Gastrointestinal motility and glycemic control in diabetes: the chicken and the egg revisited? J Clin Invest. 2006;116:299–302.
29. Vinik AI, Erbas T. Diabetic autonomic neuropathy. Handb Clin Neurol. 2013;117:279–94.
30. Martin CL, Albers JW, Pop-Busui R, DCCT/EDIC Research Group. Neuropathy and related findings in the diabetes control and complications trial/epidemiology of diabetes interventions and complications study. Diabetes Care. 2014;37:31–8.
31. Boulton AJ, Gries FA, Jervell JA. Guidelines for the diagnosis and outpatient management of diabetic peripheral neuropathy. Diabet Med. 1998;15:508–14.
32. Boulton AJ, Vinik AI, Arezzo JC, Bril V, Feldman EL, Freemaon R, Malik RA, Maser RE, Sosenko JM, Ziegler D, American Diabetes Association. Diabetic neuropathies: a statement by the American Diabetes Association. Diabetes Care. 2005;28:956–62.
33. Thomas PK. Classification, differential diagnosis, and staging of diabetic peripheral neuropathy. Diabetes. 1997;46(Suppl. 2):S54–7.
34. Kaku M, Vinik A, Simpson DM. Pathways in the diagnosis and management of diabetic polyneuropathy. Curr Diab Rep. 2015;15:609. https://doi.org/10.1007/s11892-015-0609-2.
35. Vinik A, Mehrabyan A, Colen L, Boulton A. Focal entrapment neuropathies in diabetes. Diabetes Care. 2004;27:1783–8.
36. Young RJ, Ewing DJ, Clarke BF. Chronic and remitting painful diabetic polyneuropathy. Correlations with clinical features and subsequent changes in neurophysiology. Diabetes Care. 1988;11:34–40.
37. Snyder MJ, Gibbs LM, Lindsay TJ. Treating painful diabetic peripheral neuropathy: an update. Am Fam Physician. 2016;94:227–34.
38. Spallone V. Management of painful diabetic neuropathy: guideline guidance or jungle? Curr Diab Rep. 2012;12:403–13.
39. Griebeler ML, Morey-Vargas OL, Brito JP, Tsapas A, Wang Z, Carranza Leon BG, Phung OJ, Montori VM, Murad MH. Pharmacologic interventions for painful diabetic neuropathy: an umbrella systematic review and comparative effectiveness network meta-analysis. Ann Intern Med. 2014;161:639–49.
40. Finnerup NB, Sindrup SH, Jensen TS. The evidence for pharmacological treatment of neuropathic pain. Pain. 2010;150:573–81.
41. Richter RW, Porenoy R, Sharma U, Lamoreaux L, Bockbrader H, Knapp LE. Relief of painful diabetic peripheral neuropathy with pregabalin: a randomized, placebo-controlled trial. J Pain. 2005;6:253–60.
42. Bril V, England J, Franklin GM, Backonja M, Cohen J, Del Toro D, Feldman E, Iverson DJ, Perkins B, Russell JW, Zochodne D, American Academy of Neurology, American Association of Neuromuscular and Electrodiagnostic Medicine, American Academy of Physical Medicine and Rehabilitation. Evidence-based guideline: treatment of painful diabetic neuropathy: report of the American Academy of Neurology, the American Association of Neuromuscular and Electrodiagnostic Medicine, and the American Academy of Physical Medicine and Rehabilitation. Neurology. 2011;76:1758–65.

43. Rudroju N, Bansal D, Talakokkula ST, Gudala K, Hota D, Bhansali A, Ghai B. Comparative efficacy and safety of six antidepressants and anticonvulsants in painful diabetic neuropathy: a network meta-analysis. Pain Physician. 2013;16:E705–12.
44. Chong MS, Hester J. Diabetic painful neuropathy: current and future treatment options. Drugs. 2007;67:569–85.
45. Ziegler D, Fonseca V. From guideline to patient: a review of recent recommendations for pharmacotherapy of painful diabetic neuropathy. J Diabetes Complicat. 2015;29:146–56.
46. Marks DM, Shah MJ, Patkar AA, Masand PS, Park GY, Pae CU. Serotonin-norepinephrine reuptake inhibitors for pain control: premise and promise. Curr Neuropharmacol. 2009;7:331–6.
47. Goldstein DJ, Lu Y, Detke MJ, Lee TC, Iyengar S. Duloxetine vs. placebo in patients with painful diabetic neuropathy. Pain. 2005;116:109–18.
48. Rowbotham MC, Goli V, Kunz NR, Lei D. Venlafaxine extended release in the treatment of painful diabetic neuropathy: a double-blind, placebo-controlled study. Pain. 2004;110:697–706.
49. Sindrup SH, Andersen G, Madsen C, Smith T, Brosen K, Jensen TS. Tramadol relieves pain and allodynia in polyneuropathy: a randomized, double-blind, controlled trial. Pain. 1999;83:85–90.
50. Schwartz S, Etropolski M, Shapiro DY, Okamoto A, Lange R, Haeussler J, Rauschkolb C. Safety and efficacy of tapentadol ER in patients with painful diabetic peripheral neuropathy: results of a randomized-withdrawal, placebo-controlled trial. Curr Med Res Opin. 2011;27:151–62.
51. Gilron I, Bailey JM, Tu D, Holden RR, Weaver DF, Houlden RL. Morphine, gabapentin, or their combination for neuropathic pain. N Engl J Med. 2005;352:1324–34.
52. Ko SH, Kwonn HS, Yu JM, Baik SH, Park IB, Lee JH, Ko KS, Noh JH, Kim DS, Mok JO, Park TS, Son HS, Cha BY. Comparison of the efficacy and safety of tramadol/acetaminophen combination therapy and gabapentin in the treatment of painful diabetic neuropathy. Diabet Med. 2010;27:1033–40.
53. Zhang WY, Li Wan Po A. The effectiveness of topically applied capsaicin. A meta-analysis. Eur J Clin Pharmacol. 1994;46:517–22.
54. Polydefkis M, Hauer P, Sheth S, Sidofsky M, Griffin JW, McArthur JC. The time course of epidermal nerve fiber regeneration: studies in normal controls and in people with diabetes, with and without neuropathy. Brain. 2004;127:1606–15.
55. Barbano RL, Herrmann DN, Hart-Gouleau S, Pennella-Vaughan J, Lodewick PA, Dworkin RH. Effectiveness, tolerability, and impact on quality of life of the 5% lidocaine patch in diabetic polyneuropathy. Arch Neurol. 2004;61:914–8.
56. Uluduz D, Bozluolcay M, Ince B, Kiziltan M. Simultaneous multiple cranial nerve neuropathies and intravenous immunoglobulin treatment in diabetes mellitus. Neurol India. 2006;54:308–9.
57. Ostric M, Vrca A, Kolak L, Franolic M, Vrca NB. Cranial nerve lesion in diabetic patients. Coll Antropol. 2011;35:131–6.
58. Grider JS, Manchikanti L, Carayannopoulos A, Sharma ML, Balog CC, Harned ME, Grami V, Justiz R, Nouri KH, Hayek SM, Vallejo R, Christo PJ. Effectiveness of spinal cord stimulation in chronic spinal pain: a systematic review. Pain Physician. 2016;19:E33–54.
59. Slangen R, Schaper NC, Faber CG, Joosten EA, Dirksen CD, van Dongen RT, Kessels AG, van Kleef M. Spinal cord stimulation and pain relief in painful diabetic peripheral neuropathy: a prospective two-center randomized controlled trial. Diabetes Care. 2014;37:3016–24.

Chapter 15
Phantom Limb Pain

Luminita M. Tureanu and Ljuba Stojiljkovic

More than 185,000 patients in the USA undergo limb amputations yearly. In 2005 it was estimated that 1.6 million people live without the limb, and it is projected that this number may reach 3.5 million by 2050 [1]. The most common factors associated with the limb loss are diabetes mellitus, trauma, peripheral vascular disease, and bone and joint malignancies [1]. The limb loss is associated with significant increases in healthcare costs and disability.

Postamputation sensation was first described by French military surgeon Ambroise Pare (1510–1590). He noticed that some of the patients complained of severe pain in the missing limb following amputation [2]. After Lord Nelson lost his right arm during the attack on Santa Cruz de Tenerife, he experienced phantom limb pain and wrote that this ghostly sensation is "a direct proof" of the existence of the soul. He concluded that if arm can survive physical annihilation, why not the whole person?

In 1871 Silas Weir Mitchel introduced the phrase "phantom limb," which is used to describe phantom limb sensations ever since [2, 3]. Despite centuries of the recognized phenomenon, very little is known about pathophysiological and molecular mechanisms involved in the appearance and propagation of the phantom limb sensations, including phantom limb pain.

After amputation of a limb virtually all amputees experience the sensation that the deafferented body part is still present, and these sensations are called phantom sensations.

Non-painful sensations may include specific position, shape, or movement of a phantom limb, itching, tingling, and paresthesia. Pain in the part of the body that does not exist is called phantom limb pain, which may be severe and is very difficult to treat.

L. M. Tureanu (✉) · L. Stojiljkovic
Department of Anesthesiology, Feinberg School of Medicine, Northwestern University, Chicago, IL, USA
e-mail: l-tureanu@northwestern.edu

K. Shimoji et al. (eds.), *Chronic Pain Management in General and Hospital Practice*, https://doi.org/10.1007/978-981-15-2933-7_15

15.1 Phantom Limb Pain: Clinical Aspects

15.1.1 Incidence

Early literature reported the incidence of phantom pain as low as 2%. However, most recent studies have shown that the incidence is much higher, 60–80%. The incidence is independent of gender, level, and site of amputation. Interestingly, phantom pain is far less frequent in young children and congenital amputees. The incidence is only 3.7% in congenital amputees, 20% in children less than 2 years old, 25% in 2–4 years old, 61% in 4–6 years old, and in 75% in 6–8 years old [4].

15.1.2 Onset and Duration

Onset of pain is very early after amputation and appears immediately in 75% of the cases. However, the pain may appear much later, and can be delayed for months and years. In many patients, pain is present for several days and gradually fades. In some subset of patients, pain may persist over the years and even decades [5].

15.1.3 Character and Localization

Phantom pain is commonly classified as neuropathic pain, and it is believed to be related to a damage of central or peripheral neurons. Usually it is described as squeezing, throbbing, shooting, stabbing, or burning [6].

About 30–50% of limb amputees report a phenomenon called "telescoping." Telescoping refers to fading of phantom sensation in a way that the phantom arm becomes progressively shorter until is felt as phantom hand dangling from the stump. Recent evidence suggests that telescoping and phantom limb pain are positively correlated; the presence of telescoping is associated with more phantom pain [7].

15.1.4 Animal Models of Phantom Limb Pain

Total paw denervation in rodents elicits an abnormal behavior of licking, scratching, and self-injury of the anesthetic limb ("autotomy"). Although autotomy is not a normal response by humans to total limb denervation or chronic pain, it occurs in species ranging from rodents to primates [8]. Since the same denervation produces phantom limb pain and anesthesia dolorosa in humans, autotomy has been used as a model of human phantom limb pain [9, 10].

15.1.5 *Pathophysiological Mechanisms of Phantom Limb Pain*

Mechanisms underlying development of chronic neuropathic pain conditions, as well as phantom pain sensations are still largely unknown. Many contributing factors, including systemic inflammatory mediators [11], and peripheral and central nervous system rearrangements have been proposed [12, 13]. Recently it has been shown that cognitive and emotional sensitization and pain catastrophizing (top-down modulation) may contribute to the increased nociception in this patient population [14, 15].

In a recent study, increased levels of pro-inflammatory mediators, such as TNF-α, TNF-β, IL-8, ICAM-1, and CRP were positively correlated with the intensity of phantom pain. Higher inflammatory state also correlated with more pain catastrophizing and has contributed both directly and indirectly to more severe perception of pain in these patients [11].

15.2 Peripheral Mechanisms

Nerve injuries during amputation and development of neuromas have long been associated with the development of pain in amputees. After injury, nerves undergo significant structural and functional changes, which initially lead to excessive discharges from damaged areas [16]. In addition, regenerative axonal sprouting at the stump can lead to the development of amputation neuroma, further aggravating phantom pain [17]. Sodium channels show upregulation and abnormal accumulation in injured nerve endings, which increases excitability in afferent nerve fibers, contributing to increased nerve discharge from the stump [18].

15.3 Central Sensitization

Increased discharge from injured peripheral neurons has been shown to increase activity in dorsal horn of the spinal cord, increased response to other peripheral afferent stimuli, and expansion of receptive fields. Clinically, these mechanisms lead to hyperalgesia (decreased threshold for pain) and allodynia (pain elicited by non-painful stimuli) in amputees [13]. Changes in pain thresholds have been shown to be positively related with phantom pain [19].

15.3.1 *Cortical Reorganization and Plasticity in the Somatosensory System*

One of the characteristic features of the adult primate brain is the distinct topographical "maps" representing different sense modalities [20]. In 1960s researchers believed that neuronal circuits are genetically specified and that remained stable throughout the lifetime [21]. However, the body of evidence from extensive brain research suggests this is not the case. Indeed, both animal and human studies have revealed tremendous ability of reorganization of primary sensory cortex in response to alterations of the sensory receptor surface throughout adulthood. The first clear experimental demonstration of plasticity in adult central nervous system came from the work of Wall et al. [22]. The authors showed changes in the receptive fields' size shortly after partial denervation. In a series of elegant experiments, Merzenich et al. [23] demonstrated that after amputation of the middle finger in adult monkeys, the area of cortex that corresponded to this digit started to respond to stimuli delivered to adjacent fingers. Moreover, in 1991 Pons and colleagues [24] demonstrated that after long-term deafferentation of the upper limb, the cortical area that originally corresponded to the amputated limb started to respond to sensory stimuli delivered to the face. This phenomenon of functional reorganization is called representational plasticity and signifies the form of cortical plasticity. Flor et al. [25] provided the evidence that shift of the mouth into the hand representation has a close association with phantom limb pain. The larger the shift of the mouth representation into the zone that formerly represented the amputated arm, the greater the phantom-limb pain. These data indicate that phantom limb pain may be at least in part a consequence of plastic changes in the primary somatosensory cortex [25, 26].

The studies of phantom limbs provide us with an exceptional opportunity to understand the physiology of functional reorganization and cortical plasticity as well as to further analyze the mechanisms of how the brain constructs and continuously updates the body image in response to changes in sensory inputs [27, 28].

Pain memories established before amputation are powerful contributors to phantom limb pain. Pain memories are most likely implicit memories that involve changes related to nociceptive inputs and subsequent changes in processing in the cortical somatosensory system. The primary somatosensory cortex is known to be involved in processing of pain. If the somatosensory pain memories have been established prior to amputation, the deafferentation that follows limb amputation and subsequent sensory invasion of that cortical zone by neighboring zones provides the mechanisms how non-painful stimuli from adjacent zones may preferentially lead to activation of sensation of pain. Since the cortical area coding seems to stay assigned to original receptive fields, activation of the cortical area that represents the limb by stimuli originating from adjacent areas such as face is referred to this limb and is perceived as phantom pain [29].

15.4 Molecular Mechanisms of Phantom Pain

Long-term memory of pain in somatosensory cortex is one of the most important factors involved in generation and stabilization of phantom pain. The mechanisms of how neurons and synapses encode the long-term changes that induce memory consolidation have been under intense scientific investigation in neurobiology. Recent data suggest that Erk/mitogen activated kinase (MAPK/Erk) may play a key role in these processes. Activation of cAMP response element binding protein (CREB), cAMP activated protein kinase A (PKA), and MAPK/Erk pathway not only play a critical role in cell growth and differentiation, but may also serve as evolutionary conserved regulator of memory formation. Studies indicate that MAPK/Erk signaling cascade is critical for both long-term neuronal plasticity and memory consolidation [30]. When synapses are activated, they strengthen, especially if they fire repetitively. This activity-dependent process is called long-term potentiation (LTP) and has been proposed as a cellular model for memory development. Eliciting long-term effect of LTP (L-LTP) needs de novo protein synthesis. This process is believed to be mediated by transcription activation that requires recruitment of transcriptional factors via MAPK/Erk and CREB dependent signaling [30].

Phantom sensations and phantom pain are believed to result from functional reorganization and CNS plasticity as well as alterations in long-term memory in cortical representations of amputated limbs. Because topographical somatosensory "maps" are highly conserved among species, assumptions about neuronal structures and processes involved in generation and propagation of phantom sensations and pain in humans can be made based on animal models. Rodent models have been successfully used in studies of neuropathic pain and autotomy rodent models are widely accepted as an animal model of phantom pain [8–10]. Moreover, molecular processes involving different signaling pathways leading to activation of immediate early genes (IEG) such as c-fos have been shown to be involved in central mechanism of pain and memory [31–33]. In a rat model of phantom pain, c-fos activation has been associated with the expansion of somatosensory cortical fields after non-painful stimuli were applied to adjacent areas of somatosensory cortex [34].

15.5 Diagnosis

The diagnosis of phantom limb pain is usually based on patient reporting symptoms, and a detailed history is invaluable in making appropriate treatment decisions. History should focus on characteristics of pain, including location, type, onset, associated symptoms, intensity, alleviating and aggravating factors. The severity of pain, while subjective and therefore difficult to evaluate, can be assessed by using several pain scales, such as numeric pain scales, visual analog scores, or the McGill pain questionnaire. Performing a psychological evaluation and further assessing the impact of pain on quality of life are equally important components. Patient's response to previous therapies can further guide individualized treatment [35]. A differential diagnosis including residual limb ischemia and joint sepsis should always be kept in mind. Other sources of chronic limb pain, such as stump pain, complex regional pain syndrome, and vasculitis should be ruled out. There is no specific test that would confirm the presence of phantom limb pain and further imaging, lab work, and testing are usually not necessary.

In a recent publication, Clarke et al. [36] reviewed 151 papers on residual limb pain and found that none of the studies listed specific diagnostic criteria. They proposed an algorithm for uniform classification, the Durham Pain Investigations Group, Post-Amputation Pain Algorithm (DPIG-PAPA). The correct diagnosis of the clinical entity is thought as a prerequisite for optimizing treatment strategies.

15.6 Treatment

Over the past several decades a plethora of different treatment modalities have been proposed for the treatment of phantom pain, however, given the complexity of the involved pathophysiology, treatment remains challenging. Richardson and Kulkarni [37] in their comprehensive review on the management of phantom limb pain identified thirty eight different therapies and found on overall low quality of evidence, with no particular therapy emerging as first line, evidence based therapy. Although our knowledge on the topic and proposed therapies has evolved, mechanism specific treatments are still lacking. Improved success rates have been achieved with multidisciplinary approaches. Current treatment modalities include pharmacological and non-pharmacological options, including invasive/surgical and non-invasive approaches.

15.6.1 Pre-Emptive Analgesia

The perioperative period has long been postulated as a potential window of opportunity for the prevention of further clinical manifestations consistent with phantom limb pain. Improved pain control in the pre-operative period is thought to be able to prevent noxious stimuli present at the amputation site that would activate peripheral and central sensitization.

While attempting a systematic review on the association of perioperative factors with chronic postamputation pain, Srivastava [38] ended up doing a narrative review, as the identified studies and proposed outcomes measures were too heterogeneous. He concluded that while data on chronic postamputation pain risk reduction is less robust, there seem to be some evidence that the incidence of acute perioperative pain may be reduced by optimizing perioperative analgesia. Specifically, the current evidence suggests that optimized perioperative analgesia reduces the incidence of acute perioperative pain, but no firm conclusion could be drawn on reducing the risk for chronic postamputation pain. A whole evidence based system pathway to optimize perioperative amputation pain is described, which comprises pre-emptive analgesia, intraoperative anesthesia/analgesia and optimized, individualized postoperative analgesia.

Among the analgesic modalities thought to provide pre-emptive analgesia, epidural analgesia has been studied the most. In the randomized, double-blind trial of Nikolajsen [39], patients undergoing lower limb amputation who received epidurals with bupivacaine and morphine were compared with patients who received epidurals with saline and intravenous morphine. The epidural catheters were placed a median of 18 hours preoperatively and patients were followed at 3, 6, and 12 months postoperatively. There was no difference between groups in the incidence of stump and phantom pain and the opioid consumption.

Karanikolas et al. [40] performed a prospective clinical trial including 65 patients undergoing lower limb amputation, who were randomized to five treatment groups. All patients, except controls, received epidural analgesia and intravenous patient controlled analgesia (PCA) and were blinded to the administered solution. Patients in the control group did not have an epidural catheter and received conventional analgesia per the vascular surgery department analgesic routine. To avoid bias, patients in the control group had an epidural catheter placed subcutaneously in the lumbar area and received normal saline solution through the catheter. They also received an intravenous PCA with normal saline. Patients were followed up at 1 and 6 months postamputation, and their pain severity was assessed using the visual analog scale and the McGill pain questionnaire. When epidural analgesia and intravenous PCA were started 48 hours preoperatively, optimized and continued for 48 hours postoperatively, there was a statistically significant difference in phantom limb pain at the 6 months follow-up between the intervention and the control group.

The randomized prospective trial of Lambert et al. [41] evaluated 30 patients undergoing lower limb amputation under general anesthesia who received either an epidural infusion with bupivacaine and diamorphine for 24 hours before surgery and 72 hours after surgery or a perineural infusion of 0.25% bupivacaine. Patients were followed up at 3 days, 6 and 12 months after amputation to evaluate the rate and intensity of stump and phantom limb pain, and the opioid consumption. The intervention made no difference in the rate of phantom pain when compared with the natural course of the condition, and no long-term benefits were observed. The opioid consumption was higher in the perineural group but did not reach statistical significance.

Peripheral nerve blockade has also been studied in patients with phantom limb pain. While most studies report 3 days or less of postoperative perineural local anesthetic infusion of varying analgesic concentrations, potential long-term benefits have been inconsistent.

Placement of perineural catheters under direct vision was described by Fisher [42] in 1991, and later on followed by several studies that used the same technique. A randomized clinical trial conducted by Pinzur et al. [43] on 21 patients showed that a perineural infusion of 0.5% Bupivacaine in the study group is an effective modality for postoperative analgesia in the first 72 hours. However, there was no difference between groups in the ability to reduce the phantom limb pain at the 3 and 6 months follow-up. Positive results were reported by Lennox and colleagues [44], who demonstrated improved pain control, with visual analog scores of less than 3 in 83% of cases and decreased opioid requirements during first 72 hours, in patients who received continuous perineural catheters placed intraoperatively using a similar technique.

In a prospective, observational study, Borghi et al. [45] evaluated the effect of prolonged perineural blockade in 71 patients undergoing lower extremity amputation. Patients received pre- or intra-operatively a perineural sciatic catheter with 0.5% ropivacaine. Sixty-two patients completed the study, and the median duration of catheter infusion was 30 days. In 65% of the patients the catheter infusion was continued for 1 month or longer. At the end of the 12 months evaluation period, the incidence of severe phantom limb pain was 3%, yet 39% of the patients experienced phantom limb sensations. The authors concluded that a prolonged perineural infusion with 0.5% ropivacaine appears to be an effective therapeutic option for this patient population.

In a large retrospective chart review of 198 patients, Ayling et al. [46] showed a substantial reduction of 40% in postoperative opioid consumption, when peripheral nerve catheters were used for 72 hours in lower extremity amputation patients. The perineural stump catheters were placed by surgeons at the time of amputation, under direct vision, next to the exposed sciatic or posterior tibial nerve. The study did not find a difference in pain scores at 24 hours and did not look at postamputation phantom pain in this patient population.

More recent, Ilfeld and colleagues [47] did a randomized, double masked, placebo controlled, cross over pilot study on two below knee and one below elbow amputation patients with intractable, chronic phantom limb pain of at least 12 months. The patients were randomized to receive either 0.5% ropivacaine or saline infusion as outpatients for over 6 days and had the option to repeat the same protocol, but with crossover treatment, 12–16 weeks after the initial catheter placement. They were followed for up to 52 weeks, with one patient having no phantom limb pain recurrence and another one having only small levels of baseline pain. The authors were able to show that prolonged ambulatory perineural catheter infusions are a reliable intervention for the treatment of intractable phantom limb pain.

While most of the studies to date have shown either no long-term benefits on phantom limb pain or at best inconsistent results, Ilfeld's pilot study seems to bring some long needed reassurance that long-term benefits may be obtained with longer duration of continuous perineural infusion. Given the relative low associated costs, without need for prolonged hospitalization, practically no side effects, no potential for addiction, and no impact on cognitive function, the ambulatory perineural catheters may emerge as an attractive therapeutic option for this challenging to treat patients.

Bosanquet et al. [48] in a systematic review and meta-analysis, looked at seven studies including 416 patients, who underwent lower limb amputation, and compared patients who received a perineural catheter placed intraoperatively with patients who received no treatment or placebo. Only three studies evaluated phantom limb pain as long-term outcome. The GRADE system was used to assess the quality of evidence, which was found to be very low. While there was around 50% reduction in postoperative opioid consumption, there was no effect on short- or long-term outcomes such as postoperative pain, postoperative mortality, incidence of phantom limb pain and stump pain.

A recent systematic review of Humble et al. [49] including 32 studies, on patients who underwent amputation, mastectomy or thoracotomy, showed that regional anesthesia is beneficial for reducing acute and chronic pain. Same positive effects were demonstrated by a retrospective study of Shahin et al. [50] who looked at different anesthetic techniques and their impact on phantom limb pain. While no difference was found at the 14–17 months follow-up, patients who received epidural anesthesia or peripheral nerve blocks had significant less pain during the first week after amputation.

Ypsilantis and Tang [51] in their review on pre-emptive analgesia for chronic limb pain after amputation for peripheral vascular disease retrieved eleven studies, which evaluated five different analgesic options used in the treatment of phantom limb pain: local anesthetics, opiates, NMDA receptor antagonists, alpha (2)-agonist, and GABA analogues. The drugs were given alone or in combination, and the route of administration was oral, intravenous, epidural, or perineural. The authors emphasized that well conducted, randomized control trials are few, and that the small number of patients and protocol violations are among the weaknesses of current available studies. A summary of recommendations, including level of evidence, was included in the review. For acute postoperative pain, a level A of evidence was found for the following therapeutic modalities:

- Epidural infusion of bupivacaine and morphine (with potential serious complications).
- Postoperative perineural infusion of bupivacaine.
- Epidural combination of bupivacaine/diamorphine for 72 hours was found to be more effective than perineural infusion of bupivacaine alone in treating acute perioperative pain.
- Single injection peripheral nerve block with bupivacaine and clonidine provided analgesia during the first 24 hours postoperatively.

A perioperative epidural infusion of bupivacaine combined with diamorphine and clonidine may offer potential pre-emptive analgesia for chronic stump pain and phantom limb pain (level B evidence).

15.6.2 Pharmacological Approaches

Various medications, administered by different routes, have been attempted over the years in an effort to improve pain control in phantom limb pain patients. The optimal, evidence based pharmacological approach is still uncertain.

McCormick et al. [52] conducted a recent systematic review on current literature, and organized the data from the perspective of three different compartments that are potentially implicated in the mechanisms of phantom limb pain: neuromas on the peripheral/afferent pathways, central pathways/maladaptive plasticity, and efferent sympathetic pathways. Medications which target peripheral pathways and have been studied for phantom limb pain include amitriptyline, perineural ropivacaine and bupivacaine, epidural bupivacaine and botulinum toxin (level 2, respectively level 3 evidence). Agents acting on the central pathways include antiepileptics, opioids, and NMDA receptor antagonists (level 2 and level 3 evidence). Targeted treatments for the sympathetic pathways that have been studied are few and include beta blockade and lumbar sympathetic block.

Among the most commonly used medications to treat phantom limb pain are non-steroidal anti-inflammatory drugs and acetaminophen. However, data suggest that their helpfulness ratings are low [53].

Amitriptyline is a tricyclic antidepressant that has been commonly used to treat patients with neuropathic pain, including phantom limb pain. The analgesic effect is likely based upon interference with the NMDA receptors, uptake of serotonin and norepinephrine, and blockade of sodium channels. Although amitriptyline has been used for decades in the treatment of neuropathic pain, the last Cochrane review on the topic, including 17 studies and 1342 participants, found no evidence to support its analgesic benefits, bringing out a concern for overestimation of the therapeutic effect [54]. Moreover, the 2016 Cochrane review on pharmacological interventions to treat phantom limb pain found amitriptyline to be ineffective for this type of pain [55]. Dry mouth and dizziness were listed as frequent side effects.

Gabapentin has a long history of use in chronic, neuropathic pain. It has been used as an adjunct in both children and adults with phantom limb pain [56]. The review of Abbass [57] including three randomized controlled trials and comprising a total of 89 patients found that gabapentin may decrease the intensity of phantom limb pain. In a recent Cochrane review gabapentin showed conflicting results regarding pain relief, which seem to favor the treatment vs control group [55]. However, function, depression, and sleep were not improved and several side effects, such as somnolence, dizziness, and nausea were present.

Opioids provide analgesia by binding to peripheral and central receptors. Morphine, methadone, oxycodone, and tramadol have all been used to treat various neuropathic conditions, including phantom limb pain [58]. In a double-blind, randomized, placebo controlled cross over study, Wu et al. [59] showed that sustained-release morphine treatment resulted in a decrease in pain intensity when compared with mexiletine, but was associated with a higher rate of side effects, mainly constipation. There was no difference in self-reported overall functional activity and interference of pain with daily activities. Level 2 evidence studies support the use of morphine, both oral and intravenous. McCormick and colleagues [52] in their systematic review found a level 2 evidence for tramadol and level 4 evidence for methadone. There is data to suggest that chronic opioid use before amputation increases the opioid requirements during first 3 days postoperatively, and the requirement remained increased day 7 postoperatively [60].

Ketamine, an NMDA receptor agonist, has been found to improve acute pain, while only a questionable effect was found in chronic phantom limb pain. In the small pilot study of Buvanendran et al. [61] three patients going for below knee amputation received oral ketamine (1.0 mg/kg) for 3 days perioperative and no serious side effects occurred. Oral ketamine may therefore emerge as a safe medication with potential ambulatory use. Hayes and colleagues [62] in their randomized controlled trial included 45 patients undergoing above or below knee amputation. Patients received an intravenous ketamine infusion for 3 days after a pre-induction bolus. The incidence of phantom limb pain was 47% in the ketamine group, compared with 71% in the control group. Interestingly enough, the ketamine infusion group had an increased incidence of stump pain at on day 3 post-operatively. The 2016 Cochrane review of Aviar et al. [55] confirmed the analgesic effects of ketamine in phantom limb patients, and also mentioned the presence of several side effects, including sedation, hallucinations, hearing, and position impairment.

Other NMDA receptor antagonists that have been used in the treatment of these patients are dextromethorphan and memantine. An earlier systematic review from 2014 found a level 3 evidence for both drugs [52]. Loy et al. [63] in their systematic review found that while memantine was well tolerated, in 4 out of 8 of the included studies there were no significant analgesic effects in patients with chronic phantom limb pain of over one year. More recently, when compared with placebo, dextromethorphan also had analgesic effects, but the same effects were not observed with memantine [55].

The hormone calcitonin is also among the medications which has been used in the treatment of phantom limb pain. The suggested mechanisms, although unclear, may involve central, serotoninergic pathways [64]. Available data suggest that there is level 3 evidence for intravenous calcitonin in this patient population [52].

The Cochrane review of Alviar and colleagues [55] included 14 randomized and quasi randomized clinical trials, comprising 269 patients, and evaluated the effectiveness of anticonvulsants, antidepressants, NMDA receptor antagonists, opioids, calcitonin, local anesthetics, and botulinum toxin. The review aimed to summarize the evidence of these pharmacological interventions to treat phantom limb pain, looking at several relevant outcomes, including change in pain intensity, function, sleep, mood, quality of life, adverse events, and treatment satisfaction. The authors determined that the current evidence is inconclusive and that larger, more robust clinical trials are needed to conclude which medications would be useful in clinical practice.

15.6.3 Non-pharmacological Approaches

Non-pharmacological approaches have always been part of the armamentarium used to treat phantom limb pain. Among the most commonly used therapies are transcutaneous electrical stimulation (TENS), relaxation techniques, biofeedback, hypnosis, and acupuncture.

Batsford et al. [65] performed a systematic review of randomized controlled trials of these conservative therapies and used the GRADE approach to rate the available evidence. The authors concluded that while high quality evidence is scarce, these therapies which almost lack any adverse events may show potential and deserve further research.

TENS has been used as a non-pharmacological intervention and its effectiveness has recently been evaluated in a Cochrane review [66]. The authors could not find any randomized controlled trials, and the published literature was not robust enough to draw any conclusions.

Movement representation techniques, including mirror therapy and motor imagery among others, have also been utilized to reduce certain types of neuropathic pain. In their systematic review and meta-analysis, Thieme and colleagues [67] found no evidence to support an analgesic effect of such therapies in patients with phantom limb pain. Looking at the efficacy of mirror therapy for phantom limb pain, Barbin et al. [68] reported that the available evidence is insufficient and mirror therapy cannot be recommended as first intention therapy. The latest systematic review on the effectiveness of mirror therapy, motor imagery, and virtual feedback confirmed previous findings on lack of evidence to support such therapies [69].

Acupuncture has been used to treat a variety of chronic pain conditions. There are few publications on acupuncture as adjuvant in phantom limb pain, consisting mostly of case studies [70]. Recently, Treveylan et al. [71] came up with a preliminary protocol using the Delphi approach which has been developed to address the lack of consensus regarding the recommended acupuncture treatment of phantom limb pain. The protocol consisted of a combination of body and auricular acupuncture, including sympathetic points, needling around the stump if necessary, mirroring by needling the opposite limb, and retaining needles for 20–30 min, among other options. This was followed shortly by a randomized controlled feasibility study that showed that acupuncture was perceived as effective and beneficial, and demonstrated a meaningful change in pain intensity [72]. Scalp acupuncture has been reported as being successful in the treatment of phantom limb pain after below elbow amputation [73]. Among the points used were the Sishencong points on the vertex, which can suppress the sympathetic discharge when stimulated [74]. While more robust research is needed, there seems to be preliminary evidence that acupuncture may have a role as adjuvant or alternative approach where other treatments have failed.

Non-pharmacological, invasive approaches have usually been considered after conservative treatment has failed. To name a few, neurectomy, cordotomy, thalamotomy, sympathectomy, spinal cord stimulation, and deep brain stimulation have all been tried for intractable phantom limb pain. The more invasive the procedure the higher the complication rate, including permanent nerve injury [35].

Spinal cord stimulation (SCS) has been used since the 1970s in selective phantom limb patients resistant to other therapies, as an effective neuromodulatory intervention, albeit with poor somatotopic specificity [75, 76]. The recent review of Ayier et al. [77] comprising twelve studies, each including a relatively small number of patients, found mixed results. Technological advancements in SCS, such as change from constant voltage to constant current system, may show promise in better coverage of this type of pain [78].

Dorsal root ganglion (DRG) stimulation is yet another neuromodulatory intervention that has been trialed for patients with phantom limb pain. Recent data seem to suggest that DRG may be the site where phantom limb pain is generated, and small studies seem to support the fact that DRG therapy may be an effective tool among phantom limb therapies [79].

Peripheral neuromodulation has been recently reported in one case of phantom limb pain. Complete and persistent pain relief was achieved after implantation of neuromodulation peripheral leads into the stump [80].

Targeted muscle reinnervation (TMR) is emerging as a promising surgical technique for the treatment of neuromas after limb amputation. The procedure aims to restore physiological continuity to peripheral nerves involved in amputation and support nerve reorganization. TMR has been studied in high level upper limb amputations, and more recently in lower limb amputations, and has been shown, synergistic with pattern recognition control, to improve functional prosthesis control [81]. There is evidence to support that primary TMR done at the time of amputation may not only prevent neuroma formation, but also actually act pre-emptively and contribute to the reduction of phantom limb pain, and improve functional outcomes and quality of life in these challenging to treat patients [82, 83]. A multi-institutional cohort study of 51 patients who underwent immediate TMR at the time of amputation showed that the intervention group had lower phantom and residual limb pain, and achieved a pain free rate of more than 45% [83]. In a 2019 multicenter, prospective randomized clinical trail on 28 amputees with chronic pain, Dumanian et al. [84] showed that TMR improved phantom limb pain in major limb amputees. When compared with conventional surgical treatment the study showed there was a trend towards improvement in the residual limb pain as well [84].

The latest evidence based recommendations for the treatment of phantom limb pain come from the 2016 Italian Consensus Conference on Pain in Neurorehabilitation [85]. Combination therapy among first line neuropathic pain drugs is probably more effective and has less associated side effects when compared with single drug therapy. While gabapentin, ketamine, and morphine may have short-term analgesic effects, amitriptyline was not found to be effective. For calcitonin, the current recommendation is to avoid it. The evidence to support epidural analgesia is conflicting. The consensus recommended that several non-pharmacological therapies can be considered, including mirror therapy, mental imagery, phantom exercises, progressive muscle relaxation, and non-invasive brain stimulation. Another recommendation focused on altered quality of life in patients who have phantom limb pain, and subsequent depression for which they should receive treatment. The impact of pain treatment on the functional recovery and rehabilitation outcomes has been recognized as potentially relevant and it is recommended to be assessed in this group of patients.

In summary, although substantial progress has been made in our understanding of the theoretical mechanisms of phantom limb pain, its clinical management remains a challenge to the practicing clinician. The most beneficial treatment is based on an early and aggressive multimodal approach, involving pre-emptive analgesia, pharmacological and non-pharmacological interventions, rehabilitation and possible vocational training, education, and psychotherapy.

References

1. Ziegler-Graham K, MacKenzie EJ, Ephraim PL, Travison TG, Brookmeyer R. Estimating the prevalence of limb loss in the United States: 2005–2050. Arch Phys Med Rehabil. 2008;89(3):422–9. https://doi.org/10.1016/j.apmr.2007.11.005.
2. Finger S, Hustwit MP. Five early accounts of phantom limb in context: Pare, Descartes, Lemos, Bell, and Mitchell. Neurosurgery. 2003;52(3):675–86; discussion 85-6.

3. Ohry A. The forgotten stories on patients who made history. Prog Health Sci. 2013;3(1): 134–41.
4. Simmel ML. The reality of phantom sensations. Soc Res. 1962;29(3):337–56.
5. Nikolajsen L, Jensen TS. Phantom limb pain. Br J Anaesth. 2001;87(1):107–16.
6. Ehde DM, Czerniecki JM, Smith DG, Campbell KM, Edwards WT, Jensen MP, et al. Chronic phantom sensations, phantom pain, residual limb pain, and other regional pain after lower limb amputation. Arch Phys Med Rehabil. 2000;81(8):1039–44.
7. Flor H. Phantom-limb pain: characteristics, causes, and treatment. Lancet Neurol. 2002;1(3):182–9.
8. Seltzer Z, Wu T, Max MB, Diehl SR. Mapping a gene for neuropathic pain-related behavior following peripheral neurectomy in the mouse. Pain. 2001;93(2):101–6.
9. Wall PD, Scadding JW, Tomkiewicz MM. The production and prevention of experimental anesthesia dolorosa. Pain. 1979;6(2):175–82.
10. Coderre TJ, Grimes RW, Melzack R. Deafferentation and chronic pain in animals: an evaluation of evidence suggesting autotomy is related to pain. Pain. 1986;26(1):61–84.
11. Chamessian A, Van De Ven T, Buchheit T, Hsia H-L, McDuffie M, Gamazon ER, et al. Differential expression of systemic inflammatory mediators in amputees with chronic residual limb pain. Pain. 2017;158(1):68–74.
12. Giummarra MJ, Moseley GL. Phantom limb pain and bodily awareness: current concepts and future directions. Curr Opin Anaesthesiol. 2011;24(5):524–31. https://doi.org/10.1097/ACO.0b013e32834a105f.
13. Nikolajsen L. Postamputation pain: studies on mechanisms. Dan Med J. 2012;59(10):B4527.
14. Vase L, Nikolajsen L, Christensen B, Egsgaard LL, Arendt-Nielsen L, Svensson P, et al. Cognitive-emotional sensitization contributes to wind-up-like pain in phantom limb pain patients. Pain. 2011;152(1):157–62. https://doi.org/10.1016/j.pain.2010.10.013.
15. Vase L, Egsgaard LL, Nikolajsen L, Svensson P, Jensen TS, Arendt-Nielsen L. Pain catastrophizing and cortical responses in amputees with varying levels of phantom limb pain: a high-density EEG brain-mapping study. Exp Brain Res. 2012;218(3):407–17. https://doi.org/10.1007/s00221-012-3027-6.
16. Devor M. Ectopic discharge in Abeta afferents as a source of neuropathic pain. Exp Brain Res. 2009;196(1):115–28. https://doi.org/10.1007/s00221-009-1724-6.
17. Lago N, Navarro X. Evaluation of the long-term regenerative potential in an experimental nerve amputee model. J Peripher Nerv Syst. 2007;12(2):108–20. https://doi.org/10.1111/j.1529-8027.2007.00130.x.
18. Kretschmer T, Happel LT, England JD, Nguyen DH, Tiel RL, Beuerman RW, et al. Accumulation of PN1 and PN3 sodium channels in painful human neuroma-evidence from immunocytochemistry. Acta Neurochir (Wien). 2002;144(8):803.–10; discussion 10. https://doi.org/10.1007/s00701-002-0970-1.
19. Nikolajsen L, Ilkjaer S, Jensen TS. Relationship between mechanical sensitivity and postamputation pain: a prospective study. Eur J Pain. 2000;4(4):327–34. https://doi.org/10.1053/eujp.2000.0194.
20. Penfield W. In: Penfield W, Rasmussen T, editors. The cerebral cortex of man; a clinical study of localization of function. New York: Macmillan; 1950.
21. Wiesel TN, Hubel DH. Single-cell responses in striate cortex of kittens deprived of vision in one eye. J Neurophysiol. 1963;26:1003–17.
22. Wall PD. The presence of ineffective synapses and the circumstances which unmask them. Philos Trans R Soc Lond Ser B Biol Sci. 1977;278(961):361–72.
23. Merzenich MM, Nelson RJ, Stryker MP, Cynader MS, Schoppmann A, Zook JM. Somatosensory cortical map changes following digit amputation in adult monkeys. J Comp Neurol. 1984;224(4):591–605.
24. Pons TP, Garraghty PE, Ommaya AK, Kaas JH, Taub E, Mishkin M. Massive cortical reorganization after sensory deafferentation in adult macaques. Science. 1991; 252(5014):1857–60.
25. Flor H, Elbert T, Knecht S, Wienbruch C, Pantev C, Birbaumers N, et al. Phantom-limb pain as a perceptual correlate of cortical reorganization following arm amputation. Nature. 1995;375(6531):482–4.

26. Karl A, Flor H, Birbaumer N, Lutzenberger W, Birbaumer N, Cohen LG, et al. Reorganization of motor and somatosensory cortex in upper extremity amputees with phantom limb pain. J Neurosci. 2001;21(10):3609–18.
27. Ramachandran V, Rogers-Ramachandran D. Phantom limbs and neural plasticity. Arch Neurol. 2000;57(3):317–20.
28. Ramachandran V, Hirstein W. The perception of phantom limbs. The D. O. Hebb lecture. Brain. 1998;121:1603–30.
29. Polley DB, Chen-Bee CH, Frostig RD. Two directions of plasticity in the sensory-deprived adult cortex. Neuron. 1999;24(3):623–37.
30. Impey S, Obrietan K, Storm DR. Making new connections: role of ERK/MAP kinase signaling in neuronal plasticity. Neuron. 1999;23(1):11–4.
31. Kovacs KJ. c-Fos as a transcription factor: a stressful (re)view from a functional map. Neurochem Int. 1998;33(4):287–97.
32. Narita M, Imai S, Oe K, Narita M, Kubota C, Yajima Y, et al. Induction of c-fos expression in the mouse brain associated with hyperalgesia induced by intrathecal injection of protein kinase C activator. Brain Res. 2004;1015(1–2):189–93. https://doi.org/10.1016/j.brainres.2004.04.027.
33. Narita M, Ozaki S, Narita M, Ise Y, Yajima Y, Suzuki T. Change in the expression of c-fos in the rat brain following sciatic nerve ligation. Neurosci Lett. 2003;352(3):231–3.
34. Stojiljkovic L, Glusman S, Voronov G, Sekosan M, Radulovic J. 368 Does the c-Fos activation mediate the expansion of cortical somatosensory fields in phantom pain? Eur J Pain. 2007;11(1):163.
35. Luo Y, Anderson TA. Phantom limb pain: a review. Int Anesthesiol Clin. 2016;54(2):121–39. https://doi.org/10.1097/AIA.0000000000000095.
36. Clarke C, Lindsay DR, Pyati S, Buchheit T. Residual limb pain is not a diagnosis: a proposed algorithm to classify postamputation pain. Clin J Pain. 2013;29(6):551–62. https://doi.org/10.1097/AJP.0b013e318261c9f9.
37. Richardson C, Kulkarni J. A review of the management of phantom limb pain: challenges and solutions. J Pain Res. 2017;10:1861–70. https://doi.org/10.2147/JPR.S124664.
38. Srivastava D. Chronic post-amputation pain: peri-operative management—Review. Br J Pain. 2017;11(4):192–202. https://doi.org/10.1177/2049463717736492.
39. Nikolajsen L, Ilkjaer S, Christensen JH, Krøner K, Jensen TS. Randomised trial of epidural bupivacaine and morphine in prevention of stump and phantom pain in lower-limb amputation. Lancet. 1997;350(9088):1353–7.
40. Karanikolas M, Aretha D, Tsolakis I, Monantera G, Kiekkas P, Papadoulas S, et al. Optimized perioperative analgesia reduces chronic phantom limb pain intensity, prevalence, and frequency: a prospective, randomized, clinical trial. Anesthesiology. 2011;114(5):1144–54. https://doi.org/10.1097/ALN.0b013e31820fc7d2.
41. Lambert AW, Dashfield AK, Cosgrove C, Wilkins DC, Walker AJ, Ashley S. Randomized prospective study comparing preoperative epidural and intraoperative perineural analgesia for the prevention of postoperative stump and phantom limb pain following major amputation. Reg Anesth Pain Med. 2001;26(4):316–21.
42. Fisher A, Meller Y. Continuous postoperative regional analgesia by nerve sheath block for amputation surgery–a pilot study. Anesth Analg. 1991;72:300–3.
43. Pinzur MS, Garla PG, Pluth T, Vrbos L. Continuous postoperative infusion of a regional anesthetic after an amputation of the lower extremity. A randomized clinical trial. J Bone Joint Surg Am. 1996;78(10):1501–5.
44. Lennox PH, Winkelaar GB, Umedaly H, Hsiang YN. A continuous perineural infusion of local anesthetic provides effective postoperative pain management after lower limb amputation. Can J Anaesth. 2002;49(6):639–40.
45. Borghi B, D'Addabbo M, White PF, Gallerani P, Toccaceli L, Raffaeli W, et al. The use of prolonged peripheral neural blockade after lower extremity amputation: the effect on symptoms associated with phantom limb syndrome. Anesth Analg. 2010;111(5):1308–15. https://doi.org/10.1213/ANE.0b013e3181f4e848.
46. Ayling OG, Montbriand J, Jiang J, Ladak S, Love L, Eisenberg N, et al. Continuous regional anaesthesia provides effective pain management and reduces opioid requirement following major lower limb amputation. Eur J Vasc Endovasc Surg. 2014;48(5):559–64.

47. Ilfeld BM, Moeller-Bertram T, Hanling SR, Tokarz K, Mariano ER, Loland VJ, et al. Treating intractable phantom limb pain with ambulatory continuous peripheral nerve blocks: a pilot study. Pain Med. 2013;14(6):935–42.
48. Bosanquet DC, Glasbey JC, Stimpson A, Williams IM, Twine CP. Systematic review and meta-analysis of the efficacy of perineural local anaesthetic catheters after major lower limb amputation. Eur J Vasc Endovasc Surg. 2015;50(2):241–9.
49. Humble SR, Dalton AJ, Li L. A systematic review of therapeutic interventions to reduce acute and chronic post-surgical pain after amputation, thoracotomy or mastectomy. Eur J Pain. 2015;19(4):451–65.
50. Sahin SH, Colak A, Arar C, et al. A retrospective trial comparing the effects of different anesthetic techniques on phantom pain after lower limb amputation. Curr Ther Res Clin Exp. 2011;72(3):127–37.
51. Ypsilantis E, Tang TY. Pre-emptive analgesia for chronic limb pain after amputation for peripheral vascular disease: a systematic review. Ann Vasc Surg. 2010;24(8):1139–46.
52. McCormick Z, Chang-Chien G, Marshall B, Huang M, Harden RN. Phantom limb pain: a systematic neuroanatomical-based review of pharmacologic treatment. Pain Med. 2014;15(2):292–305.
53. Hanley MA, Ehde DM, Campbell KM, Osborn B, Smith DG. Self-reported treatments used for lower-limb phantom pain: descriptive findings. Arch Phys Med Rehabil. 2006;87(2):270–7.
54. Moore RA, Derry S, Aldington D, Cole P, Wiffen PJ. Amitriptyline for neuropathic pain in adults. Cochrane Database Syst Rev. 2015;(7):CD008242. https://doi.org/10.1002/14651858.CD008242.pub3.
55. Alviar MJ, Hale T, Dungca M. Pharmacologic interventions for treating phantom limb pain. Cochrane Database Syst Rev. 2016;(12):CD006380.
56. Rusy LM, Troshynski TJ, Weisman SJ. Gabapentin in phantom limb pain management in children and young adults: report of seven cases. J Pain Symptom Manag. 2001;21(1):78–82.
57. Abbass K. Efficacy of gabapentin for treatment of adults with phantom limb pain. Ann Pharmacother. 2012;46(12):1707–11.
58. Wilder-Smith CH, Hill LT, Laurent S. Postamputation pain and sensory changes in treatment-naive patients: characteristics and responses to treatment with tramadol, amitriptyline, and placebo. Anesthesiology. 2005;103(3):619–28.
59. Wu CL, Agarwal S, Tella PK, et al. Morphine versus mexiletine for treatment of postamputation pain: a randomized, placebo-controlled, crossover trial. Anesthesiology. 2008;109:289–96.
60. Roullet S, Nouette-Gaulain K, Biais M, Bernard N, Bénard A, Revel P, et al. Preoperative opioid consumption increases morphine requirement after leg amputation. Can J Anaesth. 2009;56(12):908–13. https://doi.org/10.1007/s12630-009-9185-8.
61. Buvanendran A, Kroin JS, Rajagopal A, Robison SJ, Moric M, Tuman KJ. Oral ketamine for acute pain management after amputation surgery. Pain Med. 2017;19:1265. https://doi.org/10.1093/pm/pnx229.
62. Hayes C, Armstrong-Brown A, Burstal R. Perioperative intravenous ketamine infusion for the prevention of persistent post-amputation pain: a randomized, controlled trial. Anaesth Intensive Care. 2004;32(3):330–8.
63. Loy BM, Britt RB, Brown JN. Memantine for the treatment of phantom limb pain: a systematic review. J Pain Palliat Care Pharmacother. 2016;30(4):276–83.
64. Azria M. Possible mechanisms of the analgesic action of calcitonin. Bone. 2002;30(5 Suppl):80S–3S. Review.
65. Batsford S, Ryan CG, Martin DJ. Non-pharmacological conservative therapy for phantom limb pain: a systematic review of randomized controlled trials. Physiother Theory Pract. 2017;33(3):173–83. https://doi.org/10.1080/09593985.2017.1288283.
66. Johnson MI, Mulvey MR, Bagnall AM. Transcutaneous electrical nerve stimulation (TENS) for phantom pain and stump pain following amputation in adults. Cochrane Database Syst Rev. 2015;8:CD007264. https://doi.org/10.1002/14651858.CD007264.pub3.
67. Thieme H, Morkisch N, Rietz C, Dohle C, Borgetto B. The efficacy of movement representation techniques for treatment of limb pain—a systematic review and meta-analysis. J Pain. 2016;17(2):167–80. https://doi.org/10.1016/j.jpain.2015.10.015.

68. Barbin J, Seetha V, Casillas JM, Paysant J, Pérennou D. The effects of mirror therapy on pain and motor control of phantom limb in amputees: a systematic review. Ann Phys Rehabil Med. 2016;59(4):270–5. https://doi.org/10.1016/j.rehab.2016.04.001.
69. Herrador Colmenero L, Perez Marmol JM, Martí-García C, Querol Zaldivar MLÁ, Tapia Haro RM, Castro Sánchez AM, et al. Effectiveness of mirror therapy, motor imagery, and virtual feedback on phantom limb pain following amputation: a systematic review. Prosthetics Orthot Int. 2017;42:288. https://doi.org/10.1177/0309364617740230.
70. Hu X, Trevelyan E, Yang G, Lee MS, Lorenc A, Liu J, et al. The effectiveness of acupuncture or TENS for phantom limb syndrome. II: a narrative review of case studies. Eur J Integr Med. 2014;6(3):365–81.
71. Trevelyan EG, Turner WA, Robinson N. Developing an acupuncture protocol for treating phantom limb pain: a Delphi consensus study. Acupunct Med. 2015;33(1):42–50. https://doi.org/10.1136/acupmed-2014-010668.
72. Trevelyan EG, Turner WA, Summerfield-Mann L, Robinson N. Acupuncture for the treatment of phantom limb syndrome in lower limb amputees: a randomised controlled feasibility study. Trials. 2016;17(1):519. https://doi.org/10.1186/s13063-015-0668-3.
73. Tseng CC, Chen PY, Lee YC. Successful treatment of phantom limb pain and phantom limb sensation in the traumatic amputee using scalp acupuncture. Acupunct Med. 2014;32(4):356–8. https://doi.org/10.1136/acupmed-2014-010556.
74. Wang JD, Kuo TB, Yang CC. An alternative method to enhance vagal activities and suppress sympathetic activities in humans. Auton Neurosci. 2002;100(1–2):90–5.
75. McAuley J, van Gröningen R, Green C. Spinal cord stimulation for intractable pain following limb amputation. Neuromodulation. 2013;16:530–6. https://doi.org/10.1111/j.1525-1403.2012.00513.x.
76. Viswanathan A, Phan PC, Burton AW. Use of spinal cord stimulation in the treatment of phantom limb pain: case series and review of the literature. Pain Pract. 2010;10(5):479–84. https://doi.org/10.1111/j.1533-2500.2010.00374.x.
77. Aiyer R, Barkin RL, Bhatia A, Gungor S. A systematic review on the treatment of phantom limb pain with spinal cord stimulation. Pain Manag. 2017;7(1):59–69. https://doi.org/10.2217/pmt-2016-0041.
78. Bunch JR, Goldstein HV, Hurley RW. Complete coverage of phantom limb and stump pain with constant current SCS system: a case report and review of the literature. Pain Pract. 2015;15(1):E20–6. https://doi.org/10.1111/papr.12226.
79. Eldabe S, Burger K, Moser H, Klase D, Schu S, Wahlstedt A, et al. Dorsal root ganglion (DRG) stimulation in the treatment of phantom limb pain (PLP). Neuromodulation. 2015;18(7):610–6. https://doi.org/10.1111/ner.12338.
80. Cornish P, Wall C. Successful peripheral neuromodulation for phantom limb pain. Pain Med. 2015;16(4):761–4. https://doi.org/10.1111/pme.12532.
81. Kuiken TA, Barlow AK, Hargrove L, Dumanian GA. Targeted muscle reinnervation for the upper and lower extremity. Tech Orthop. 2017;32(2):109–16. https://doi.org/10.1097/BTO.0000000000000194.
82. Bowen JB, Wee CE, Kalik J, Valerio IL. Targeted muscle reinnervation to improve pain, prosthetic tolerance, and bioprosthetic outcomes in the amputee. Adv Wound Care. 2017;6(8):261–7. https://doi.org/10.1089/wound.2016.0717.
83. Valerio IL, Dumanian GA, Jordan SW, Mioton LM, Bowen JB, West JM, et al. Preemptive treatment of phantom and residual limb pain with targeted muscle reinnervation at the time of major limb amputation. J Am Coll Surg. 2019;228(3):217–26. https://doi.org/10.1016/j.jamcollsurg.2018.12.015. Epub 2019 Jan 8.
84. Dumanian GA, Potter BK, Mioton LM, Ko JH, Cheesborough JE, Souza JM, et al. Targeted muscle reinnervation treats neuroma and phantom pain in major limb amputees: A randomized clinical trial. Ann Surg. 2019;270(2):238-46. https://doi.org/10.1097/SLA.0000000000003088.
85. Ferraro F, Jacopetti M, Spallone V, Padua L, Traballesi M, Brunelli S, et al. Italian Consensus Conference on Pain in Neurorehabilitation (ICCPN). Diagnosis and treatment of pain in plexopathy, radiculopathy, peripheral neuropathy and phantom limb pain. Evidence and recommendations from the Italian Consensus Conference on Pain on Neurorehabilitation. Eur J Phys Rehabil Med. 2016;52(6):855–66.

Chapter 16
Neuropathic Pain Syndromes. 5: Other Neurological Conditions

Soshi Iwasaki and Michiaki Yamakage

In the Chap. 5, we describe other neurological conditions without research on postherpetic neuralgia, CRPS, diabetic and other neuropathies, and phantom limb pain, or the unique issues associated with them. Hence, Chaps. 1–4, written by Antoun Nader, Taruna Penmetcha, Michiaki Yamakage, and Wolfgang Hamann are described in detail. Depending on the site to be impaired, neuropathic pain can be divided into peripheral neuropathic pain or central neuropathic pain [1] and cancer-associated neuropathic pain. The four diseases mentioned in Chaps.1–4 are classified as peripheral neuropathic pain: carpal tunnel syndrome, meralgia paresthesia, trigeminal neuralgia, and post-thoracotomy pain and so on are residual diseases of peripheral neuropathic pain to be described in this chapter. Central neuropathic pain includes central post-stroke pain, multiple sclerosis pain, Parkinson's disease pain, spinal cord injury pain, and syringomyelia. Cancer-associated neuropathic pain contains chemotherapy-induced polyneuropathy, neuropathy secondary to tumor infiltration or nerve compression, phantom breast pain, postmastectomy pain, and post-radiation plexopathy and myelopathy. Classifications of "definite," "possible," and "unlikely" have been proposed when neuropathic pain is clinically diagnosed [2].

16.1 Peripheral Neuropathic Pain

16.1.1 Causes of Pain

Carpal tunnel syndrome (CTS) [3], meralgia paresthesia (MP) [4], and trigeminal neuralgia (TN) [5] cause nerve entrapment or compression resulting in pain, paresthesias, and sensory loss within the distribution of the ulnar nerve, lateral cutaneous

S. Iwasaki (✉) · M. Yamakage
Department of Anesthesiology, Sapporo Medical University, Sapporo-shi, Hokkaido, Japan

K. Shimoji et al. (eds.), *Chronic Pain Management in General and Hospital Practice*, https://doi.org/10.1007/978-981-15-2933-7_16

nerve of the thigh (LCNT), and the trigeminal nerve, respectively. Post-thoracotomy pain syndrome (PTPS) is an intercostal nerve injury resulting in pain, allodynia, paresthesia for more than 2 months after thoracotomy [6]. Readers should be aware that not only the mechanisms of these peripheral mechanisms but also the central mechanisms are more or less involved in those peripheral neuropathic pains.

16.1.2 Pain Management

The treatment of CTS, MP, and TN falls under two categories: surgical intervention and non-surgical (conservative) intervention [3–5].

Surgical intervention of CTS is a carpal tunnel release (CTR) ; about 70–90% of patients have good to excellent long-term outcomes with open carpal tunnel release [7]. On the other hand, minimal invasive surgery is preferred per se for surgical treatment for pain, using an endoscopic technique for faster relief of pain and faster improvement in functional abilities for the first 2 weeks, at 1 year postoperatively. Both open and endoscopic procedures are equivalently efficient [8]. Neurolysis and resection of LCNT are surgical interventions when non-surgical interventions have failed [3]. Neurolysis of LCNT may be considered first, because it may relieve symptoms, but there is a possibility of recurrence. Resection of LCNT is then recommended secondarily [4]. The surgical treatment of TN is microvascular decompression (MVD). In MRI findings, it is more effective when nerve compression is evident (sometimes neurosurgeons call it "pure MVD"; according to the aforementioned clinical diagnostic criteria, it corresponds to definite) [9].

16.1.3 Other Signs and Symptoms Related to Pain

In CTS, symptoms worsen at night or at bedtime (nocturnal wake), and numbness is present at the middle finger side half of the ring finger, middle finger, index finger, and thumb [3]. Patients with MP complain of pain, burning, numbness, muscle aches, coldness, lightening pain, or buzzing in their lateral or anterolateral thigh [4]. Painful symptoms associated with TN are virtually always unilateral; bilateral TN is very rare except for TN caused by multiple sclerosis (MS) (see central neuropathic pain). Typical characterizations include notions of brief, sudden, stabbing, electric shock-like, and severe pain attacks. The paroxysms may last up to 2 min, but their duration is usually limited to a few seconds [5]. Over 75% of thoracotomy patients report a constant severe ache in the ipsilateral shoulder post surgery. This pain is resistant to intravenous opioids and is only partially relieved by NSAIDs [10] and could subsequently develop into multiple implications including respiratory failure resulting in pneumonia.

16.1.4 Diagnosis

For the diagnosis and differential diagnosis of CTS, it is indispensable to take into account a detailed medical history (Fig. 16.1) [11]. Nerve conduction studies, ultrasound testing, and MRI are used to confirm the neurophysiological severity by using a scale to show, respectively, a thickening of the median nerve [3], swelling of the median nerve, and increased signal intensity on T2-weighted images [12]. Tinel's test and Phalen's test are commonly made in clinically setting, the sensitivity of each test is limited in the range of 48–73% and 67–83%, respectively, and their specificity is 30–94% [13–15]. As well as being useful for diagnosis of CTS, the findings of clinical tests and nerve conduction velocity measurements, Tinel's signs, and MRI are useful in the diagnosis of MP [4]. A pelvic compression test has also been used with a sensitivity of 95% and a specificity of 93.3% [16].

In recent years, Cruccu et al. have proposed the classification and diagnosis of TA categorized from complaints, the medical history, inquiries, clinical laboratory findings, and MRI findings (Fig. 16.2) [4] into 3 diagnostic categories: classical TN, secondary TN, and idiopathic TN. The former needs to show vascular compression of the trigeminal nerve root besides proper clinical findings (pure MVC).

Diagnosis of post-thoracotomy pain is not difficult because of its surgical history and sustained burning pain or allodynia along the wound.

Medical history

- symptom onset - which in the early stage is mainly nocturnal paresthesias.
- provocative factors - such as hand positions and repeated movements.
- working activity - instrument use, vibrating tools.
- pain localisation and irradiation - in the cutaneous median nerve region with ascending, sometimes up to the shoulder, or descending irradiation.
- manoeuvres which alleviate symptoms - e.g. hand shaking, position changes.
- presence of predisposing factors - e.g. diabetes, adiposity, chronic polyarthritis, myxoedema, acromegaly, pregnancy.
- sports activity - e.g. baseball, body-building.

Differential diagnosis

- Cervical radiculopathy (especially C6-C7)
- Brachial plexopathy (in particular of the upper trunk)
- Proximal median neuropathy (especially at the pronator teres level)
- Thoracic outlet syndrome
- CNS disorders (multiple sclerosis, small cerebral infarction)

Fig. 16.1 Required medical history and differential diagnosis about CTS [10]

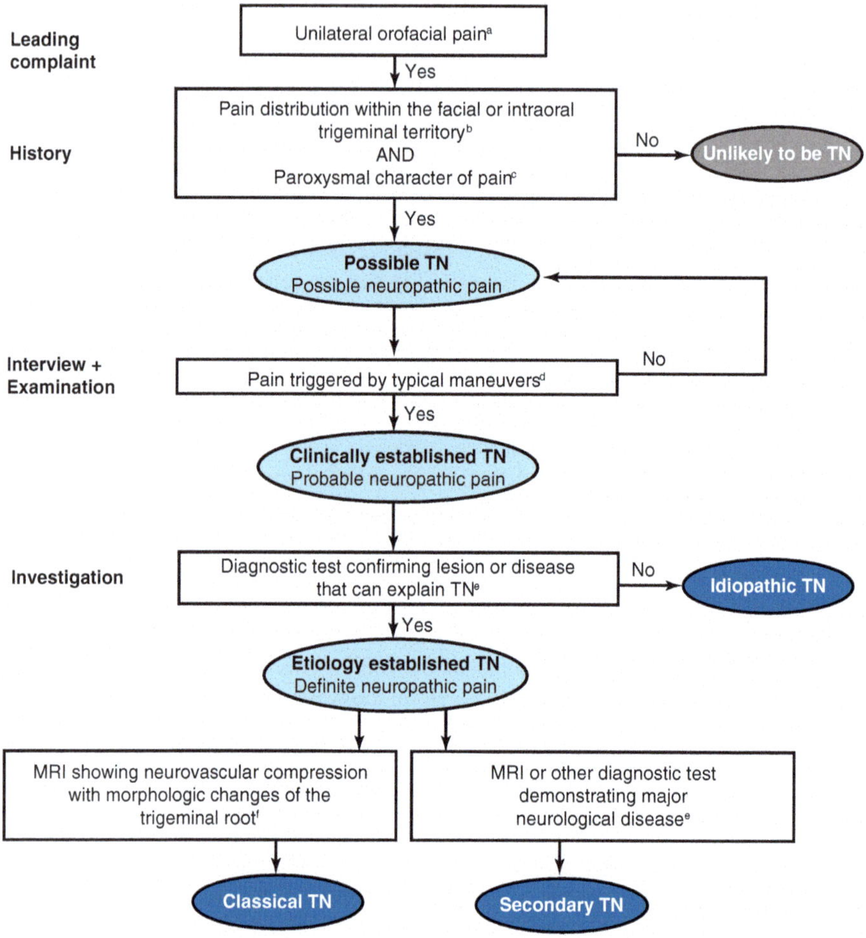

Fig. 16.2 New classification and diagnostic grading of TA [4]

16.1.5 General Treatments (Medical, Surgical, and Others) and Prognosis

In most CTS and MP cases, before surgical intervention, conservative therapy is the primary choice in patients with mild or moderate symptoms because of the high natural cure rate. These treatments include oral and intravenous steroids, vitamin B6 [17] and B12, nonsteroidal anti-inflammatory drugs (NSAIDs), and the use of hand splints, but evidence of the effectiveness of these treatments is low.

For the treatment of trigeminal neuralgia, neural blocks, MVD [18], and a γ knife can be used in addition to evidence based drug therapy [19, 20]. The most widely used treatment for the pain of trigeminal neuralgia is carmazepine [21] and oxycarmazepine [22]. The latter has less efficacy and fewer adverse events than the former. NTT (number needed to treat) and NTH (number needed to harm) of carmazepine are 1.8 [21] and 3.7 [23]. Hence, we need to pay attention to its unique adverse events: pancytopenia and eruption and so on. Baclofen, an agonist of GABA receptor, has a lower evidence level than carmazepine, but the NTT is as low as 1.4 [24]; it is considered as a second choice.

In addition, pregabalin, gabapentin, phenytoin, clonazepam, and valproic acid are used alone or in combination, but the evidence level is low [19]. In cases where these medications are ineffective or in cases intolerable due to adverse events, and with the patient's request, MVD is indicated. Depending on the affected branches, and whether the lower orbital nerve block, the superior orbit block, the chord nerve block, the maxillary nerve block, the mandibular nerve block, and the Gussel ganglion block are used properly, nerve destruction by nerve destruction drugs or radiofrequency thermal coagulation will be enforced. But the enforcement of the latter is increasing because of its safety and effective rate [25].

PTPS has proven to be very challenging to prevent, because it develops even following continuous thoracic epidural analgesia managed by a dedicated acute pain service utilizing multimodal adjuvant therapies including acetaminophen, nonsteroidal analgesics, opioids, and gabapentin [26]. If the epidural block and the intercostal nerve block are effective, then high frequency thermocoagulation therapy is subsequently applied. Spinal cord stimulation therapy is also applied while confirming the effect of sympathetic block.

16.1.6 Case Reports

A 76-year-old female patient had undergone surgery for left lung cancer with video assisted thoracotomy surgery 6 months previously. Pain along the video-port of surgery continued after surgery, as a clinical finding.

CT and PET did not recognize the recurrence of cancer, so she was introduced to the pain clinic. After admission, a thoracic epidural catheter was introduced, and oral pregabalin was gradually increased from 100 mg/day to 300 mg/day. She experienced a loss of motivation and insomnia due to pain, but she was improving with 15 mg oral mirtazapine.

16.1.7 Summary

Peripheral neuropathic pain can be caused by nerve entrapment or nerve injury in the peripheral tissues. Conservative or drug therapy is primarily chosen, but nerve decompression surgery may be needed depending on the strength of symptoms or according to nerve compression findings.

16.2 Central Neuropathic Pain

16.2.1 *Causes of Pain*

Central neuropathic pain (CNP) is chronic pain that is common among stroke survivors, amputees, spinal cord injury patients, and patients with multiple sclerosis. It occurs after several months of these diseases. This condition can be caused by a lesion or disease affecting the somatosensory system [27]. Pain appearing after a cerebrovascular disorder such as cerebral infarction or cerebral hemorrhage includes central post-stroke pain (CPSP) such as thalamic pain and peripheral pain of each part of the body secondary to the onset [28]. CPSP is a refractory disorder, and pain arises in a sensory disorder site consistent with the site of brain injury.

16.2.2 *Pain Management*

Because treatment takes a long time, we need to consult with a patient's family and set goals, and a multifaceted approach including rehabilitation and a psychological approach in addition to pain treatment is necessary [28]. For CPSP, antidepressant drugs, antiepileptic drugs, drug therapies such as pregabalin, and non-drug therapies such as neural stimulation therapy are considered.

16.2.3 *Other Signs and Symptoms Related to Pain*

CPSP may accompany shoulder pain and shoulder hand syndrome and pain due to spasticity [29]. CPSP may be accompanied by a muscle tension type headache and is induced by mental stress.

16.2.4 *Diagnosis*

Some of the pain is recognized by comparing one hand to the other, but it is easier to detect the pain in the periphery of the limb than in the trunk. In a thalamic lesion, pain occurs in the opposite half of the body, and in a medulla oblong lesion, pain occurs in the ipsilateral side and the opposite side of the body. We frequently recognize allodynia and abnormal sensation due to tactile stimulation. Then, by image diagnosis, we confirm that the site of sensory disorder and the site of pain coincide with the site of brain injury [30].

16.2.5 General Treatments (Medical, Surgical, and Others) and Prognosis

There is no established drug therapy for CPSP, but pregabalin, amitriptin as an antidepressant, lamotrigine as an antiepileptic drug, SNRI, valproic acid, opioids, and carmazepine are used alone or in combination [31, 32]. Initially, patients with a cerebrovascular disorder are prone to falls and attention should be paid to adverse events such as delirium, drowsiness, and a dry mouth. Motor cortex stimulation (MCS), repetitive transcranial magnetic stimulation (rTMS), SCS, and deep burst stimulation (DBS) have been tried in a few cases of drug-resistant CPSP [33]. Botulinum therapy reduces spasticity and increases the range of motion of the joint as well as providing pain relief and may be used in conjunction with rehabilitation therapy [34].

16.2.6 Case Reports

A 78-year-old woman had a cerebral infarction of the left basal ganglia, accompanied by a right hemiplegia and aphasia. Physical findings at the first visit were accompanied by swelling of the right upper limb, a hot sensation, pain, and aphasia of aphasia. Complex words frequently occurred, and communication was difficult. A slight disorder was recognized in a superficial sense. Maintaining a sitting position provided a mild level of assistance, and walking was assisted by parallel bars and wearing of a long limb orthosis. Oral duloxetine was started from 30 mg and was increased to 60 mg. Due to the spasticity of the right upper limb, Botulinus was administered once, and rehabilitation continued. Fluctuation in the range of movement due to heat sensation, swelling, and pain of the upper limbs was alleviated. In addition, discontent and complaints that changed the subject's emotions decreased, and refusal of rehabilitation, anger towards pain, frequent occurrences of complex words also reduced. As a result, cooperative action was obtained in the ADL, turnover, rising up, and sitting position maintenance, and a reduction in the amount of assistance for standing was observed.

16.2.7 Summary

Cognitive dysfunction and psychogenic responses associated with cerebrovascular disorders make pain assessment difficult. Pain varies from central to peripheral and is often resistant to drugs. With cooperation from other professions, we can set goals with patients' families and plan a treatment.

16.3 Cancer-Associated Neuropathic Pain

16.3.1 Causes of Pain

Secondary neuropathy occurs when a tumor infiltrates or compresses a nerve. Neuropathic pain develops in cancer patients. In addition, chemotherapy-induced polyneuropathy (CIPN) and post-radiation plexopathy and myelopathy are generated by anti-cancer drugs and radiotherapy, respectively [35, 36].

16.3.2 Pain Management

Treatment of cancer pain is performed using the WHO pain ladder, but an analgesic adjuvant (antidepressant, antiepileptic drug, or antiarrhythmic drug) is used for neuropathic pain. A celiac plexus block or saddle block can be an option.

16.3.3 Other Signs and Symptoms Related to Pain.

Normal pain is often localized, and nighttime pain and persistent pain tend to be exacerbated [37]. Appeal weight loss as a past medical history. Anorexia nervosa and nausea are seen, and depressive symptoms during treatment are directly related to the patient's life prognosis [38, 39]. Knowledge of the effect of opioids on activating the descending pain suppression system is necessary for understanding such symptoms [40]. For pain shown in internal organs, it is necessary to consider any related pain.

16.3.4 Diagnosis

The cause of pain is evaluated by referring to morphological information from PET, CT, and MRI. Not all pain from cancer patients is cancer-derived.

16.3.5 General Treatments (Medical, Surgical, and Others) and Prognosis

Non-opioids analgesics and opioids (Fig. 16.3) are usually used for cancer pain. Neuropathic pain with cancer may be relatively less responsive to these opioid drugs than other pains. Such cases may be indicated for adjuvant analgesics including

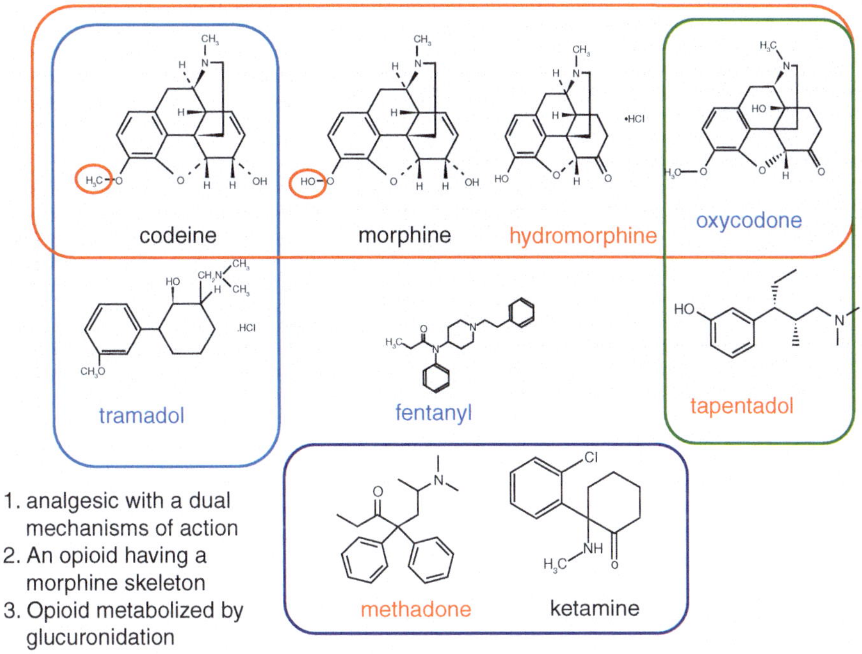

Fig. 16.3 The opioids in palliative medicine

antidepressants and radiotherapy. For the treatment of chronic pain, an analgesic adjuvant and antidepressant are often used alone, but often they are prescribed along with opioids for cancer pain.

As analgesic adjuvants, antidepressants, antiepileptics, corticosteroids, alpha 2 agonists, sodium blockers, anticholinergics, octreotide, and the like are frequently used. As antidepressant drugs, tricyclic antidepressants, SNRI, bupropion, and mirtazapine are used, but in the palliative care field, attention must be paid to symptoms such as nausea caused by serotonin excess and anticholinergic action [41, 42].

16.3.6 Case Reports

A 68-year-old man, after renal pelvic carcinoma of the left renal pelvic malignant tumor radical curative surgery, local recurrence and undergoing GC therapy, myelosuppression of grade 4 was seen, treatment ceased, and palliative care was taken. Pain in the left lower limb was experienced during the course of treatment, and image findings showed malignant iliopsoid syndrome (Fig. 16.4). The physical findings showed signs of iliopsoas. Delirium was caused by increased oxycodone, but the pain was unbearable, and the pain score was 8–9 points/10. The opioid was switched from oxycodone to methadone, and the iliopsoas muscle was irradiated

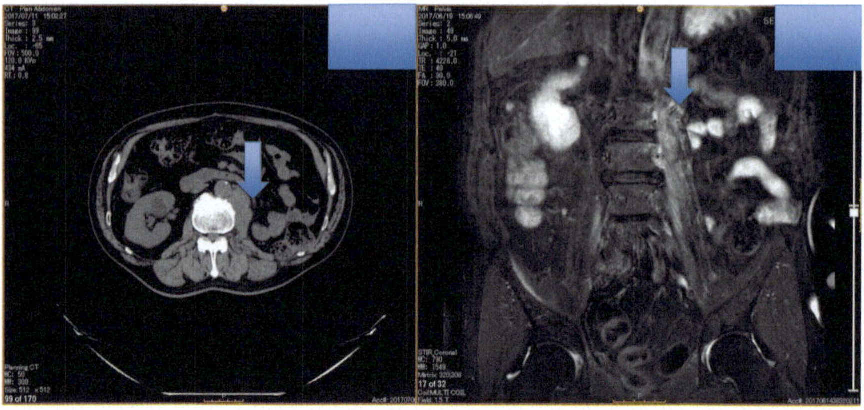

Fig. 16.4 A case of malignant iliopsoid syndrome. On the left renal carcinoma, left nephrectomy was performed, but it recurred locally and infiltrated into the iliopsoas muscle resulting severe leg pain and muscle weakness in the left limb. Left transverse CT, right coronal MRI. Arrow indicates tumor

with 30 Gy. As the use of quick-release oxycodone formulations became unnecessary, the pain improved and palliative care ceased.

16.3.7 Summary

Cancer-related neuropathic pain is difficult to treat. In addition to selecting the appropriate opioid and adjusting the volume, it is desirable to use an analgesic adjuvant and radiation therapy in combination.

References

1. Dworkin RH, O'Connor AB, Backonja M, et al. Pharmacologic management of neuropathic pain: evidence-based recommendations. Pain. 2007;132:237–51.
2. Rasmussen PV, Sindrup SH, Jensen TS, et al. Symptoms and signs in patients with suspected neuropathic pain. Pain. 2004;110:461–9.
3. Ibrahim I, Khan WS, Goddard N, et al. Carpal tunnel syndrome: a review of the recent literature. Open Orthop J. 2012;6:69–76.
4. Cheatham SW, Kolber MJ, Salamh PA. Meralgia paresthetica: a review of the literature. Int J Sports Phys Ther. 2013;8:883–93.
5. Cruccu G, Finnerup NB, Jensen TS, et al. Trigeminal neuralgia: new classification and diagnostic grading for practice and research. Neurology. 2016;87:220–8.
6. Gerner P. Post-thoracotomy pain management problems. Anesthesiol Clin. 2008;26:355–67.
7. Turner A, Kimble F, Ball J. Can the outcome of open carpal tunnel release be predicted?: a review of the literature. ANZ J Surg. 2010;80:50–4.
8. Vasiliadis HS, Xenakis TA, Mitsionis G, et al. Endoscopic versus open carpal tunnel release. Arthroscopy. 2010;26:26–33.

9. Sindou M, Leston J, Decullier E, Chapuis F. Microvascular decompression for primary trigeminal neuralgia: long-term effectiveness and prognostic factors in a series of 362 consecutive patients with clear-cut neurovascular conflicts who underwent pure decompression. J Neurosurg. 2007;107:1144–53.
10. Burgess FW. Epidural versus intravenous fentanyl following thoracotomy. Anesthesiology. 1993;79:621–3.
11. Alfonso C, Jann S, Massa R, et al. Diagnosis, treatment and follow-up of the carpal tunnel syndrome: a review. Neurol Sci. 2010;31:243–52.
12. Radack DM, Schweitzer ME, Taras J. Carpal tunnel syndrome: are the MR findings a result of population selection bias? Am J Roentgenol. 1997;169:1649–53.
13. Kuhlman KA. Sensitivity and specificity of carpal tunnel syndrome sign. Am J Phys Med Rehabil. 1997;76:451–7.
14. Naranjo A, Ojeda S, Mendoza D, et al. What is the diagnostic value of ultrasonography compared to physical evaluation in patients with idiopathic carpal tunnel syndrome? Clin Exp Rhemutatol. 2007;25:853–9.
15. Amirfeyz R, Gozzard C, Leslie IJ. Hand elevation test for assessment of carpal tunnel syndrome. J Hand Surg (Br). 2005;30:361–4.
16. Lundborg G. Intraneural microcirculation. Orthop Clin North Am. 1988;19:1–12.
17. Sato Y, Honda Y, Iwamoto J, et al. Amelioration by mecobalamin of subclinical carpal tunnel syndrome involving unaffected limbs in stroke patients. J Neurol Sci. 2005;231:13–8.
18. Devor M, Govrin-Lippmann R, Rappaport ZH. Mechanism of trigeminal neuralgia: an ultrastructural analysis of trigeminal root specimens obtained during microvascular decompression surgery. J Neurosurg. 2002;96:532–43.
19. Cruccu G, Gronseth G, Alksne J, American Academy of Neurology Society, European Federation of Neurological Society, et al. AAN-EFNS guidelines on trigeminal neuralgia management. Eur J Neurol. 2008;15:1013–28.
20. Jorns TP, Zakrzewska JM. Evidence-based approach to the medical management of trigeminal neuralgia. Br J Neurosurg. 2007;21:253–61.
21. Wiffen PJ, Derry S, Moore R, et al. Carbamazepine for acute and chronic pain in adults. Cochrane Database Syst Rev. 2011;(1):CD005451.
22. Nasreddine W, Beydoun A. Oxcarbazepine in neuropathic pain. Expert Opin Investig Drugs. 2007;16:1615–25.
23. Taylor JC, Brauer S, Espir ML. Long-term treatment of trigeminal neuralgia with carbamazepine. Postgrad Med J. 1981;57:16–8.
24. Fromm GH, Terrence CF, Maroon JC. Trigeminal neuralgia. Current concepts regarding etiology and pathogenesis. Arch Neurol. 1984;41:1204–7.
25. Zakrzewska JM, Akram H. Neurosurgical interventions for the treatment of classical trigeminal neuralgia. Cochrane Database Syst Rev. 2011;(9):CD007312.
26. Kinney MAO, Jacob AK, Passe MA, et al. Increased risk of postthoracotomy pain syndrome in patients with prolonged hospitalization and increased postoperative opioid use. Pain Res Treat. 2016;2016:7945145.
27. Rowbotham MC, Twilling L, Davies PS, Reisner L, Taylor K, Mohr D. Oral opioid therapy for chronic peripheral and central neuropathic pain. N Engl J Med. 2003;348:1223–32.
28. Harrison RA, Field TS. Post stroke pain: identification, assessment, and therapy. Cerebrovasc Dis. 2015;39:190–201.
29. Paolucci S, Iosa M, Toni D, et al. Prevalence and time course of post-stroke pain: a multicenter prospective hospital-based study. Pain Med. 2016;17(5):924–30.
30. Flaster M, Meresh E, Rao M, Biller J. Central poststroke pain: current diagnosis and treatment. Top Stroke Rehabil. 2013;20:116–23.
31. Kim JS. Pharmacological management of central post-stroke pain: a practical guide. CNS Drugs. 2014;28(9):787–97.
32. Frese A, Husstedt IW, Ringelstein EB, Evers S. Pharmacologic treatment of central post-stroke pain. Clin J Pain. 2006;22:252–60.

33. Garcia JBS, Neto JOB, Amâncio EJ, et al. Central neuropathic pain. Rev Dor São Paulo. 2016;17:67–71.
34. Intiso D, Basciani M, Santamato A, et al. Botulinum toxin type A for the treatment of neuropathic pain in neuro-rehabilitation. Toxins (Basel). 2015;7:2454–80.
35. Fallon MT. Neuropathic pain in cancer. Br J Anaesth. 2013;111:105–11.
36. Esin E, Yalcin S. Neuropathic cancer pain: what we are dealing with? How to manage it? Onco Targets Ther. 2014;7:599–618.
37. Garzón-Rodríguez C, Lyras L, Gayoso LO, et al. Cancer-related neuropathic pain in out-patient oncology clinics: a European survey. BMC Palliat Care. 2013;12:41.
38. Smith HR. Depression in cancer patients: pathogenesis, implications and treatment. Oncol Lett. 2015;9:1509–14.
39. Sullivan DR, Forsberg CW, Ganzini L, et al. Longitudinal changes in depression symptoms and survival among patients with lung cancer: a national cohort assessment. J Clin Oncol. 2016;34:3984–91.
40. Blondell RD, Azadfard M, Wisniewski M. Pharmacologic therapy for acute pain. Am Fam Physician. 2013;87:766–72.
41. Holbech JV, Jung A, Jonsson T, Wanning M, Bredahl C, Bach FW. Combination treatment of neuropathic pain: Danish expert recommendations based on a Delphi process. J Pain Res. 2017;10:1467–75.
42. Nersesyan H, Slavin KV. Current approach to cancer pain management: availability and implications of different treatment options. Ther Clin Risk Manag. 2007;3:381–400.

Chapter 17
Psychological and Psychiatric Pain Conditions

Yukari Shindo and Michiaki Yamakage

17.1 The Association Between Pain and Psychiatric Disorders

Chronic pain patients with many also having a psychiatric disorder are either pre-existing or consequential [1]. A majority (64%) of patients with chronic work-related musculoskeletal pain were diagnosed with at least one mental disorder [2].

Several psychiatric syndromes are described below.

17.1.1 Depression

All individuals experience psychological states such as anxiety, fear, intimidation, sadness, and anger from time to time. However, when patients experience these feelings on a constant basis, feelings of hopelessness, powerlessness, or helplessness can develop, causing the patient to fall into a depressive state or in some cases, develop depression. Current data indicate that between 16% and 64% of patients with chronic pain fulfill the diagnostic criteria for major depression [3, 4]. It is also estimated that 56–72% of patients treated in pain clinics display symptoms of depression [5, 6].

Studies show that depression is an important psychological factor involved in the pathogenesis of chronic pain [7]. In addition, depression is now recognized as a

Y. Shindo (✉)
Japan Health Care College, Sapporo, Hokkaido, Japan
e-mail: y_shindo@nihoniryo-c.ac.jp

M. Yamakage
Sapporo Medical University, School of Medicine, Sapporo, Hokkaido, Japan
e-mail: yamakage@sapmed.ac.jp

K. Shimoji et al. (eds.), *Chronic Pain Management in General and Hospital Practice*, https://doi.org/10.1007/978-981-15-2933-7_17

potential comorbidity of chronic pain [8]. When considering the relationship between chronic pain and depression, there may be cases in which depression precedes chronic pain, and cases in which depression occurs as a consequence of the patient's pain. In the former case, pain is considered a symptom of the mood disorder, while in the latter case (as described by Pincus et al. [9]), pain results from the interaction between patient vulnerabilities, such as pain, negative emotions (including depression), social stress, and helplessness.

It was a cross-sectional telephone survey of random sample of 18,980 subjects representative of the general populations of the United Kingdom, Germany, Italy, Portugal, and Spain. Major depressive disorder was diagnosed in 4.0% of subjects; 43.4% of these subjects had at least one chronically painful physical condition, which was four times more often than in subjects without major depressive disorder [10]. Similarly, in a study of 573 patients with depression by Bair et al. [11], 69% of patients reported severe pain, 30% reported moderate pain, and 25% reported mild pain. Ohayonet and Schatzberg [12] also reported that 66.3% of the patients with depression in their study had chronic pain, with more than half (57.1%) reporting pain originating before the start of their depression.

Because patients with chronic pain often report depression, and because the pain can be modulated by depression, treatment of the depressive state through antidepressant medication, etc., is also essential to treat chronic pain. In a recent random longitudinal study of patients with chronic pain and comorbid depression, it was reported that a depression treatment program alleviated chronic pain [13].

17.1.2 Anxiety Disorders

Anxiety disorders can also be associated with chronic pain, and each can reinforce the other [14]. An estimated 11–60% of patients with chronic pain report the co-occurrence of various anxiety disorders [15].

Patients with chronic pain can also experience a variety of pain-related anxieties, including anxiety related to (1) severe pain/prolonged pain, (2) pain of an unknown etiology, and (3) the treatment of the chronic pain. If the anxiety being caused their pain is severe or continues for an extended period of time, it can have a major effect on the pain they experience.

Some patients with chronic pain have perfectionist ideas and think that "the pain has not been completely alleviated," have an "all or none" point-of-view, or have hypochondriac tendencies. In particular, when patients display negative thoughts or are desperate to escape their pain, they can exhibit avoidant behavior, refusing to move the area affected by pain for fear of causing more pain. If patients continue this behavior for long periods of time, issues such as amyotrophia (loss of muscle tissue due to disuse) and arthrogryposis (contracture of the joints due to disuse) can occur, causing further pain. This vicious cycle of anxiety, avoidance, disuse, and more pain is known as the fear-avoidance model [16, 17].

In order to help patients avoid this vicious cycle of fear, avoidance, and pain, care providers need to help patients overcome their fear of activity, of getting hurt again, or both. In addition, for helping patients avoid the cycle of fear and avoidance, providers need to counsel patients on how to interpret the pain they are experiencing and help them understand that pain does not necessarily signify a catastrophic event.

17.1.3 Post-Traumatic Stress Disorder (PTSD)

Post-traumatic stress disorder (PTSD) is a disorder characterized by re-experience, evasive behavior, apathy, and hyperarousal caused by a traumatic event. In recent years, research on PTSD in patients with chronic pain has been increasing [18–20]. Research shows that PTSD can not only influence whether trauma survivors will develop chronic pain [21], but also how long the pain they develop with last [22] and the extent to which their pain will interfere with their ability to function [23].

Studies also show that the risk of developing chronic pain is high for patients with PTSD [24, 25]. Pain is the most prominent symptom reported by patients with PTSD, especially by patients who have served in the military. In these patients, the symptom is especially prominent [26, 27]. Studies also show that pain that occurs after a traumatic event is a risk factor for the onset of PTSD [28].

There are also many reports on the relationship between the experience of abuse during childhood and chronic pain in adulthood [29, 30]. For example, Davis et al. [31] reported in meta-analysis that (1) individuals who reported being abused or neglected in childhood also reported more pain symptoms and related conditions than those not abused or neglected in childhood; (2) patients with chronic pain were more likely to report having been abused or neglected in childhood than healthy controls; (3) patients with chronic pain were more likely to report having been abused or neglected in childhood than no patients with chronic pain identified from the community; and (4) individuals from the community reporting pain were more likely to report having been abused or neglected than the individuals from the community not reporting pain.

Thus, experiencing both severe pain and trauma could lead to an increase in the chance of both coexisting. It may be necessary to pay attention to PTSD as a contributing factor when pain becomes chronic or is exacerbated, as well as to provide proper care.

17.1.4 Attention Deficit Hyperactivity Disorder (ADHD)

In recent years, research has shown that patients with chronic pain are more likely to experience repeated car accidents and to be forgetful than patients without chronic pain [32, 33]. It has been suggested that issues with attention are the cause of both of these outcomes. Cases of attention deficit hyperactivity disorder (ADHD) have been reported in the scientific literature as early as 1902 [34]. The diagnosis of ADHD is based around three core symptoms—inattention, hyperactivity, and impulsivity—which impair the patient's ability to perform activities of daily living. Results of a report by the World Health Organization (WHO) estimate the prevalence of ADHD among adults at 3.4% [35]. However, a recent study of 123 patients with another form of chronic pain, fibromyalgia syndrome (FMS), the authors found that 44.72% ($N = 55$) of adults they screened met the criteria for ADHD [36]. These results suggest that in adults, ADHD may co-occur with FMS, and may impact the severity of FMS. Patients with FMS should be assessed for the presence of adult ADHD.

It is thought that because of a distraction-related disorder, there is an excessive focus on pain. In addition, impairments in executive function associated with ADHD may also cause difficulty in adjusting to daily life, which may lead to additional comorbidities with chronic pain. Thus, identifying ADHD in patients with chronic pain and initiating proper treatment is important for the normalization of activities of daily living, reducing pain-focused behaviors, and is crucial for enhancing the therapeutic effects of treatment.

17.2 Chronic Pain, Substance Abuse, and Dependence

Preventing substance abuse is a particularly difficult challenge for patients with chronic pain. The prevalence of substance abuse (incidence rate) in patients with chronic pain is estimated to be 15–40% [37]. In recent years, the efficacy of opioids for non-malignant pain (neuropathic and musculoskeletal pain) [38, 39] has contributed to the widespread use of opioids for chronic pain. However, studies show that the risk of opiate-dependence is high in chronic pain patients with comorbid psychiatric disorders [40]. Studies also show that opioids may less be effective for managing chronic pain when comorbid psychological factors are present [41]. In the USA, the abuse and dependence of opioids in patients with chronic pain has become a serious problem [42–44].

Risk factors for opioid abuse in chronic pain patients with comorbid psychiatric disorders include:

- A personal or family history of substance abuse, youth, history of sexual abuse before puberty, psychiatric disorder [44].
- Portenoy [45] reported that in chronic pain patients who have experienced opioid abuse or dependence, there is a high risk of further abuse or dependence on other substances. Both genetic and environmental risks contribute to a family history of substance abuse [46].
- Daily drug use, psychological stress [43].
- Abuse of numerous substances, inadequate social support (from family members, etc.) [47].

- Tobacco addiction (difficulty regarding smoking cessation), history of rehabilitation regarding substance or alcohol dependence [48].
- Addiction to opioids [49].
- Opioid dependence in the case of chronic pain is often triggered by opioid analgesics prescribed from a medical institution, whereas triggers are spontaneous in general substance dependence [50].

There are many cases in which high-dose opioids are being prescribed for the management of chronic pain [51, 52]. Prolonged use of opiates can lead to the need for higher and higher doses of the pain-relieving agents to achieve the same level of relief (a phenomenon known as tolerance). This can pose problems for patients with chronic pain. In particular, patients with chronic pain using high-dose, prolonged opioid therapy can develop side effects not experienced in the management of other chronic forms of pain such as cancer-related pain, bowel dysfunction, gonadal dysfunction, cognitive dysfunction, impaired immune function, substance abuse, substance dependence, and analgesic tolerance/hyperalgesia [50].

Risk factors for prolonged use of high-dose opiates to treat chronic pain include [53]:

1. Pain with no identifiable etiology.
2. Pain with no effective treatment.
3. Pain that limits activity or function in which the following concerns are present:
   (a) Pain may not be alleviated.
   (b) It may not be possible to control pain.
   (c) The existence of the underlying cause of pain makes it impossible to regain normal life.
4. Pain that is diffuse (generalized).
5. Pain that co-occurs with clinically apparent depression/anxiety.

To avoid potentially serious problems during opioid treatment, providers should be familiar with the characteristics of patients who are at risk for substance abuse, as well as the patients in whom high-dose, long-term opiate therapy is likely to be used, and not initiate opioid treatment carelessly for such patients.

17.3 Somatic Symptom and Related Disorders (SSD)

In the psychiatric field, there has been a focus on the psychiatric aspect of chronic pain, and pain disorders were often attempted to be understood through the concepts of persistent somatoform pain disorder in ICD-10 or somatoform disorder in DSM-IV. In the newly released DSM-V (revised in 2013), the category "somatoform disorder" listed in the previous version, the DSM-IV, was renamed as "somatic symptom and related disorders" in the DSM-V [54]. Accordingly, all the disorders categorized as "somatoform disorders" listed in the DSM-IV were also changed.

The diagnosis of somatic symptom disorders in the DSM-V is based on the presence of (1) somatic symptoms which have a significant negative effect on daily functions, (2) excessive thinking by the patient concerning these somatic symptoms, and (3) associated emotional and behavioral characteristics. Somatic symptom disorders are a substitute for somatization disorder, pain disorder, and undifferentiated somatoform disorders, which were included in previously the DSM-IV. Somatic symptom disorders included in the current version of the DMS-V include: (1) somatic symptom disorder, (2) illness anxiety disorder, (3) conversion disorder (functional neurological symptom disorder), (4) psychological factors affecting other medical condition, (5) factitious disorder, (6) other specified somatic symptom and related disorder, (7) unspecified somatic symptom and related disorder. The diagnoses of somatoform disorders are characterized by whether there is a medical explanation for somatic symptoms, such as whether the chief complaint (somatic complaints) is related to another medical condition [55].

The changes to the concept of somatoform disorders in the latest version of the DSM-IV were added in the hope that these diagnoses would be of use to healthcare providers in the primary care setting, a majority of whom do not have a background in psychiatry. In addition, while the somatic disorders included in the DSM-IV apply to symptoms with no obvious medical explanation, the new definition of somatic symptom disorders included in the DSM-V shifts the focus to the inappropriateness and degree of excessiveness of the patient's symptom-related thoughts, emotions, and behaviors. However, there has been some criticism that, under these new definitions, "patients with many somatic symptoms receive a misdiagnosis of mental illness due to somatic symptom disorder" [56]. Furthermore, because the new definitions for somatic symptom disorders are not mutually exclusive from other psychiatric disorders, there is concern that this new definition may result in increased prevalence of psychiatric disorders in patients with chronic pain.

17.3.1 Somatic Symptom Disorder (Pain Disorder)

The diagnostic criteria of DSM-5 define somatic symptom disorder as follows:

Criteria for somatic symptom disorder
(a) One or more somatic symptoms that are distressing or result in significant disruption of daily life
(b) Excessive thoughts, feelings, or behaviors related to the somatic symptoms or associated health concerns as manifested by at least one of the following:
1. Disproportionate and persistent thoughts about the seriousness of one's symptoms
2. Persistently high level of anxiety about health or symptoms
3. Excessive time and energy devoted to these symptoms or health concerns
(c) Although any one somatic symptom may not be continuously present, the state of being symptomatic is persistent (typically more than 6 months)

American Psychiatric Association [54]

In the case of somatic symptoms, there are cases in which treatment is requested with excessive attention to worrisome physical concerns. However, there is no evidence that they provide false information or perform actions to cheat others.

17.3.2 Illness Anxiety Disorder (IAD)

In the DSM-IV, a diagnosis of hypochondriasis was reserved for cases in which the patient (1) presents with worry, but no complaint concerning somatic symptoms, or (2) if symptoms are present, they are very mild in nature. Conversely, even if the patient has a hypochondriacal complaint, if the patient's somatic symptoms are above a certain level of severity, it is no longer considered to be an illness anxiety disorder, and must be treated as somatic symptom disorder [57]. Many diagnoses which fell under the category "somatoform disorder" in the DSM-IV have been reclassified as somatic symptom disorder or illness anxiety disorders (IAD) in the DSM-V.

17.3.3 Conversion Disorder (Functional Neurological Symptom Disorder)

Furthermore, the requirement that patients display "presence of conflict and other stress factors prior to onset or worsening of symptoms" listed as a criterion in the DSM-IV was deleted in the newly published DSM-V. However, this does not signify that psychological factors are still not relevant in the diagnosis of the patient's physical symptoms. In practice, even if psychological factors are suspected, in many cases it is not possible to determine the relationship, and diagnosis has become possible even in such cases.

17.3.4 Factitious Disorders

The classification "factitious disorder" was moved from its status as an independent classification in the DSM-IV to a type of somatic symptom and related disorder in the DSM-V. But, this does not indicate that the symptoms that fall under this definition are limited to physical symptoms the patient presents. In addition to the diagnosis "factitious disorder imposed on self," the diagnosis "factitious disorder imposed on others" in which patients project states of illness onto others (e.g., children, parents, pets) is also listed. Patients with factitious disorder complain of pain, even though no pain is present. In some cases, the patient has a clear external motivation for this behavior, such as gaining money or furthering an economic interest, rather than an intrinsic motivation such as gaining attention from playing the role of a sick person. In this case of patient pretending to be sick to gain money or some other external gain, the patient would be excluded from factitious disorder and classified instead as malingering.

The difference between these two examples is that with fraudulent diseases, there is no external motivation for reporting the disease. For such patients, the principal aim is to play the role of a sick person in order to obtain the attention and sympathy of surrounding persons. If the patient presents with signs and symptoms of a disease not consistent with an identifiable medical disease or a psychiatric disorder, the likelihood of being a factitious disorder increases. When factitious disorder is suspected, it is important to avoid invasive examination and treatment as much as possible. Even with minimally invasive nerve blocks such as trigger point blocks, the needs of the patient tend to escalate gradually, and caution should be exercised.

17.3.5 What Is the Cause of Headache in Troublesome Patients, Patients with Troublesome Problems, and Patients with Pain-in-the-Neck Chronic Pain?

Psychiatric comorbidity is often hidden in patients with chronic pain, even when the patient's chief complaint is pain. Therefore, by first suspecting comorbidity and noticing the condition, it is possible to proceed with appropriate treatment. Ideally, treating the patient's comorbid psychiatric issues will relieve their pain, but in patients with chronic pain, patients often continue to report pain regardless of the success or failure of their psychiatric treatment. Because of this, for patients to be able to manage their pain successfully, it is important that therapists listen to their complaints carefully. It is important to understand the symptoms in terms of the living conditions and lives of patients, and somatic symptoms may indicate loneliness and the status and position in family/society. Complaints of somatic symptoms are often the only method patients have to connect with the people around them, and if they lose this, there is a possibility that there may be no way for them to connect with others.

The goal of psychosomatic treatment of chronic pain is not to eliminate pain completely, but rather to help patients accept their pain, regain a sense of self-control, broaden the range of daily activities they can perform, and improve their adaptation to social life. Psychiatrics can play a key role in helping patients achieve these goals. Thus, long-term psychiatric treatment may be necessary for patients experiencing chronic pain, and an unrelenting attitude is required. As the name implies, chronic pain is a chronic disease, and while patients may experience periodic remissions and exacerbations of their pain, providers should aim for long-term remission using a holistic approach which incorporates interpersonal relationships and emphasizes patient's quality of life.

References

1. Dworkin RH, Caligor E. Psychiatric diagnosis and chronic pain: DSM-III-R and beyond. J Pain Symptom Manag. 1988;3(2):87–98.
2. Dersh J, Gatchel RJ, Polatin P, et al. Prevalence of psychiatric disorders in patients with chronic work-related musculoskeletal pain disability. J Occup Environ Med. 2002;44(5):459–68.
3. Magni G, Marchetti M, Moreschi C, et al. Chronic musculoskeletal pain and depressive symptoms in the National Health and Nutrition Examination. I. Epidemiologic follow-up study. Pain. 1993;53(2):163–8.
4. Polatin PB, Kinney RK, Gatchel RJ, et al. Psychiatric illness and chronic low-back pain. Spine. 1993;18(1):66–71.
5. Gallagher RM, Moore P, Chernoff I. The reliability of depression diagnosis in chronic low back pain. Gen Hosp Psychiatry. 1995;17(6):399–413.
6. Korff MV, Simon G. The relationship between pain and depression. British Journal of Psychiatry. 1996;168(30):101–8.
7. Magni G, Moreschi C, Rigatti-Luchini S, et al. Prospective study on the relationship between depressive symptoms and chronic musculoskeletal pain. Pain. 1994;56:289–97.
8. Kaufman J, Charney D. Comorbidity of mood and anxiety disorders. Depress Anxiety. 2000;12(1):69–76.
9. Pincus T, Williams A. Models and measurements of depression in chronic pain. J Psychosom Res. 1999;47(3):211–9.
10. Ohayon MM, Schatzberg AF. Using chronic pain to predict depressive morbidity in the general population. Arch Gen Psychiatry. 2003;60(1):39–47.
11. Bair MJ, Robinson RL, Eckert GJ, et al. Impact of pain on depression treatment response in primary care. Psychosom Med. 2004;66:17–22.
12. Ohayon MM, Schatzberg AF. Chronic pain and major depression disorder in the general population. J Psychiatr Res. 2010;44:454–61.
13. Ang DC, Bair MJ, Damush TM, et al. Predictors of pain outcomes in patients with chronic musculoskeletal pain co-morbid with depression: results from a randomized controlled trial. Pain Med. 2010;11(4):482–91. https://doi.org/10.1111/j.1526-4637.2009.00759.x.
14. Curtin KB, Norris D. The relationship between chronic musculoskeletal pain, anxiety and mindfulness: adjustments to the fear-avoidance model of chronic pain. Scand J Pain. 2017;17:156–66.
15. Roy-Byrne PP, Davidson KW, Kessler RC, et al. Anxiety disorders and comorbid medical illness. Gen Hosp Psychiatry. 2008;30(3):208–25.
16. Boselie JJL, Vlaeyen JW. Broadening the fear-avoidance model of chronic pain? Scand J Pain. 2017;17:176–7.
17. Vlaeyen JW, Linton SJ. Fear-avoidance and its consequences in chronic musculoskeletal pain: a state of the art. Pain. 2000;85(3):317–332.
18. Beck JG, Clapp JD. A different kind of co-morbidity: understanding posttraumatic stress disorder and chronic pain. Psychol Trauma. 2011;3(2):101–8.
19. Beckham JC, Crawford AL, Feldman ME, et al. Chronic posttraumatic stress disorder and chronic pain in Vietnam combat veterans. J Psychosom Res. 1997;43(4):379–89.
20. Moeller-Bertram T, Keltner J, Strigo IA. Pain and post traumatic stress disorder—review of clinical and experimental evidence. Neuropharmacology. 2012;62(2):586–97.
21. Wuest J, Ford-Gilboe M, Merritt-Gray M, et al. Abuse-related injury and symptoms of posttraumatic stress disorder as mechanisms of chronic pain in survivors of intimate partner violence. Pain Med. 2009;10(4):739–47.
22. Kongsted A, Bebdix T, Qerama E, et al. Acute stress response and recovery after whiplash injuries. A one-year prospective study. Eur J Pain. 2008;12(4):455–63.
23. Katz J, Asmundson GJ, McRae K, et al. Emotional numbing and pain intensity predict the development of pain disability up to one year after lateral thoracotomy. Eur J Pain. 2009;13(8):870–8.

24. Atwoli L, Platt JM, Basu A, et al. Associations between lifetime potentially traumatic events and chronic physical conditions in the South African Stress and Health Survey: a cross-sectional study. BMC Psychiatry. 2016;16(1):214. https://doi.org/10.1186/s12888-016-0929-z.
25. Avdibegovic E, Delic A, Hadzibeganovic K, et al. Somatic diseases in patients with posttraumatic stress disorder. Med Arh. 2010;64(3):154–7.
26. Dobie DJ, Kivlahan DR, Maynard C, et al. Posttraumatic stress disorder in female veterans. Arch Intern Med. 2004;164:394–400.
27. Jakupcak M, Osborne T, Michsel S, et al. Anxiety senstivity and depression: mechanisms in veterans with posttrau,atic stress disorder. J Trauma Stress. 2006;19(4):471–9.
28. Norman SB, Stein MB, Dimsdale JE, et al. Pain in the aftermath of trauma is a risk factor for post-traumatic stress disorder. Psychol Med. 2008;38(4):533–42.
29. Raphael KG, Chandler HK, Ciccone DS. Is childhood abuse a risk factor for chronic pain in adulthood? Curr Pain Headache Rep. 2004;8(2):99–110.
30. Raphael KG, Widom CS. Post-traumatic stress disorder moderates the relation between documented childhood victimization and pain 30 years later. Pain. 2011;152(1):163–9.
31. Davis DA, Luecken LJ, Zautra AJ. Are reports of childhood abuse related to the experience of chronic pain in adulthood? A meta-analytic review of the literature. Clin J Pain. 2005;21(5):398–405.
32. Young JL, Redmond JC. Fibromyalgia, chronic fatigue, and adult attention deficit hyperactivity disorder in the adult: a case study. Psychopharmacol Bull. 2007;40(1):118–26.
33. Young JL. Chronic fatigue syndrome: 3 cases and a discussion of the natural history of attention-deficit/hyperactivity disorder. Postgrad Med. 2013;125(1):162–8.
34. Still GF. Some abnormal psychical conditions in children: excerpts from three lectures. J Atten Disord. 2006;10(2):126–36.
35. Fayyad J, De Graaf R, Kessler R, et al. Cross-national prevalence and correlates of adult attention-deficit hyperactivity disorder. Br J Psychiatry. 2007;190(5):402–9.
36. Van Rensburg R, Meyer HP, Hitchcock SA, et al. Screening for adult ADHD in patients with fibromyalgia syndrome. Pain Med. 2018;19:1825–31. https://doi.org/10.1093/pm/pnx275.
37. Cohen E, Henkin I. Substance abuse and lifestyle among an urban schizophrenic population: some observations. Psychiatry. 1995:58(2):113–20.
38. Finnerup NB, Otto M, McQuay HJ, et al. Algorithm for neuropathic pain treatment: an evidence based proposal. Pain. 2005;118(3):289–305.
39. Kalso E, Edwards JE, Moore RA, et al. Opioids in chronic non-cancer pain: systematic review of efficacy and safety. Pain. 2004;112(3):372–80.
40. Edlund MJ, Steffick D, Hudson T, et al. Risk factors for clinically recognized opioid abuse and dependence among veterans using opioids for chronic non-cancer pain. Pain. 2007;129(3):355–62.
41. Chelminski PR, Ives TJ, Felix KM, et al. A primary care, multi-disciplinary disease management program for opioid-treated patients with chronic non-cancer pain and a high burden of psychiatric comorbidity. BMC Health Serv Res. 2005;5(1):3. https://doi.org/10.1186/1472-6963-5-3.
42. Manchikanti L, Pampati V, Damron KS, et al. Prevalence of opioid abuse in interventional pain medicine practice settings: a randomized clinical evaluation. Pain Physician. 2001;4(4):358–65.
43. Savage SR. Assessment for addiction in pain-treatment settings. Clin J Pain. 2002;18(4 Suppl):S28–38.
44. Webster LR, Webster RM. Predicting aberrant behaviors in opioid-treated patients: preliminary validation of the Opioid Risk Tool. Pain Med. 2005;6(6):432–42.
45. Portenoy RK. Opioid therapy for chronic nonmalignant pain: a review of the critical issues. J Pain Symptom Manag. 1996;11(4):203–17.
46. Meller WH, Rinehart R, Cadoret RJ, et al. Specific familial transmission in substance abuse. Int J Addict. 1998;23(10):1029–39.
47. Dunbar SA, Katz NP. Chronic opioid therapy for nonmalignant pain in patients with a history of substance abuse: report of 20 cases. J Pain Symptom Manag. 1996;11(3):163–71.

48. Friedman R, Li V, Mehrotra D. Treating pain patients at risk: evaluation of a screening tool in opioid-treated pain patients with and without addiction. Pain Med. 2003;4(2):182–5.
49. Athuri S, Sudarshan G. Development of a screening tool to detect the risk of inappropriate prescription opioid use in patients with chronic pain. Pain Physician. 2004;7(3):333–8.
50. Ballantyne JC, Mao J. Opioid therapy for chronic pain. N Engl J Med. 2003;349(20):1943–53.
51. Dunn KT, Saunders KW, Rutther CM, et al. Overdose and prescribed opioids: Associations among chronic non-cancer pain patients. Ann Intern Med. 2010;152(2):85–92.
52. McLellan AT, Turner BJ. Chronic noncancer pain management and opioid overdose: time to change prescribing practices. Ann Intern Med. 2010;152(2):123–4.
53. Alford DP. Chronic back pain with possible prescription opioid misuse. JAMA. 2013; 309(9):919–25.
54. American Psychiatric Association. Diagnostic and statistical manual of mental disorders. 5th ed. Washington, DC: American Psychiatric Association; 2013.
55. A Division of American Psychiatric Association. DSM-5 Fact Sheets, updated disorders, Somatic Symptom Disorder. 2017. https://www.psychiatry.org/psychiatrists/practice/dsm/educational-resources/dsm-5-fact-sheets. Accessed 06 Dec 2017.
56. Frances A. The new somatic symptom disorder in DSM-5 risks mislabeling many people as mentally ill. Br Med J. 2013;346:f1580. https://doi.org/10.1136/bmj.f1580.
57. Dimsdale JE, Creed F, Escobar J, et al. Somatic symptom disorder: an important change in DSM. J Psychosom Res. 2013;75(3):223–8.

Chapter 18
Headache

Oluseyi Fadayomi and Antoun Nader

Headache is a ubiquitous disorder, affecting almost half of the adult population globally. It is the most common form of pain and a major reason people miss days at work or school or visit the doctor.

In adults aged 18–65 years of age, throughout the world, half to three quarters of adults in this group have had a headache in the last year, with about 30% reporting migraine headache [1].

18.1 Classification of Headaches

According to the International Headache Society, headaches can be classified as follows:

Primary Headaches

1. Migraine
2. Tension-type headache
3. Trigeminal autonomic cephalalgias
4. Other primary headache disorders

Secondary Headaches

1. Headache attributed to trauma or injury to the head and/or neck
2. Headache attributed to cranial or cervical vascular disorder
3. Headache attributed to non-vascular intracranial disorder
4. Headache attributed to a substance or its withdrawal
5. Headache attributed to infection

O. Fadayomi (✉) · A. Nader
Northwestern Memorial Hospital, Chicago, IL, USA

K. Shimoji et al. (eds.), *Chronic Pain Management in General and Hospital Practice*, https://doi.org/10.1007/978-981-15-2933-7_18

6. Headache attributed to disorder of homoeostasis
7. Headache or facial pain attributed to disorder of the cranium, neck, eyes, ears, nose, sinuses, teeth, mouth, or other facial or cervical structure
8. Headache attributed to psychiatric disorder

In this chapter we will be focusing more on the primary headaches.

18.2 Migraine Headaches

Migraine is a common disabling primary headache disorder. It is sometimes referred to as a vascular headache. Epidemiological studies have documented its high prevalence and high socio-economic and personal impacts. In the Global Burden of Disease Survey 2010, it was ranked as the third most prevalent disorder and seventh-highest specific cause of disability worldwide [2].

Approximately two-thirds of migraines occur in women. The prevalence in North America ascertained through epidemiological studies is 12–17.6% in females and 4–6% in males. Prior to puberty the prevalence of migraine in boys and girls is similar, during and after adolescence, the incidence increases more rapidly in girls. In females, prevalence increases up to about the age of 40 after which it decreases, the decrease becomes steeper as women approach menopause [3].

More than 80% of patients with severe migraines experience headache related disability, which ranges from decreased productivity to time off work during an attack. The cost in productivity may exceed $20 billion per year in the USA. The risk if suffering from migraines is about 50% higher among those with first degree relative with migraines; however, genetic factors appear to account for less than 50% of all migraines [3].

18.2.1 Pathophysiology

The now widely accepted neurovascular hypothesis posits that migraine is a disorder of the endogenous pain modulating system, and can be viewed as an inherited dysfunction of sensory modulatory network with homeostatic perturbations causing abnormal processing of essentially normal neural traffic [4].

The advancement in the understanding of migraine pathophysiology over the last 2 decades has not only allowed the development of novel target-based therapeutic approaches, but it is also contributing to clarification of the rationale for several current pharmacotherapeutic approaches that have been used in the acute treatment of migraine [5].

The pain generating structures of the head include the venous sinuses, meninges and large cerebral arteries, basal meninges, muscles, skin, and cranial nerves V, IX, and X. A plexus of largely unmyelinated fibers arises from the trigeminal ganglion (cranial nerve V) and innervates the cerebral and pial arteries, the venous sinuses, and the dura mater; this plexus is referred to as the trigeminovascular system. A similar plexus arises from the dorsal roots of the upper three cervical nerves and innervates comparable structures in the posterior fossa [3].

There is substantial evidence that diencephalic and brainstem nuclei are involved in the modulation of trigeminovascular activation [4, 6], which consists of efferent projections innervating duro-vascular structures, and afferent projections from these structures back to the trigeminal nucleus caudalis. The activation of these pathways culminates in meningeal vasodilation, neurogenic inflammation, central sensitization, and is eventually perceived as head pain [7, 8]. In addition, many neuropeptides are purported to be involved in the migraine circuitry both peripherally and centrally [9].

The neurons in the trigeminovascular system contain substance P, one of the major nociceptive neurotransmitters of primary sensory neurons, calcitonin gene related peptide (CGRP), which causes vasodilation and when infused intravenously into susceptible individuals, triggers headache; neurokinin A, which is similar in structure and function to substance P. When the trigeminal ganglion is stimulated and causes antidromic activation of the trigeminovascular system, these peptide neurotransmitters are released near the blood vessels they innervate; this results in vasodilatation with consequent extravasation of plasma, or the so-called sterile neurogenic inflammation. Leakage of plasma proteins from the dilated blood vessels in turn stimulates the trigeminal nerve endings and causes nociceptive orthodromic signals to the trigeminal ganglion; the end result of this sterile neurogenic inflammation is the perception of pain in and around the head [3].

18.2.2 Classification of Migraines

Migraine has two major subtypes:

1. Migraine without aura
2. Migraine with aura

18.2.2.1 Migraine Without Aura

Recurrent headache disorder manifesting in attacks lasting 4–72 h. Typical characteristics of the headache are unilateral location, pulsating quality, moderate or severe intensity, aggravation by routine physical activity, and association with nausea and/or photophobia and phonophobia [2].

Diagnostic criteria:

(i) At least five attacks fulfilling criteria (ii)–(iv)
(ii) Headache attacks lasting 4–72 h (untreated or unsuccessfully treated)
(iii) Headache has at least two of the following four characteristics:

- Unilateral location
- Pulsating quality
- Moderate or severe pain intensity
- Aggravation by or causing avoidance of routine physical activity (e.g., walking or climbing stairs)

(iv) During headache at least one of the following:

- Nausea and/or vomiting
- Photophobia and phonophobia

(v) Not better accounted for by another ICHD-3 diagnosis [2]

18.2.2.2 Migraine with Aura

They are recurrent attacks, lasting minutes, of unilateral fully reversible visual, sensory, or other central nervous system symptoms that usually develop gradually and are usually followed by headache and associated migraine symptoms [2].

Diagnostic criteria:

(i) At least two attacks fulfilling criteria (i) and (iii)
(ii) One or more of the following fully reversible aura symptoms:

- Visual
- Sensory
- Speech and/or language
- Motor
- Brainstem
- Retinal

(iii) At least two of the following four characteristics:

- At least one aura symptom spreads gradually and lasts for over 5 min, and/or two or more symptoms occur in succession
- Each individual aura symptom lasts 5–60 min
- At least one aura symptom is unilateral
- The aura is accompanied, or followed within 60 min, by headache

(iv) Not better accounted for by another ICHD-3 diagnosis, and transient ischemic attack has been excluded.

18.2.3 Treatment

Migraines can be treated abortively or prophylactically. The aims of acute pharmacological treatment are to rapidly restore function with minimal recurrence, with the avoidance of side effects. The choice of pharmacological treatment is individualized, and is based on the consideration of the characteristics of the migraine attack, the patient's concomitant medical problems, and treatment preferences. Notwithstanding, a good understanding of the pharmacodynamic and pharmacokinetic properties of the various drug options is essential to guide therapy [5].

The following drugs are useful for the treatment of acute migraines headaches (abortive treatment).

18.2.3.1 Triptans (Imitrex, Maxalt, Zomig, Frova, Relpax, Amerge) are 5-HT 1D/1B receptor agonists. Triptans are effective medicines used to treat migraine headaches. They significantly reduce pain within 2 h for most people. Complete relief is less common, but the likelihood may be greater if you take a triptan early during a migraine attack. Triptans also help relieve other migraine symptoms, such as nausea, vomiting, and sensitivity to light, noise, and motion [10]

These drugs are available in a variety of forms. For example: as an auto-injector, tablet, and nasal spray. Injectable preparations have a quicker onset of action, followed by nasal sprays and oral disintegrating tablets and tablets that must be swallowed. These allow for treatment to be tailored to the patients' needs. Approximately 60–80% of patients achieve significant relief from a triptan; however, the headache will recur in up to one-third of patients. A second dose of the same preparation, taken 2–24 h after the first, may again provide significant relief. A triptan should not be used again for at least 24 h after the second dose [3].

18.2.3.2 Ergotamine Tartrate

This drug is first isolated by Stoll and has been used in the acute treatment of migraine since 1926. It has 5-HT agonist activity that also is very effective for migraines. One to two tablets are taken at the onset of the headache or aura, followed by 1 tablet every 30 min until the headache is gone or until a maximum of 5 tablets per headache or 10 tablets per week have been consumed, and if consumed in excess, they can cause vasospastic complications and are emetogenic [3].

Most physicians feel that there is some place for ergotamine in the acute treatment of migraine. However, there is no consensus as to its place in clinical practice. Tfelt-Hansen et al. reviewed 18 randomized controlled clinical trials involving oral ergotamine, or oral ergotamine plus caffeine (e.g., cafergot), at an initial ergotamine dose ranging from 1 to 5 mg [11]. After assessing the quality of the evidence, they concluded that there was non-uniformity pertaining to the utility of oral ergotamine in the treatment of migraine based on the conflicting outcomes of these trials [11]. Despite their findings, consensus recommendations on the role of ergotamine in the acute treatment of migraine have been suggested.

18.2.3.3 Isometheptene (Midrin)

It is an older drug with 5-HT agonist and sympathomimetic activity. It also contains dichloralphenazone, a mild sedative-hypnotic drug similar to chloral hydrate. It has fewer vasospastic complications than ergotamine [3].

18.2.3.4 Butalbital (Fioricet [Acetaminophen and Caffeine], Fiorinal [Aspirin and Caffeine])

They are effective and can be used alone or together with one of the vasoconstricting abortive drugs (triptan, ergotamine). Barbiturate containing preparations causes drowsiness and can be habit forming if used excessively [3].

18.2.3.5 Narcotic-Containing Preparations

Codeine, hydromorphone, hydrocodone, in combination with aspirin or acetaminophen, are used too frequently, particularly in emergency rooms and should be used only as a last resort. Narcotics bind opiate receptors and mask pain, but they do not bind serotonin receptors and therefore do not interrupt the putative pathophysiologic mechanism of migraine [3].

Narcotics also have significant side effects, such as sedation, nausea, vomiting, respiratory depression, addictive effects, so their overuse in the setting of migraine is not appropriate [10].

Opiates, barbiturates, and combination analgesics containing either of these drugs should ideally not be chosen as first-line treatments. In the majority of patients, these medications are less effective than other options, and their frequent administration increases the propensity to develop medication overuse headache [5].

18.2.3.6 Dihydroergotamine

Generally administered via the parenteral route (IV/IM), but also available as a nasal spray. Remains the drug of choice for status migrainosus [3].

18.2.4 Non-Specific Pharmacological Treatments for Acute Migraines

18.2.4.1 NSAIDs

The NSAIDs are a class of drugs widely used for the treatment of pain, fever, and inflammation. Generally, NSAIDs show their anti-inflammatory effects at higher doses than their analgesic and antipyretic properties. NSAIDs are grouped in several chemical classes and this chemical diversity leads to a range of pharmacokinetic characteristics.

NSAIDs are widely used for acute migraine treatment. Their action is mainly to inhibit neurogenic inflammation and the reversal of central sensitization associated with migraine [12]. Several double blind, randomized controlled studies have shown the efficacy for ibuprofen [13], naproxen sodium, ASA, and diclofenac potassium for the treatment of migraine.

It works for some patients with mild to moderate migraines.

Categorically, NSAIDs are contraindicated in patients with peptic ulcer disease, inflammatory bowel disease, gastric bypass surgery, ASA allergy, renal dysfunction, and those on concomitant anticoagulants. In order to decrease the risk for the development of MOH, the use of NSAIDs should be limited to 14 days a month or fewer [5].

18.2.4.2 Acetaminophen

Acetaminophen, commonly known as paracetamol, was developed in the nineteenth century. It became available by prescription in the UK in 1956, and subsequently over the counter in 1963. The active components of paracetamol are the 2 antipyretic active metabolites—acetanilide and phenacetin. The mechanism of action of paracetamol is still not completely understood, but its effects are probably achieved through the central inhibition of prostaglandin synthesis [14]. Differently from the NSAIDs, paracetamol does not directly inhibit COX functions outside the central nervous system, and its central action is not through direct blockage of an active site but rather through reduction of COX activity. Paracetamol is a very commonly used medication, and has evidence of efficacy in migraine as well [15]. It is usually used for migraine attacks of mild or moderate severity. For the treatment of episodic tension-type headache or migraine attacks, Diener et al. [16] reported that, at 2 h, administration of paracetamol 1000 mg resulted in greater pain reduction, from moderate or severe to no pain (19% and 10%, respectively) versus placebo. Similarly, pain intensity went from moderate or severe to no worse than mild pain (56% and 36%, respectively).

Acetaminophen may also be used in combination with other drugs. The combination of aspirin/paracetamol/caffeine has been demonstrated to have greater efficacy than any one of its components in comparable doses when administered alone [16]. Combinations that include opioids (e.g., paracetamol/codeine) should not be routinely used in migraine treatment owing to the poor evidence for efficacy beyond that provided by NSAIDs, and to the risk of developing MOH. If the use of opioids is necessary, a combination of analgesic with tramadol may be the preferred option.

18.2.4.3 Corticosteroids

The role of corticosteroids in acute migraine treatment has not been firmly established. Findings from animal experiments indicate that migraine pain may be partly caused by a sterile neurogenic inflammatory process in the dura mater [17].

The evidence for the role of corticosteroids in the prevention of migraine recurrence has been conflicting. Several trials attempted to address this issue, and found, for example, that dexamethasone failed to reduce headache relapse after ED discharge [18–20]. On the contrary, there is some support for its usage in the prevention of headache recurrence, especially if the migraine attack has lasted longer than 72 h [21].

18.2.5 Preventive Treatment

As with acute therapies, little overall change has occurred in migraine preventive therapy since 2012. Beta blockers, tricyclic antidepressants, anticonvulsants including topiramate and divalproex sodium, onabotulinum toxin A (for chronic migraine), and flunarizine (outside the USA) continue to be standard therapies for migraine prevention [22, 23]. A randomized placebo-controlled study[94] of candesartan as an effective preventive therapy in 72 patients with migraine has led to increasing use of this treatment, particularly because of its generally excellent tolerability. Unfortunately, clinical criteria or biomarkers that predict which specific preventive therapy might be most effective for an individual patient are not available, and the choice of preventive therapy is therefore often based on tolerability or comorbid conditions. Injections of local anesthetics with or without steroids, particularly in the region of occipital nerves, are routinely done in headache centers as preventive therapy for patients with migraine. These procedures are often described as nerve blocks, although blockade of nerve sensory function as evidenced by anesthesia in the distribution of the nerve might not be required for therapeutic efficacy. Clinical experience indicates that these procedures are particularly beneficial for patients with very frequent migraine or status migrainosus. An observational study [24] and clinical experience have indicated that tenderness over the occipital nerve and forward radiation of pain on pressure over the occipital nerve are predictors of benefit from occipital injections. Results from randomized placebo-controlled studies have been mixed: one study [25] of 69 patients with episodic or chronic migraine showed no benefit, whereas two studies [26, 27] of 84 and 36 patients with chronic migraine did show benefit. Positive responses to occipital nerve injections were also reported in patients with prolonged or persistent migraine aura [28], as well as in those with triptan overuse headache [29]. Because the occipital nerve is believed to be composed primarily of C2 and C3 afferents, occipital injection could therefore miss the C1 nerve, which is also a potential modulator of migraine pain [30]. Occipital nerve injections are relatively easy to do, with low complication rates and, thus, are a reasonable approach to try in selected patients, despite mixed supporting evidence. Clinical trials with refinement of predictive clinical criteria would be helpful in guiding appropriate use of occipital injections in the future [31].

18.3 Tension-Type Headache

Tension-type headache (TTH) has a very high socio-economic impact, and its life-time prevalence is reported to be between 30% and 78% in different studies. It is widely acknowledged that noninvasive management with a multidisciplinary approach should be considered for the treatment of tension-type headache [32].

Tension-type headache is very common, with a life-time prevalence in the general population ranging between 30% and 78% in different studies, and it has a very high socio-economic impact [2].

The 1-year prevalence rate for chronic tension-type headache in the general population is about 3% in women and 1.5% in men [33, 34] with just less than half of those with chronic tension-type headache reporting headache-related impairment in work performance. Chronic tension-type headaches are a risk factor for the overuse of analgesic medications and thus the development of analgesic abuse headaches [34–37], continuous headaches and frequent comorbid psychiatric or analgesic use problems.

18.3.1 Pathophysiology of Tension-Type Headache

The pathophysiologic basis is mostly unknown. Some investigators believe that TTH lies at the end of a spectrum that includes severe migraine and cluster at one end and TTH at the other. Under this assumption, at least to some degree, the underlying mechanism of most chronic, recurring headache syndromes would be shared [3].

The muscle contraction theory of TTH relates pain to prolonged contraction, or spasm, of cervical or peri-cranial muscles but no objective data to support the theory.

TTH is the most common headache type and most difficult to classify [3]. Many different and equally vague terms have been applied to this headache. Based on the HIS, the classifications are as follows:

1. Infrequent episodic tension-type headache
2. Frequent episodic tension-type headache
3. Chronic tension-type headache
4. Probable tension-type headache

18.3.1.1 Infrequent Episodic Tension-Type Headache

They are typically bilateral, pressing or tightening in quality and of mild to moderate intensity, lasting minutes to days. The pain does not worsen with routine physical activity and is not associated with nausea, but photophobia or phonophobia may be present [2].

Diagnostic criteria:

(i) At least 10 episodes of headache occurring on <1 day per month on average (<12 days per year) and fulfilling criteria (ii)–(iv)
(ii) Lasting from 30 min to 7 days
(iii) At least two of the following four characteristics:

- Bilateral location
- Pressing or tightening (non-pulsating) quality
- Mild or moderate intensity
- Not aggravated by routine physical activity such as walking or climbing stairs

(iv) Both of the following:

- No nausea or vomiting
- No more than one of photophobia or phonophobia

(v) Not better accounted for by another ICHD-3 diagnosis

18.3.1.2 Frequent Episodic Tension-Type Headache

Frequent episodes of headache, typically bilateral, pressing or tightening in quality and of mild to moderate intensity, lasting minutes to days. The pain does not worsen with routine physical activity and is not associated with nausea, but photophobia or phonophobia may be present [2].

Diagnostic criteria:

(i) At least 10 episodes of headache occurring on 1–14 days per month on average for >3 months (12 and <180 days per year) and fulfilling criteria (ii)–(iv).
(ii) Lasting from 30 min to 7 days
(iii) At least two of the following four characteristics:

- Bilateral location
- Pressing or tightening (non-pulsating) quality mild or moderate intensity
- Not aggravated by routine physical activity such as walking or climbing stairs

(iv) Both of the following:

- No nausea or vomiting
- No more than one of photophobia or phonophobia

(v) Not better accounted for by another ICHD-3 diagnosis

18.3.1.3 Chronic Tension-Type Headache

A disorder evolving from frequent episodic tension-type headache, with daily or very frequent episodes of headache, typically bilateral, pressing or tightening in quality and of mild to moderate intensity, lasting hours to days, or unremitting. The pain does not worsen with routine physical activity, but may be associated with mild nausea, photophobia, or phonophobia [2].

Diagnostic criteria:

(i) Headache occurring on 15 days per month on average for >3 months (180 days per year), fulfilling criteria (ii)–(iv)
(ii) Lasting hours to days, or unremitting.
(iii) At least two of the following four characteristics:

- Bilateral location
- Pressing or tightening (non-pulsating) quality
- Mild or moderate intensity
- Not aggravated by routine physical activity such as walking or climbing stairs

(iv) Both of the following:

- No more than one of photophobia, phonophobia, or mild nausea.
- Neither moderate or severe nausea nor vomiting

(v) Not better accounted for by another ICHD-3 diagnosis.

18.3.1.4 Probable Chronic Tension-Type Headache

Diagnostic criteria:

(i) Headache fulfilling all but one of criteria i–iv for chronic episodic tension-type headache.
(ii) Not fulfilling ICHD-3 criteria for any other headache disorder.
(iii) Not better accounted for by another ICHD-3 diagnosis.

18.3.2 Treatment

This can be divided into abortive and prophylactic treatment.

18.3.2.1 Abortive Treatment Strategies

Over the counter analgesic preparations—aspirin, acetaminophen, or combination of both with or without caffeine. Caffeine combined with analgesics such as aspirin. Acetaminophen, ibuprofen enhance their analgesic efficacy [3]. Stronger headaches may require aspirin, acetaminophen, and ibuprofen with codeine or butalbital.

Other NSAIDs can also be used:

- Carboxylic acids (aspirin).
- Propionic acids (ibuprofen, naproxen, ketoprofen, and fenoprofen).
- Aryl and heterocyclic acid (indomethacin, diclofenac).
- Fenamic acids (mefenamic acid and meclofenamate).
- Enolic acids (piroxicam and phenylbutazone).
- Pyrrolo (pyrolle-ketorolac).
- COX-2 inhibitors (celecoxib).

It is worthwhile to try stress management modalities or acupuncture. It is difficult to predict in whom these modalities are likely to be beneficial [3].

18.3.2.2 Prophylactic Treatment Strategies

Many of the medications used for migraine prophylaxis are useful in preventing episodes of tension headaches. This might reflect their common pathophysiology.

- Antidepressants: amitriptyline, nortriptyline, imipramine, desipramine (25–200 mg at bedtime). TCAs help induce sleep, which may constitute one of the mechanisms by which they help. They have anticholinergic effects that include dry mouth, excessive daytime sleepiness, dizziness, urinary retention, glaucoma, cardiac arrhythmias, and photosensitization; they can also cause weight gain.
- Serotonin reuptake inhibitors (SSRIs) and serotonin-norepinephrine reuptake inhibitors (SNRIs) can be used in patients that cannot tolerate the side effects of TCAs. The major side effects of SSRIs are decreased libido and erectile dysfunction. Care should be taken in patients using triptans as this can precipitate a serotonin syndrome.
- Beta blockers: propranolol, metoprolol, atenolol, timolol, and nadolol.
- Anticonvulsants such as valproic acid (Depakote and Depakote ER).
- Botulinum toxin A injection into the most tender peri-cranial muscle(s) or directly into a trigger point has been reported to increase significantly the number of headache-free days in patients with CTTH [3].

18.4 Trigeminal Autonomic Cephalalgias (TACs)

They represent a group of three headache disorders characterized by the occurrence of pain in the distribution of the first division of the trigeminal nerve accompanied by prominent parasympathetic autonomic features in the same distribution [3].

They are primary headache disorders with core similarities. The primary feature common to all is attacks of severe unilateral headache of varying duration, accompanied by cranial autonomic symptoms (CAS). The group contains some of the most painful conditions known to man [38]. They can be divided into the following categories:

1. Cluster headache
2. Hemicrania (Paroxysmal hemicranias, Hemicrania Continua)
3. Short-lasting unilateral neuralgiform headache attacks with conjunctival injection and tearing (SUNCT).

These disorders are highly disabling, some with onset early in life and persisting for many years, resulting in considerable economic and social burden [39]. Although occasionally described as rare, the prevalence of CH, the most prevalent of the TACs, is 0.1%, comparable to Parkinson's disease [40]. The TACs share many clinical features; nevertheless, there are also key differences, including treatment response, making clinical differentiation crucially important. With their stereotypical presentation, it may be surprising that a correct initial diagnosis is made in only 21% of CH patients, and the diagnostic delay is 6 years [41, 42].

18.4.1 Cluster Headache

Named for the tendency for attacks to cluster together at specific times of the year, CH has the longest average attack duration among the TACs, lasting around 45 min. Occurring up to eight times a day, the pain is extreme, probably the worst of all headaches, and biorhythmic features are highly pronounced, with both circadian and circannual attack patterns [43, 44].

18.4.1.1 Pathophysiology

The pathophysiologic mechanism of cluster headaches is not known. Some investigators believe that cluster headache lies within a continuum of head pains that include cluster and severe migraine at one extreme and tension-type headache at the other [3].

While our understanding of the TACs remains imperfect, there is strong proof that similarities extend from clinical phenotype to pathophysiological mechanisms. Different theories have been postulated. Vasodilation in intracranial arteries and increases in particular neuropeptides measured in jugular blood are well documented, but are non-specific and are also seen in other circumstances, suggesting that these phenomena are secondary in nature [45].

18.4.2 Treatment

In general, the drugs that are used to treat migraine are useful in cluster except that the role for treatment aimed at aborting an acute headache is limited because the attack has usually run its course by the time the agent has exerted its effect [3]. Therefore, cluster is best treated early on with prophylactic drugs with the aim of interrupting the cluster. The major limitations of drugs aimed at interrupting the cluster (drugs used in migraine prophylaxis) are their slow onset of action, with the most requiring 2–4 weeks to demonstrate activity at the initial dose, and similar intervals for subsequent dose adjustments [3].

CH treatment can be divided into three groups: abortive, preventive, and transitional/bridge therapy [38].

18.4.2.1 Abortive

Oxygen delivered via a facemask at 8–15 L/min as abortive therapy to end the attack [46]. 100% oxygen given via face mask at 12 L/min over 15 min generally results in the cessation of the CH within 15 min [47]. Note that there is a clinical suspicion that overuse of oxygen will increase the frequency of CH [48].

Sumatriptan (6 mg, SQ) is a first-line abortive agent for CH. It is well considered for CH, but some patients do well with other triptans such as rizatriptan [49]. An intranasal triptan (Sumatriptan or Zolmitriptan) is also considered first line therapy [50].

A 4% aqueous solution of lidocaine applied by a dropper or a pledget to the sphenopalatine ganglion (via the ipsilateral nostril) is another useful abortive agent. In the past, the sympathomimetic agent, cocaine was used in this fashion and gave good relief from CH. The intranasal use of lidocaine in CH patients demands that the patient must lie down and get into a proper position with their head to enable the medication to reach the ipsilateral sphenopalatine ganglion [51].

A rapidly acting dihydroergotamine (DHE) given intranasally is an effective abortive agent, but should not be used within 24 h of a triptan. Taking two DHE sprays or an oral triptan immediately before going to sleep will enable the medication to reach a peak plasma level and typically abort this headache [48].

Intranasal butorphanol, an opioid mixed agonist–antagonist, antagonist at μ(mu) opioid receptor, and agonist at Kappa opioid receptor, is an effective abortive agent, but caution must be used to avoid rebound headaches. Adverse events from this medication include a burning feeling in the sinuses to "weird" and "hyper" feelings and dysphoria. Some patients may experience hallucinations. Butorphanol's addiction potential is significantly underrated. The intranasal solution may be diluted to 50% without a loss in stability [48].

18.4.2.2 Preventive

First-choice preventive treatment is the calcium channel blocker verapamil, administered with the aim of reducing the duration, frequency, and severity of attacks [46]. It is used for both the episodic and chronic CH patients [48].

Lithium, the second-choice preventive therapy for CH [38], excellent prophylactic treatment, and blood levels should be monitored. Lithium carbonate may be used as a single drug, and if efficacy is lost, a second drug such as verapamil may be added [48].

Topiramate, methysergide, prednisone, baclofen, gabapentin, and melatonin can be used in CH, but are typically used only as third-choice preventives [46].

As with migraine patients, medication overuse headache (MOH) has been seen in CH patients who may abuse opioids, ergots, and triptans as well as simple analgesics, developing both analgesic and vasoconstrictor rebound headache [52].

18.4.2.3 Transitional

Oral glucocorticoids can be used as transitional therapy, administered for a rapid preventive effect, while verapamil or lithium is being titrated [46]. If the side effects are tolerable, glucocorticoids work very well in CH and some of the other TACs [53]. Another option for transitional therapy is the greater occipital nerve (GON) block using a local anesthetic either alone or combined with injectable glucocorticoids. Surgery is not widely used, due to inconsistent results and adverse events. When it is used, the target is parasympathetic or sensory pathways (gangliolysis, neurectomy, resection) [54]. A more promising approach, however, is the use of neurostimulation targeting the posterior hypothalamus, sphenopalatine ganglion, occipital and vagal nerves, which has demonstrated positive effects in a growing number of studies conducted over the past two decades [55]. The effects of the available modes of neurostimulation are not directly comparable, since occipital nerve and deep brain stimulation seem to have solely a preventive effect, whereas sphenopalatine ganglion and vagal nerve stimulation have both acute and preventive effects [38].

18.4.3 Hemicrania (Paroxysmal Hemicranias, Hemicrania Continua)

Paroxysmal hemicrania consists of frequent, unremitting, unilateral headaches exhibiting a frequency of a few to more than 20 per day; the headaches last 5–45 min each [3].

It may in some presentations resemble CH, the main differences being shorter, more frequent attacks, and fewer predilections for nocturnal occurrence [56].

Oxygen is not effective, possibly due to the shorter attacks and the somewhat delayed onset of effect, but attacks can be completely prevented by the NSAIDs such as indomethacin [57]. Using the same criteria as for CH, PH is classified as either episodic (20–35%) or chronic (65–80%). It is not known why most PH patients experience chronic symptoms, while most CH patients experience episodic events, and why PH attacks do not show as marked a circadian rhythm. While most attacks in PH arise spontaneously, it does appear that 10% are triggered mechanically, the C2–C3 region of the neck being particularly sensitive. There appears to be no preponderance by sex [58].

Given the high frequency of short attacks, therapeutic focus should be on prevention. The first choice for PH is indomethacin, typically in doses of 150–225 mg [58]. Although the response is described as absolute, very high doses of around 300 mg may be needed, and timing may also play a role, some patients requiring 10 days of maintenance therapy before any effect sets in, or needing to take the medication at a specific time of day [59]. When the patient is attack-free, tapering can be attempted at regular intervals, and with the episodic sub-form, medication can be stopped between attack periods. Gastro protective measures should always be considered, and not all patients can tolerate indomethacin in the doses required for efficacy; kidney function may also need to be monitored. Other treatment options include topiramate and GON blocks [24].

18.4.4 Short-Lasting Unilateral Neuralgiform Headache Attacks with Conjunctival Injection and Tearing (SUNCT)

SUNCT is a rare headache that occurs almost exclusively in males. Bursts of stabbing, throbbing, or burning pain around the eye or temple lasts 5 s to 5 min and occurs in paroxysms of up to 30/h (with an average of 5–6/h) [3].

SUNCT is characterized by still shorter and more frequent attacks than PH. These are, per definition, accompanied by conjunctival injection and lacrimation and last 1–600 s, occurring with a very high frequency of up to 30/h [60]. They can be triggered by mechanical stimuli to the skin and can also occur as repetitive stabs [61]. The pain distribution is typically orbital or peri-orbital, and the character can be electric or shock-like, hence the name neuralgiform. Between attacks, most patients are completely pain-free, and only seldom do attacks occur at night. The concept of abortive therapy in a headache disorder characterized by attacks whose duration is measured in seconds is not realistic, and there are no controlled trials investigating preventive treatment. Treatment is therefore a specialist task, with evidence based on one large and several small case series [62]. Preventive first-choice medication is lamotrigine, with topiramate and gabapentin second. Extra efficacy may be gained by combination with corticosteroids. However, as with all TACs, some cases are medically refractory, and patients do not respond to or cannot tolerate effective dosages. Magnetic resonance imaging may show evidence of neurovascular compression in some patients, and some of these may respond to microvascular decompression of the trigeminal nerve [63].

References

1. Headache disorders. World Health Organization; 2016.
2. International Headache Society 2017 Guidelines. The international classification of headache disorders. 3rd ed. London: International Headache Society; 2017.
3. Benzon HT, Raja SN, Liu SS, Fishman SM, Cohen SP. Essentials of pain medicine. 3rd ed; 2011. p. 260–71.
4. Goadsby PJ, Holland PR, Martins-Oliveira M, Hoffmann J, Schankin C, Akerman S. Pathophysiology of migraine: a disorder of sensory processing. Physiol Rev. 2017;97(2):553–622.
5. Ong JJY, De Felice M. Migraine treatment: current acute medications and their potential mechanisms of action. Neurotherapeutics. 2018;15:274. https://doi.org/10.1007/s13311-017-0592-1.
6. Akerman S, Holland PR, Goadsby PJ. Diencephalic and brainstem mechanisms in migraine. Nat Rev Neurosci. 2011;12(10):570–84.
7. Charles A. Advances in the basic and clinical science of migraine. Ann Neurol. 2009;65(5):491–8.
8. Pietrobon D, Striessnig J. Neurobiology of migraine. Nat Rev Neurosci. 2003;4(5):386–98.
9. Noseda R, Borsook D, Burstein R. Neuropeptides and neurotransmitters that modulate thalamocortical pathways relevant to migraine headache. Headache. 2017;57(Suppl. 2):97–111.
10. Holroyd KA, O'Donnell FJ, Stensland M, Lipchik GL, Cordingley GE, Carlson BW. Management of chronic tension-type headache with tricyclic antidepressant medication, stress management therapy, and their combination: a randomized controlled trial. JAMA. 2001;285(17):2208–15.
11. Tfelt-Hansen P, Saxena PR, Dahlöf C, Pascual J, Láinez M, Henry P, Diener H, Schoenen J, Ferrari MD, Goadsby PJ. Ergotamine in the acute treatment of migraine: a review and European consensus. Brain. 2000;123(Pt 1):9–18.
12. Tepper DE. Non-steroidal anti-inflammatories for the acute treatment of migraine. Headache. 2013;53(1):225–6.
13. Suthisisang C, Poolsup N, Kittikulsuth W, Pudchakan P, Wiwatpanich P. Efficacy of low-dose ibuprofen in acute migraine treatment: systematic review and meta-analysis. Ann Pharmacother. 2007;41(11):1782–91.
14. Graham GG, Scott KF. Mechanisms of action of paracetamol and related analgesics. Inflammopharmacology. 2003;11(4):401–13.
15. Lipton RB, Baggish JS, Stewart WF, Codispoti JR, Fu M. Efficacy and safety of acetaminophen in the treatment of migraine: results of a randomized, double blind, placebo-controlled, population based study. Arch Intern Med. 2000;160(22):3486–92.
16. Diener HC, Pfaffenrath V, Pageler L, Peil H, Aicher B. The fixed combination of acetylsalicylic acid, paracetamol and caffeine is more effective than single substances and dual combination for the treatment of headache: a multicentre, randomized, double blind, single-dose, placebo-controlled parallel group study. Cephalalgia. 2005;25(10):776–87.
17. Markowitz S, Saito K, Moskowitz MA. Neurogenically mediated plasma extravasation in dura mater: effect of ergot alkaloids. A possible mechanism of action in vascular headache. Cephalalgia. 1988;8(2):83–91.
18. Donaldson D, Sundermann R, Jackson R, Bastani A. Intravenous dexamethasone vs. placebo as adjunctive therapy to reduce the recurrence rate of acute migraine headaches: a mul-

ticenter, double-blinded, placebo-controlled randomized clinical trial. Am J Emerg Med. 2008;26(2):124–30.
19. Rowe BH, Colman I, Edmonds ML, Blitz S, Walker A, Wiens S. Randomized controlled trial of intravenous dexamethasone to prevent relapse in acute migraine headache. Headache. 2008;48(3):333–40.
20. Fiesseler FW, Shih R, Szucs P, et al. Steroids for migraine headaches: a randomized double blind, two-armed, placebo-controlled trial. J Emerg Med. 2011;40(4):463–8.
21. Friedman BW, Greenwald P, Bania TC, et al. Randomized trial of IV dexamethasone for acute migraine in the emergency department. Neurology. 2007;69(22):2038–44.
22. Silberstein SD, Holland S, Freitag F, et al. Evidence-based guideline update: pharmacologic treatment for episodic migraine prevention in adults: report of the Quality Standards Subcommittee of the American Academy of Neurology and the American Headache Society. Neurology. 2012;78:1337–45.
23. Pringsheim T, Davenport W, Mackie G, et al. Canadian headache society guideline for migraine prophylaxis. Can J Neurol Sci. 2012;39:S1–59.
24. Afridi SK, Shields KG, Bhola R, Goadsby PJ. Greater occipital nerve injection in primary headache syndromes—prolonged effects from a single injection. Pain. 2006;122:126–9.
25. Dilli E, Halker R, Vargas B, et al. Occipital nerve block for the short-term preventive treatment of migraine: a randomized, double-blinded, placebo-controlled study. Cephalalgia. 2015;35(11):959–68. https://doi.org/10.1177/0333102414561872.
26. Inan LE, Inan N, Karadaş Ö, et al. Greater occipital nerve blockade for the treatment of chronic migraine: a randomized, multicenter, double blind, and placebo-controlled study. Acta Neurol Scand. 2015;132(4):270–7. https://doi.org/10.1111/ane.12393.
27. Cuadrado ML, Aledo-Serrano A, Navarro P, et al. Short-term effects of greater occipital nerve blocks in chronic migraine: a double blind, randomised, placebo-controlled clinical trial. Cephalalgia. 2017;37(9):864–72. https://doi.org/10.1177/0333102416655159.
28. Cuadrado ML, Aledo-Serrano A, López-Ruiz P, et al. Greater occipital nerve block for the acute treatment of prolonged or persistent migraine aura. Cephalalgia. 2017;37(8):812–8. https://doi.org/10.1177/0333102416655160.
29. Karadaş Ö, Özön A, Özcelik F, Özge A. Greater occipital nerve block in the treatment of triptan-overuse headache: a randomized comparative study. Acta Neurol Scand. 2017;135(4):426–33. https://doi.org/10.1111/ane.12692.
30. Johnston MM, Jordan SE, Charles AC. Pain referral patterns of the C1 to C3 nerves: implications for headache disorders. Ann Neurol. 2013;74:145–8.
31. Charles A. The pathophysiology of migraine: implications for clinical management. Lancet Neurol. 2017;17:174. https://doi.org/10.1016/S1474-4422(17)30435-0.
32. Salman İB, Sertel Berk HÖ. Cognitive behavioral therapy for tension-type headache: a case report. Agri. 2017;29(4):177–84. https://doi.org/10.5505/agri.2017.35582.
33. Schwartz BS, Stewart WF, Simon MS, Lipton RB. A population-based study of the epidemiology of tension-type headache. JAMA. 1998;279:381–3.
34. Rasmussen BK, Lipton RB. Epidemiology of tension-type headache. In: Olesen J, Tfelt-Hansen P, Welch KMA, editors. The headaches. 2nd ed. Philadelphia, PA: Lippincott Williams & Wilkins; 2000. p. 545–50.
35. Schoenen J, Wang W. Tension-type headache. In: Goadsby PJ, Silberstein SD, editors. Headache. Boston, MA: Butterworth-Heinemann; 1997. p. 177–200.
36. Olesen JC for the Headache Classification Committee of the International Headache Society. Classification and diagnostic criteria for headache disorders, cranial neuralgias, and facial pain. Cephalalgia. 1988;8(suppl 7):1–96.
37. Granella F, Farina S, Malferrari G, Manzoni GC. Drug abuse in chronic headache: a clinic-epidemiologic study. Cephalalgia. 1987;7:15–9.
38. Barloese MCJ. The pathophysiology of the trigeminal autonomic cephalalgias, with clinical implications. Clin Auton Res. 2018;28:315. https://doi.org/10.1007/s10286-017-0468-9.
39. Jensen RM, Lyngberg A, Jensen RH. Burden of cluster headache. Cephalalgia. 2007;27:535–41.

40. Fischera M, Marziniak M, Gralow I, Evers S. The incidence and prevalence of cluster headache: a meta-analysis of population-based studies. Cephalalgia. 2008;28:614–8.
41. Lund N, Barloese M, Petersen A, Haddock B, Jensen R. Chronobiology differs between men and women with cluster headache, clinical phenotype does not. Neurology. 2017;88(11):1069–76. https://doi.org/10.1212/WNL.0000000000003715.
42. Rozen TD, Fishman RS. Cluster headache in the United States of America: demographics, clinical characteristics, triggers, suicidality, and personal burden. Headache. 2012;52(1):99–113. https://doi.org/10.1111/j.1526-4610.2011.02028.x.
43. Kudrow L. The cyclic relationship of natural illumination to cluster period frequency. Cephalalgia. 1987;7(Suppl 6):76–8.
44. Barloese M, Lund N, Petersen A, et al. Sleep and chronobiology in cluster headache. Cephalalgia. 2015;35:969–78.
45. May A, Büchel C, Turner R, Goadsby PJ. Magnetic resonance angiography in facial and other pain: neurovascular mechanisms of trigeminal sensation. J Cereb Blood Flow Metab. 2001;21:1171–6.
46. May A, Leone M, Afra J, et al. EFNS guidelines on the treatment of cluster headache and other trigeminal-autonomic cephalalgias. Eur J Neurol. 2006;13:1066–77.
47. Schoenen J. Deficient habituation of evoked cortical potentials in migraine: a link between brain biology, behavior and trigeminovascular activation? Biomed Pharmacother. 1996;50(2):71–8.
48. Jay GW, Barkin RL. Primary headache disorders part I-migraine and the trigeminal autonomic cephalalgias. Dis Mon. 2017;63(11):308–38. https://doi.org/10.1016/j.disamonth.2017.04.001.
49. Law S, Derry S, Moore RA. Triptans for acute cluster headache. Cochrane Database Syst Rev. 2010;(4):CD008042. https://doi.org/10.1002/14651858.CD008042.pub2.
50. Cittadini E, May A, Straube A, Evers S, Bussone G, Goadsby PJ. Effectiveness of intranasal zolmitriptan in acute cluster headache: a randomized, placebo controlled, double blind crossover study. Arch Neurol. 2006;63(11):1537–42.
51. Bakbak B, Gedik S, Kiktekir BE, Okka M. Cluster headache with ptosis responsive to intranasal lidocaine application: a case report. J Med Case Rep. 2012;6:64.
52. Paemeleire K, Bahra A, Evers S, Matharu MS, Goadsby PJ. Medication overuse headache in patients with cluster headache. Neurology. 2006;67(1):109–13.
53. Maihöfner C, Speck V, Sperling W, Giede-Jeppe A. Complete remission of SUNCT syndrome by intravenous glucocorticoid treatment. Neurol Sci. 2013;34:1811–2.
54. Jarrar RG, Black DF, Dodick DW, Davis DH. Outcome of trigeminal nerve section in the treatment of chronic cluster headache. Neurology. 2003;60:1360–2.
55. Láinez MJ, Guillamón E. Cluster headache and other TACs: pathophysiology and neurostimulation options. Headache. 2017;57:327–35.
56. Antonaci F, Sjaastad O. Chronic paroxysmal hemicrania (CPH): a review of the clinical manifestations. Headache. 1989;29:648–56.
57. Summ O, Evers S. Mechanism of action of indomethacin in indomethacin-responsive headaches. Curr Pain Headache Rep. 2013;17:327.
58. Cittadini E, Matharu MS, Goadsby PJ. Paroxysmal hemicrania: a prospective clinical study of 31 cases. Brain. 2008;131:1142–55.
59. Goadsby PJ. Trigeminal autonomic cephalalgias: fancy term or constructive change to the IHS classification? J Neurol Neurosurg Psychiatry. 2005;76:301–5.
60. Williams MH, Broadley SA. SUNCT and SUNA: clinical features and medical treatment. J Clin Neurosci. 2008;15:526–34.
61. Cohen AS, Matharu MS, Goadsby PJ. Short-lasting unilateral neuralgiform headache attacks with conjunctival injection and tearing (SUNCT) or cranial autonomic features (SUNA)—a prospective clinical study of SUNCT and SUNA. Brain. 2006;129:2746–60.
62. Matharu MS, Cohen AS, Boes CJ, Goadsby PJ. Short-lasting unilateral neuralgiform headache with conjunctival injection and tearing syndrome: a review. Curr Pain Headache Rep. 2003;7:308–18.
63. Favoni V, Grimaldi D, Pierangeli G, et al. SUNCT/SUNA and neurovascular compression: new cases and critical literature review. Cephalalgia. 2013;33:1337–48.

Chapter 19
Trigeminal Neuralgia

Kim Nguyen

19.1 Introduction

Trigeminal neuralgia is a chronic neuropathic pain syndrome. It is also known as suicide disease or tic doulourex, after the characteristic facial wince made while experiencing a pain paroxysm [1]. This syndrome is characterized as brief episodes of severe, sudden, shock-like pain unilaterally in the distribution of the trigeminal nerve. The onset and termination of the pain episodes is abrupt in nature [1]. Trigeminal neuralgia can be divided into classical or secondary trigeminal neuralgia.

It typically affects women more than men with a prevalence ratio approximately 1:1.5–1:17 [2, 3]. There are approximately 4.3–27 new diagnosed cases per 100,000 adults each year [4, 5]. Trigeminal neuralgia is typically seen in adults over the age of 40 and increases with age [1, 2, 5–7]. The average age of onset for classical trigeminal neuralgia is 53 years old, while the average age for secondary trigeminal neuralgia is 43 years old [1]. Although it has a low incidence, it is one of the more commonly seen neuralgias in the older population [7]. Trigeminal neuralgia is rarely seen in children and a low percentage of patients experience onset in the second and third decades. The majority of cases are sporadic with only a few rare familial cases being reported [8]. It is unclear what risk factors make patients prone to trigeminal neuralgia. It has been noted that hypertension and migraines may be associated with the development of trigeminal neuralgia although data has been inconsistent [2].

K. Nguyen (✉)
Northwestern University Feinberg School of Medicine, Chicago, IL, USA
e-mail: kim.nguyen@northwestern.edu

K. Shimoji et al. (eds.), *Chronic Pain Management in General and Hospital Practice*, https://doi.org/10.1007/978-981-15-2933-7_19

19.2 Clinical Features

Trigeminal neuralgia is defined as attacks of intense, electrical, shock-like, sharp, or stabbing pain within the distribution of the trigeminal nerve. It typically affects the maxillary or mandibular branches. It is described as sudden and brief lasting seconds to a couple minutes associated with recurrent episodes [4, 9]. It is paroxysmal in natural and the maximal pain is at or near onset. In some cases of severe pain, facial muscle spasms can also occur.

Facial pain associated with trigeminal neuralgia is usually unilateral. If trigeminal neuralgia is present bilaterally, it is rare to experience attacks on both sides of the face simultaneously. The pain typically involves the V2 and V3 distribution of the trigeminal nerve. In rare cases where trigeminal neuralgia has isolated involvement of V1, mild autonomic symptoms may also be present [3]. This includes rhinorrhea, lacrimation, and conjunctival injection.

Many patients have trigger zones along the affected nerve. This leads to patients protecting these areas to avoid onset of attacks. Trigger zones is one of the most defining features to help diagnosis trigeminal neuralgia from other cause of facial pain. These zones are in the trigeminal territory which also includes the oral cavity [10]. In most patients with this clinical feature, pain is triggered by light, non-noxious mechanical stimulus, or facial movements [3]. These movements include chewing, smiling, talking, brushing teeth, shaving, and grimacing [11]. In some cases, even air movement can trigger an attack. The site of pain can differ from the site of stimulation causing some patients to describe the pain as radiating, similar to sciatica. It is rare for patients to only have spontaneous attacks [11]. The presentation of trigeminal neuralgia may originate with spontaneous attacks but later are in response to a defined trigger or a movement that the patient may not be aware of. This may even include blinking of the eye or a twitch of a different facial muscle [11].

"Pretrigeminal neuralgia" has been described in some patients as a dull, aching, continuous pain in the lower face and jaw that evolves into trigeminal neuralgia [12, 13]. Sometimes, this pain is thought to be due to a dental origin leading to unnecessary procedures [14].

Some patients may experience continuous pain between attacks which vary in quality and intensity. This is seen in as many as half of the trigeminal neuralgia patients and is more commonly seen in women [1]. Typically the pain is dull, tingling, or burning, and differs from the paroxysmal pain experienced during attacks [11]. The continuous pain is experienced in the same distribution as the paroxysmal pain [15]. Currently, there is no standardize term for trigeminal neuralgia with the addition of continuous pain but terms such as atypical, trigeminal neuralgia type 2, or trigeminal neuralgia with concomitant continuous pain have been used [11]. This continuous pain is thought to be unrelated to the etiology and can be an additional component in classical or secondary types of trigeminal neuralgia. The etiology of the continuous pain is unclear. It has been suggested that this pain may be the result of central mechanisms or prolonged compression leading to progressive root damage [16, 17]. Regardless of the etiology, patients with continuous pain report poorer outcomes after surgical treatment.

Following a paroxysmal attack, many patients may experience a refractory period where new attacks are unable to be elicited [1]. It has been suggested that this refractory period is due to hyperpolarization of the sensory nerve [18]. The characteristics such as intensity and duration of the preceding attack may contribute to the presence and duration of this refractory period seen in some patients [10]. Similarly, some patients may experience unpredictable periods of time with complete remission. This may span from months to even years. It is proposed that this is due to partial demyelination and reduction in excitability [18].

Additionally, some patients may report mild sensory loss and therefore does not fit exactly into the description of trigeminal neuralgia [4]. These patients with atypical pain often times are more refractory to treatment compared to those with typical symptoms of trigeminal neuralgia.

Some patients may experience autonomic symptoms associated with their facial pain. This includes miosis, ptosis, eyelid edema, conjunctival injection, lacrimation, nasal congestion, rhinorrhea, and sweating [1, 19] Traditionally, autonomic symptoms were not associated with trigeminal neuralgia; however, it has been found that a small subset may experience these additional symptoms [3, 19]. These symptoms are likely associated with the trigeminovascular reflex which can be elicited with severe facial pain.

19.3 Etiology and Pathophysiology

The pathophysiology of trigeminal neuralgia is unclear. One mechanism involves focal demyelination of the nerve near its entry and connection with the pons. It is thought that this area has higher susceptibility or lower resistance to damage due to oligodendroglia being substituted for Schwann cells as the myelin sheath [11]. This is referred to as locus minoris resistentiae [11]. Enlarged blood vessels in this area can compress and throb against the microvasculature of the afferent nerves injuring the myelin sheath and causing this demyelination. As a result, this can lead to hyperactivity and erratic functioning of the trigeminal nerve making it sensitive to stimulation [11].

There are a number of potential causes for this compression. The superior cerebellar artery can have an aberrant branch that can lie on the trigeminal nerve [20]. In addition, aneurysm or cerebellopontine angle tumors can lead to compression. Especially in younger patients, workup for these underlying lesions is essential. Strokes that can cause brainstem disease can also result to neuronal injury in this area.

A second theory proposes that ectopic activity is the result of hyperexcitability due to axonal resting potential being at a level closer to depolarization [21]. The demyelination allows for easier passage of ions and therefore requires more energy to re-establish the resting potential. Since the axons are unable to have enough energy to do so, the rest potential moves closer to the depolarization threshold [21]. Therefore, it makes the axons hyperactive and can spontaneously or with little stimulus trigger an action potential.

19.4 Diagnosis

Diagnosis of trigeminal neuralgia is based on clinical features as described above. The patient's history and description of the pain attacks and triggers are most important in making the diagnosis. A history of unilateral, paroxysmal, severe, electric shock-like pain following a trigger can lead to the diagnosis of clinically established trigeminal neuralgia. It is key to note the onset of pain can assist in making the diagnosis [1]. Once trigeminal neuralgia is suspected, secondary causes of facial pain should be ruled out prior to making the final diagnosis.

MRI can be used to detect tumors, multiple sclerosis, arteriovenous malformations, or abnormalities of the skull base. This accounts for the etiology for approximately 5–10% of cases [22]. Therefore, the threshold to obtain imaging should be low [4]. Additionally, MRI should be considered in younger patients and those with atypical features. This could include dull, constant pain between attacks, or sensory loss. Patients who do not respond to initial medical treatment should also consider neuroimaging [4]. Benefits of MRI also include the ability to help explore surgical options in patients with trigeminal neuralgia.

There are two types of trigeminal neuralgia, classic and secondary. Once other causes of facial pain have been ruled out, neuroimaging can be done to determine between the two. Classic trigeminal neuralgia involves idiopathic trigeminal neuralgia or due to vascular compression of the trigeminal nerve [9]. Classic trigeminal neuralgia is seen in approximately 80–90% of cases [4]. This form of neuralgia requires evidence of no clinically significant neurologic deficits [9]. MRA may be able to identify vascular compressions as the cause of classic trigeminal neuralgia. Compression is typically seen by an aberrant artery or vein at the root entry zone [20].

Secondary trigeminal neuralgia involves painful neuropathy due to a major neurologic disease or structural brain lesion [11]. Examples of these lesions include tumor in the cerebellopontine angle, abnormalities of the skull base, and demyelinating lesions in multiple sclerosis [9]. Approximately 15% of patients with typical pain attacks have symptoms as a result of these benign tumors at this location or MS [9].

Tumors associated with trigeminal neuralgia most often affects the trigeminal root as it enters the pons and is usually benign in nature [11]. Tumors that are infiltrative can result in axonal degeneration, whereas compression causes focal demyelination leading to ectopic discharges. These tumors may be cholesteatomas, acoustic neuromas, epidermoid cysts, or meningioma [11]. Symptoms of malignant tumors typically are associated hyperesthesia and persistent pain differing from the presentation of trigeminal neuralgia [11]. Neuroimaging with MRI with and without contrasts allows for higher resolution compared to CT and can help identify these causes. It has been found that trigeminal neuromas rarely cause trigeminal neuralgia in patients.

Patients with multiple sclerosis have a 20 fold increased risk of developing trigeminal neuralgia [2]. Approximately 1–5% of multiple sclerosis patients will eventually develop trigeminal neuralgia [20]. It is believed that these patients experience both demyelination due to plaques in the pons and neurovascular compression therefore producing an additive mechanism of injury [23]. With this double crush syndrome near the trigeminal root's entry into the pons, these patients are at a high risk of developing trigeminal neuralgia [24]. In some patients, trigeminal neuralgia may be the only presentation of multiple sclerosis. This would lead to further workup likely showing areas of demyelination on MRI and abnormal neurophysiologic tests. In this subset, patients are more likely to experience insufficient relief with pharmacological treatments or require high doses resulting in increased side effects. Therefore, these patients often times require surgical intervention sooner than patient's with classic trigeminal neuralgia [11].

Trigeminal neuropathy can also result in trigeminal neuralgia in some patients [11]. These patients typically present with sensory loss with or without episodes of paroxysmal pain. These attacks can be longer with an additional component of continuous pain [25]. These neuropathies can be post-traumatic. In these cases, patients may report recent facial trauma or dental, maxillofacial or neurosurgical procedures. Additionally, neuropathy can be associated with connective tissue diseases either idiopathic or genetic. For these cases, patients are more likely to have bilateral symptoms as compared to classic trigeminal neuralgia. When diagnosing this form of trigeminal neuralgia, MRI may appear normal but the patient may have delayed or absent trigeminal reflexes [26].

Other workup includes laboratory testing to evaluate renal and liver function as well as sodium levels prior to initiating medical therapy. In addition, an ECG can be done to rule out atrioventricular block since this is a contraindication for first line drug therapy. Electrophysiological testing does not have an established role in diagnosing trigeminal neuralgia. It is unable to clearly distinguish classic from secondary trigeminal neuralgia (Table 19.1).

19.4.1 *Differential Diagnosis*

Other causes of facial pain are more common than trigeminal neuralgia, therefore a through history and physical is necessary. It is essential to determine the time of onset of the facial pain since this will help make the diagnosis. Facial pain preceding or coinciding with a herpes zoster rash in the same distribution is likely secondary to an acute herpes zoster [1]. Painful post-traumatic neuropathy (PPTN) can be the result from facial trauma or invasive dental procedures. This is often times associated with loss or gain of function and other sensory abnormalities that is typically

Table 19.1 Diagnostic criteria of trigeminal neuralgia according to the IHS Classification International Classification of Headache Disorders (ICHD3-beta)

Diagnostic criteria
A. At least three attacks of unilateral facial pain fulfilling criteria B and C
B. Occurring in one or more divisions of the trigeminal nerve, with no radiation beyond the trigeminal distribution
C. Pain has at least three of the following four characteristics:
1. recurring in paroxysmal attacks lasting from a fraction of a second to 2 min
2. severe intensity
3. electric shock-like, shooting, stabbing, or sharp in quality
4. precipitated by innocuous stimuli to the affected side of the face
D. No clinically evident neurological deficit
E. Not better accounted for by another ICHD-3 diagnosis

not seen in trigeminal neuralgia. These additional symptoms in PPTN are associated with damaged peripheral nerve from the injury [27].

Trigeminal neuralgia can also be confused with dental pain therefore location where the pain originates from is important. Trigeminal neuralgia can be triggered by brushing the teeth, chewing, and other oral manipulations leading to a dental concern. Additionally, some patients may have atypical symptoms of trigeminal neuralgia such as tooth or jaw pain which can mimic dental pain. This results in presentation for dental care prior to medical evaluation. On careful history, trigeminal neuralgia can be described as intermittent sharp pain, whereas dental pain is typically described as dull or throbbing.

Patients with bilateral constant pain should be evaluated for various types of headaches. This includes tension-type headaches and cluster-tic syndrome which involves both cluster headaches with coexisting trigeminal neuralgia. Additionally, primary stabbing headache can result in similar symptoms to trigeminal neuralgia. This presents as a sharp and jabbing transient pain often times in the trigeminal and cervical dermatomes. These episodes last a few seconds and can occur at variable times. This is typically differentiated from trigeminal neuralgia due to occasional episodes outside of the trigeminal dermatome. Temporomandibular joint disorder can also have similar characteristics as trigeminal neuralgia but is typically bilateral. Glossopharyngeal neuralgia should be considered in patients with stabbing pain in the back of the tongue, soft palate, pharynx, or deep in the ear. Triggers from this type of neuralgia include sneezing, coughing, and swallowing [1].

Consideration for uncommon causes of craniofacial pain and headache can be made if autonomic symptoms are also present. A differential diagnosis with these symptoms is short-lasting unilateral neuralgiform headache. This can be associated with conjunctival injection and tearing (SUNCT) or with autonomic symptoms (SUNA) [28]. This type of headache involves unilateral sudden brief attacks of head pain. Similar to trigeminal neuralgia, these episodes can be triggered by facial touch. Given the similarities of the presentation and triggers, it can be difficult to differentiate SUNCT, SUNA, and trigeminal neuralgia [28] (Table 19.2).

Table 19.2 Differential diagnosis in trigeminal neuralgia

It is important to get a thorough history and physical when diagnosis trigeminal neuralgia. The patient's facial pain may be associated with precipitating events or others symptoms that may lead to other diagnosis which includes:
Previous trauma
Painful post-traumatic trigeminal neuropathy
Dental-related pain
Musculoskeletal-related pain
Associated with a rash or facial lesions
Acute herpes zosters causing trigeminal neuropathy
Odontogenic differential diagnosis
Dental caries or pulpitis
Dental infection
Cracked tooth
Jaw pain or back of the mouth pain
Dental-related pain
Temporomandibular joint disorders
Glossopharyngeal neuralgia
Bilateral symptoms or forehead pain
Persistent idiopathic pain (previously known as atypical facial pain)
Primary stabbing headache
Tension-type headaches
Cluster headaches or cluster-tic syndrome
Migraines
Occipital neuralgia
Paroxysmal hemicranias (?)
Associated with autonomic symptoms
Short-lasting unilateral neuralgiform headache with conjunctival injection and tearing (SUNCT)
Short-lasting unilateral neuralgiform headache attacks autonomic symptoms (SUNA)
Paroxysmal hemicranias

19.5 Treatment

19.5.1 Medical Treatment

Pharmacologic therapy is the first line treatment for patients with trigeminal neuralgia. Carbamazepine is the initial drug and demonstrates effective medical therapy [4, 9]. It is the best studied and established treatment for classic trigeminal neuralgia. Studies have found complete or near complete pain relief in almost 60% of studied patients compared to 0–40% patients receiving the placebo [9]. The number needed to treat is 1.7 [29, 30]. The mechanism of action of carbamazepine is by acting as a voltage-gated sodium channel blocker [1]. Once ionized in the intracellular fluid, it targets activated voltage-gated sodium channels and prevents action potentials from repetitive and sustained firing. This results in diminished propagation of synaptic impulses. While the drug is bound, this causes the cells to be less excitable. In addition, carbamazepine is known to be a GABA receptor agonist. This additional site of action may contribute to its effective use for neuropathic pain. The initial dose of carbamazepine is 100–200 mg twice daily and is titrated to attain sufficient pain relief. Most patients require 600–800 mg daily as a total maintenance dose with 1200 mg daily being the maximum suggested dose [31]. The drug has slow but good absorption after oral administration.

Although carbamazepine is a known effective drug for medical management of trigeminal neuralgia, there are a number of adverse side effects. Some of these side effects are generally manageable but others are intolerable to some patients. The number needed to harm for severe side effects is 24 and is 3.4 for minor side effects [32]. The most common side effects include drowsiness, nausea, vomiting, and dizziness [31]. This is typically avoided with slow titration. Additionally, carbamazepine is a known CYP450 inducer resulting in drug interaction and increased clearance of other drugs [31]. Leukopenia is not an uncommon side effect of carbamazepine. This results in changes in the production of red blood cells, white blood cells, and platelets. Rarely, these effects can result in aplastic anemia. Other side effects include increased risk of suicide, hyponatremia, and SIADH. With quick discontinuation of the medication, patients have an increased risk of seizures [31]. The most serious and potentially fatal adverse effects include dangerous skin reactions such as Stevens–Johnson syndrome and toxic epidermal necrolysis [31, 33]. There is an increased risk of development of these fatal skin reactions with patients on carbamazepine who have the HLA-B∗15:02 allele. This human leukocyte antigen allele is almost exclusively in patients of Asian descent so screening is recommended in this population prior to initiating carbamazepine therapy [33]. Even if one copy of the HLA-B∗15:02 allele is identified on genetic testing, this drug should be avoided.

If carbamazepine is ineffective, incomplete, or intolerable, adding a second drug or switching drugs may be the next option [11]. Oxcarbazepine is an alternative medication used in treatment of trigeminal neuralgia. It is a prodrug of carbamazepine and studies have been shown that it has similar efficiency. It is structurally similar to carbamazepine and therefore has the same mechanism of action but has shown to have fewer side effects [34]. This includes a lesser impact on the liver during metabolism and less severe forms of agranulocytosis. Nevertheless, due to it similar structure, it is important to screen patients of Asian descent for HLA-B∗1502 allele due to the increased risk of developing fatal skin reactions [34]. Furthermore, oxcarbazepine has a 25% risk of allergic cross reactivity and should be avoided in carbamazepine allergy [4].

Gabapentin is widely used and effective for neuropathic pain although evidence is lacking for its use in trigeminal neuralgia [4]. Gabapentin is used based on the fact that trigeminal neuralgia is a neuropathic pain and is familiar for providers. Other medical treatment options include baclofen, lamotrigine, and pimozide. In patients who failed monotherapy with carbamazepine, a combination of these alternative medications may be beneficial. Patients with trigeminal neuralgia refractory to pharmacologic therapy, botulinum toxin injections may be an option although there is limited data.

In cases of severe exacerbations, patients may require inpatient treatment with hydration and titration of antiepileptic medication. Some patients may be treated with an intravenous loading dose of fosphenytoin although there is limited evidence for this practice [1].

19.5.2 Image-Guided Nerve Block

Injections of local anesthetic and steroids can be done for immediate and long-term pain relief. These are typically performed under image-guidance with fluoroscopy, computed tomography, or ultrasound. The target is the pterygopalatine fossa which allows spread of the injectate to Meckel's cave [35, 36]. This is the location of the trigeminal ganglion within the middle cranial fossa [35]. The result is sensory analgesia or a numbness sensation in the distribution of the trigeminal nerve. Side effects include a facial droop due to the close proximity of the motor nucleus of the facial nerve [35] (Fig. 19.1).

19.5.3 Surgical Treatment

Patients who fail conservative management may be candidates for surgical intervention after review of the diagnosis and etiology. Although surgical treatment has been found to be more effective for trigeminal neuralgia compared to other neuropathic

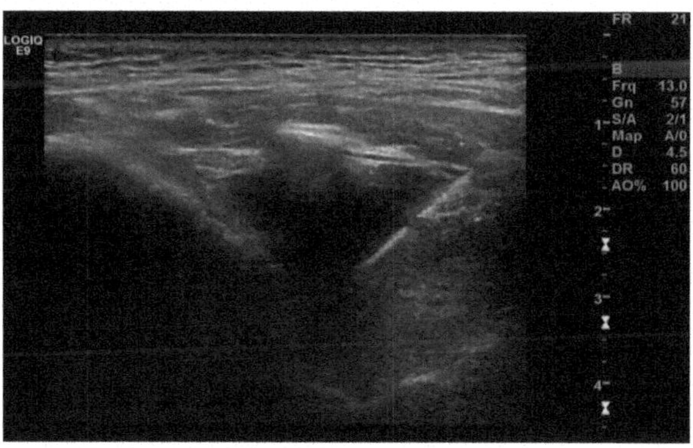

Fig. 19.1 Ultrasound image of a nerve block with the needle in place to inject into the pterygopalatine fossa. The ultrasound probe is placed below the zygomatic bone, superior to the mandibular notch, and anterior to the mandibular condyle. The medication is injected anterior to the lateral pterygoid plate and below the lateral pterygoid muscle into the desired fossa. Image by Dr. Antoun Nader at Northwestern Memorial Hospital

pain syndromes, medical management remains the first line. Patients who continue to have severe symptoms despite usual doses of medication or experience severe side effects should begin discussion about surgical intervention [4]. In some cases, given the possibility of long-lasting pain relief, patient may opt for early surgical treatment.

Surgical treatment involves microvascular decompression or ablative treatment which involves lesioning of the trigeminal nerve. The location of the targeted lesion must be considered when choosing the type of surgical procedure. The four locations to consider include interventions in the posterior fossa, at the level of the trigeminal ganglion, at the root of the nerve, and areas distal to the ganglion.

19.5.3.1 Microvascular Decompression

Within the posterior fossa, microvascular decompression involves the separation or removal of vascular structures surrounding the trigeminal nerve [37]. Microvascular decompression is the first choice treatment if indicated [1]. This is a major neurosurgical procedure involving craniotomy, access into the dura, cerebellar hemisphere shifting, and microscopy in order to visualize the desired structures. The cerebellopontine angle is identified which is where the nerve emerges. Often times an ectatic superior cerebellar artery is extricated and separated from the trigeminal root [37].

Studies suggest that this procedure provides the longest duration of pain control among the surgical options [11]. According to the AAN/EFNS guidelines, microvascular depression is the most efficacious and up to 90% of patients achieve pain relief [9]. As many as 80% of patients remain symptom free at 1 year and approximately 73% were pain free at 5 years [11].

The most common complication is aseptic meningitis (11%) [11]. Major complications include cerebrospinal fluid leaks, hematoma, and infarction which account for up to 4% of patients. Other complications include long-term hearing loss and sensory loss [9]. The average mortality for this procedure is 0.2% [11]. There is also a chance that the neurosurgeons do not find significant damage of the nerve from neurovascular compression. Given this possibility of failure, it is essential to identify morphologic changes of the nerve root on MRI. Therefore, it is important to have a collaborative approach with the neurosurgeon, neurologist, and patient to determine the best treatment modality (Fig. 19.2).

19.5.3.2 Percutaneous Procedures

Percutaneous procedures are typically done in patients with recurrent pain following microvascular decompression or have high surgical risk from other medical comorbidities. These less invasive procedures are more likely to be done in patients age 65 years or older although studies show that outcomes from microvascular decompression are similar in this population compared to younger patients [39].

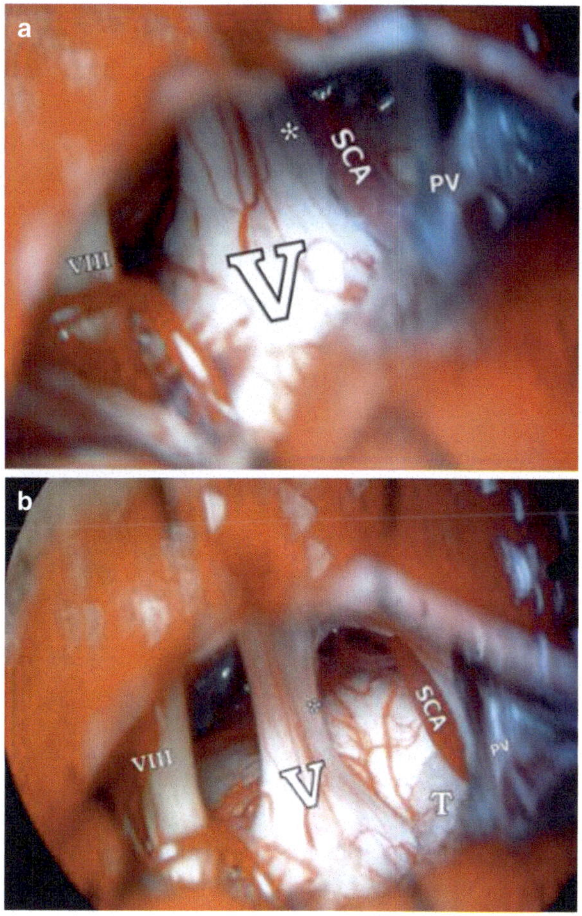

Fig. 19.2 The goal of microvascular decompression is separation of the neurovascular interaction irritating the trigeminal nerve (V). A prosthesis can be inserted to keep the vascular structure away from the nerve. (**a**) This image shows the superior cerebellar artery (SCA) in contact with the trigeminal nerve. (**b**) After separation of the SCA from the trigeminal nerve, a Teflon wadding (T) was placed to help secure the SCA and prevent further interaction. VIII vestibulocochlear nerve, PV petrosal vein. Reproduced with permission from Surgical Technique of Microvascular Decompression Surgery for Trigeminal Neuralgia [38]

Additionally, patients with multiple sclerosis are usually offered percutaneous procedures due to the etiology of pain and higher chance of satisfaction following this type of surgical intervention [40]. In general, percutaneous procedures involve producing injury to the trigeminal nerve.

To treat at the level of the trigeminal ganglion or the nerve root, rhizotomy is the surgical treatment of choice. Rhizotomy is a percutaneous surgical procedure that allows for lesioning at this specific site. It is performed using a cannula or electrode first inserted through the cheek [11]. It is then passed between the maxillary bone and mandibular arch to the infratemporal fossa. The target is the foramen ovale which is used to reach the location of the trigeminal ganglion [11]. These procedures are typically done under fluoroscopy although using computed tomography (CT) has been suggested [41] (Fig. 19.3).

Radiofrequency thermocoagulation uses heat to create a lesion of the trigeminal ganglion or nerve. This has been found to be beneficial for lesioning small pain fibers [11]. Anesthesia is required for placement of the electrode at the desired target

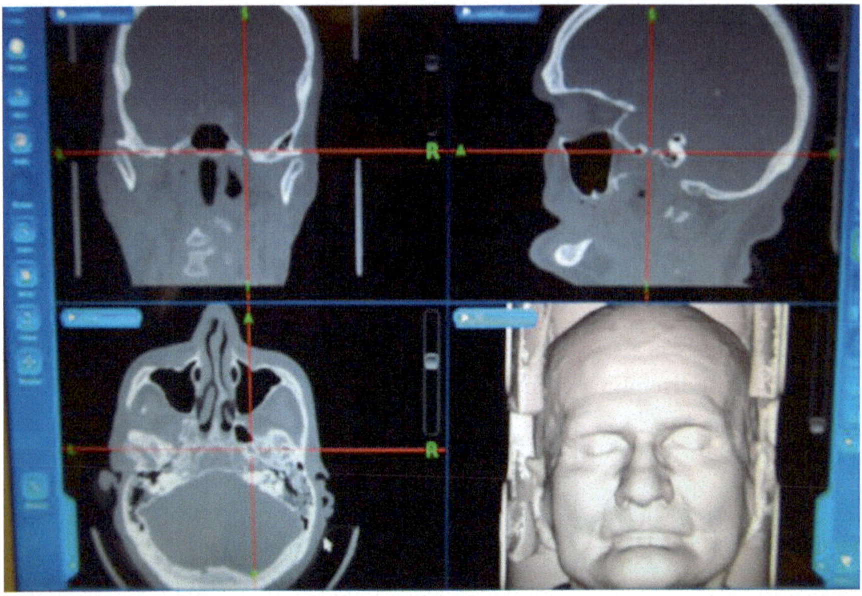

Fig. 19.3 CT based images in the coronal, axial, and sagittal views showing the foramen ovale. Reproduced with permission from Interventional Management of Head and Face Pain [41]

and at the time of lesioning. Between these moments, patients must be awake in order to report any paresthesia evoked by the tip of the electrode. This is necessary in order to prevent lesioning the wrong division of the trigeminal nerve [11]. The electrode is advanced slowly until paresthesia is evoked at the distribution of his or her symptoms. The patient is then anesthetized again in order to perform the thermocoagulation. The thermal lesion is produced by an alternating electrical field with an oscillating frequency [42].

This method cannot target the first trigeminal division due to the risk of damaging small fibers leading to complications involving corneal deafferentation and keratitis [11]. Benefits of percutaneous interventions are immediate and complete relief in the majority of cases. Risks include injury to the maxillary artery or the dura mater that covers the Meckel's cave [11]. Additionally, some patients may experience sensory deficits within the distribution of the trigeminal nerve that is more lasting and severe following radiofrequency than the other methods [11].

Mechanical balloon compression compresses the ganglion using a Fogarty catheter. The procedure is done under general anesthesia and does not require the patient to be awakened. Once the area has been reached under fluoroscopy, the balloon is introduced and inflated for approximately 1–2 min [43]. There have been reports of compression time as long as 10 min [44]. The usual limited compression time decreases the risk of severe numbness or masseter muscle weakness [45]. Following compression, the catheter used to reach the desired target and the balloon are removed. Patients typically experience pain relief immediately following surgery. Side effects more specific to balloon compression is permanent motor root weakness seen in approximately 3% of cases [46].

Chemical rhizolysis causes a lesion by injecting glycerol, a mild neurolytic, into the trigeminal cistern [47]. This procedure is based on the patient's anatomy. It is not necessary for the patient to be awakened during the procedure although some surgeons may prefer it [43]. Once the trigeminal cistern is identified, glycerol is injected under continuous fluoroscopy. The glycerol remains in contact with the nerve for 1–2 h as the patient is kept in the same position. Patients typically experience pain relief immediately or within a couple days following surgery. In some cases, it may take up to 2 weeks while others recommend a repeat procedure if there is no pain relief within one week [48]. Side effects include mild numbness to profound sensory loss. In patients with treatment to the V1 division, a side effect could be corneal hypoesthesia [43].

Both mechanical balloon compression and glycerol injection are used to block triggering impulses by targeting the large myelinated fibers. By avoiding small fibers, this decreases the risk of corneal keratitis as seen with radiofrequency thermocoagulation [11].

Lesions may be located distal to the trigeminal ganglion at the site of emergence from the facial bones. For these lesions, options include radiofrequency lesions, neurectomy, alcohol injections, or cryolesions [11]. These procedures are able to target the branches of the trigeminal nerve. These branches include the lingual, alveolar, infraorbital, and supraorbital nerves.

Rare complications from percutaneous procedures for treatment of trigeminal neuralgia include stroke, hemorrhage, CSF rhinorrhea, and pseudomeningocele. Additionally, permanent hearing loss, facial weakness or trochlear nerve, or abducens nerve palsy causing diplopia may also occur [43, 46] (Fig. 19.4).

19.5.3.3 Radiosurgery

Radiosurgery is another treatment option that uses focused gamma radiation to produce lesions. This is referred to as stereotactic radiosurgery or gamma knife. Using MRI and a stereotactic frame, beams are directed at the proximal trigeminal root,

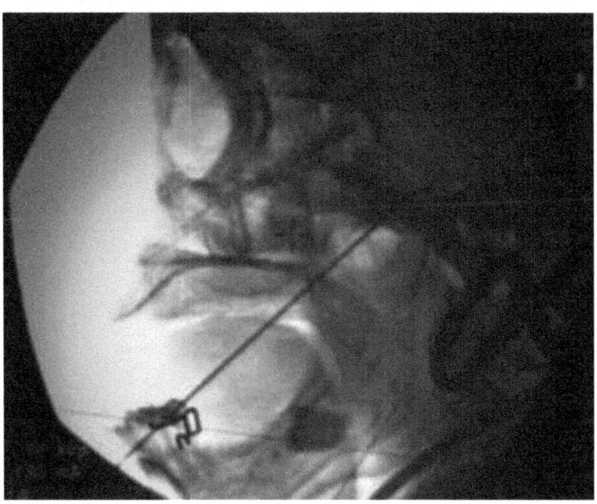

Fig. 19.4 Lateral view of a radiofrequency ablation of the trigeminal ganglion. The tip of the needle is over the petrous bone and is seen going through the foramen ovale. Reproduced with permission from Interventional Management of Head and Face Pain [49]

nerve, or ganglion [20]. This causes lesions in the form of axonal degeneration and necrosis [20]. Like other stereotactic radiosurgery interventions, the major issue is finding the exact location of the trigeminal root to direct the radiation beams [11]. Unlike other interventions that provide immediate relief, patient typically experience pain relief within 4–8 weeks, with maximal relief within 3 months. Many report a decrease in pain relief by 3 years [9]. In a subset of patients who do not achieve pain relief lasting one year, repeat radiation may be required. With additional procedures, findings show the time of pain free and the rate of success significantly increases. The risk of facial hypesthesia also increases with more interventions and should be considered during management.

Side effects of stereotactic radiosurgery include new or worsened sensory loss, paresthesia or pain but anesthesia dolorosa has rarely been reported [9]. Some patients report that these symptoms following the procedure may be more bothersome than the initial symptoms of trigeminal neuralgia.

19.5.3.4 Anesthesia Dolorosa

A major side effect and feared complication of surgical intervention is anesthesia dolorosa, a painful post-traumatic neuropathy [50]. Although surgical intervention is typically well-tolerated, some patients may experience a painful, persistent anesthesia, or hypesthesia in the region of denervation. In some cases, this sensory change can be more intolerable than the initial symptoms of trigeminal neuralgia [9]. This complication is more commonly seen with rhizotomy or thermocoagulation.

19.5.3.5 Considerations

The risks must be considered when deciding what procedure to do. Except for stereotactic radiosurgery due its delayed onset of relief, the other surgical options have a high initial response rate [4]. Microvascular decompression has been found to have the highest chance of pain relief long term. It has a very low risk of minor complications and sensory loss but has a 0.4% risk of death [39]. Long term, ablative procedures are less effective and facial numbness and minor complications are more likely to occur. However, the effectiveness of the procedure is greatest in patients who develop these additional symptoms [51]. Ablative procedures have much lower risk of major complications or death and therefore are used for those with high operative risk or in those with atypical features.

19.6 Prognosis

Trigeminal neuralgia is a waxing and waning syndrome and differs among patients. Patients may experience intermittent episodes lasting as long as weeks or months then have periods of pain-free intervals. Some patients may have persistent facial pain between episodes and recurrence is common [4]. Medication therapy can provide pain relief for many although there is a high risk of side effects. Others require surgical intervention depending on their etiology. Case series shows that patients with classical trigeminal neuralgia with evidence of vascular compression respond better to surgical management. Those with no prior surgeries and a shorter duration of disease were also found to have better outcomes with surgical intervention [4].

19.7 Case Report #1

A 58-year-old female presented to the pain medicine clinic with 6 weeks of facial pain. She described the pain on the left side of her face that is intermittent. She described the pain as sharp and like a "zing" that suddenly comes on. Between the episodes, she does not experience pain. She noticed that the pain usually comes on when she is eating. She initially thought it was dental pain but recently had an unremarkable dentist appointment. The patient saw her primary care doctor who prescribed pain medications but this did not result in resolution of her symptoms.

On exam, cranial nerves I–XII were intact. She did grimace when pressure was applied to the left side of her face. Given that her symptoms were consistent with trigeminal neuralgia, she was prescribed carbamazepine. Additionally, she was scheduled for MRI of her brain to rule out major neurologic diseases. The patient also received orders for a CBC and CMP blood work.

The patient returned to clinic one month later and reported that her symptoms have resolved. The MRI of her brain showed neurovascular compression at the trigeminal root. She instructed to continue the carbamazepine, since she has adequate pain relief.

Comment This patient presented to the pain clinic with typical symptoms of trigeminal neuralgia. She described electrical pain that was triggered with movement. In addition, she did not get relief with pain medicine and she recently had a dental appointment with no abnormalities. Given the clinical features the patient presented with, it is appropriate to begin medical treatment for trigeminal neuralgia prior to obtaining imaging or lab reports. The etiology of the trigeminal neuralgia should be investigated but medical therapy should not be delayed.

19.8 Case Report #2

The patient was continued on carbamazepine for three years with adequate relief of her symptoms until recently. She has noticed that her symptoms have become more severe and frequent within the last couple months. She initially had her dose of carbamazepine increased but she had drowsiness and nausea that was affecting her daily activities. She had an MRI done showing vascular structures in close proximity of her trigeminal ganglion. She was offered a second line drug in combination with a lower dose of carbamazepine but she was hesitant given her symptoms.

Due to the etiology of her trigeminal neuralgia as seen in the MRI, microvascular decompression was discussed. It was explained that this is a major surgical procedure but it could possibly provide long-term relief. Her other past medical history includes hypertension and reports that she walks several miles regularly for exercise. She was deemed an appropriate candidate for the procedure and risks and benefits were explained. The patient proceeded with surgery.

On her 3 months follow-up appointment, she stated that she no longer has any symptoms and is able to live her life without worrying about having a trigeminal neuralgia pain attack. She was happy she underwent the procedure and hopes that she will continue to remain pain free.

Comment: It is not uncommon for patients to have difficulty tolerating medical therapy and continue to have severe pain. If this is the case, surgical intervention may be an option. It is important to determine the etiology of the trigeminal neuralgia to help guide management. Microvascular decompression is the most common and has the possibility of providing the longest duration of pain relief. Despite this, it is a major neurological surgery so it is essential to consider a patient's comorbidities and risks for surgery.

19.9 Summary

Trigeminal neuralgia is a chronic neuropathic pain syndrome that typically affects adults over the age of 40. It is described as pain episodes of brief, severe, sudden, shock-like unilateral facial pain. It can last from seconds to minutes and can be repetitive. The pain attacks can be triggered by light touch, movement of the jaw, or even air flow. Management includes medical therapy with carbamazepine being the first line medication. Surgical options are also available for microvascular decompression or ablative treatment. This pain syndrome can cause a significant impact on a patient's quality of life.

References

1. Maarbjerg S, Di Stefano G, Bendtsen L, Cruccu G. Trigeminal neuralgia—diagnosis and treatment. Cephalalgia. 2017;37(7):648–57.
2. Katusic S, Beard CM, Bergstralh E, Kurland LT. Incidence and clinical features of trigeminal neuralgia, Rochester, Minnesota, 1945–1984. Ann Neurol. 1990;27(1):89–95.
3. Maarbjerg S, Gozalov A, Olesen J, Bendtsen L. Trigeminal neuralgia--a prospective systematic study of clinical characteristics in 158 patients. Headache. 2014;54(10):1574–82.
4. Bennetto L, Patel NK, Fuller G. Trigeminal neuralgia and its management. BMJ. 2007;334(7586):201–5.
5. MacDonald BK, Cockerell OC, Sander JW, Shorvon SD. The incidence and lifetime prevalence of neurological disorders in a prospective community-based study in the UK. Brain J Neurol. 2000;123(Pt 4):665–76.

6. Mueller D, Obermann M, Yoon M-S, Poitz F, Hansen N, Slomke M-A, et al. Prevalence of trigeminal neuralgia and persistent idiopathic facial pain: a population-based study. Cephalalgia. 2011;31(15):1542–8.
7. Childs AM, Meaney JF, Ferrie CD, Holland PC. Neurovascular compression of the trigeminal and glossopharyngeal nerve: three case reports. Arch Dis Child. 2000;82(4):311–5.
8. Fleetwood IG, Innes AM, Hansen SR, Steinberg GK. Familial trigeminal neuralgia. Case report and review of the literature. J Neurosurg. 2001;95(3):513–7.
9. Gronseth G, Cruccu G, Alksne J, Argoff C, Brainin M, Burchiel K, et al. Practice parameter: the diagnostic evaluation and treatment of trigeminal neuralgia (an evidence-based review): report of the Quality Standards Subcommittee of the American Academy of Neurology and the European Federation of Neurological Societies. Neurology. 2008;71(15):1183–90.
10. Kugelberg E, Lindblom U. The mechanism of the pain in trigeminal neuralgia. J Neurol Neurosurg Psychiatry. 1959;22(1):36–43.
11. Cruccu G. Trigeminal Neuralgia. Contin Minneap Minn. 2017;23(2):396–420.
12. Fromm GH, Graff-Radford SB, Terrence CF, Sweet WH. Pre-trigeminal neuralgia. Neurology. 1990;40(10):1493–5.
13. Evans RW, Graff-Radford SB, Bassiur JP. Pretrigeminal neuralgia. Headache. 2005;45(3):242–4.
14. von Eckardstein KL, Keil M, Rohde V. Unnecessary dental procedures as a consequence of trigeminal neuralgia. Neurosurg Rev. 2015;38(2):355–60. discussion 360.
15. Brisman R. Typical versus atypical trigeminal neuralgia and other factors that may affect results of neurosurgical treatment. World Neurosurg. 2013;79(5–6):649–50.
16. Burchiel KJ. A new classification for facial pain. Neurosurgery. 2003;53(5):1164–6. discussion 1166–1167.
17. Obermann M, Yoon M-S, Ese D, Maschke M, Kaube H, Diener H-C, et al. Impaired trigeminal nociceptive processing in patients with trigeminal neuralgia. Neurology. 2007;69(9):835–41.
18. Devor M, Amir R, Rappaport ZH. Pathophysiology of trigeminal neuralgia: the ignition hypothesis. Clin J Pain. 2002;18(1):4–13.
19. Simms HN, Honey CR. The importance of autonomic symptoms in trigeminal neuralgia. Clinical article. J Neurosurg. 2011;115(2):210–6.
20. Nurmikko TJ, Eldridge PR. Trigeminal neuralgia—pathophysiology, diagnosis and current treatment. Br J Anaesth. 20011;87(1):117–32.
21. Burchiel KJ. Abnormal impulse generation in focally demyelinated trigeminal roots. J Neurosurg. 1980;53(5):674–83.
22. Cheng TM, Cascino TL, Onofrio BM. Comprehensive study of diagnosis and treatment of trigeminal neuralgia secondary to tumors. Neurology. 1993;43(11):2298–302.
23. Love S, Coakham HB. Trigeminal neuralgia: pathology and pathogenesis. Brain J Neurol. 2001;124(Pt 12):2347–60.
24. Truini A, Barbanti P, Pozzilli C, Cruccu G. A mechanism-based classification of pain in multiple sclerosis. J Neurol. 2013;260(2):351–67.
25. Benoliel R, Zadik Y, Eliav E, Sharav Y. Peripheral painful traumatic trigeminal neuropathy: clinical features in 91 cases and proposal of novel diagnostic criteria. J Orofac Pain. 2012;26(1):49–58.
26. Cruccu G, Pennisi EM, Antonini G, Biasiotta A, di Stefano G, La Cesa S, et al. Trigeminal isolated sensory neuropathy (TISN) and FOSMN syndrome: despite a dissimilar disease course do they share common pathophysiological mechanisms? BMC Neurol. 2014;14:248.
27. Ramesh VG, Premkumar G. An anatomical study of the neurovascular relationships at the trigeminal root entry zone. J Clin Neurosci Off J Neurosurg Soc Australas. 2009;16(7): 934–6.
28. Lambru G, Matharu MS. SUNCT, SUNA and trigeminal neuralgia: different disorders or variants of the same disorder? Curr Opin Neurol. 2014;27(3):325–31.
29. Killian JM, Fromm GH. Carbamazepine in the treatment of neuralgia. Use of side effects. Arch Neurol. 1968;19(2):129–36.
30. Wiffen PJ, Derry S, Moore RA, Kalso EA. Carbamazepine for chronic neuropathic pain and fibromyalgia in adults. Cochrane Database Syst Rev. 2014;4:CD005451.

31. Label: Carbamazepine—carbamazepine capsule, extended release [Internet]. Available from: https://dailymed.nlm.nih.gov/dailymed/drugInfo.cfm?setid=7a1e523a-b377-43dc-b231-7591c4c888ea.
32. Cruccu G, Gronseth G, Alksne J, Argoff C, Brainin M, Burchiel K, et al. AAN-EFNS guidelines on trigeminal neuralgia management. Eur J Neurol. 2008;15(10):1013–28.
33. Leckband SG, Kelsoe JR, Dunnenberger HM, George AL, Tran E, Berger R, et al. Clinical Pharmacogenetics Implementation Consortium guidelines for HLA-B genotype and carbamazepine dosing. Clin Pharmacol Ther. 2013;94(3):324–8.
34. Label: Oxcarbazepine—oxcarbazepine tablet [Internet]. Available from: https://dailymed.nlm.nih.gov/dailymed/drugInfo.cfm?setid=17325a80-fb9c-4a83-b4b4-98e0b999d852.
35. Nader A, Kendall MC, De Oliveria GS, Chen JQ, Vanderby B, Rosenow JM, et al. Ultrasound-guided trigeminal nerve block via the pterygopalatine fossa: an effective treatment for trigeminal neuralgia and atypical facial pain. Pain Physician. 2013;16(5):E537–45.
36. Nader A, Schittek H, Kendall MC. Lateral pterygoid muscle and maxillary artery are key anatomical landmarks for ultrasound-guided trigeminal nerve block. Anesthesiology. 2013;118(4):957.
37. Jannetta PJ. Microsurgical management of trigeminal neuralgia. Arch Neurol. 1985;42(8):800.
38. Zhong J, Sun H. Surgical technique of microvascular decompression surgery for trigeminal neuralgia. In: Li S-T, Zhong J, Sekula RF, editors. Microvascular decompression surgery [Internet]. Dordrecht: Springer; 2016. p. 67–77. Available from: http://link.springer.com/10.1007/978-94-017-7366-9_6.
39. Ashkan K, Marsh H. Microvascular decompression for trigeminal neuralgia in the elderly: a review of the safety and efficacy. Neurosurgery. 2004;55(4):840–8. discussion 848–850.
40. Brisman R. Treatment of trigeminal neuralgia associated with multiple sclerosis. World Neurosurg. 2014;81(3–4):497–8.
41. Van Buyten JP. Interventional treatment for trigeminal neuralgia: radiofrequency and neuromodulation. In: Narouze S, editor. Interventional management of head and face pain [Internet]. New York, NY: Springer; 2014. p. 59–64. Available from: http://link.springer.com/10.1007/978-1-4614-8951-1_9.
42. Sluijter M, Racz G. Technical aspects of radiofrequency. Pain Pract Off J World Inst Pain. 2002;2(3):195–200.
43. Winn HR, Youmans JR, editors. Youmans and Winn neurological surgery. 7th ed. Philadelphia, PA: Elsevier; 2017. p. 1405–11.
44. Skirving DJ, Dan NG. A 20-year review of percutaneous balloon compression of the trigeminal ganglion. J Neurosurg. 2001;94(6):913–7.
45. Brown JA, Pilitsis JG. Percutaneous balloon compression for the treatment of trigeminal neuralgia: results in 56 patients based on balloon compression pressure monitoring. Neurosurg Focus. 2005;18(5):E10.
46. Taha J. Trigeminal neuralgia: percutaneous procedures. Semin Neurosurg. 2004;15(2–3):115–34.
47. Håkanson S. Trigeminal neuralgia treated by the injection of glycerol into the trigeminal cistern. Neurosurgery. 1981;9(6):638–46.
48. Liu JK, Apfelbaum RI. Treatment of trigeminal neuralgia. Neurosurg Clin N Am. 2004;15(3):319–34.
49. Narouze SN. Trigeminal (Gasserian) ganglion, maxillary nerve, and mandibular nerve blocks. In: Interventional management of head and face pain [Internet]. New York, NY: Springer; 2014. p. 53–7. Available from: http://link.springer.com/10.1007/978-1-4614-8951-1_8.
50. Headache Classification Committee of the International Headache Society (IHS). The international classification of headache disorders, 3rd edition (beta version). Cephalalgia. 2013;133(9):629–808.
51. Lopez BC, Hamlyn PJ, Zakrzewska JM. Systematic review of ablative neurosurgical techniques for the treatment of trigeminal neuralgia. Neurosurgery. 2004;54(4):973–82. discussion 982–983.

Chapter 20
Orofacial Pain

Maxim S. Eckmann and Antoun Nader

20.1 Introduction

Facial pain is defined as pain between the orbitomeatal line and the neck, anterior to the ear pinne. The face includes the oral and nasal cavity, the sinuses, the orbital cavity, and the temporomandibular joint. Chronic and acute facial pain cause a high degree of suffering and health care costs world-wide, with a prevalence of approximately 3–4% [1]. Facial pain can be a challenging disorder to diagnose and treat for many reasons. A diversity of anatomic structures in the head and neck contribute to facial pain, to include the upper cervical spine, teeth, jaw, sinuses, blood vessels, and soft tissue structures. The nervous system can also become diseased, therefore neuralgias of these pathways create pain that can be perceived in any of the aforementioned structures. Lifetime prevalence of pain stemming from trigeminal neuralgia has been estimated at 0.3% [2]; however, specialists in referral centers such as pain physicians, neurologists, and neurosurgeons are likely to encounter a disproportionate number of cases. Persistent idiopathic facial pain, or atypical facial pain, also has about a 0.3% lifetime prevalence [2].

Complicating the understanding of facial pain is the diversity of classifications throughout history [3]. Pain can be defined by the specific anatomic structure involved (e.g., temporomandibular joint), by underlying pathology and pathophysiology including malignancy, infection, neuropathy, or inflammatory. Additionally temporal and regional qualifiers, as in other pain states, have been used to classify orofacial pain. Often, patients present to both physicians and dentists for this reason; therefore, both fields require significant crossover of awareness to adequately assess orofacial pain.

M. S. Eckmann (✉)
Executive Medical Director of Pain Medicine Director, Interventional Pain Therapy at St. Lukes Baptist Hospital Director, Translational Research Professor, Department of Anesthesiology UT Health San Antonio, Texas, USA
e-mail: eckmann@uthscsa.edu

A. Nader
Feinberg School of Medicine, Northwestern University, Chicago, IL, USA
e-mail: anader@nm.org

K. Shimoji et al. (eds.), *Chronic Pain Management in General and Hospital Practice*, https://doi.org/10.1007/978-981-15-2933-7_20

20.2 Neuroanatomy of Facial Pain

Primary afferent neurons project from the mouth and face mostly via the trigeminal (cranial nerve V; ophthalmic, maxillary, and mandibular divisions) through the trigeminal (a.k.a. Gasserian) ganglion to second order neurons in the trigeminocervical brain stem complex and trigeminal sensory nuclei. These second order neurons then project to cortical and subcortical areas including the reticular formation, thalamus, and cranial nerve nuclei. Afferents also come from cranial nerve VII (facial), IX (glossopharyngeal), X (vagus), and XII (hypoglossal) to the trigeminocervical brain stem complex. Cranial nerves VII, IX, and X send nociceptive fibers with CN VII through the geniculate ganglion towards the trigeminal nucleus in the middle cranial fossa. The nucleus caudalis portion of the trigeminal sensory nucleus is particularly involved in pathways of craniofacial pain. These second order neurons then travel and synapse with third order neurons in the ventral posteromedial nucleus (VPM), where connections between the ventral trigeminothalamic tract and dorsal trigeminothalamic tract occur. Third order neurons then project to the postcentral gyrus.

Pain sensitive structures in the face or affecting the face include skin, subcutaneous tissue, muscles, periosteum, dura, nerves, and ganglia (trigeminal, glossopharyngeal, vagus, hypoglossal, spinal nerves C1–C3). The complexity and preponderance of neural innervation of the face leads to a diversity of neuralgias from any diseases, trauma, or surgery that invade them. Therefore, facial pain can be caused by several neuralgias including trigeminal neuralgia, glossopharyngeal neuralgia, geniculate neuralgia (e.g., post-herpetic neuralgia/Ramsay Hunt syndrome type 2), and cervical spine disease or radiculopathy at C2 or above. Generally, treatment of pain stemming from these neuropathies includes membrane stabilizing anti-neuropathic pain medications, possible definitive surgical interventions where warranted, control of systemic causes (e.g., autoimmune), and percutaneous injections or ablation procedures where available for accessible structures.

20.3 Trigeminal Neuralgia

Trigeminal neuralgia (TN) is an often severely painful condition that causes significant suffering and reduced quality of life. If untreated or sub-optimally controlled, it can be highly associated with depression and even suicidal ideation. The trigeminal nerve has mixed motor and sensory function and is the largest cranial nerve. The description of the condition was originally credited to Drs. Johannes Michael Fehr and Elias Schmidt in the 1600s, and philosopher John Locke who wrote a detailed letter in 1677 [4]. However, translations of Persian writings dating back to 1000 AD also appear to describe TN. The shooting nature of TN was captured in the term coined by Nicolas Andrade as *tic douloureux*; it was accompanied by obvious outward signs of distress and appeared to be like a convulsion. It was not until the early

1800s that the trigeminal nerve was identified as the anatomic source of the condition. Trigeminal mediated pain is now classified as typical and atypical TN, or TN and TN type 2; typical or classic symptoms are characterized by severe unilateral shooting or shock-like pain in usually one of the dermatomal or sclerotomal distributions of the trigeminal divisions. Over 95% of the time V2 (maxillary) or V3 (mandibular) are involved. Attacks may last seconds to minutes and can be triggered by facial stimulus including light touch, temperature changes, talking, and chewing. However, TN attacks may also be paroxysmal. Patients who have recalcitrant TN may report weight loss due to aversion to eating. In the clinic office, patients with talking triggers may sound as if their voice is muffled due to compensation for the trigger. TN2, by comparison, is a constant dull or burning pain, possibly associated with prickling. TN2 notably has a significant background pain element that is present over 50% of the time [5]. Trigeminal neuropathy also can cause neuropathic pain but is differentiated by signs of impaired neurologic function and can stem from a host of specific causes such as trauma, tumor, or systemic disease. Trigeminal deafferentation pain (TDP), or *anesthesia dolorosa*, is pain in the distribution of an ablated or destroyed trigeminal nerve that has lost sensory function.

20.3.1 Pathophysiology

The common pathophysiologic process of trigeminal pain syndromes is thought to be the segmental demyelination of the ganglion or dorsal root [6]; in classic TN, this occurs near the dorsal root entry zone, but it could occur more peripherally as well for trigeminal pain. TN was observed to be associated with the presence of nearby vascular loops and it was proposed [7] pressure from the superior cerebellar artery was a common culprit. The anterior inferior cerebellar artery may also be involved to a lesser degree. Decompression of this artery, for which a microscopic procedure was developed by Dr. Peter Jannetta [8], remains an effective surgical technique in the event of vascular abutment of the nerve near the connection with the pons. Atrophy or nerve distortion, however, are considered to be necessary to form a causal relationship between pain and blood vessel contact. Overall typical TN is thought to be caused by neurovascular conflict in 80–90% of cases [9].

Several other diseases may cause trigeminal pain that is reminiscent of TN. Bilateral symptoms should be very uncommon, so the evaluating provider should be alerted to a possible systemic cause. It is estimated that multiple sclerosis (MS) is seen in 2–4% of patients with trigeminal pain or TN, and the pain may be the presenting symptom of the disease [10]. V1 distribution pain can be more commonly seen in MS as well. MS patients are 20 times more likely to develop TN than the general population [9]. Atypical TN may in some cases reflect a posterior fossa meningioma or other neoplasm. Post-herpetic neuralgia can also present in the V1 distribution and is usually preceded by viral vesicles. In some cases, the cause of TN cannot be determined and is otherwise idiopathic.

20.3.2 Imaging Evaluation

MRI is the most useful single imaging examination to evaluate causes of TN [9]. Most facilities have specific protocols to evaluate the trigeminal nerve pathway so orders should reflect the indication for the exam. If an inflammatory, infectious, or malignant process is suspected, then contrast enhancement may be indicated. MRI may detect not only vascular impingement with nerve geometry changes, but may also detect other lesions in the brain and cranial vault that may explain symptoms. Primary and metastatic neoplasms of the aforementioned tracts in the brain stem may cause facial pain. Infarcts, infectious neuritis, cavernous malformations, schwannomas, and extracranial malignancies or processes (more peripherally) also may be culprits.

20.3.3 Treatment

After thorough evaluation to include history and pain qualities, neurologic exam, and review of cranial imaging (MRI), formal pharmacotherapy can be initiated especially considering frequently severe pain burden and functional impairment. Brief trials of non-steroidal anti-inflammatory agents (if not contraindicated) can be attempted; however, membrane stabilizing medications active at voltage-sensitive sodium channels are standard treatment for TN. Carbamazepine [11] has been an effective standard treatment historically; however, there are possible severe adverse effects such as Stevens-Johnson syndrome, hepatitis, and leukopenia. Oxcarbazepine [11] is a newer agent that can be effective and possibly better tolerated, though it also can have severe side effects including hyponatremia. Antidepressants and baclofen may also be effective, as well as gabapentin or pregabalin, phenytoin, or clonazepam [12]. If herpes zoster reactivation (a.k.a. Shingles disease) is suspected, antiviral therapy early in the course of the disease such as valacyclovir or acyclovir [13] may reduce the severity of pain and nerve injury while also reducing the chance of post-herpetic neuralgia. Patients should be assessed for emotional distress, mood disorders, and fear-avoidance behaviors as with other chronic or severe pain syndromes. Psychological and psychiatric support may be indicated for these patients.

20.3.4 Injections

Injection procedures can be of benefit in some patients with TN or TN2, when delivered to peripheral trigeminal branches or the trigeminal ganglion, particularly if mass effects or nerve invasion are not part of the pathology. Combinations of local anesthetic and possibly steroids can provide short to intermediate term pain improvement (hours–weeks or more) which can potentially be substantial in patients already on systemic therapy. Injections of the head and neck should be performed under monitored conditions with the availability of resuscitation equipment due to the high level of vascularity and potential local anesthetic toxicity or vasovagal response. Patients should be appropriately prepared medically and have fasted; sterile precautions are employed. Seizures are possible even with low volume injections if there is arterial vascular uptake or backflow into the perfusion of the brain. Non-particular steroids probably have a role over particular steroids in these injections to reduce the potential for embolic phenomena. Peripheral injections at the supraorbital, infraorbital, or mental foramena have somewhat less risk should be performed with a small volume and thin gauge needle (25 g or less) with the concept of skin safety in mind. These can be reserved for very distal/superficial pain of the face that falls into cutaneous distribution covered by those peripheral branches.

Trigeminal branches may also be blocked at deeper locations closer to the ganglion. The mandibular nerve is accessible posteriorly to the lateral pterygoid plate from a lateral approach or just outside the foramen ovale in a foraminal view (Fig. 20.1). Although classically performed blindly, fluoroscopy is among the most practically available and functional imaging modalities for this procedure. If available, CT guidance can be used but is unnecessary. The maxillary nerve is accessible as it exits the foramen rotundum in the pterygomaxillary fissure, anterior to the lateral pterygoid plate (Fig. 20.2). The needle trajectory may begin just superior to the mandibular notch and inferior to the zygomatic arch, moving in a posterior to anterior direction until contact is made with the bony boundaries of the fissure. In some patients the needle may more practically be advanced just anteriorly to the coronoid process in a more direct approach to the fissure. An ultrasound technique for maxillary block has been described [14]. A transocular approach to the ophthalmic division is possible but uncommonly performed for TN treatment.

Trigeminal or Gasserian ganglion block is an advanced interventional technique that can be readily performed with fluoroscopy, although CT guidance has been used where available. The depth of the block often exceeds 2–2.5 in., so the practitioner should be skilled in driving a thin gauge needle with precision to avoid patient discomfort and multiple passes. The fluoroscopic view of the foramen ovale is

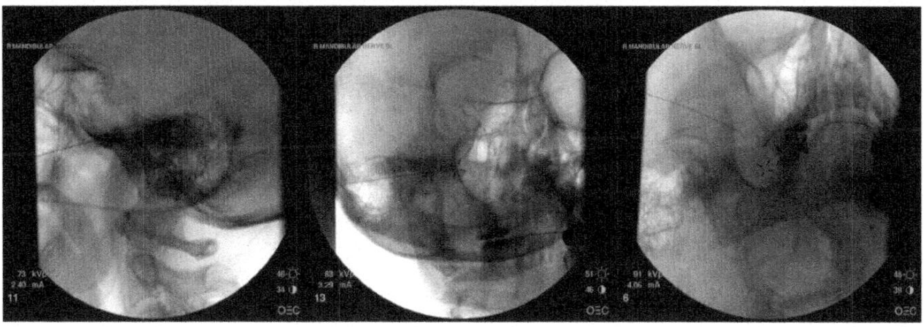

Fig. 20.1 Mandibular block with fluoroscopic guidance

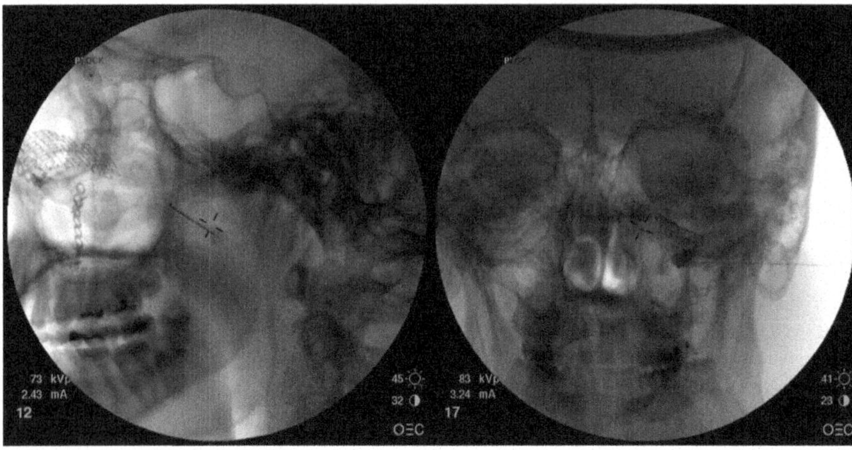

Fig. 20.2 Maxillary block with fluoroscopic guidance

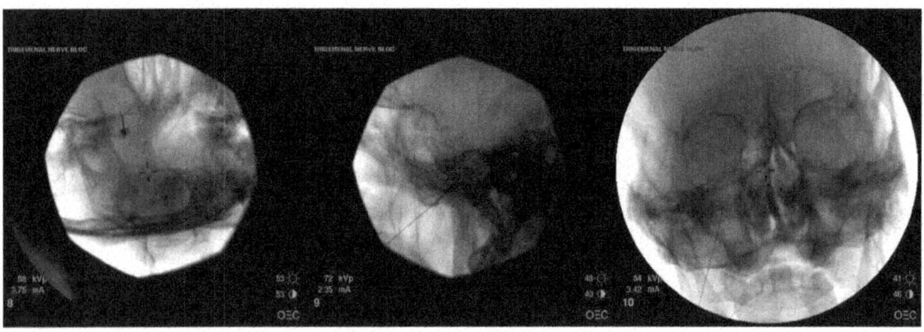

Fig. 20.3 Trigeminal (Gasserian) ganglion block with fluoroscopic guidance

obtained in a multiple step process that starts with identification of the petrous ridge [15]. The fluoroscopic C-arm is declined progressively until the petrous ridge vertically drops to the lower third of the maxillary sinus. Then, the C-arm is rotated ipsilaterally about 10–15°. The lucency of the foramen ovale should be seen adjacent or overlapping the shadow of the petrous bone, just lateral to the upper last molar and medial to the mandible (Fig. 20.3). The needle approach is coaxial in this view to the edge of the foramen; if contact is made with periosteum, the needle can be gently redirected into the foramen and advanced in a lateral view into the sphenoid bone with care not to pass the level of the clivus. AP view should demonstrate needle tip near the mid-pupillary line and contrast injection should be devoid of vascular uptake. CSF aspiration or injection is possible due to the dural sleeve in Meckel's cave. Digital subtraction angiography can be utilized if available to confirm proper contrast location and absence of vascular injection. Post-injection precautions include vigilance for hematoma formation. Facial swelling can be initially treated at bedside with a cool compress and manual pressure.

20.3.5 Decompression and Ablation

Patients who continue to have TN despite conservative management may require invasive procedures. When trigeminal vascular compression is the leading diagnosis, microvascular decompression (MVD) is an established technique with reported 90% response rate and durable relief [16] up to years in duration. It gained favor over ganglionectomy due to general avoidance of motor dysfunction and facial/corneal anesthesia as well as anesthesia dolorosa.

Several other procedures are available to offer relief of intractable pain through varying degrees of nerve destruction. These include balloon microcompression, percutaneous radiofrequency ablation, stereotactic radiosurgery (SRS), and glycerol chemoneurolysis [4, 17]. These techniques are reserved for etiologies not associated with vascular compression or where MVD has not been successful and no other operative procedure is likely to help. Radiofrequency ablation appears to have the best efficacy based on available literature [17] All of these techniques can result in sensory loss in the trigeminal distribution; corneal anesthesia can lead to morbidity if not properly managed. Permanent sensory loss may affect up to 30% of patients and can be distressing. Masseter weakness is also possible, and nearly all patients have transient weakness. Radiofrequency ablation has the highest rate of overall complications (29.2%), while SRS has a lower rate at 12% [17]. Dysesthesias may affect up to 10% of patients; anesthesia dolorosa is least likely in SRS. Pulsed radiofrequency is a non-destructive percutaneous treatment that can also provide some pain relief for TN with less side effects; however, the amplitude and duration of pain relief is shorter than for conventional radiofrequency ablation. Meningitis, hematoma formation, and fistula formation are possible with percutaneous procedures.

20.4 Trigeminal Autonomic Cephalalgias and Other Neuralgias

Trigeminal autonomic cephalalgias (TAC) are considered headache disorders according to the International Headache Society (IHS), International Classification of Headache Disorders (ICHD). While they are characterized by pain in the trigeminal distribution, they are also accompanied by dysautonomic features [3]. The mechanism of TACs is thought to be dysfunction in the trigeminal-autonomic reflex and facial nerve parasympathetic outflow system involving the brainstem, superior salivary nucleus, and sphenopalatine ganglion (SPG) [18]. Syndromes in this class include short-lasting unilateral neuralgiform headache attacks with cranial autonomic symptoms (SUNA), cluster headache (CH), paroxysmal hemicrania, hemicrania continua. Cluster headaches feature up to eight daily attacks lasting up to 180 min in a unilateral supraorbital, orbital, and temporal pain on a circadian rhythm timing. Autonomic features such as ipsilateral lacrimation, conjunctival redness, nasal congestion, ptosis, and miosis are possible. Paroxysmal hemicrania (PH) has somewhat more frequent attacks than CH, but may also involve ipsilateral photophobia/phonophobia and uniquely may be responsive to treatment with indomethacin. Hemicrania continua shares these features with PH but the pain intensity waxes and wanes without a pain-free interval. SUNA features unilateral, frequent, possibly brief attacks that may occur up to hundreds of times per day, with autonomic symptoms such as conjunctival injection and tearing. Triggers can be similar to those for classic TN; however, there is an absence of a refractory period [19].

Other than aforementioned multimodal pharmacologic therapy including indomethacin for responsive syndromes, nerve blocks and neuromodulation methods can be used to treat refractory pain. The sphenopalatine ganglion (SPG) is a classic target for treatment of TAC with nerve blocks, ablation, and neuromodulation options [20]. SPG block appears to best be suited for acute pain management or diagnostic injection, especially for CH, maxillary distribution TN, and pain for sinus surgery. There may be a role for post-dural puncture headache. Sphenopalatine block can be performed with mucosal topicalization or direct injection in a transnasal approach in which an applicator is placed to the superior border of the middle turbinate and posterior wall of the nasopharynx. Local anesthetic such as viscous and aqueous lidocaine will take about 15–30 min to take full effect. If a sheath and needle system are used, then a small volume of local anesthetic can achieve the block although care should be taken against vascular injection. If effective for aborting severe headache, it can be considered a home management strategy in well-selected patients who can be trained to self-apply nasal lidocaine spray or drops in a supine position.

Percutaneous SPG block can be accurately and practically be performed with fluoroscopic guidance (Fig. 20.4). A lateral approach, analogous to that used for maxillary block, can be used. The needle trajectory may begin just superior to the mandibular notch and inferior to the zygomatic arch, moving in a posterior to anterior direction until contact is made with the bony boundaries of the fissure. In

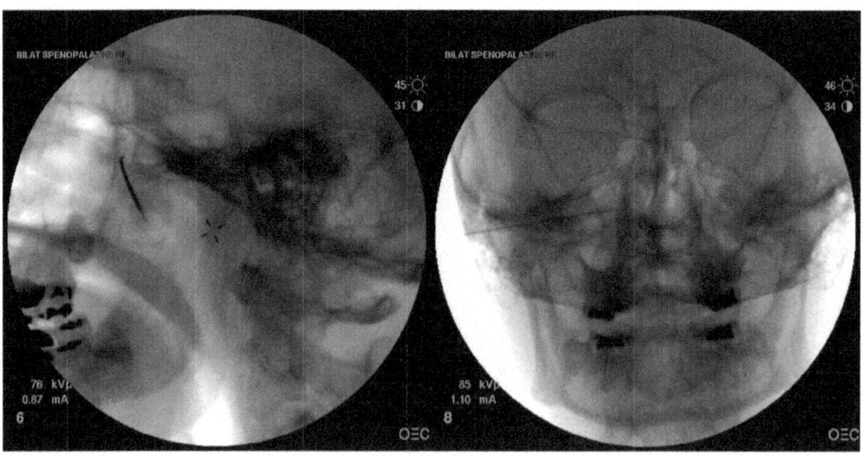

Fig. 20.4 Sphenopalatine ganglion radiofrequency ablation approach

some patients the needle may more practically be advanced just anteriorly to the coronoid process in a more direct approach to the fissure. In comparison to the maxillary block, the final needle position is more inferior. A maxillary block may also occur secondary to spread of the local anesthetic, which can often be comfortably achieved with 2–3 ml of solution. Ablation can be performed, but comes with the risk of numbness in the maxillary trigeminal distribution.

Neuromodulation options at many areas in the nervous system may be used for severe refractory pain from TAC. A small number of case reports and series of pulsed radiofrequency suggest possible benefit. No randomized controlled trials yet exist for SPG radiofrequency ablation but the largest case series available suggests up to 60% long-term response beyond 12 months [21] for CH. One randomized controlled trial for implanted SPG neurostimulation therapy showed a positive effect [22] on medication use and abortion of headache pain. Due to the invasive nature of the technique it remains an uncommon option but it has a small amount of high quality evidence to support its use. Peripheral, neuraxial, and deep brain neurostimulation can be performed at other central nervous system targets along the entire facial pain pathway to include the occipital area, high cervical epidural area, vagus nerve, and hypothalamus [23].

20.5 Other Related Pain Syndromes

20.5.1 Nervous Intermedius Neuralgia

Nervous intermedius neuralgia (NIN) is also known as geniculate or otic neuralgia and is a rare pain syndrome. It features deep paroxysmal pain in the auditory canal, and may be triggered by touch to the posterior auditory canal. It can accompany trigeminal and glossopharyngeal neuralgia due to common facial pain neural pathways. Management similar to that for TN, trigeminal and glossopharyngeal nerve blocks may be indicated to isolate a triggering source. If the nervous intermedius is thought to be under vascular compression after relevant MRI study, microvascular decompression of this nerve can be performed. Ramsay Hunt syndrome is a related disorder that stems from herpes zoster reactivation in the geniculate ganglion. It is associated with vesicular formation in the auditory canal and the auricle as well as acute facial nerve neuropathy. Antiviral therapy and prophylaxis with vaccine, topical lidocaine, and aforementioned nerve blocks may help manage the pain along with the usual anti-neuropathic pain medications used in TN.

20.5.2 Glossopharyngeal Neuralgia

Glossopharyngeal nerve distribution pain may be caused by vascular compression or by stylohyoid syndrome (a.k.a. Eagle syndrome). If vascular compression is the culprit, the posterior inferior cerebellar artery (or PICA) is the most common cause.

Pain is unilateral and paroxysmal, radiating to the posterior tongue, tonsillar fossa, pharynx, ear, and lower jaw. Triggers are analogous to TN and include swallowing, coughing, yawning, chewing, and talking. Foreign body sensation in the throat is sometimes experienced, especially in stylohyoid syndrome. Styloid resection may be required if it is the pain generator, while vascular compression if applicable is the treatment for refractory symptoms. Otherwise the treatment pathway is similar to that for TN and TACs.

20.5.3 Persistent Idiopathic Facial Pain

Persistent idiopathic facial pain (PIFP) does not follow an expected neuroanatomic distribution and cannot otherwise be attributed to known etiologies for TN, TN 2, TACs, dentoalveolar pain, or temporomandibular joint pain. Patients with PIFP are more likely to also have other chronic pain conditions such as irritable bowel syndrome, have significant psychological distress and mood disturbance, and may demonstrate a more diffuse pattern of pain over time [24, 25]. Antidepressant pharmacotherapy is the most rational initial medical option coupled with appropriate psychological support and cognitive behavioral therapy. There is limited evidence for interventions though SPG directed treatments have been tried.

20.5.4 Temporomandibular Joint Disorders

Temporomandibular joint disorders (TMDs) are a very common cause of facial and dental pain. Pain can occur with prolonged opening or with mastication. Diagnostic criteria include: recurrent pain in one or more regions of the head and/or face; X-ray, MRI, and/or bone scintigraphy demonstrating TMJ disorder; TMD signs of pain precipitated by jaw movements and/or chewing of hard or tough food, reduced range of or irregular jaw opening, noise from one or both TMJs during jaw movements, or tenderness of the joint capsule(s) of one or both TMJs. Headache generally resolves within 3 months after successful treatment of the TMJ disorder.

For pain from prolonged opening, myofascial pain may be the etiology, and it may be managed with transition to a softer diet until symptoms resolve [24, 25]. Problems with the articular disc of the temporomandibular joint (TMJ) may cause locking, clicking, limited active and passive mouth opening, and masticatory pain. If there is joint laxity, subluxation may occur. With advanced degeneration, crepitus may be appreciated. Surgery is an advanced option for disease of the TMJ; however, the foundation of treatment is patient self-management which may include physical therapy and awareness, diet changes, and splints. Splints are a first line treatment, while behavioral management may employ biofeedback, relaxation, and training to achieve better functional speech and chewing coordination. Analgesic medications may alleviate pain symptoms and psychological treatments may be required in patients who develop a chronic pain syndrome. Auricotemporal nerve blocks or TMJ injections can provide acute pain relief but may not be practical as sole treatments for chronic pain from TMD.

20.5.5 Nonodontogenic Toothache and Persistent Dentoalveolar Pain

Pain perceived in the teeth often presents to the endodontist or maxillofacial specialist. When this pain is not clearly emanating from periodontitis or other specific dental disease, other conditions present a diagnostic challenge [26]. TN and atypical TN can potentially radiate into the teeth and give the perception of toothache. Nonodontogenic toothache (NT) may have diverse other causes besides TN including myofascial pain of the masseter, digastric, temporalis muscles, and sinus disease. Persistent dentoalveolar pain (PDAP) represents a subset of NT where pain is perceived to be in a present or missing tooth and there is no imaging evidence of tissue pathology. The cause of PDAP is unclear but possibly due to a neuropathic condition. Somatosensory testing shows delayed blink reflex, increased sensitivity of capsaicin, and unilateral quantitative and qualitative sensory testing changes in a high percentage (>70%) of affected individuals [26]. Peripheral and central mechanisms are believed to be involved. PDAP may be differentiated from periodontitis in that there is almost universal report of constant pain. Antidepressant therapy, topical anesthesia, local anesthetic injection, and botulinum toxin have all been reported in the treatment of PDAP but a large amount of high quality data is not available.

20.5.6 Burning Mouth Syndrome

Pain from burning mouth syndrome is confined to the oral cavity and mucosa. The condition is associated with high levels of anxiety and depression, sensory changes of the tongue, and brain changes on fMRI [25]. The condition is rare but may respond to cognitive behavioral therapy and clonazepam.

20.6 Summary

Orofacial pain represents a diverse group of pain syndromes and can present a diagnostic challenge to medical providers. Knowledge of the presentation and neuroanatomy responsible for mediating facial pain pathways is paramount to understanding the evaluation and treatment which may include interventions and surgery. Thorough evaluation is required to guide interventions toward peripheral nerves, the trigeminal ganglion, or autonomic nervous system (SPG). Pain disorders of neurologic origin do have common pathways of management however and even though a large body of evidence is not available for more rare conditions, rational use of anti-neuropathic pain medications and targeted percutaneous nerve blocks or ablation may be required for highly chronic and debilitating cases.

References

1. Macfarlane TV, Macfarlane GJ. Self-reported facial pain in a nationwide study: UK Biobank. Int J Epidemiol. 2015;44(1):i112.
2. Mueller D, Obermann M, Yoon MS, Poitz F, Hansen N, Slomke MA, Dommes P, Gizewski E, Diener HC, Katsarava Z. Prevalence of trigeminal neuralgia and persistent idiopathic facial pain: a population-based study. Cephalalgia. 2011;31(15):1542–8.
3. Zakrzewska JM, Jensen TS. History of facial pain diagnosis. Cephalalgia. 2017;37(7):604–8.
4. Patel SK, Liu JK. Overview and history of trigeminal neuralgia. Neurosurg Clin N Am. 2016;27(3):265–76.
5. Burchiel KJ. A new classification for facial pain. Neurosurgery. 2003;53(5):1164–6. discussion 1166–7.
6. Okeson JP, Bell WE, Harmon L. Bell's orofacial pains: the clinical management of orofacial pain. Carol Stream, IL: Quintessence Publishing; 2005. p. 115.
7. Dandy WE. Trigeminal neuralgia and trigeminal tic douloureux. In: Lewis D, editor. Practice of surgery. Hagerstown, MD: WF Prior CO; 1932. p. 177–200.
8. Jannetta PJ. Arterial compression of the trigeminal nerve at the pons in patients with trigeminal neuralgia. 1967. J Neurosurg. 2007;107(1):216–9.
9. Kontzialis M, Kocak M. Imaging evaluation of trigeminal neuralgia. J Istanb Univ Fac Dent. 2017;51(3):S62–8.
10. Jensen TS, Rasmussen P, Reske-Nielsen E. Association of trigeminal neuralgia with multiple sclerosis: clinical and pathological features. Acta Neurol Scand. 1982;65(3):182–9.
11. Di Stefano G, La Cesa S, Truini A, Cruccu G. Natural history and outcome of 200 outpatients with classical trigeminal neuralgia treated with carbamazepine or oxcarbazepine in a tertiary centre for neuropathic pain. J Headache Pain. 2014;15:34.
12. Oomens MA, Forouzanfar T. Pharmaceutical management of trigeminal neuralgia in the elderly. Drugs Aging. 2015;32(9):717–26.
13. Feller L, Khammissa RAG, Fourie J, Bouckaert M, Lemmer J. Postherpetic neuralgia and trigeminal neuralgia. Pain Res Treat. 2017;2017:1681765.
14. Nader A, Schittek H, Kendall MC. Lateral pterygoid muscle and maxillary artery are key anatomical landmarks for ultrasound-guided trigeminal nerve block. Anesthesiology. 2013;118(4):957.
15. Fluoro Flip. In: Garza R, Eckmann MS, Xu R, editors. A pocket guide to fluoroscopic spinal and peripheral pain procedures. 1st ed. Delhi: Jaypee Publishing; 2017.
16. Sindou M, Leston J, Decullier E, Chapuis F. Microvascular decompression for primary trigeminal neuralgia: long-term effectiveness and prognostic factors in a series of 362 consecutive patients with clear-cut neurovascular conflicts who underwent pure decompression. J Neurosurg. 2007;107(6):1144–53.
17. Lopez BC, Hamlyn PJ, Zakrzewska JM. Systematic review of ablative neurosurgical techniques for the treatment of trigeminal neuralgia. Neurosurgery. 2004;54(4):973–82. discussion 982–3.
18. Wei DY, Jensen RH. Therapeutic approaches for the management of trigeminal autonomic cephalalgias. Neurotherapeutics. 2018;15(2):346–60.

19. Weng HY, Cohen AS, Schankin C, Goadsby PJ. Phenotypic and treatment outcome data on SUNCT and SUNA, including a randomised placebo-controlled trial. Cephalalgia. 2018;38(9):1554–63.
20. Ho KWD, Przkora R, Kumar S. Sphenopalatine ganglion: block, radiofrequency ablation and neurostimulation—a systematic review. J Headache Pain. 2017;18(1):118.
21. Sanders M, Zuurmond WW. Efficacy of sphenopalatine ganglion blockade in 66 patients suffering from cluster headache: a 12- to 70-month follow-up evaluation. J Neurosurg. 1997;87(6):876–80.
22. Schoenen J, Jensen RH, Lantéri-Minet M, Láinez MJ, Gaul C, Goodman AM, Caparso A, May A. Stimulation of the sphenopalatine ganglion (SPG) for cluster headache treatment. Pathway CH-1: a randomized, sham-controlled study. Cephalalgia. 2013;33(10):816–30.
23. Wei DY, Jensen RH. Therapeutic approaches for the management of trigeminal autonomic cephalalgias. Neurotherapeutics. 2018;15(2):346–60.
24. Zakrzewska JM. Differential diagnosis of facial pain and guidelines for management. Br J Anaesth. 2013;111(1):95–104.
25. Zakrzewska JM. Multi-dimensionality of chronic pain of the oral cavity and face. J Headache Pain. 2013;14:37.
26. Malacarne A, Spierings ELH, Lu C, Maloney GE. Persistent dentoalveolar pain disorder: a comprehensive review. J Endod. 2018;44(2):206–11.

Chapter 21
Myofascial Pain Syndrome and Fibromyalgia

Maria M. Cristancho, Gunar B. Subieta, and Maria L. Torres

21.1 Historic Overview of Soft Tissue Pain

The description of musculoskeletal pain goes back to the early 1800s, and over the years different terms have been used, including muscular rheumatism, non-articular rheumatism, psychogenic rheumatism, and fibrositis among others [1]. With a better understanding of the etiology and associated symptoms in patients with soft tissue pain (STP), two distinct clinical terms were accepted as MPS and FM.

The combined work of pioneers like Steindler and Travell in the 1940s provided a better diagnostic criteria and coined the term MPS [2]. This included findings of taut bands in the specific muscle groups, which produced pain to a referred area, combined with Travell's description of a reproducible pattern of pain, upon pressuring the trigger points in individual muscle groups.

FM, in contrast, was described by Graham in 1950 [1] in patients exhibiting diffuse tender points, associated with other multiple systemic comorbidities. It was not until 1990 that the American College of Rheumatology (ACR) proposed a uniform classification system for FM [1], which required a history of widespread pain for 3 months, and pain on digital pressure at 11 of 18 anatomically defined tender points. This classification was useful for the research community, but clinically very challenging for physicians, due to many factors, including the different results obtained, depending on the examiner, and lack of objectivity of these findings. A revised classification system was published in 2010, using two scoring systems known as WPI (widespread pain index) and SSS (symptom severity score), in an attempt to standardize and help physicians better diagnose FM [3] (Fig. 21.1).

M. M. Cristancho · G. B. Subieta
Anesthesia and Pain Management, Cook County Hospital, Chicago, IL, USA
e-mail: mcristancho@cookcountyhhs.org; gsubieta@cookcountyhhs.org

M. L. Torres (✉)
Pain Management Department, Cook County Hospital, Chicago, IL, USA
e-mail: mtorres4@cookocunt6yhhs.org; mtorres4@cookcountyhhs.org

K. Shimoji et al. (eds.), *Chronic Pain Management in General and Hospital Practice*, https://doi.org/10.1007/978-981-15-2933-7_21

LOCAL	REGIONAL	GENERALIZED
Bursitis	Myofascial Pain Syndrome	Fibromyalgia Syndrome
Tendonitis	Complex Regional Pain Syndrome	Chronic Fatigue Syndrome
Synovitis	Referred visceral pain to a musculoskeletal region	Hypermobility Syndrome

Fig. 21.1 Proposed classification of soft tissue pain syndromes. Adapted from Russell [1]

21.2 Myofascial Pain Syndrome

21.2.1 Introduction

Myofascial pain syndrome (MPS) is a clinical entity that affects the musculoskeletal system, localized to the muscle fiber itself, and its overlying fascia causing significant pain and disability. It is highly prevalent in patients presenting with chronic musculoskeletal pain. The onset of their pain could be related to a specific event or injury, or it may have developed over time. Patients can also present with sensory, motor, and autonomic complaints [2]. Patients describe their pain as constant, dull, and deep aching, sometimes associated with hyperalgesia or allodynia. Motor symptoms present as weakness on the region supplied by the muscular group, and autonomic findings like vasoconstriction, erythema, sweating, and piloerection in the area of referred pain.

MPS is a very broad term, which describes identifiable and localized regional muscle groups producing pain upon pressure defined as a trigger point (TP). It also encompasses a diverse, non-specific group of clinical entities, which share in common localization of trigger points, resulting in syndromes like tension headache, temporomandibular joint disturbances, neck pain, forearm and hand pain, postural pain, and pelvic/urogenital pain syndromes [4]. It is characterized as a local or regional pain, comprising a single or more than one muscle, and clear evidence of a taut muscular band in the skeletal muscle affected, a trigger point, and a referred pain pattern distribution of the pain.

The main component of MPS is the trigger point, described by Travell and Simons as a "hyperirritable spot, usually within a taut band of skeletal muscle or in the muscle fascia, which is painful on compression, and can give rise to characteristic referred pain, motor dysfunction, and autonomic phenomena" [2]. The characteristic features of a trigger point (TP) are: focal tenderness to palpation of the muscle involved, reproduction of pain with 4 kg of pressure over the TP, presence of an associated taut band, restricted range of movement in the muscle affected, pseudo weakness of the muscle affected, and referred pain on continued pressure for approximately 5 s over the TP [2]. TPs are classified as active, latent, primary, secondary, or satellite. An active TP is the one directly causing pain spontaneously

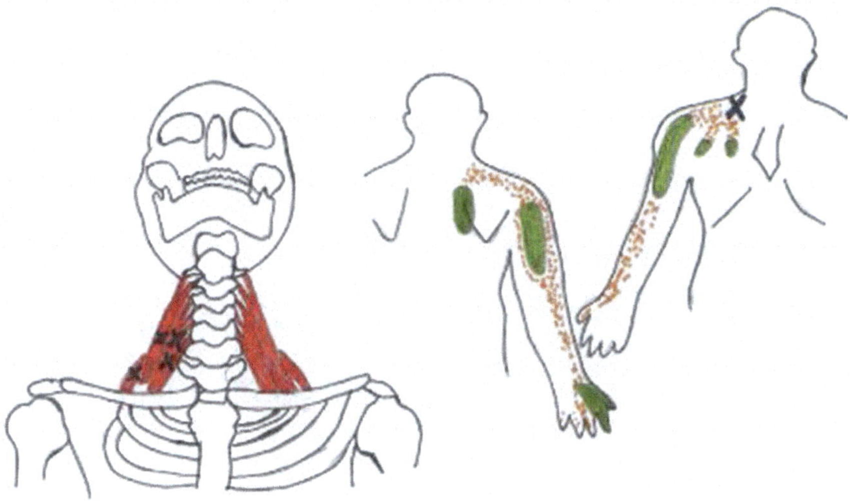

Fig. 21.2 Example of cervical myofascial pain trigger points labeled with the "X" on the right and their referred pattern in green and orange. Green bold areas showing main area of referral and orange dots representing associated referral areas

at rest, and the one that can be associated with motor, or autonomic dysfunction, as well as referred pain [5, 6]. A latent TP is the most prevalent type of trigger point and is described as a focal area of tenderness, with muscle contraction, not spontaneously like the active TP; it is not painful at rest, but pain is elicited with certain movement. It can become active with stress, overuse, or stretching. Primary TPs are those that do not have an underlying cause, whereas secondary TPs have an origin, like nerve entrapments or radiculopathies. Satellite TPs, are TPs that without treatment, end up compromising adjacent structures that were not originally affected. The taut band, as the second component of MPS, is a group of muscular or fascial fibers of increased consistency, that extend along the muscle affected from origin to insertion. It is caused by an abnormal state of muscular tension, produced by palpation of the TP. It cannot be seen on physical exam, but can be detected only with careful palpation over the muscle affected. The third component of MPS is the referred pain produced by palpation of a TP. This referred pain does not follow a dermatomal distribution, but it usually has a very consistent pattern once elicited (Fig. 21.2).

21.2.2 Etiology

There are several precipitating factors associated with the development of MPS, including the main etiology accepted as acute muscular stress, repetitive microtrauma, overuse, lack of exercise, radiculopathy, neuralgias, nerve compression, postural disorders, thyroid dysfunction, vitamin or mineral deficiencies, sleep disturbances, and even psychological or emotional distress [2, 5, 7]. The main theory accepts that TPs develop after an inciting injury to the muscle fibers. If the stress to the muscle persists or any of the abovementioned factors are added to this initial injury, then the syndrome develops. This theory is known as the "injury pool theory."

21.2.3 Pathophysiology

There have been several theories that explain how MPS develops, but there is a lack of scientific evidence that proves it fully, and it is not entirely understood. Travell and Simons, in their integrated hypothesis [8], described an overall dysfunction of the motor endplate, in which an abnormal depolarization is present, due to excessive release of acetylcholine, defects of the acetylcholinesterase enzyme, and an increase in the activity of the nicotinic acetylcholine receptor. These factors of hyper contractility and repetitive sustained muscular contraction produce an inflammatory response; hence, pain completing Simon's circle of integrated hypothesis. A local twitch response (LTR) model has also been proposed [2], where an electrical stimuli is produced over the tender site, and this would be considered the "sensitive locus." An active locus would be the site where spontaneous electrical activity is recorded, without any stimuli, as demonstrated by Hubbard and Berkoff [2]. This active locus was proposed to be the motor end plate. They concluded that the sum of the sensitive locus, plus the active locus, as well as the nociceptor, constituted the actual trigger point. Another theory proposed is one that describes an autonomic component and the development of central sensitization [5]. In this model there is an inciting trauma, edema, or ischemia, which triggers a local inflammatory response releasing neuropeptides, inflammatory and vasoactive substances that act upon sensory and sympathetic fibers, causing more ischemia, leading to peripheral sensitization. If left untreated, multiple changes occur at the level of the peripheral, as well as the central nervous system, which eventually leads to the development of central sensitization.

21.2.4 Diagnosis

The diagnosis of MPS is mainly clinical, as there are no laboratory exams or radiologic studies that can diagnose this entity. This is where a complete clinical history and thorough physical exam are necessary to diagnose. Patients describe their pain as localized or regional, dull, constant, and deep over the muscle, or muscle group affected, ranging from mild to severe intensity, and the pain and associated symptoms are elicited when the TP is palpated. According to the region of the body affected, the associated symptoms may include headache, dizziness, tinnitus, temporomandibular joint pain, lacrimation, or neck pain. Associated autonomic symptoms and signs can be elicited like sweating, lacrimation, erythema, vasomotor, and temperature changes. The main concern for the patient is the potential for temporal, or permanent disability, when the symptoms become severe. It can also be functionally disabling when significant levels of fatigue, weakness, decrease in endurance, or joint rigidity occur, impairing their daily activities. The development of psychological and sleep disturbances, and the associated emotional burden, can exacerbate and worsen the clinical picture.

A thorough physical exam and review of their clinical history can help guide the clinician's diagnosis, which could include the identification of a palpable tender trigger point (TP), a palpable taut band, and the presence of referred pain on palpation of the TP. The physical exam must include a thorough general, neurological, and musculoskeletal survey. Digital pressure of 4 kg, enough to blanch the nailbed, over the trigger point for 5 s [2, 9]. The patient's reaction to palpation of the TP is described as the "jump sign" [8], an involuntary reflex often disproportionate to the pressure applied. Simons and colleagues [9] described eight characteristics that had to be present to diagnose MPS, including the onset description and immediate cause of pain, the pain distribution pattern, restricted motion with increased sensitivity to stretching, weakened muscle due to pain with no muscular atrophy, compression causing pain similar to the patient's chief complaint, a palpable taut band of muscle correlating with the patient's TP, and a LTR (local twitch response) elicited by snapping palpation or rapid insertion of a needle, and reproduction of the referred pain, with mechanical stimulation of the TP.

21.2.5 *Diagnostic Testing*

Although there is no specific laboratory exam or radiographic test to confirm the diagnosis of MPS, laboratory testing should be done if other diagnoses are suspected, or if there are other concerning symptoms. In MPS, there is an absence of laboratory abnormalities in blood chemistry or hematologic studies. For purely research purposes, electromyography confirms the abnormal excess of spontaneous electrical activity inside the trigger point, but this study is not required to diagnose the condition [2, 5]. There are also methods for pressure measurement, in which pressure is recorded within the trigger point, and then compared to the contralateral non-affected muscle and a difference of 2 kg/cm^2 is considered an abnormal reading [2]. Again, these methods may be useful in research studies but not necessary for a diagnosis in our regular clinical practice.

21.2.6 *Differential Diagnosis*

Other clinical entities that should be considered include myositis, arthritis, bursitis, tendonitis, connective tissue disorders, metabolic and endocrine derangements, neuropathic disorders, radiculopathies, psychiatric disorders, and FM.

21.2.7 Treatment

Treatment of a patient, with the diagnosis of MPS, is to be approached on an individual basis, taking into account the patient's past medical history or related comorbidities, their functional status, lifestyle, and occupation. It is also very important to discuss the patient's expectations of treatment results [10–12]. On first evaluation, a clear understanding of the disease, its associated symptoms, precipitating factors, and treatment plan with goals and time oriented expectations should be fully discussed with the patient, empowering them to take ownership of their disease.

Of utmost importance is taking a multi-disciplinary approach [6], which frequently requires consultation and treatment from specialists like pain medicine, rheumatology, physical therapy, and psychology. Better outcomes are seen in settings where these different specialties are housed together, where treatment modalities can not only follow each other, but also be discussed among providers working towards a common goal. The initiation of treatment has to be in a progressive manner, which requires arrangement of clinic visits at the same time, to ensure maximal patient compliance and overall treatment success. An initial psychological evaluation and further support is very beneficial in the majority of these patients, since chronic muscle pain is frequently accompanied by depression. Many patients report exacerbation of their symptoms, with increasing stress, anxiety, lack of sleep, anger, and worsening depression. Some patients have reported benefits from cognitive behavioral therapy and meditation.

Treatment modalities include non-invasive and invasive procedures, as well as non-pharmacologic and pharmacologic regimens [10–12]. The goal is to minimize pain, restore patient's functional status, shorten disability periods, and improve their quality of life. The main intervention for the treatment of MPS is to control the triggering etiology, be it excessive microtrauma with repetitive movements of the muscle group affected, stretching, or avoidance of stress on the muscle groups.

21.2.8 Non-Pharmacologic Treatment

Treatment of MPS is mostly non-pharmacologic. In the non-pharmacologic modalities, the main goal is to restore the muscle fibers length at rest; therefore, physical rehabilitation and supervised specific stretching exercises are mainstay. The physical therapist has different means of providing relief, such as hot and cold therapy, localized freezing sprays followed with immediate stretching, ultrasound, infrared light, localized massage, relaxation, postural exercises, ergonomic and body mechanics changes, acupressure, laser, and TENS [2]. Travell and Simons advocated for the passive stretching of the affected muscle after freezing spray was applied [2]. Simons et al. [9] described the massaging technique as "deep stroking" or "stripping" massage. The treatment of the trigger points is also very important in patients who have failed the multiple, non-invasive means of treatment. It consists of identifying the trigger point itself and injecting it, via a single puncture, creating a "fanlike" pattern to cover it as much as possible [2, 9, 13, 14]. Different injection techniques have been described over the years, including dry injections, or dry needling, or the administration of local anesthetics, with or without corticosteroids, normal saline, sterile water, or Botox. Cummings et al. [13] reported a systematic revision of 23 clinical studies of MPS treatment with injection of the trigger point, concluding that regardless of the injectate, or whether one was injected or not, there is no difference in control of pain after the needling procedure. In fact, some studies suggest that dry needling alone could potentially be more effective, as compared to injection of medications.

When clinically indicated and in selected challenging cases such as TP injection in obese patients, patients with distorted muscular anatomy and for deeper targets, the use of ultrasound has been suggested as an evolving and adjuvant modality in an attempt to technically improve identification of TPs, enhance needle visualization [15], improve overall efficacy and safety of injection, and decrease the incidence of complications such as pneumothorax, epidural abscess, hematoma formation, skeletal muscle toxicity, or intrathecal injection [16]. The use of ultrasound has been described with some success for reported cases of TP injection of the cervicothoracic region [17], the anterior abdominal musculature, and the subscapularis and pectoralis status post-mastectomy [18] to decrease the incidence of implant puncture.

21.2.9 Pharmacologic Treatment

21.2.9.1 Topical Agents

Although there are no specific randomized control studies, topical anti-inflammatories, such as salicylic acid, menthol, diclofenac creams, as well as local anesthetic creams and patches, are effective in a small subset of patients. Preparations of local topical agents, IE: lidocaine patch, are also effective, due to local penetration with limited systemic absorption, and have been effective in a small subset of patients. This was confirmed in a small randomized controlled trial, which found that although pain reduction was suboptimal, patients were satisfied with the analgesic effect, and also with avoiding any penetrating trauma.

Non-prescription topical agents may also be effective. Examples include Biofreeze, Salonpas, Icy-hot, and many other preparations that have as their main active ingredient methyl salicylate or menthol, and they are believed to activate peripheral receptors with minimal side effects.

Systemically, we can address the pain at the periphery by the use of anti-inflammatories, such as NSAIDs and toxins like botulinum neurotoxin; and centrally, by using adjuvant medications, acetaminophen, muscle relaxants, anticonvulsants, opioids, and antidepressants. Although multiple studies have shown different degrees of effectiveness for these systemic medications, we will review them by relevance.

21.2.9.2 Systemic Pharmacologic Agents

Although there is limited evidence for the effectiveness of NSAIDs, they are often the initial treatment for MPS [19]. The specific anti-inflammatory to be used depends on the patient's comorbidities, interaction with other medications, and potential side effects. They are usually initiated by the patient due to their easy availability as an over-the-counter medication. The main concern for the practitioner and patient is that these medications have an extensive profile of interactions and potential side effects. Hence, it is advisable that the practitioner should select one of them based on a patient by patient criteria. They may be too risky for geriatric patients or those with significant comorbidities, and their use should be limited to acute flair ups.

In healthy patients, should one of the medications in this group be found to be ineffective, it is always wise to rotate through different preparations, such as the propionic acid, salicylic acid, acetic acid, enolic acid, and non-acidic and Cox 2 derivatives. Once the patient has failed such rotation, then one can clearly remove them from the therapeutic arsenal [19].

21.2.9.3 Muscle Relaxants

Just like with the NSAIDs, chronic use of these medications is discouraged [20, 21]. The pharmacological properties of this group vary depending on the medication. The majority of the ones used in outpatient practice provide relaxation via a central mechanism. This should be taken into account prior to initiating them with other medications that exacerbate this central sedative effect. Although its mechanism of action is not clear, of potential interest is cyclobenzaprine, which will cause muscle relaxation without affecting muscle function. When compared to clonazepam, it had more noticeable relaxation properties. Currently, there are no studies supporting enough evidence for its use for MPS [22, 23].

21.2.9.4 Antidepressants

Antidepressants, such as tricyclic antidepressants, have been extensively studied more for fibromyalgia with acceptable results. Even though the pathophysiological mechanism for both MPS and fibromyalgia is different, the prevention of central sensitization and the potentiation of descending inhibitory pain pathways may promote symptom improvement. These medications are also very effective for patients with associated tension headache. Amitriptyline has been the TCA with more scientific background and clinicians should pick the choice of TCA according to their side effect profile [20, 21].

Newer antidepressant medications such as selective serotonin reuptake inhibitors (SSRIs) and selective norepinephrine reuptake inhibitors (SNRIs) have also been studied extensively for fibromyalgia but not as much for MPS. Recent literature shows the beneficial effects of SNRI as an adjuvant therapy for MPS but there are no studies that prove that MPS can be treated by only using an SNRI alone [22, 23].

21.2.9.5 Anticonvulsants and Membrane Stabilizers

In patients with MPS that exhibit symptoms of neuropathic pain, anticonvulsants have demonstrated effectiveness. It should be noted that the majority of research has been performed to address fibromyalgia, and there is a paucity in research studies promoting gabapentin, pregabalin, or any other anticonvulsant as a first-line treatment for MPS [22].

21.2.9.6 Alpha-2 Adrenergic Agonists

Tizanidine is thought to act centrally, at the level of the spinal cord, inhibiting postsynaptic pathways and decreasing substance P. Tizanidine is used primarily as a muscle relaxant, and it is also believed that it may contribute by decreasing free neuroexcitatory neurotransmitters, promoting less central sensitization. Tizanidine's side effect profile includes sedation and may also cause hypotension by itself, or compound hypotension on a patient taking other blood pressure medications.

21.2.9.7 Benzodiazepines

Benzodiazepines are the gold standard for the acute management of muscle spasm, and given their anxiolytic and anticonvulsant properties, they may be very effective managing MPS. There has been extensive research on their use on myofascial subsets of temporomandibular syndromes with good outcomes. Clinical concerns with these medications are their known addictive properties, as well as their extensive central side effect profile that includes cognitive impairment, issues with recall, antegrade memory loss, fatigue, and withdrawal symptoms.

21.2.9.8 Opioids

Due to their lack of efficacy, and serious side effect profile, opioids have no demonstrated role in chronic myofascial pain syndrome.

21.2.9.9 Botox

Onabotulinum toxin A (Botox) is thought to be a therapeutic option, due to how it interferes with muscle contraction, by preventing the release of acetylcholine at the level of the motor nerve, ending in the neuromuscular junction. Many medical societies have explored its use for the treatment of MPS on different anatomical sites, yet its use still remains controversial. Although Botox has been shown to reduce contraction at the level of the trigger point, there seems to be inter-clinician variability due to different results. There is insufficient clinical evidence to support the effectiveness of Botox in the treatment of MPS [24–27].

21.3 Fibromyalgia

21.3.1 Introduction

Fibromyalgia commonly presents with widespread chronic musculoskeletal pain, in contrast to MPS, which typically is limited to a certain anatomical region. Fibromyalgia patients characteristically have diffuse pain and symmetrical tender points, not corresponding to a dermatomal distribution [28]. Associated symptoms are fatigue, insomnia, anxiety, depression, and cognitive impairment. Additional symptoms of Raynaud's phenomenon, irritable bowel disease, heat, and cold intolerance can be also associated with this condition [1]. Fibromyalgia etiology remains unknown. Some authors consider this entity as an advanced form of MPS spectrum, while others believe that it is completely a different entity, and at times the two may overlap. Fibromyalgia is a common source of chronic pain, and it is the most common source of generalized musculoskeletal pain in women between the ages of 20 and 55 years [28]. Fibromyalgia was first described in France and England in the mid-nineteenth century [1]. Its incidence has been described from 2% to 4% of the general population between 18 and 65 years of age, [1] most commonly in females, and it is one of the more common etiologies of musculoskeletal pain seen by rheumatologists in clinical practice.

21.3.2 Etiology

Etiology of this disease is multifactorial and not fully understood [1, 28, 29]. Most of what has been published on FM's etiology and risk factors demonstrate the main role that the central autonomic nervous system (CNS) plays. A common finding in FM is central sensitization, where an amplified response to pain is exhibited after a period of time of continuous peripheral noxious stimuli. This together with a "wind up" phenomena (hyperexcitability of the spinal cord neurons) are abnormally increased in FM [29].

The descending inhibitory pathways have been shown to also be involved, and the mechanism is through impairment of their response to noxious stimuli. Apart from the abnormalities seen in the pain conduction pathways and their ultimate target in the CNS, an added exacerbated glial cell activation with subsequent persistent and amplified inflammation cascade has also been demonstrated. In terms of neurotransmitters involved in the etiology of FM and involvement of the autonomic nervous system, there have been studies that include serotonin (5-HT) which has been shown to be low in patients with FM, explaining the disturbances in the sleep patterns and other neurotransmitters such as dopamine, norepinephrine, endorphins, metenkephalins, and substance P, which have been shown to be high in patients with FM, causing hyperactivity of the sympathetic nervous system and dysautonomy, disrupting pain modulation itself [29].

The neuroendocrine axis imbalance etiologic mechanism has also been proposed. FM patients exhibit a hyperactivity of the hypothalamic-hypophyseal axis (HHA), and thus increased level of circulating corticosteroids and ACTH, exacerbating the dysautonomy. Low levels of GH have also been described, mostly due to sleep pattern disruption [1].

Psychological risk factors or associations have also been described, since these patients exhibit depression, anxiety, or high levels of physical and emotional stress, linked to the etiology or triggering factor of the disease. It has been noted that there is a genetic predisposition, and about 30% of affected patients have another family member with the diagnosis. Some viral infections such as HIV, HCV, EBV, Parvovirus, Coxsackie B, and HSV-6 have been implicated, and may explain the chronic fatigue component of the syndrome. Others have proposed an autoimmune etiology, since some patients develop systemic lupus erythematosus, rheumatoid arthritis, and Sjögren syndrome. Myopathy, local tissue factors, and physical trauma have also been proposed as other contributing factors in the etiology of FM [5].

Other etiologic theories have been described as mentioned above and while their direct causative mechanism has not been definitively linked to the origin of FM, they may be the result of the condition itself. An example of this is sleep disturbances and fatigue. It has been documented that many patients with FM also have non-REM sleep pattern which leads them to experience non-restorative sleep subsequently to fatigue, muscular rigidity, and hyperalgesia [5].

21.3.3 Diagnosis

The FM diagnosis is usually clinical. A thorough history, detailed physical examination, and psychological assessment are required to identify precipitating or associated factors. Chronic widespread musculoskeletal pain is the main clinical symptom, usually associated with hyperalgesia, dysesthesia, or allodynia. Other associated symptoms are fatigue which is present in 80% of patients, chronic headaches, sleep disturbances, dizziness, cognitive and memory impairment, anxiety, depression, PTSD, temporomandibular joint pain, morning stiffness, vision problems, interstitial cystitis, restless legs syndrome, irritable bowel syndrome, and dysmenorrhea [1]. In 1990 the American College of Rheumatology (ACR) proposed a set of diagnostic criteria which included: widespread pain lasting more than 3 months affecting all four quadrants of the body (both sides and above and below the waist, axial skeletal pain present in the cervical spine or anterior chest or thoracic spine and low back), and tender points in at least 11 of the 18 locations on digital palpation [1]. Over the years, this criteria was revised in 2010 [3] to also include an objective assessment of the disease severity. The widespread pain index (WPI) and symptom severity score (SSS) were developed. The preliminary diagnostic criteria suggests that FM is present if the patient has a widespread pain index (WPI) ≥7 and symptom severity (SS) scale score ≥ 5 or WPI between 3 and 6 and SS ≥9; the symptoms to be present at a similar level for at least 3 months and no other associated disorder that would explain the pain. The WPI is the number of areas in which the patient had pain over the last week (right and left shoulder girdle, right and left upper arm, right and left lower arm, right and left hip, buttock, trochanter), right and left upper leg, right and left lower leg, right and left jaw, right and left chest abdomen, right and left back, and neck with a total score between 0 and 19) (Fig. 21.3). The symptom severity score is the sum of the severity of the 3 core symptoms (fatigue, waking up unrefreshed, cognitive symptoms) and each of the three symptoms is to be rated by the patient as 0—no problem; 1—slight or mild problems, intermittent; 2—moderate, considerable; and 3—usually severe, pervasive, continuous, life-disturbing problems. The other component of SSS is the somatic symptom group that rates the extent (severity) of somatic symptoms in general (final score between 0 and 12). Somatic symptoms are also rated from 0 with no symptoms to 1 with few symptoms, 2 moderate, and 3 severe. They include muscle pain, fatigue, weakness, headache, dizziness, insomnia, constipation,

3 Criteria to be met 1. WPI ≥7 and SSS ≥5 or WPI 3-6 and SS ≥9 2. Symptoms at a similar level for at least 3 months 3. No other disorder present to explain the symptoms
WPI Score is 0 to 19 giving 1 point to each area in which the patient has had pain over the last week - Shoulder girdle right and left respectively (1 point each) - Right upper arm and left upper arm (1 point each) - Right lower arm and left lower arm (1 point each) - Right and left Hip (buttock, trochanter) (1 point for each side) - Right upper leg and left upper leg (1 point each) - Right lower left and left lower leg (1 point each) - Right and left jaw (1 point each) - Chest - Abdomen - Upper back - Lower back - Neck
SS Scale Score -"3 symptoms": Fatigue, waking unrefreshed, cognitive symptoms The patient rates each of the 3 symptoms above, indicating their severity from 0 to 3 (0=no problem, 1= slight or mild problems, generally mild or intermittent, 2=moderate, considerable problems, often present and/or at a moderate level and 3=severe, pervasive, continuous, life-disturbing problems) -Somatic symptoms * are rated by the patient from 0 to 3 (0=no symptoms, 1=few symptoms, 2=moderate number of symptoms and 3=a great deal of symptoms) SS is the sum of the severity of the "3 symptoms" plus the severity of somatic symptoms in general. Final score is between 0-12
Somatic symptoms*: muscle pain, irritable bowel syndrome, fatigue/tiredness, thinking or remembering problem, muscle weakness, headache, pain/cramps in the abdomen, numbness/tingling, dizziness, insomnia, depression, constipation, pain in the upper abdomen, nausea, nervousness, chest pain, blurred vision, fever, diarrhea, dry mouth, itching, wheezing, Raynaud's phenomenon, hives/welts, ringing in ears, vomiting, heartburn, oral ulcers, loss of/change in taste, seizures, dry eyes, shortness of breath, loss of appetite, rash, sun sensitivity, hearing difficulties, easy bruising, hair loss, frequent urination, painful urination, and bladder spasms.

Fig. 21.3 Diagnostic criteria for fibromyalgia: WPI and SSS scales. Adapted from Wolfe et al. [3]

abdominal pain, nausea, nervousness, chest pain, blurred vision, fever, diarrhea, dry mouth, itching, wheezing, Raynaud's phenomenon, hives/welts, ringing in ears, vomiting, heartburn, irritable bowel syndrome, oral ulcers, loss of/change in taste, seizures, dry eyes, shortness of breath, loss of appetite, rash, sun sensitivity, hearing difficulties, easy bruising, hair loss, frequent urination, painful urination, and bladder spasms.

A 2016 revision to the 2010 guidelines has been published [19], and it incorporates minor changes to the WPI and SSS score criteria (WPI $\geq$7 and SSS $\geq$5 or WPI 4–6, as opposed to 3–6 in the 2010 criteria and SSS $\geq$9). This new revision includes generalized pain criteria, where pain has to present in at least 4 of 5 regions (right upper, left upper, right lower, left lower, and axial). Another addition is the fibromyalgia symptom (FS) or polysymptomatic distress (PSD) scale that is the sum of WPI and SSS. The symptom presence for at least 3 months diagnostic criteria remains the same, and the diagnosis of FM can be made irrespective of other diagnoses, not excluding other clinical relevant disorders.

On physical exam, FM patients exhibit tenderness in specific, soft tissue anatomic locations, as described. Hence, the term "tender point examination" of the nine pairs of tender points is used to identify the areas affected [5]. In order to be able to reproduce the findings on physical exam, the point palpation to elicit tenderness has to have a certain amount of pressure equal to 4 kg/cm^2, which is often described as pressure enough to blanch the examiner's nail bed [1]. There are "control points" that have been identified, and they should be included in the physical exam, because these locations normally do not exhibit tenderness to palpation. These control point's locations include thumb, mid forearm, and forehead. In general, neurologic exam does not reveal any abnormality in the absence of major organic disease [5].

Laboratory testing and imaging studies are often found to be normal in these patients, and often do not offer much to the diagnosis. They should be included in the workup to rule out any other significant major organic cause, which could be responsible for the patient's source of pain.

21.3.4 Treatment

The treatment of fibromyalgia is mainly supportive, and as similar to the MPS multi-disciplinary approach. Patient education on the nature of the disease is important, since this condition does not have a cure, but can be kept under control with proper avoidance of triggering factors, such as anxiety or stress. It is important for the provider to validate the patient's symptoms, since most of these patients are frustrated from their unexplained symptoms and disability. Patients who understand and engage actively in their treatment plan have the best outcomes. The goal of therapy, as with MPS, is to decrease pain and associated symptoms, restore the patient's functional status, and improve their quality of life. Physical therapy and psychological therapy such as cognitive behavioral therapy and biofeedback, lifestyle modifications, nutritional therapy, sleep hygiene, exercise, relaxation therapies, strengthening and stretching exercises, hydrotherapy, and acupuncture have all been proposed, by multiple society guidelines, as supported treatment modalities.

Pharmacologic therapy should focus on reducing the activity of excitatory neurotransmitters and increasing the activity of inhibitory pain pathways. Medications that have shown best efficacy include tricyclic antidepressants (TCA) (amitriptyline), SSRIs (fluoxetine, sertraline), SNRIs (milnacipran, duloxetine, venlafaxine), anticonvulsants (gabapentin, pregabalin), muscle relaxants (cyclobenzaprine, tizanidine), and central acting agents (tramadol, tapentadol).

Amitriptyline has been studied in more than 20 trials against placebo. It is known to improve pain and sleep disturbances, but its extensive side effect and anticholinergic profile, plus the worsened fatigue, hinder the potential usefulness of this medication [20–22].

Newer antidepressants, such as duloxetine and milnacipran, have shown significant improvement on a patient's symptomatology, and are FDA approved drugs for this condition [23]. Both of these drugs are better tolerated when they are taken with food. The patient should be warned of initial nausea during the initiation and titration period, but symptoms usually resolve within 1 week. The maximum FDA approved dose for duloxetine is 60 mg a day, but trials are ongoing that titrated the dose up to 120 mg without adverse outcomes. The usual dose for milnacipran is 100 mg a day. Clinical trials showed further benefit with doses as high as 200 mg/day, but issues observed with this dosage level included new or worsening hypertension, which was attributed to its higher adrenergic receptor affinity. Interestingly, this higher dose also seems to improve fatigue significantly. Both duloxetine and milnacipran have not been shown to improve sleep quality.

Antiepileptics, such as pregabalin and gabapentin, which exert their effect by binding to the presynaptic alpha 2 subunit voltage gated calcium channels, had limited placebo controlled trials, but were proven effective, especially with pregabalin, which is now FDA approved for the treatment of FMS. Pregabalin has been used at doses as high as 450 mg a day, with some trials going to as high as 600 mg a day, proving it to be safe and efficient. Gabapentin was only effective at high doses (1800–2400 mg a day). Other antiepileptics, such as valproic acid, have not been as effective, and have shown increased side effects and complications. The only exception is clonazepam, which was found to be useful for temporomandibular disorder. The use of gabapentinoids results in a small, but significant improvement, in sleep quality; but there was no improvement in fatigue [20–22].

Muscle relaxants can be used in FMS, and the relaxant of choice would be cyclobenzaprine. This molecule is an analog to imipramine and amitriptyline (TCAs), with receptor mediated effect, resulting in norepinephrine and serotonin reuptake blockade and some anticholinergic effects. Another muscle relaxant that is chemically an antihistamine (orphenadrine) has been anecdotally mentioned to have very good results for FMS, but there are no studies to validate this finding [20].

Tramadol, a centrally acting agent with dual mechanisms of action (weak opioid agonist and norepinephrine and serotonin reuptake inhibitor) has been found beneficial. Tapentadol is also a centrally acting opioid agonist, with a binary mechanism of action not only providing mu receptor activity, but also providing descending inhibition, via norepinephrine reuptake inhibitors, yielding similar or better results. The main advantage of this medication, when compared to tramadol, is that when abruptly stopped, at least 80% of subjects did not have any withdrawal symptoms, unlike those with tramadol. There have not been any studies focusing on the topic of fibromyalgia specifically, but other chronic pain studies compare its efficacy to that of oxycodone [30, 31].

Cannabinoids are an emerging class in the treatment for fibromyalgia. There have been a couple of randomized controlled trials, using nabilone, with promising results. Given the nature of central hyperactivity as one of the main factors in FMS, it is not surprising that the use of this depressant would yield positive effects.

Dopaminergic agonists used in Parkinson's disease, such as pramipexole, which is also used for restless legs syndrome, have shown in one study to improve both the quality of sleep and the pain in fibromyalgia patients. This effect is not replicated by any other analog medication that might work by the same mechanism on the same receptor.

Pure opioid agonists are not recommended for fibromyalgia. As further evidence emerges, there might be some similarities between opioid induced hyperalgesia (OIH) and fibromyalgia. One current thought suggests that neuroglia is activated, and remains in a constant state of alert after high dose opioid therapy [30, 31].

Unlike MPS, the use of anti-inflammatories is controversial, due to the chronicity of FMS. Numerous studies failed to confirm the effectiveness of NSAIDS in the treatment of fibromyalgia, yet some patients may experience enhanced analgesia while using these medications as an adjuvant for flare ups.

Specific NMDA receptor antagonists, such as ketamine and dextromethorphan, were found to exhibit beneficial effects for the fatigue and depressive components [32]. A potential issue emerges when ketamine is used chronically in a frequent manner, given that no studies in humans have been able to rule out the toxicity that has been found in animal studies. Dextromethorphan, which has a better side effect profile, has much less potency, and might be a good option as an adjuvant, when other therapies are ineffective, and the patient has had a good response to ketamine infusions.

Over the counter supplementation with 5-hydroxytryptamine, S-adenosyl-L-methionine (SAMe) revealed some symptom improvement, given that both these supplements are used for insomnia and depression, respectively; clinical evidence of results, however, are lacking [33, 34].

In summary, the management for both MPS and FMS depends not only on multimodal pharmacological therapies, but also on the physical and psychological modification of the patient's environment, to maximize the relief of symptoms.

21.4 Conclusion

Patients with myofascial pain syndrome and fibromyalgia are commonly observed in the clinical practices of general medicine, rheumatologists, and pain specialist's physicians. The diagnosis of both of these conditions is often delayed, due to its lack of objective physical findings or confirmatory laboratory tests. A multidisciplinary team approach, that addresses the patient's main complaints, which often includes pain specialists, physical therapy and rehabilitation specialists, pain psychologists, and rheumatologists, can have the best outcome for the patient. Patients also need to understand their disease, in order to achieve satisfactory treatment results, which includes restoring their functionality and productivity in life.

References

1. Russell I. Fibromyalgia syndrome and Myofascial pain syndrome. In: Wall and Melzack's textbook of pain. 6th ed. Philadelphia, PA: Elsevier; 2013. p. 658–82.
2. Demers Lavelle E, Lavelle W, Smith H. Myofascial trigger points. Anesthesiol Clin. 2007;25:841–51.
3. Wolfe F, et al. The American College of Rheumatology Preliminary Diagnostic Criteria for fibromyalgia and measurement of symptom severity. Arthritis Care Res. 2010;62(5):600–10.
4. Bennett R. Myofascial pain syndromes and their evaluation. Best Pract Res Clin Rheumatol. 2007;21(3):427–41.
5. Ruiz M, Nadador V, Fernandez-Alcantud J, Hernandez-Salvan J, et al. Dolor de origen muscular: dolor miofascial y fibromialgia. Revista Sociedad Española de Dolor. 2007;1:36–44.
6. Francisco Hernandez F. Sindromes miofasciales. Reumatologia Clinica. 2009;5(52):36–9.
7. Segura-Pérez M, Hernández-Criado T, Calvo-Lobo C, Vega-Piris L, Fernandez-Martin R, Rodriguez-Sanz D. A multimodal approach for myofascial pain syndrome: a prospective study. J Manipulative Physiol Ther. 2017;40(6):397–403. https://doi.org/10.1016/j.jmpt.2017.06.001.
8. Han S, Harrison P. Myofascial pain syndrome and trigger point management. Reg Anesth. 1997;22(1):89–101.
9. Simons DG. Understanding effective treatments of myofascial trigger points. J Bodyw Mov Ther. 2002;6(2):81–8.
10. Whitehouse MW. Anti-inflammatory glucocorticoid drugs: reflections after 60 years. Inflammopharmacology. 2011;19(1):1–19.
11. Uhl R, Roberts TT, Papaliodis DN, Mulligan MT, et al. Management of chronic musculoskeletal pain. J Am Acad Orthop Surg. 2014;22(2):101–10.
12. Ramsook R, Malanga GA. Myofascial low back pain. Curr Pain Headache Rep. 2012;16(5):423–32.
13. Cummings TM, White AR. Needling therapies in the management of myofascial trigger point pain: a systematic review. Arch Phys Med Rehabil. 2001;82:986–92.
14. Liu L, Huang Q-M. Evidence of dry needling in the management of myofascial trigger points associated with low back pain: a systematic review and meta-analysis. Arch Phys Med Rehabil. 2017;99(1):144–52. https://doi.org/10.1016/j.apmr.2017.06.0018.
15. Khumbare D, Singh D, Rathbone A, et al. Ultrasound-guided interventional procedures myofascial trigger points with structured literature review. Reg Anesth Pain Med. 2017;42(3):407–12.
16. Chim D, Cheng P. Ultrasound-guided trigger point injections. Tech Reg Anaesth Pain Manage. 2009;13(3):179–83.
17. Botwin KP, Sharma K, Saliba R, et al. Ultrasound-guided trigger point injections in the cervicothoracic musculature: a new and unreported technique. Pain Physician. 2008;11(6):885–9.
18. Shin HJ, Shin JC, Kim WS, et al. Application of ultrasound-guided trigger point injection for myofascial trigger points in the subscapularis and pectoralis muscles to post-mastectomy patients: a pilot study. Yonsei Med J. 2014;55(3):792–9.

19. Wolfe F, Clauw DJ, et al. 2016 revisions to the 2010/2011 fibromyalgia diagnostic criteria. Semin Arthritis Rheum. 2016;46(3):319–29.
20. Zhang T, Adatia A, Zarin W, et al. The efficacy of botulinum toxin type a in managing chronic musculoskeletal pain: a systematic review and meta analysis. Inflammopharmacology. 2011;19(1):21–34.
21. Smith H, Barkin R. Fibromyalgia syndrome: a discussion of the syndrome and pharmacotherapy. Am J Ther. 2010;17(4):418–39.
22. Clauw D. Fibromyalgia: a clinical review. JAMA. 2014;311(15):1547–55.
23. Chinn S, Caldwell W, Gritsenko K. Fibromyalgia pathogenesis and treatment options update. Curr Pain Headache Rep. 2016;20(4):25.
24. Borg-Stein J, Iaccarino MA. Myofascial pain syndrome treatments. Phys Med Rehab Clin. 2014;25(2):357–74.
25. Miller D, Richardson D, Mahmood E, Bajwa RJ, Jabbari B. Botulinum neurotoxin-A for treatment of refractory neck pain: a randomized, double-blind study. Pain Med. 2009;10(6):1012–7.
26. Ferrante F, Bearn L, Rothcock R, King L. Evidence against trigger point injection technique for the treatment of cervicothoracic myofascial pain with botulinum toxin type A. J Am Soc Anesthesiol. 2005;103(2):377–83.
27. Gerwin R. Botulinum toxin treatment of myofascial pain: a critical review of the literature. Curr Pain Headache Rep. 2012;16(5):413–22.
28. Goldenberg D. Clinical manifestations and diagnosis of fibromyalgia in adults. UpToDate. 2017:1–23.
29. Bellato E, Marini E, Castoldi F, et al. Fibromyalgia syndrome, etiology, pathogenesis, diagnosis, and treatment. Pain Res Treat. 2012;2012:1–17. https://doi.org/10.1155/2012/426130.
30. Ngian G-S, Guymer EK, Littlejohn GO. The use of opioids in fibromyalgia. Int J Rheum Dis. 2011;14(1):6–11.
31. Afilalo M, Okamoto I, Van Hove I, et al. Tapentadol immediate release compared with oxycodone immediate release for the relief of moderate-to-severe pain in patients with end stage joint disease. J Pain. 2008;9(4):32.
32. Cohen SP, Verdolin MH, Chang AS, et al. The intravenous ketamine test predicts subsequent response to an oral dextromethorphan treatment regimen in fibromyalgia patients. J Pain. 2006;7(6):391–8.
33. Seidel MF, Müller W. Differential pharmacotherapy for subgroups of fibromyalgia patients with specific consideration of 5-HT3 receptor antagonists. Expert Opin Pharmacother. 2011;12(9):1381–91.
34. Grothe D, Scheckner B, Albano D. Treatment of pain syndromes with venlafaxine. Pharmacotherapy. 2004;24(5):621–9.

Chapter 22
Urogenital Pain Including Pelvic Pain

Maged Mina, Jonathan Benfield, Sylvia Botros-Brey, and Cyril Mina

22.1 Causes and Etiology of Chronic Pelvic Pain

Chronic pelvic pain (CPP) is defined as noncyclical pain below the umbilicus for at least 6 months' duration involving the pelvis, anterior abdominal wall, lower back, and/or buttocks severe enough to cause functional disability or require treatment. It has been reported to affect up to 15% of women with an estimated annual cost of \$2.8 billion [1]. Proper diagnosis and treatment are elusive: While 70% of women with CPP will receive proper diagnosis and treatment plans, 61% of patients will remain undiagnosed [2, 3]. Many of these patients subsequently develop chronic pain with depression, pain out of proportion to pathology that adversely affects roles in marriage, family, and career [1, 2]. Early and appropriate diagnosis and intervention is important. CPP is multifactorial with several possible sources of pain originating within the gastrointestinal, urinary, reproductive, musculoskeletal, or neurological structures [4]. One study found the distribution of sources of pain to include gastrointestinal disorders (37%), followed by urological (31%), gynecological disorders (20%), and myofascial disorders (12%) [5]. Additionally, there often exists more than one etiology of pain—a thorough evaluation for additional sources of pain is necessary when assessing patients. In at least one-half of cases, there are one or more associated entities, such as irritable bowel syndrome, interstitial cystitis/painful bladder syndrome, endometriosis, or pelvic adhesions [1, 6–8]. The presence of concomitant

M. Mina (✉)
Department of Anesthesia Pain Clinic, UT Health San Antonio, San Antonio, TX, USA

J. Benfield
South Texas Spine Clinic, San Antonio, TX, USA

S. Botros-Brey
Department of Urology, UT Health San Antonio, San Antonio, TX, USA

C. Mina
University of Texas, Dallas, TX, USA

K. Shimoji et al. (eds.), *Chronic Pain Management in General and Hospital Practice*, https://doi.org/10.1007/978-981-15-2933-7_22

endometriosis with bladder pain/interstitial cystitis occurs (PBS/IC) 48% of the time, hypertonic pelvic floor dysfunction with PBS/IC 50–78% of the time, and concomitant vulvodynia 25% of the time [8]. Concomitant myofascial disorders are more common than once thought. Tu et al. estimated the prevalence of musculoskeletal disorders to be as high 22% among patients with CPP [9]. A focused pelvic exam assessing the muscles of the pelvic floor for pain, trigger points, and high tone should be part of the evaluation for CPP. The absence of abnormal findings and the lack of evidence of infectious, allergic, or oncological causes suggest a psychological origin of this condition [4]. Expert opinion suggests that without a single clear etiology, CPP can be conceptualized as a complex neuromuscular-psychosocial disorder consistent with either a chronic regional pain syndrome such as reflex sympathetic dystrophy or a functional somatic pain syndrome such as irritable bowel syndrome [10–12]. The pathophysiology is unclear, but it may include aspects of hyperesthesia/allodynia and pelvic floor dysfunction [10, 12]. It is important to assess the psychosocial context of the patient. Nearly 50% of women seeking care for CPP report a history of sexual, physical, or emotional trauma, and 30% have positive screening results for post-traumatic stress disorder [10, 13].

Sources of pain that should be considered when evaluating CPP are:

1. *GI/Anorectal*: Over one-third of patients presenting with CPP will have GI symptoms/origin. These patients will typically present with symptoms of pain associated with abdominal cramps, constipation, loose stools, and defecation. Causes include: irritable bowel syndrome, proctitis or proctalgia fugax, anorectal pain syndrome, anal fissure, and hemorrhoids.
2. *Urological*: About one-third of patients presenting with CPP will have urological symptoms/origin. These patients will typically present with urgency/frequency/nighttime voiding. They will often have lower abdominal/pelvic pain associated with perceived bladder fullness or bladder emptying. Causes include: prostate pain syndrome, interstitial cystitis, painful bladder syndrome, urethral pain syndrome, and urethral diverticulum.
3. *Gynecological*: About 20% of patients presenting with CPP will have a gynecological origin to their pain. This pain varies in presentation, but may get worse with periods or can localize to the vulva. Not all patients with endometriosis or adenomyosis (endometrial tissue found outside of the lining of the uterus, or within the lining of the uterus) will have pain and often the pain is not proportional to physical findings. Causes include: endometriosis, adenomyosis, vaginal pain syndrome, vulvar pain syndrome, generalized vulvar pain syndrome, localized vulvar pain syndrome: vestibular or clitoral pain, pelvic inflammatory disease, pelvic adhesions, and pelvic congestion syndrome.
4. *Muscular*: About 12% of patients with CPP will have pelvic floor dysfunction. These patients often present with vague pain that they have difficulty localizing, or sharp shooting pain that lasts for short or longer bouts. They may present with pain during intercourse, pain with constipation, urination or urgency/frequency. The pain can often be reproduced on exam. Causes include: high tone pelvic floor dysfunction, pelvic floor muscle pain syndrome, piriformis muscle syndrome, pelvic

floor muscle spasm, abdominal wall myofascial pain (trigger point), muscular strains and sprains, rectus tendon strain, and faulty or poor posture.

5. *Neurological*: Peripheral nerve involvement involves changes both in the peripheral and the central nervous system causing heightened reaction between stimulus and the response on the long term. The development of neuromas in the peripheral nervous system as they become sensitive to light touch and pressure where sympathetic fibers can also grow into the neuromas as well as the dorsal root ganglia and further progressing into the windup phenomenon which becomes centrally mediated. Pathology along the course of the nerves such as neoplasms, injection, trauma, surgical incisions, and postoperative adhesions may cause nerve impingement. The anterior groin nerves include the iliohypogastric nerve, ilioinguinal nerve, genitofemoral, lateral femoral cutaneous nerve, and the obturator nerve. Posterior subgluteal triangle nerves include: (1) sciatic nerve (SN), (2) posterior femoral cutaneous nerve (branching into the posterior cutaneous perineal branch and the cluneal nerves), (3) the nerve to the obturator internus muscle, (4) pudendal nerve S2-S4. (PN) Pudendal neuralgia: Anatomical variations may predispose the patient to developing pudendal neuralgia over time or with repeated low-grade trauma (such as sitting for prolonged periods of time or cycling) [14]. The autonomic nervous system shares innervation to the pelvic organs via the parasympathetic and the sympathetic nerves accompanying the sacral and thoracolumbar nerve roots as they travel towards the spine. Pathology involving the ganglion impar, superior hypogastric plexus and the inferior hypogastric plexus could be contributing factors in Chronic Pelvic pain and possible target sites for nerve blocks.
6. *Musculoskeletal* conditions contributing to chronic pelvic pain include the following: fibromyalgia, compression of lumbar vertebrae, early articular hip disorders, acetabular labral tears, developmental hip dysplasia, hip osteoarthritis, low back pain, neoplasia of the spinal cord or sacral nerve, spondylosis, degenerative joint disease, chronic coccygeal pain, and femoral acetabular impingement.
7. *Psychological*: Psychogenic factors could play a role in development and the maintenance of chronic pelvic pain yet the data are not consistent if these were as a consequence or existing independently. Factors that were searched include sexual or physical abuse, anxiety and depression, post-traumatic stress disorder related to rape, somatization, and early trauma in childhood ages [15].

22.2 General Treatment of Chronic Pelvic Pain

22.2.1 Road Map for the Diagnosis and Treatment of Chronic Pelvic Pain

A detailed history and physical exam are required to identify the presence of a specific organ system disease, which will be addressed by the appropriate specialist. If there is none present, then treat it as chronic pelvic pain syndrome ruling out other diseases treated by multidisciplinary pain clinic, which includes physical therapy modalities, behavioral therapy modalities, pharmacological modalities, interventional modalities, and complementary alternative medicine.

22.2.1.1 Physical Exam and Diagnosis

Examining a patient with chronic pelvic pain is preceded by obtaining a thorough pain history, timeline, associated signs and symptoms, and pertinent past medical, surgical, and social history. This includes but is not limited to prior abdominal, gynecological, or psychological conditions (including child, physical, or sexual abuse) and/or surgeries preceding the pain onset. Additionally, basic lab work, age and gender appropriate cancer screens, gynecologic exam in females, and testicular and/or prostate examinations for male patients should be completed prior to a pain physician consultation. Attention to co-existing bowel or bladder incontinence; penile, vaginal, or rectal pain or discharge accompanying the pelvic pain is critical to identify neurologic, infectious, visceral or oncologic conditions or disease [16–18]. Abdominal, hip, lumbar spine, and sacral-iliac joint evaluations should accompany pelvic examinations [16]. For brevity, this section pays direct attention to the pelvic floor examination. Pelvic floor examination requires a chaperone to insure patient and provider comfort. Verbal consent should be obtained from the patient [16]. Pelvic floor anatomy and thus examination differ between genders. Pelvic floor examination consists of an external and internal evaluation of several structures. This includes surface anatomy; muscles: puborectalis, pubococcygeus, iliococcygeus, coccygeus, piriformis, obturator internus, and levator ani; neurological structures: ilioinguinal, iliohypogastric genitofemoral, lateral femoral cutaneous (LCFN), obturator, pudendal, and thoraco-sacral nerve roots T12-S5 in their respective dermatomes [16–18]. The external examination screens for cysts, osseous, or soft tissue abnormalities or masses, surgical scars, swelling, skin color changes, or other anatomic abnormalities or variants [16]. An involuntary and voluntary contraction via a Kegel maneuver and cough or Valsalva maneuver are performed by the patient to verify the appropriate lift and descent of external perineal organs [16]. Women will require evaluation for vulvodynia, vaginal or rectal prolapse. Men will require evaluation for testicular descent, varicoceles and rectal prolapse along with sensory nerve examination including sensory testing of thoraco-sacral dermatomes, ilioinguinal, iliohypogastric, genitofemoral, LCFN, obturator and pudendal nerve and an anal wink response [16–19]. Next, the internal exam will require gloving the exam hand and applying lubricant for patient comfort. Female exams include insertion of a gloved finger into the vagina and anus. Male exams require similar technique with one to palpate musculature under the scrotum and the other hand inserted into the anus [16–19]. Keeping correct anatomic orientation during examination can be difficult. It is suggested to visualize pelvic musculature using the face of a clock [16]. The "pelvic clock" is oriented into 12 o'clock represents anterior orientation with the pubic bone; 6 o'clock is posterior and represents the anus. The right and left Internal Obturator muscles are located at 3 and 9 o'clock, respectively. Levator ani are found between 3–5 o'clock on the left and 7–9 o'clock on the right [16]. These muscles can be graded on a Modified Oxford scale. This is a 0–5 scale with 0 being the lowest or weakest and 5 being the highest or strong on the scale. 0/5 = no contraction or tightening, 1/5 = flicker contraction with no lift or tightening, 2/5 weak contract with no lift or tightening, 3/5 moderate contraction with soft lift or tightening, 4/5 good contraction with ability to lift or tighten pelvic floor muscles for 5+ seconds, and 5/5 with strong contraction and lift or tighten for 10+ seconds [16, 20, 21]. The Brink scale [22] is another commonly used scale to grade muscle strength testing for the pelvic floor. There is variability in manual muscle strength testing based upon scale and position used during the exam. Digital palpation for muscle strength testing is validated and comparable to manometry [20]. However, neither is a gold standard. Unfortunately, there is no gold standard diagnostic test or provocative maneuver to diagnose chronic pelvic pain or to differentiate if a myofascial component of pelvic pain is the provoking etiology or resultant sign or symptom of a different pathology. Provocative maneuvers for pelvic examination outside of testing for specific pelvic floor dysfunction are similar to those found in lumbar spine, sacroiliac and hip provocative maneuvers. They include posture testing for increased or decreased lumbar lordosis, Trendelenburg sign, hip range of motion, Patrick or FABER test, posterior pelvic pain provocation test, abdominal muscle testing, and pelvic floor testing including strength and tenderness. Nevile et al. [23] suggested that there is 100% specificity in identifying women with chronic pelvic pain when using the forced FABER test and pelvic floor muscle palpation. Tu et al. [24] agreed with these findings that the higher frequency of positive pelvic provocative maneuvers correlated with a higher likelihood of a somatic or myofascial cause of the chronic pelvic pain. Both authors Nevile and Tu confirmed the use of both exams but there was no one maneuver that provided a gold standard [23, 24]. Patients with increased tenderness and decreased strength on pelvic muscle floor testing accompanied by asymmetric anatomical osseous structures like iliac crest and pubic symphysis heights and a negative work-up for a visceral etiology justify treatment for myofascial induced pelvic pain [23, 24]. As an extension and aid to physical evaluation, diagnostic electromyography, manometry, and imaging can also be performed [25].

22.2.1.2 Multidisciplinary Approaches

Physical Therapy Modalities

Physical therapy, including Kegel exercise and myofascial treatments, accompanied with biofeedback, behavioral modifications, and acupuncture is an evidence based approach to treating chronic pelvic pain in men and women [16]. A multi-modal comprehensive physical therapy program uses manual therapy with myofascial release techniques of pelvic floor and abdominal musculature with a range of motion exercises that focuses on flexibility and strength of weak pelvic floor and abdominal muscles and biofeedback to improve relaxation and strength [26]. Within physical therapy modalities, myofascial release techniques targeted to weak or restricted pelvic floor muscles are more effective than general therapeutic massage [27]. Improved results can be seen when biofeedback and relaxation techniques are adjuvants to a comprehensive myofascial physical therapy program [27, 28]. One study reported results with as few as 6 days of therapy even if the therapy and or relaxation techniques were self-administered [29]. Chronic pelvic pain requires thorough and thoughtful examination with the use of a respectful exam of pelvic floor muscles using standardized and validated scales like the Modified Oxford or Brink scale or manometry. The exam can be aided by electro diagnostic testing of further imaging. First-line treatment options include relaxation and stress management accompanied by patient education and improved self-care. If no improvement, a manual myofascial therapy as described above should be prescribed. Further treatment modalities would include with biofeedback, real-time ultrasound, electrical stimulation, and vaginal expanders. Select modalities can be included in home exercise programs. In summary, treatment plans should include a multi-model approach of myofascial focused physical therapy, biofeedback, and relaxation techniques independent of or adjuvant to pharmacologic or interventional treatments. Importantly, patients should be referred to appropriate physicians if age and gender specific cancer screenings and visceral work-up have not been completed to rule out oncologic, infectious, neurologic, or visceral pathology.

Behavioral Therapy Modalities

Several studies have demonstrated the importance of psychological interventions in patients with chronic pelvic pain with great positive outcomes. Relaxation and biofeedback have been extensively used to control the pain and reduce muscle tone particularly pelvic floor pathology. Other modalities included patient education, cognitive therapy, and mood coping exercises [30].

Pharmacological Modalities

Using different combinations of medications to improve quality of life may provide better efficacy than single agents by allowing lower dosages and hence reducing side effects. Dose titration might be required to achieve the best effective dose with the least amount of side effects. Medications involve multiple routes such as systemic, topical transdermal, and suppository.

A. *Analgesics*

1. Paracetamol (acetaminophen)

   The mechanism of action of paracetamol is unclear; however, it is believed to work by inhibiting central prostaglandin synthesis, and potentiating other analgesic medications. When combined with NSAIDs or caffeine, paracetamol has been shown to provide pain relief in pelvic pain. Hepatotoxicity is a known risk of acetaminophen with dose related effects.

2. Non-steroidal anti-inflammatory agents (NSAIDs)

   These are anti-inflammatory, antipyretic analgesics that act by inhibiting the enzyme cyclooxygenase (COX) have proven to be more effective than paracetamol, but with a higher incidence of side effects. Selective COX-2 inhibitors have also been successfully used in the management of primary dysmenorrhea, endometriosis, and CPP specifically, though the risk of scheduled use of NSAIDS remains high with effects on the hepatic, renal, cardiovascular and gastrointestinal systems.
3. Opioids

   Opioids have a limited role in chronic nonmalignant pelvic pain and their use remains controversial. Opioid analgesics provide pain relief through their effect on opioid receptors located in the brain (cortex, thalamus, and periaqueductal gray) and the spinal cord mostly the μ or the δ receptors although activating δ receptors contribute to their side effect profile. The long-term use of opioids should be taken into consideration due to the risks of opioid abuse, misuse, and diversion.

B. *Antidepressants*

1. Tricyclic antidepressants (TCAs) are considered first-line treatment of many neuropathic chronic pain conditions, where amitriptyline, nortriptyline, and imipramine have been studied in patients with CPP with positive improvement of pain symptoms [31].
2. Serotonin reuptake inhibitors (sertraline) and selective serotonin norepinephrine reuptake inhibitors have been used successfully in the treatment of patients with CPP by increasing the availability of serotonin and norepinephrine. Duloxetine has been identified as an effective pain modulator in patients with pelvic pain [32].

C. *Membrane Stabilizers*

1. Calcium Channel Blockers

   Both gabapentin and pregabalin act as calcium channel blockers and exert their effects by decreasing the reuptake of norepinephrine, glutamate, and substance P and function as membrane stabilizers both centrally and peripherally. Being traditionally prescribed for neuropathic pain, these agents have been used successfully in nonspecific pain conditions. Gabapentin has been studied more with evidence backing its efficacy in CPP where the dose was titrated up to 2700 mg per day to achieve 50% reduction in pain scores [33].
2. Sodium Channel Blockers

   These anticonvulsants agents work by decreasing global neuronal membrane excitability and reduce the spontaneous firing of sensory neurons. Examples are phenytoin, carbamazepine, oxcarbazepine, lamotrigine, tiagabine, and topiramate which have been studied and found to be effective in many neuropathic pain conditions [34].

D. *Topical Medications*

Lidocaine in the form of topical 5% patches provides relief in patients with great tolerability in patients with neuropathic pain and allodynia. Lidocaine exerts its actions by blocking of the voltage-gated sodium channels that are expressed by nerve fibers, hence delaying the propagation of action potentials. Its efficacy has been documented in cases of neuropathic pain, including post-surgical and incisional pain [35].

Other topical medications, such as capsaicin, that selectively bind to the ion channel receptor, vanilloid receptor subtype 1 (TRPV1) receptors, have been identified as pain modulators in individuals with endometriosis and CPP. Its proposed mechanism of action is by desensitization of the unmyelinated C nerve fibers that contribute to the pelvic pain.

E. *Treatments Used in Specific Pelvic Syndromes*

1. Prostatic Pain Syndrome

   Alpha blockers, antibiotics, and NSAIDS play a therapeutic role in prostatic pain syndrome [36]. The mechanism of action of alpha-antagonists is by blocking the alpha-receptors of the bladder neck and prostate and by direct action on alpha1A/1D receptors in the CNS with significant improvement in total symptom, pain, voiding, and QOL scores [37]. Combination therapy of antibiotics with alpha-blockers has shown even better outcomes in prostatic pain syndrome.
2. Bladder pain syndrome may respond to oral pentosan polysulfate sodium and amitriptyline, which are effective for pain related symptoms [38].

Interventional Modalities

For CPP due to neuropathic pain, validated questionnaires should be utilized to screen for neuropathic pain conditions, such as the Leeds Assessment of Neuropathic Symptoms and Signs (LANSS). All patients experiencing chronic pelvic pain should be given benefits of comprehensive multimodal and multidisciplinary pain management, which refers to interventional nerve blocks, surgical interventions.

A. *Peripheral Nerve Block Injections*

The role of injections may be divided into two. First, providing therapeutic relief by injecting a mixture of local anesthetic and steroid at the area of nerve entrapment as the steroids to help reduce inflammation and swelling at the site of nerve irritation, also by blocking of sodium channels reduce irritable firing from the nerve [39]. The second possible benefit of local infiltration is diagnostic peripheral nerves involved (divided into thoracolumbar and sacral root afferents).

Thoracolumbar nerves:

1. The iliohypogastric (IH) nerve arises from L1.
2. The ilioinguinal (IL) nerve it also arises from L1.

3. The genitofemoral (GFN) nerve arises from L1 and L2.
4. The lateral femoral cutaneous nerve (LFCN) of the thigh arises from L2 and L3.
5. The obturator nerve (ON) arises from L2-L4.

   Posterior subgluteal triangle nerves:

1. sciatic nerve (SN),
2. posterior femoral cutaneous nerve (branching into the posterior cutaneous perineal branch and the cluneal nerves),
3. the nerve to the obturator internus muscle,
4. pudendal nerve S2-S4. (PN).

   These nerves pass deep to the piriformis muscle and superficial to the superior gemellus and obturator internus muscles.

1. Ilioinguinal and Iliohypogastric Nerve Blocks.

   For patients suffering from chronic post-surgical neuropathic pain in the groin, pain extends to the scrotum or the testicle in men, the labia majora in women, and the medial aspect of the thigh.

   Ultrasound-guided techniques with 95% accuracy in localizing both nerves have been validated. A linear probe of high frequency (6–13 MHz) is used to visualize the superficial nerves orienting the probe perpendicular to the inguinal line joining pubic tubercle to the ASIS, with the lateral end of the probe just above or posterior to the ASIS to view the three layers of abdominal muscles and the IL and IH nerves in the fascial split between internal oblique and transversus abdominis muscles. An out-of-plane or an in-plane technique has been described to deposit a mixture of local anesthetic and steroids into the fascial plane [40].
2. Genitofemoral Nerve Block.

   A linear probe of high frequency (6–13 MHz) is used for blocking the genital branch of the GF nerve under ultrasound guidance described by scanning at the level of the internal inguinal ring viewing the femoral artery in the long axis then sliding the probe cephalad, tracing the artery as it dives toward the inguinal ligament to become the external iliac artery. The probe is finally situated perpendicular to the inguinal line and lateral to the pubic tubercle. At this level the spermatic cord in males (which contains the testicular artery, the artery to the vas deferens and the vas deferens) or the round ligament of the uterus in females can be seen as oval or round figures superficial to the external iliac artery. The spermatic cord or round ligament is then traced by sliding the probe medially. The key structure is the spermatic cord (round ligament of the uterus in a female), which is oval or circular in shape with 1 or 2 arteries within it (the testicular artery and the artery to the vas deferens). The vas deferens is often seen as a thick tubular structure also found within the spermatic cord. At this point, an oval or circular structure can easily be seen superficial to the external iliac artery just opposite to the internal inguinal ring. The probe is then moved slightly in the medial direction away from the femoral artery in an attempt to trace the spermatic cord or round ligament. An out-of-plane technique is also used, with the needle approaching the skin from the lateral aspect of the probe. An in-plane and out-of-plane can be used to infiltrate the injectate without epinephrine to avoid vasospastic effects inside and outside the spermatic cord [41].

3. Pudendal nerve injections.

   It has already been indicated that when the pudendal nerve is injured there are several sites where this may occur. Differential block of the pudendal nerve helps to provide information in relation to the site where the nerve may be trapped [41]. Pudendal nerve blocks can be performed in patients with CPP due to pudendal neuralgia providing both diagnostic and therapeutic effects.

   A low-frequency, 2–5 MHz, curved array ultrasound probe is used to scan at the lateral border of the sciatic notch in a transverse view to locate the ischial spine seen as a sharp hyperechoic line caudal to the ischium which is viewed as a curved line with the sacrospinous ligament attached as a hyperechoic line connecting it to the sacrum. Lateral to the tip of the ischial spine the sciatic nerve can be visualized accompanied very closely by the inferior gluteal artery then more lateral is the internal pudendal artery followed by the pudendal nerve usually not visualized hence the target is medial to the internal pudendal artery using color Doppler to identify the vessels [41].

B. *Neurolytic Sympathetic Blocks*

1. Superior Hypogastric Plexus

   The caudal portion of the paravertebral sympathetic chain forms the superior hypogastric plexus (SHP) anterior to the L5–S1 junction. As the fibers descend towards the S1 levels, they begin to divide into the hypogastric nerves where they become medial to the iliac vessels and ventral to the psoas muscle. Sympathetically mediated pain via the superior hypogastric plexus can be determined through diagnostic blocks also providing therapeutic relief in patients with CPP that is nociceptive, visceral, or neuropathic related.

   Approaches

   (a) Posterior traditional approach for bilateral percutaneous neurolytic blocks of SHP using 10% phenol has been described by Plancarte in 1997 that was preceded by successful diagnostic blocks using 0.25% bupivacaine [42].
   (b) Anterior transdiscal approach through L5-S1 also has been described [43].
   (c) Anterior ultrasound-guided superior hypogastric plexus neurolysis [44].

2. Ganglion Impar (GI) Block

   The terminal portion of the paravertebral sympathetic chain fuses together to form a single retroperitoneal ganglion posterior to the rectum at the sacrococcygeal junction called the ganglion impar (GI), also known as the sacrococcygeal ganglion or the ganglion of Walther. It extends to the second coccygeal vertebrae sending gray rami communicates fibers with the sacral nerves to pelvic viscera.

Approaches

(a) Plancarte described the anococcygeal landmark approach to perform the block in 1990 treating patients with pelvic pain related to the perineum, distal rectum, the distal thirds of the urethra, and the vagina also used for coccydynia. The block is performed with a spinal needle that is angled being aiming cephalad through the anococcygeal ligament.
(b) Due to the high risk of rectal perforation this approach did not gain much support.
(c) CT-guided ganglion impar blocks using ethanol described for the ganglion impar in patients with perineal pain [45].
(d) Vertical transsacrococcygeal approach to ganglion impar has been used to avoid needle passage through the perineum [46].
(e) Paracoccygeal approach achieves a shorter passage to the ganglion impar [47].
(f) Needle-in-needle technique using fluoroscopy has some advantages as reducing the risk of infection, injury to intervertebral discs and needle breaking [48].
(g) Ultrasound assisted approach in conjunction with fluoroscopy to view needle tip once passes through the sacrum [47].
(h) A combined neurolytic SHGP block with GI block can be used for reducing pain in patients presenting with pelvic and/or perineal pain [49].

C. *Neuromodulation Interventions*

1. Sacral Neuromodulation (SNM)

   The technique was introduced in the 1980s for intractable pelvic pain and dysfunction after failed conservative approaches, before escalating to more invasive restorative bladder surgeries in cases of bladder pain syndrome, interstitial cystitis, and CPP. Although the mechanism of symptom relief through SNM is still not fully understood yet it may play a role to inhibit the transmission of afferent sensory signals to the spinal cord and brain. Using bilateral or unilateral leads cannot be fully determined due to little evidence to support on or the other [50]. In patients with pudendal neuralgia patients may respond to neuromodulation particularly if the stimulation is perceived at the same site as the perceived pain [51].

2. Spinal Cord Dorsal Column Neuromodulation

   Initially introduced in 1967, dorsal column stimulation (DCS) for the treatment of intractable pain continues to evolve to cover patients with neuropathic pain, visceral pain, and recently nociceptive pain in patients that have chronic, intractable pain that have failed other conservative modalities. Multiple studies have shown the visceral pathways through the dorsal column which may explain the effectiveness of DCS in cases of refractory pelvic pain with a history of dyspareunia, endometriosis, and surgical adhesions due to multiple abdominal surgeries. Neuromodulation of the midline dorsal column pathway that is recently described to be involved in the perception of pelvic pain may have a role in pain reduction. Implanting the leads seems optimal at T11–T12 levels using dual compact or quad leads after a successful trial [52].

D. *Pulsed Radiofrequency Interventions*

Pulsed radiofrequency (PRF) uses short bursts of thermal energy rather than continuous lesioning used in traditional radiofrequency ablation techniques, hence may cause neuromodulation by transient inhibition of evoked synaptic activity lesioning with less neuronal damage. More studies are showing the effectiveness of PRF in cases of intractable peripheral neuropathic pain.

Cases series have been described for PRF of the pudendal nerve and the ilio-inguinal nerves [53, 54].

E. *Pelvic Floor Muscles Trigger Point Interventions*

1. Piriformis syndrome in patients with CPP and may benefit from injecting the piriformis muscle with local anesthetic and steroids or using botulinum toxin [55].

   Ultrasound-guided piriformis muscle injection has been described using a curved array probe low frequency (2–5 Hz) with the patient prone scanning in the transverse plane starting at the posterior superior iliac spine moving the probe caudally to view the ischium which is a curved hyperechoic line which then becomes the ischial spine seen as a sharp straight line on the medial part of the image representing lower border of the piriformis and superficial to it is the gluteus maximus muscle [41].
2. Trigger point injections of the pelvic floor may help in cases of myofascial pain although studies have not shown great difference between dry and wet needling into the trigger points.

   Botulinum A toxin (BTX-A) has a paralyzing effect on striated muscles by inhibiting the release of acetylcholine at the neuromuscular junction. Other proposed mechanisms of actions include blocking of other pain regulating neurotransmitters including glutamate, substance P, and calcitonin gene-related peptide adding to its analgesic effect. Pelvic floor muscle over activity plays a role in CPP where BTX-A may be injected to reduce the resting pressure in the pelvic floor muscles in patients with elevated resting pressure in the pelvic floor muscles. It has been found that BTX-A lowers this pressure significantly providing symptom relief [56].
3. Sphincter injections with BTX-A can be used to relax sphincter tone to be injected at the sphincter level improving functionality and reducing pain scores in patients with urethral and anal sphincter dystonia [57].

References

1. Gyang A, Hartman M, Lamvu G. Musculoskeletal causes of chronic pelvic pain: what a gynecologist should know. Obstet Gynecol. 2013;121:645–50.
2. Scialli AR, Barbieri RL, Glasser MH, Olive DL, Winkel CA. Chronic pelvic pain: an integrated approach. Washington, DC: APGO; 2000.

3. Crofton MD. Medical Education Collaborative, Association of Professors of Gynecology and Obstetrics. 2000:3–9.
4. Dalpiaz O, Kerschbaumer A, Mitterberger M, Pinggera G, Bartsch G, Strasser H. Chronic pelvic pain in women—still a challenge. BJUI. 2001;102:1061–106.
5. Ahangari A. Prevalence of chronic pelvic pain among women: an updated review. Pain Phys. 2014;17(2):E141–7.
6. Williams RE, Hartmann KE, Sandler RS, Miller WC, Steege JF. Prevalence and characteristics of irritable bowel syndrome among women with chronic pelvic pain. Obstet Gynecol. 2004;104(3):452–8.
7. Haggerty CL, Peipert JF, Weitzen S, et al. PID evaluation and clinical health (PEACH) study investigators. Predictors of chronic pelvic pain in an urban population of women with symptoms and signs of pelvic inflammatory disease. Sex Transm Dis. 2005;32(5):293–9.
8. Cervigni M, Natale F. Gynecological disorders in bladder pain syndrome/interstitial cystitis patients. Int J Urol. 2014;21:85–8.
9. Tu FF, As-Sanie S, Steege J. Prevalence of pelvic musculoskeletal disorders in a female chronic pelvic pain clinic. J Reprod Med. 2006;51:185–9.
10. Speer LM, Mushkbar S, Erbele T. Chronic pelvic pain in women. Am Fam Physician. 2016;93(5):380–7.
11. Engeler DS, Baranowski AP, Dinis-Oliveira P, et al. The 2013 EAU guidelines on chronic pelvic pain: is management of chronic pelvic pain a habit, a philosophy, or a science? 10 years of development. Eur Urol. 2013;64(3):431–9.
12. Potts JM, Payne CK. Urologic chronic pelvic pain. Pain. 2012;153(4):755–8.
13. Meltzer-Brody S, Leserman J, Zolnoun D, Steege J, Green E, Teich A. Trauma and post-traumatic stress disorder in women with chronic pelvic pain. Obstet Gynecol. 2007;109(4):902–8.
14. Mahakkanukrauh P, Surin P, Vaidhayakarn P. Anatomical study of the pudendal nerve adjacent to the sacrospinous ligament. Clin Anat. 2005;18(3):200–5.
15. Leserman J, Zolnoun D, Meltzer-Brody S, et al. Identification of diagnostic subtypes of chronic pelvic pain and how subtypes differ in health status and trauma history. Am J Obstet Gynecol. 2006;195(2):554–60. discussion 560–1.
16. Cifu DX, Kaelin DL, Kowalske KJ, Lew HL, Miller MA, Ragnarsson KT, Worsowicz GM. Pelvic floor disorders. In: Braddom's physical medicine & rehabilitation, vol. 38. 5th ed. Philadelphia, PA: Elsevier; 2016. p. 835–49.
17. Apte G, et al. Chronic female pelvic pain—part 1: clinical pathoanatomy and examination of the pelvic region. Pain Pract. 2011;12(2):88–110.
18. Nelson P, et al. Chronic female pelvic pain—part 2: differential diagnosis and management. Pain Pract. 2011;12(2):111–41.
19. Wyandaele J, Eetvelde BV. Reproducibility of digital testing of the pelvic muscles in men. Arch Med Rehabil. 1996;77:1179–81.
20. Da Roza T, et al. Oxford Grading Scale vs manometer for assessment of pelvic floor strength in nulliparous sports students. Physiotherapy. 2013;99(3):207–11.
21. Frawley H. Pelvic floor muscle strength testing. Aust J Physiother. 2005;25:263–42.
22. Brink CA, Sampselle CM, Wells TJ. A digital test for pelvic muscle strength in older women with urinary incontinence. Nurs Res. 1989;38:196–9.
23. Nevile CE, et al. A preliminary report of musculoskeletal dysfunction in female chronic pelvic pain: a blinded study of examination findings. J Bodyw Movement Ther. 2012;16:50–6.
24. Tu FF, et al. Physical therapy evaluation of patients with chronic pelvic pain: a controlled study. Am J Obstet Gynecol. 2008;198:272e1–7.
25. Aguilar V, White A, Rogers R. Updates on the diagnostic tools for evaluation of pelvic floor disorders. Curr Opin Obstet Gynecol. 2017;29:458–64.
26. Masterson TA, et al. Comprehensive pelvic floor physical therapy program for men with idiopathic chronic pelvic pain syndrome: a prospective study. Transl Androl Urol. 2017;6(5):910–5.
27. FitzGerald MP, et al. Randomized multicenter feasibility trial of myofascial physical therapy for the treatment of urological chronic pelvic pain syndromes. J Urol. 2009;182:570–80.

28. Cornel EB, et al. The effect of biofeedback physical therapy in men with chronic pelvic pain syndrome type III. Eur Urol. 2005;47:607–11.
29. Anderson RU, et al. 6-day intensive treatment protocol for refractory chronic prostatitis/chronic pelvic pain syndrome using myofascial release and paradoxical relaxation training. J Urol. 2011;185:1294–9.
30. Haugstad GK, Haugstad TS, Kirste UM, et al. Mensendieck somatocognitive therapy as treatment approach to chronic pelvic pain: results of a randomized controlled intervention study. Am J Obstet Gynecol. 2006;194(5):1303–10.
31. An update on the drug treatment of neuropathic pain. Part 1: antidepressants. Drug Ther Bull. 2012;50(10):114–7. https://www.ncbi.nlm.nih.gov/pubmed/23065751.
32. Lunn MP, Hughes RA, Wiffen PJ. Duloxetine for treating painful neuropathy, chronic pain or fibromyalgia. Cochrane Database Syst Rev. 2014;1:CD007115.
33. Lewis SC, Bhattacharya S, Wu O, et al. Gabapentin for the management of chronic pelvic pain in women (GaPP1): a pilot randomized controlled trial. PLoS One. 2016;11(4):e0153037.
34. Bhattacharya A, Wickenden AD, Chaplan SR. Sodium channel blockers for the treatment of neuropathic pain. Neurotherapeutics. 2009;6(4):663–78.
35. Baron R, Allegri M, Correa-Illanes G, et al. The 5% lidocaine-medicated plaster: its inclusion in international treatment guidelines for treating localized neuropathic pain, and clinical evidence supporting its use. Pain Ther. 2016;5:149–69. https://doi.org/10.1007/s40122-016-00603.
36. Turner JA, Ciol MA, Von Korff M, et al. Prognosis of patients with new prostatitis/pelvic pain syndrome episodes. J Urol. 2004;172(2):538–41.
37. Anothaisintawee T, Attia J, Nickel JC, et al. Management of chronic prostatitis/chronic pelvic pain syndrome: a systematic review and network meta-analysis. JAMA. 2011;305(1):78–86.
38. Engeler D, Baranowski AP, Borovicka J, Cottrell A, Dinis-Oliveira P, Elneil S, Hughes J, Messelink EJ, van Ophoven A, Reisman Y, de C. Williams AC. Guidelines on chronic pelvic pain. Arnhem: European Association of Urology; 2014.
39. Eker HE, Cok OY, Aribogan A, et al. Management of neuropathic pain with methylprednisolone at the site of nerve injury. Pain Med. 2012;13(3):443–51.
40. Eichenberger U, Greher M, Kirchmair L, Curatolo M, Morigg B. Ultrasound-guided blocks of the ilioinguinal and iliohypogastric nerve: accuracy of a selective new technique confirmed by anatomical dissection. Br J Anaesth. 2006;97:238–43.
41. Peng PWH, Tumber PS. Ultrasound-guided interventional procedures for patients with chronic pelvic pain-a description of techniques and review of the literature. Pain Phys. 2008;11:215–24.
42. Plancarte R, Amescua C, Patt R, Aldrete A. Superior hypogastric plexus block for pelvic cancer pain. Anesthesiology. 1990;73:236–9.
43. Gamal G, Helaly M, Labib Y. Superior hypogastric block: transdiscal versus classic posterior approach in pelvic cancer pain. Clin J Pain. 2006;22:544–7.
44. Mishra S, Bhatnagar S, Rana SP, Khurana D, Thulkar S. Efficacy of the anterior ultrasound-guided superior hypogastric plexus neurolysis in pelvic cancer pain in advanced gynecological cancer patients. Pain Med. 2013;14:837–42.
45. Agarwal-Kozlowski K, Lorke DE, Habermann CR, Am Esch JS, Beck H. CT-guided blocks and neuroablation of the ganglion impar (Walther) in perineal pain: anatomy, technique, safety, and efficacy. Clin J Pain. 2009;25:570–6.
46. Eker HE, Cok OY, Kocum A, Acil M, Turkoz A. Transsacrococcygeal approach to ganglion impar for pelvic cancer pain: a report of 3 cases. Reg Anesth Pain Med. 2008;33:381–2.
47. Lin CS, Cheng JK, Hsu YW, et al. Ultrasound-guided ganglion impar block: a technical report. Pain Med. 2010;11:390–4.
48. Munir MA, Zhang J, Ahmad M. A modified needle-inside- needle technique for the ganglion impar block. Can J Anaesth. 2004;51:915–7.
49. Ahmed DG, Mohamed MF, Mohamed SA. Superior hypogastric plexus combined with ganglion impar neurolytic blocks for pelvic and/or perineal cancer pain relief. Pain Phys. 2015;18(1):E49–56.

50. Engeler DS, et al. The 2013 EAU guidelines on chronic pelvic pain: is management of chronic pelvic pain a habit, a philosophy, or a science? 10 years of development. Eur Urol. 2013;64:431–9. https://doi.org/10.1016/j.eururo.2013.04.035.
51. Carmel M, Lebel M, Tu le M. Pudendal nerve neuromodulation with neurophysiology guidance: a potential treatment option for refractory chronic pelvi-perineal pain. Int Urogynecol J. 2010;21(5):613–6.
52. Kapural L, Narouze SN, Janicki TI, Mekhail N. Spinal cord stimulation is an effective treatment for the chronic intractable visceral pelvic pain. Pain Med. 2006;7(5):440–3.
53. Petrov-Kondratov V, Chhabra A, Jones S. Pain Phys. 2017;20(3):E451–4.
54. Kim JH, Kim E, Kim BI. Pulsed radiofrequency treatment of the superior hypogastric plexus in an interstitial cystitis patient with chronic pain and symptoms refractory to oral and intravesical medications and bladder hydrodistension: a case report. Medicine (Baltimore). 2016;95(49):e5549.
55. Fishman LM, Anderson C, Rosner B. Botox and physical therapy in the treatment of piriformis syndrome. Am J Phys Med Rehabil. 2002;81:936–42.
56. Abbott JA, Jarvis SK, Lyons SD, et al. Botulinum toxin type a for chronic pain and pelvic floor spasm in women: a randomized controlled trial. Obstet Gynecol. 2006;108(4):915–23.
57. Zermann D, Ishigooka M, Schubert J, et al. Perisphincteric injection of botulinum toxin type A. A treatment option for patients with chronic prostatic pain? Eur Urol. 2000;38(4):393–9.

Chapter 23
Chest Pain

Ju Mizuno and Kazuo Hanaoka

Abbreviation

ACS	Acute coronary syndrome
af	Atrial fibrillation
AF	Atrial flutter
AR	Aortic valve regurgitation
AS	Aortic valve stenosis
CABG	Coronary artery bypass grafting
CAD	Coronary artery disease
CP	Chest pain
CRPS	Complex regional pain syndrome
CT	Computerized tomography
DCM	Dilated cardiomyopathy
ECG	Electrocardiography
EMD	Esophageal motor disorder
ER	Emergency room
FBSS	Failed-back surgery syndrome
GERD	Gastroesophageal reflux disease
HCM	Hypertrophic cardiomyopathy
HZ	Herpes zoster
ICM	Ischemic cardiomyopathy

J. Mizuno
Department of Anesthesiology and Pain Medicine, Juntendo University Faculty of Medicine, Tokyo, Japan
e-mail: jmizuno@juntendo.ac.jp

K. Hanaoka (✉)
Department of Anesthesiology and Pain Relief Center, JR Tokyo General Hospital, Tokyo, Japan
e-mail: kazuo-hanaoka@jreast.co.jp

K. Shimoji et al. (eds.), *Chronic Pain Management in General and Hospital Practice*, https://doi.org/10.1007/978-981-15-2933-7_23

LV	Left ventricular
MI	Myocardial infarction
MR	Mitral valve regurgitation
MRI	Magnetic resonance imaging
MS	Mitral valve stenosis
MVP	Mitral valve prolapse
NSAID	Non-steroidal anti-inflammatory drug
PE	Pulmonary embolism
PH	Pulmonary hypertension
PVD	Peripheral vascular disease
QOL	Quality of life
RACPC	Rapid access chest pain clinics
SCS	Spinal cord stimulation
SLE	Systemic lupus erythematosus
SSRI	Selective serotonin reuptake inhibitor
TB	Tuberculosis

23.1 Chest Pain (CP)

Chest pain (CP) is a somatic symptom of emotional disorder in ambulatory care. Various schemes have been used to classify the etiologies of CP, but the most useful is to distinguish between acute and chronic patterns of pain [1].

23.2 Acute Chest Pain (Acute CP)

Patients with acute CP include those whose episodes are of recent onset or those who have had a recent increase in the intensity or frequency of recurrent pain. The first thing which the patients may think of for acute CP will be myocardial infarction (MI). While acute CP is a well-established sign of MI, there are various other severe conditions that can cause severe symptoms such as chest discomfort and breathing difficulty.

The tests to help diagnose may be ordered or heart-related problems as a cause of acute CP may be eliminated. Some of the initial examinations of the patient with acute CP may include electrocardiography (ECG) which records the electrical activity of the heart, blood tests to measure enzyme levels, and chest X-ray to examine the heart, lungs, and blood vessels. ECG records the electrical activity of the heart through electrodes attached to the skin. ECG interpretation in acute CP can be highly specific for diagnosing MI [1]. Resting ECG and exercise ECG are of only limited value in the diagnosis of coronary artery disease (CAD). Once patients are diagnosed, additional treatments to manage conditions can be recommended.

Because injured heart muscle does not conduct electrical impulses normally, the ECG may show that MI has occurred or is in progress. Blood tests may be ordered to check for increased levels of certain enzymes normally found in heart muscle. Damage to heart cells from MI may allow these enzymes to leak into the blood over a period of hours. Point of care testing with troponins is cost-effective in the triaging of patients with suspected acute coronary syndrome (ACS). Chest X-ray allows to check the condition of the lungs and the size and shape of the heart and major blood vessels. Chest X-ray can also reveal lung-related problems such as pneumonia and pneumothorax.

Depending upon the results of these initial examinations, the patient may need follow-up detail examinations, which may include echocardiography, computerized tomography (CT) scan, magnetic resonance imaging (MRI), and stress tests. Echocardiography uses sound waves to produce a video image of the heart in motion and to record moving images of the heart. In some cases, transesophageal echocardiography may be passed down the throat to obtain better views of different parts of the heart. The CT scan can be used to look for a blood clot in pulmonary embolism (PE) or to check the aorta to make sure the patient is not having aortic dissection. Enhanced CT scans can be used to check the coronary arteries for signs of calcium, which indicate areas where thrombolytic agents are accumulating. The enhanced CT scans can also be done to check the coronary and pulmonary arteries for blockages and other problems. The MRI can look for damage to the heart or aorta. Stress tests measure heart function after exertion, i.e., how the heart and blood vessels respond to exertion, which may indicate if the pain is related to the heart. The patient may be asked to walk on a treadmill or pedal a stationary bike while hooked up to an ECG. The patient may be given a drug intravenously to stimulate the heart in a way similar to exercise.

Coronary catheterization or angiography helps doctors identify individual arteries to the heart that may be narrowed or blocked. In primary care, more than 80% of patients are found to have no organic etiology for CP. Even among selected patients referred for coronary arteriography, 10–30% have little or no evidence of CAD.

Acute CP is one of the most common reasons that people visit the emergency room (ER). Acute CP does not always signal MI. ER doctors will test for first because it is potentially the most immediate threat to life. ER doctors may also check for life-threatening lung conditions such as pneumothorax and PE. Immediate management decisions must be made for patients having new onset of acute CP or an increase in the frequency or severity of recurrent CP. Because some of the disorders are life threatening, it must be decided whether to admit the patient. Any types of acute CP, chest discomfort, and breathing difficulty are serious symptoms those are likely to put the patients first in the queue at the ER. Where an ACS is suspected, emergency referral is justified. If the patients may be experiencing MI and especially if acute CP is unexplained, or lasts more than a few moments, urgent treatment in the ER is needed immediately.

Rapid access chest pain clinics (RACPCs) may be associated with reduced hospital admission of patients with non-cardiac CP, better recognition of ACS, earlier specialist assessment of exertional angina, and earlier diagnosis of non-cardiac

CP. RACPCs were predicted to result in earlier diagnosis of both confirmed CAD and non-cardiac CP than models of care based around open access exercise tests or routine cardiology outpatients. The potential advantages of RACPC are lost if there are long waiting times for further investigation. Recommendations for further research include the following: determining the most appropriate model of care to ensure accurate triage of patients with suspected ACS; establishing the cost-effectiveness of pre-hospital thrombolysis in rural areas; determining the relative cost-effectiveness of RACPCs compared with other innovative models of care; investigating how RACPCs should be managed; and establishing the long-term outcome of patients discharged from RACPCs.

Acute CP may be treated with medications, non-invasive procedures, surgeries, or a combination of these methods depending on the cause and severity of CP.

23.3 Chronic Chest Pain (Chronic CP)

Patients with chronic CP include those who have recurrent episodes of pain occurring in a relatively stable pattern. It varies in quality, intensity, duration, location, and person. It has a prevalence of 12% and is associated with high utilization of health care. Of patients with chronic CP who are referred to a cardiac clinic, but subsequently they have not shown the heart disease.

The patients may feel chronic CP anywhere from the neck to the upper abdomen. Chronic CP in certain patients travels up the neck, into the jaw, and then radiates through to the back or down one or both arms. It comes in many varieties, ranging from a sharp, aching, stabbing to a dull ache. Some chronic CP is described as tight, squeezing, crushing, or burning sensation. It varies depending on the person. The pain may be transmitted by intercostal, sympathetic, vagus, and phrenic nerves. The innervations of the deep structures of the thorax follow common pathways to the central nervous system, making it difficult to localize the source of pain.

There are various causes of chronic CP. It may be a sign of a serious heart-related problem [2]. It may occur due to one of many common causes that are not life threatening. Not surprisingly, the patients with a history of MI are likely to be found to have CAD as the cause of recurrent episodes of pain. Some of chronic CP is not related to the heart and without evidence of myocardial ischemia or MI [3]. The pain may originate from several different structures within the chest, including the skin, ribs, intercostal muscles, pleura, esophagus, heart, aorta, diaphragm, or thoracic vertebrae. Chronic CP may be caused by problems in the lungs, esophagus, muscles, ribs, or nerves. Other conditions that should be asked about include valvular or rheumatic heart disease, hypertension, chronic lung disease, peptic disorders, esophageal disorders such as achalasia, rheumatologic disease, hyperventilation syndrome, and anxiety states. The patients who meet specific criteria for non-ischemic CP are followed to determine the cause of pain [4].

Chronic CP can arise from a variety of etiologies [5]. The etiologies of chronic CP are classified into cardiac CP and non-cardiac CP. Chronic cardiac CP may be caused either by ischemia or atherosclerotic CAD or by other cardiac-related etiologies, such as pericardial disease. Chronic non-cardiac CP is most commonly related to gastroesophageal reflux disease (GERD) or other esophageal diseases. It may be related to costochondritis, arthritic or degenerative diseases, old trauma, primary or metastatic tumors, or pleural disease. It may be referred pain from organ systems below the diaphragm, such as the stomach, duodenum, liver, gallbladder, and pancreas.

Because the probable etiology of chronic CP often can be determined from the history alone, the doctors should systematically evaluate characteristics of the pain. Some of chronic CP can represent a serious and life-threatening emergency. Chronic CP needs to be diagnosed by a medical professional. The most life-threatening ones involve the heart or lungs. Because it can be difficult to determine the exact cause of CP, it is best to seek immediate medical help. Chronic CP has many possible causes, all of which deserve medical attention. If unexplained chronic CP is presented, the only way to confirm its cause is to have a medical specialist evaluate the patients.

In pursuing the cause of CP, a probabilistic approach to diagnosis will aid in making decisions about patients. The patients are asked to describe the temporal relationship between the pain and associated symptoms. Accompanying symptoms are most helpful diagnostically when the patients occur in close proximity to the episodes of CP.

The probability of a particular diagnosis for a particular patient can be estimated by the medical specialist. While several studies have provided data for estimating the risk of CAD, there has been less investigation of the prevalence of other disease in patients with CP. Precise definition of chronic CP allows the list of possible causes to be narrowed and guides the physical examination and choice of diagnostic tests.

Classic coronary pain or angina involves a substernal pressure that commonly begins with exertion and is relieved by rest [6]. Some patients experience angina in the absence of physical exertion or emotional stress, and not all CP that begins after exertion is angina. Atypical CP must be differentiated from other types of CP, including chest wall pain, pleurisy, gallbladder pain, hiatal hernia, and CP associated with anxiety disorders. Careful examination of the chest wall is essential, and abnormal heart sounds can tell the patients a great deal.

An exercise ECG is important in identifying the presence of ischemic heart disease and the amount of myocardium at risk. Resting ECG features in patients with chronic CP are not found to be very useful [1]. The exercise ECG does not result in dramatic improvements. If the ECG is abnormal at rest, the patients should undergo a thallium stress test or exercise echocardiography. A coronary angiography is indicated if the exercise test or an ECG during pain shows that a lot of live heart muscle is at risk.

Atypical CP is cause of office consultations or functional disability. The diagnosis should be established on the basis of positive evidence of psychiatric illness rather than by exclusion [7]. The etiology is multifactorial, and management is aimed at treating the underlying psychosocial problems or psychiatric illness. Cognitive-behavioral treatments are probably as effective as drug treatments in the short-term, and the care of these patients would be improved by a more detailed explanation of non-cardiac causes and a greater opportunity for patients to discuss their fears.

23.4 Heart

23.4.1 Cardiac or Cardiovascular Disorders

Pain, pressure, tightness, or other discomfort originating in or radiating to the chest constitutes an important indicator of potentially serious cardiac or cardiovascular disorders. The heart-related problems cause chronic CP.

Treatments for heart-related causes of acute CP include medications including nitroglycerin and other medications, thrombolytic agents, or cardiac catheterization, which involves using balloons or stents to open partially blocked arteries, surgical repair of the arteries which is also known as coronary artery bypass grafting (CABG).

23.4.2 Dyslimidemia

Blood lipids are fatty substances, such as triglycerides and cholesterol. Dyslipidemia is defined as having blood lipid levels that are too high or low. Cholesterol is a natural substance, but too much of it can clog blood vessels and lead to MI.

23.4.3 Atherosclerosis

Atherosclerosis is narrowing and hardening of the arteries caused by a buildup of plaque. Atherosclerosis is the common pathological substrate of chronic stable angina as well as ACS.

Atherosclerosis is also a chronic disease which mainly represents an inflammatory response in the vessels. Endothelial dysfunction is now considered to be an important early event in the development of atherosclerosis, while in the absence of angiographically obstructive CAD, anginal CP is often attributed to microvascular coronary dysfunction [8]. Moreover, atheroma formation and in turn, atherosclerotic plaques seem to affect coronary flow, given that multivessel flow-limiting obstructions are observed in patients with chronic coronary syndrome. Morphological changes of diseased arteries related to significant atherosclerosis, such as vascular remodeling may also result in stable angina or claudication.

23.4.4 Coronary Artery Disease (CAD)

CP is one of the perceptible symptoms of CAD and plausible risk factors for CAD. The leading diagnostic consideration in patients with chronic CP is CAD. A central goal is to determine whether the pain is likely caused by myocardial ischemia. The most common clinical presentation of CAD is recurrent angina. With respect to case definition of CAD, diagnostically most useful tests are history of CAD, known acute MI, typical angina, history of diabetes mellitus, exertional pain, history of angina pectoris, and male sex for diagnosing stable CAD; pain radiating to the right arm or shoulder and palpitation for diagnosing MI; visceral pain for diagnosing ACS; and typical angina and pain reproducible by palpation for predicting major cardiac event [9].

Patients with CAD frequently report CP brought on by emotional stress or sexual intercourse. Angina pectoris usually becomes worse with exertion and is relieved by rest. The patients occasionally attribute CP to exertion, but careful questioning reveals that CP comes and goes with deep breaths or body movements during heavy exercise. If the patient notes that less exertion is required to cause CP when going out in cold weather or after eating a large meal, then CP is likely to be caused by CAD. It is important to clarify the amount of exertion required to cause CP. Its severity may provide a clue to its etiology. CP that is pleuritic or is brought on by moving the arms or torso is less likely to be caused by CAD.

The frequency and duration of CP should be defined, although the data are less helpful in distinguishing the cause of MI. Episodes of CP caused by CAD usually last less than an hour. CP caused by CAD is more likely to require the patients to stop their usual activities. CAD rarely causes episodes lasting more than 12 h without ECG changes of acute MI.

Integrating high-density lipoprotein cholesterol, aspartate aminotransferase, and high-sensitivity C-reactive protein levels with common clinical variables has a higher prediction accuracy for functionally significant CAD [10].

Advancing age, female sex, no exercise, and reduced HDL are significantly hazardous predictors throughout the duration from CP to diagnosis of CAD [11]. Age, sex, exercise, and HDL can be variables of concern to deteriorate hazards of CAD in patients with CP.

Imaging plays a central role in the diagnosis and management of CAD. Imaging is used for the detection of underlying coronary artery stenoses in patients with stable or chronic CP, for the assessment of myocardial scar and viability, for assessing prognosis, or for predicting complications [12]. Echocardiography, nuclear imaging, cardiac MRI, and more recently CT are powerful tools to provide answers to these questions. Imaging is valuable in determining the presence, extent, and severity of myocardial ischemia and the severity of obstructive coronary lesions in patients with chronic CP in the setting of high probability of CAD [13]. Imaging is critical for defining patients best suited for medical therapy or intervention, and findings can be used to predict long-term prognosis and the likely benefit from various therapeutic options. Chest radiography, radionuclide single photon-emission CT, radionuclide ventriculography, and conventional coronary angiography are the imaging modalities historically used in evaluating suspected chronic myocardial ischemia. Stress echocardiography, positron emission tomography, cardiac MRI, and multidetector cardiac CT scan have all been more recently shown to be valuable in the evaluation of ischemic heart disease.

Several studies of coronary arteriography in patients referred for evaluation of recurrent CP have quantified the prevalence of CAD in different CP syndromes. Disease prevalence in patients evaluated at referral centers, and the selected populations have a higher prevalence of CAD than the general population. Women have a lower prevalence of CAD than men. The patients with pain typical of angina are more likely to have obstructive coronary disease than are patients with atypical pain syndromes [14]. Diagnostic coronary arteriography may identify a subset of patients in whom a finding of non-critical CAD leads to a reduction in doctor visits for evaluation of CP syndromes and reduced use of nitrates. A helpful diagnostic feature of CAD is that the pain usually improves with specific medications.

In patients with chronic CP in the setting of high probability of CAD, imaging has major and diverse roles [15]. Imaging is valuable in determining and documenting the presence, extent, and severity of myocardial ischemia, hibernation, scarring, and/or the presence, site, and severity of obstructive coronary lesions. Imaging findings are important in determining the course of management of patients with suspected chronic myocardial ischemia and better defining those patients best suited for medical therapy, angioplasty, stenting, or surgery. Imaging is also necessary to determine the long-term prognosis and likely benefit from various therapeutic options by evaluating ventricular function, diastolic relaxation, end-systolic volume, and end-diastolic volume. Imaging studies are also required to demonstrate other abnormalities, such as congenital or acquired coronary anomalies and severe left ventricular (LV) hypertrophy, that can produce angina in the absence of symptomatic coronary obstructive disease due to atherosclerosis.

The diagnostic evaluation of patients without known CAD presenting with chronic stable CP or angina equivalent is complex. Imaging often plays a role in diagnosis and risk stratification, and a variety of techniques are available, each with inherent and situation-specific advantages and disadvantages. Coronary CT angiography has been proposed as a fast, non-invasive, reliable test to rule out disease in this population, with potential improvements in costs and outcomes compared with alternative strategies [16]. The relatively rapid rise in coronary CT angiography utilization, however, has led to strong calls from doctors and health care policy organizations alike to provide high-level evidence supporting its use.

Global longitudinal strain measurements at rest only have a modest diagnostic accuracy in predicting significant coronary artery stenosis among patients presenting with acute or chronic CP [17].

Patients with a history of recurrent CP that now occurs with decreasing levels of exertion may require urgent treatment. Improving exercise tolerance is strong evidence that a treatment regimen has been effective. Relief of anginal pain within 3 min of taking sublingual nitroglycerin is strong evidence that CAD has caused the pain. Decreased frequency of attacks after starting a beta-blocker, calcium channel blocker, or long-acting nitrate preparation suggests that CAD is the cause.

23.4.5 *Myocardial Infarction (MI)*

MI is a blockage of blood flow to the heart [18]. MI is a result of a blood clot that is blocking blood flow to heart muscle. Thick plaques can gradually build up on the inner walls of the coronary arteries. These plaques narrow the coronary arteries and restrict the heart's blood supply, particularly during exertion. A blockage in the blood vessels in the heart reduces blood flow and oxygen to the heart muscle itself. This reduction in blood flow through heart blood vessels causes the death of heart muscle cells. As the blood supply that normally nourishes the heart with oxygen is cut off, the heart muscle begins to die.

Though CP of MI is similar in quality and location to angina, MI is usually more intense, severe, crushing, and longer-lasting, the pain is usually in the center or left side of the chest and is not relieved by rest. The most important part of the pain history is to define what aggravates and relieves the pain. CP may spread to the arm, shoulder, jaw, or back. It may feel like a pressure or squeezing sensation. Sweating, nausea, shortness of breath, or severe weakness may accompany the pain. CP may be accompanied by diaphoresis, dyspnea, or nausea.

The initial ECG shows new Q waves or ST segment elevations in only 70% of patients, so absence of these findings does not exclude MI.

The pain often occurs at rest and is not relieved by nitroglycerin. The leading diagnostic consideration in acute CP, MI is a life-threatening condition requiring immediate medical management. The condition is considered a medical emergency and urgent care may be required.

23.4.6 *Angina*

Angina causes CP due to blockages in the blood vessels leading to the heart and results from reduced blood flow to the heart. A lack of blood flow means the heart muscle is not getting enough oxygen. Myocardial ischemia manifested by angina can be either acute or chronic and usually is a result of imbalance between myocardial oxygen supply and myocardial oxygen demand. Angina can be triggered by exercise, excitement, or emotional distress and is relieved by rest.

CP is a symptom of heart disease, but typically does not cause permanent damage to the heart. The pain is often triggered by physical activity or emotional stress. CP is a sign that the patient will be a candidate for MI at some point in the future. Angina is a recognizable pain syndrome, and careful attention to the features of the history aids the doctors in determining whether the pain is typical of angina.

23.4.6.1 Stable Angina

Stable angina, also called angina pectoris, is the most common type of angina. Chronic stable angina is chest discomfort attributed to myocardial ischemia without the presence of necrosis and is the most common symptom encountered by ER doctors.

Stable angina represents the main symptom of established CAD. Stable angina is a predictable pattern of CP. Tracking stable angina can help the patient manage the symptoms more easily. The stable CAD population is a heterogeneous group of patients both for clinical presentations and for different underlying mechanisms [19].

In the coronary artery surgery study, men with typical angina pectoris have a 93% prevalence of significant CAD, whereas women with typical angina have a 72% prevalence. Furthermore, the prevalence of CAD is strongly influenced by age. In men, the risk of CAD increases steadily between the ages of 30 and 70, with little further increase above age 70. In women, the risk rises gradually until age 60 and then increases more rapidly between ages 60 and 80.

Patients with atypical angina have a 50–60% prevalence of CAD, while the prevalence in patients with non-anginal pain is 20–30%.

Percutaneous coronary intervention and coronary surgery have not been shown to improve hard end points and routine use of invasive revascularization should be avoided in patients with chronic stable angina [20].

23.4.6.2 Unstable Angina

Unstable angina occurs suddenly and gets worse over time and may eventually lead to MI. Though stable angina is less serious than unstable angina, unstable angina can be painful and uncomfortable. Various pathophysiologic mechanisms may be responsible for unstable angina. Both types of angina are usually signs of an underlying heart condition, so it is important to see as soon as the patients have CP.

The most common mechanism is a progression of the severity of atherosclerotic disease. Vasospasm aggravating atherosclerotic disease can also cause unstable angina.

The syndrome of unstable angina includes a diverse group of patients having crushing CP due to CAD. Anginal pain is due to inadequate blood supply to the heart muscle, which deprives the heart of oxygen. The pain occurs at a lower level of exertion or at rest. Anginal pain is typically described as dull, heavy, or crushing. The patient may describe a pressure sensation rather than a true pain. Sharp, stabbing, or burning pain is less typical of angina.

Anginal pain is usually located substernally or across the anterior chest. The pain located exclusively in either the left or right chest is atypical. While radiation of the pain to the left arm is typical of angina, patients with CAD also frequently have the pain that radiates to the right arm or neck.

It is difficult to differentiate between unstable angina and acute MI. Hospitalization is often required to clarify the diagnosis and facilitate treatment interventions. Serial ECGs and cardiac enzymes will confirm or exclude MI. Further diagnostic evaluation with imaging studies or coronary arteriography may be necessary. Several studies of coronary arteriography have found that 90% of patients with typical exertional angina have significant anatomic CAD. Non-invasive multislice CT coronary angiography is a potentially useful tool in the diagnostic work-up of patients with stable angina owing to its capability to detect or exclude significant CAD [21].

Myocardial ischemia sometimes occurs in the absence of fixed obstructions of the coronary arteries, resulting in recurrent CP. Obstructive disease of the intramural small vessels can cause ischemia. Although such lesions occur more frequently in diabetics, small vessel disease is an infrequent cause of CP.

Aortic valve stenosis (AS), hypertrophic cardiomyopathy (HCM), and thyrotoxicosis can also cause myocardial ischemia. The quality and pattern of pain in these conditions usually are similar to that of CAD.

Patients with unstable angina have a short-term risk of MI. The patients have exertional pain relieved by rest or sublingual nitroglycerin. Nitroglycerin may become outdated and ineffective and be no longer provide relief. If CP episodes do not improve substantially with cardiac medications, then the patient has either refractory CAD pre-infarction angina or another cause of CP. A careful review of the patient's medications can provide clues. If MI is excluded, the patient's response to medications should be carefully evaluated. An important cause of unstable angina in patients with prior stable angina is an alteration of the patient's medication. Therapeutic interventions have been shown to reduce this risk.

The aim of stable angina management is the symptomatic relief and the secondary prevention [22]. Lifestyle modification and pharmacological therapy are the cornerstones of chronic CAD management irrespectively of possible surgical or percutaneous revascularization. Optimal medical therapy is a combination of anti-anginal or anti-ischemic drugs and disease modifying agents, including nitrates, beta-blockers, calcium channel blockers, anti-platelets, statins, and angiotensin converting enzyme inhibitors. Novel classes of treatment with different mechanisms of action have been developed in the last years, including nicorandil, ivabradine, trimetazidine, and ranolazine.

23.4.7 Coronary Vasospasm

Coronary vasospasm can cause myocardial ischemia in the absence of obstructive coronary disease [23]. Coronary artery spasm, an intense vasoconstriction of coronary arteries that causes total or subtotal vessel occlusion, plays an important role in myocardial ischemic syndromes, including stable and unstable angina, acute MI, and sudden cardiac death. Some patients report emotional stress as a trigger. CP usually has a quality similar to the pain of obstructive coronary disease, but it tends to occur in an unpredictable pattern. CP typically is not induced by exertion and may awaken the patient from sleep. Coronary artery spasm rarely worsens from single-vessel to simultaneous multivessel coronary artery spasm naturally, and simultaneous multivessel coronary artery spasm leads to serious conditions such as cardiopulmonary arrest.

Approximately 90% of patients with coronary vasospasm have ECG changes during episodes of pain. The absence of ECG changes during the pain makes coronary vasospasm unlikely.

CP frequently responds to sublingual nitroglycerin, and the frequency of episodes decreases after therapy with calcium channel blockers or long-acting nitrates.

23.4.8 Aortic Dissection

Aortic dissection is a rare condition involving a tear of the aorta, the large vessel that comes off of the heart [24]. This life-threatening condition involves the main artery leading from the heart to the aorta. Aortic dissection may cause a sudden severe pain with a tearing or ripping sensation that goes up into the neck, back, or abdomen. Nearly all patients with acute MI have anterior CP, but the majority of patients with distal dissection have posterior CP. Dissection of the thoracic aorta is a serious and potentially catastrophic cause of acute CP. A variety of factors can cause this rare but deadly condition, which results when a tear develops in the coronary artery. If the inner layers of this blood vessel separate, blood will be forced between the layers and can cause the aorta to rupture. A dissection of the aorta means that blood has entered the wall of the artery between the inner and middle layers. Dissection of the thoracic aorta occurs predominantly in men older than age 40 who have a history of hypertension, a group also at risk for acute MI.

The two primary types of dissection have different clinical presentations. Proximal dissections arise in the ascending aorta, but sometimes extend beyond the aortic arch. Nearly all patients with proximal dissection have pain in the anterior chest, and approximately half report radiation to the posterior chest. Approximately two-thirds have evidence of previous hypertension. Most have pulse deficits, a murmur of aortic valve regurgitation (AR), or neurologic deficits, and so the physical examination is important when considering this diagnosis. Distal dissection of the thoracic aorta arises in the descending aorta below the great vessels. The pain of distal dissection may be described as tearing or ripping and does not improve with nitroglycerin. Physical findings are less frequent in distal than in proximal dissection, so the diagnosis of distal dissection may be subtle and should be considered in patients who have histories of hypertension, are hypertensive at the time of pain, or have atypical pain.

The condition of aortic dissection is considered a medical emergency and urgent care may be required. Because dissection requires immediate, specific treatment, the doctors must exclude this diagnosis early. Radiographic studies of the aorta may be necessary to exclude the diagnosis.

23.4.9 Cardiac Tamponade

Cardiac tamponade is a very serious condition in which blood or fluids fill the space between the sac that encases the heart and the heart muscle [25]. This places extreme pressure on the heart. The pressure prevents the heart's ventricles from expanding fully and keeps the heart from functioning properly. The heart cannot pump enough blood to the rest of the body due to fluid buildup around the heart. This can lead to organ failure, shock, and even death. This condition is considered a medical emergency and urgent care may be required.

23.4.10 Myocarditis

Myocarditis is inflammation of the heart muscle, myocardium [26]. In addition to CP, an inflammation of the heart muscle may cause fever, general fatigue, tachycardia, and dyspnea. Myocarditis is one of the leading causes of sudden cardiac death and dilated cardiomyopathy (DCM) in young adults, and is an important cause of symptoms such as CP, dyspnea, and palpitations [27]. Myocarditis is a rare condition that can be caused by any number of autoimmune diseases, viral, bacterial, or fungal infections. Although no blockage exists, the symptoms of myocarditis can resemble those of MI [28]. The pathophysiological process of disease progression leading to DCM involves an ongoing inflammation as a result of a viral-induced auto-immune response or a persisting viral infection. It is therefore crucial to detect myocarditis early in its course and prevent persisting inflammation that may lead to DCM and end-stage heart failure.

23.4.11 Pericarditis

Pericarditis is an inflammation of the sac surrounding the heart. Pericarditis is a moderately common disorder, and CP is a frequent symptom. The symptoms of pericarditis are generally sharp and steady pain along the upper neck and shoulder muscle, and the pain is getting worse by deep breathing, swallowing food, or lying on the back. The pain is usually pleuritic or affected by body position, however, aggravated by lying down and relieved by sitting up. Pericarditis can cause CP similar to that caused by angina. The pain is often retrosternal and may radiate to the left arm, suggesting an ischemic etiology. Sharp CP occurs when the inflamed pericardium rubs against the chest wall. The clinical diagnosis is based on recurrent CP and additional objective evidence of disease activity such as pericardial rub, ECG changes, pericardial effusion, elevation of markers of inflammation, and imaging evidence of pericardial inflammation by CT scan or cardiac MRI [29].

Acute pericarditis occurs most frequently after a viral attack [30]. Other causes are autoimmune conditions, infection, chest trauma, cardiac surgery, or cardiac procedure. The presenting symptom is retrosternal CP.

A characteristic pericardial friction rub suggests the diagnosis of pericarditis, but a rub may be absent. The ECG can show ST elevations in multiple leads, a finding that may be confused with acute MI. Not all patients with pericarditis have ECG changes, and uremic pericarditis is notable, for the absence of ECG findings. Chest X-ray often shows a normal cardiac silhouette. Because of its diverse presentation, pericarditis is difficult to exclude by routine clinical examination, but the diagnosis should be suspected if the patient does not have other likely causes of CP and has clinical evidence of a precipitating cause.

23.4.12 Hypertrophic Cardiomyopathy (HCM)

HCM is the most common inherited cardiovascular disease. The genetic disease of HCM causes the autosomal dominant heart muscle to grow abnormally thicker than normal [31]. HCM sometimes leads to problems with blood flow out of the heart. HCM makes the heart work harder to pump blood. HCM can interfere with the heart's ability to pump blood. HCM is characterized by an increase in LV wall thickness, which causes LV outflow obstruction, diastolic dysfunction, myocardial ischemia, and mitral valve regurgitation (MR).

HCM is characterized by increased LV wall thickness and is highly complex due to its heterogeneous clinical presentation, several phenotypes, large number of associated causal mutations, and broad spectrum of complications. HCM is caused by mutations in sarcomeric protein genes which encodes for elements of the contractile machinery of the heart, which are identified in up to 60% of cases of the disease.

The structural and functional abnormalities of HCM can produce clinical manifestations at all ages including CP, shortness of breath, fatigue, dyspnea, palpitations, and syncope, which are related to the onset of diastolic dysfunction, LV outflow tract obstruction, ischemia, atrial fibrillation (af), and abnormal vascular responses. CP and shortness of breath often occur with exercise. Along with CP, HCM may cause dizziness, lightheadedness, and fainting.

HCM is associated with an increased risk of sudden cardiac death, heart failure, and thromboembolic events. HCM is a myocardial disease characterized by myocardial hypertrophy, disorganization of cardiac myocytes, and fibrosis. Twenty-five percent of patients have a dynamic LV outflow tract gradient caused by the combined effects of rapid ventricular ejection, a narrowed outflow tract, and systolic anterior motion of the mitral valve. Most cases are caused by mutations in genes that encode cardiac sarcomeric proteins. Over time, heart failure may occur when the heart muscle becomes too thickened. The most important complications of the disease are sudden cardiac death, heart failure, and thromboembolism. Sudden cardiac death can represent the most devastating presenting manifestation, especially in young athletes.

23.4.13 Ischemic Cardiomyopathy (ICM)

Ischemic cardiomyopathy (ICM) is usually caused by MI or CAD. ICM is a condition that occurs when the heart muscle is weakened. Patients with ICM may continue to experience persistent CP or dyspnea despite pharmacologic therapy and revascularization [32]. In optimally treated ICM patients with continued CP or dyspnea, ranolazine possibly had a positive impact on quality of life (QOL), a reduction in anginal frequency.

23.4.14 Aortic Valve Stenosis (AS)

Severe AS, when accompanied by symptoms of angina, syncope, or heart failure, is associated with high mortality rates [33]. Elderly patients with AS have an increased prevalence of coronary risk factors, of CAD and evidence of other atherosclerotic vascular diseases [34].

23.4.15 Mitral Valve Prolapse (MVP)

Mitral valve prolapse (MVP) is a controversial etiology of chronic CP. In MVP the flaps of the mitral valve do not close correctly, which can make blood leak from the left ventricle into the left atrium. MVP is a condition in which mitral valve in the heart fails to close properly. Of cardiac conditions commonly linked to CP in childhood, MVP is the most prevalent [35]. Idiopathic MVP occurs predominantly in females, often at a young age, and may be associated with CP, dyspnea, fatigue, presyncope, syncope, or sudden death [36].

A variety of symptoms have been associated with MVP, including CP, palpitations, and dizziness, although it can also have no symptoms, especially if the prolapse is mild. The incidence of CP is no higher in individuals with MVP than in those without the disorder. There have been numerous clinical reports of patients in whom MVP was the only identifiable etiology of recurrent CP. The patients with MVP have CP with various qualities and patterns, and there is no typical CP syndrome of MVP.

Clinical and echocardiographic studies have demonstrated that MVP is a common finding in otherwise healthy adults. The patients who develop serious complications have either a late systolic murmur or abnormal ECG in conjunction with the midsystolic click. The MVP should be considered as a cause of recurrent CP only after more likely causes have been excluded, since there is no specific treatment for the disorder. The major value of diagnosing MVP is to identify those patients at risk of endocarditis and arrhythmias. It is unnecessary to obtain echocardiography to exclude MVP unless a patient has findings on physical examination or ECG that suggest a risk of complications.

23.4.16 Mitral Valve Stenosis (MS)

Mitral valve stenosis (MS) is a valvular heart disease characterized by the narrowing of the orifice of the mitral valve of the heart. This means that enough blood cannot flow through the mitral valve. Signs and symptoms of mitral stenosis include the following: heart failure symptoms, such as dyspnea on exertion, orthopnea and paroxysmal nocturnal dyspnea, palpitations, CP, hemoptysis, thromboembolism in later stages when the left atrial volume is increased, i.e., dilation. The latter leads to increased risk of af, which increases the risk of blood stasis, i.e., motionless. This increases the risk of coagulation. Ascites, edema and hepatomegaly may occur, if right heart failure develops.

23.4.17 Atrial Fibrillation (af) and Atrial Flutter (AF)

An abnormal heart rhythm, arrhythmia, is when the heart beats too fast, slow, or irregularly. Af and atrial flutter (AF) are irregular heart rhythms that occur when atriums of the heart beat irregularly or too fast [37, 38]. Af is associated with a higher incidence of mortality, stroke, and coronary events than is sinus rhythm. Af with a rapid ventricular rate may cause a tachycardia-related cardiomyopathy. Immediate direct-current cardioversion should be performed in patients with af and acute MI, CP due to myocardial ischemia, hypotension, severe heart failure, or syncope.

23.4.18 Hypertensive Heart Disease

Hypertensive heart disease refers to heart conditions caused by high blood pressure. Possible symptoms of acute hypertension include sweating and chills [39].

23.4.19 Pulmonary Hypertension (PH)

Pulmonary hypertension (PH) is a spectrum disorder with multiple causes of the elevation of pressure in the lungs [40]. High blood pressure in the pulmonary arteries carrying blood to the lungs can produce CP. With the CP resembling that of angina, this abnormally makes the right side of the heart work too hard. PH often is difficult to diagnose, because it mimics many commonly reported symptoms such as CP, dyspnea, and exercise intolerance.

23.4.20 Rheumatic Fever

Rheumatic fever is a complication of an infection of the oral pharynx and tonsils by streptococcus. If rheumatic fever is left untreated, it can cause permanent damage to the heart. The patients present the CP mimicking ACS [26, 41].

23.5 Lung Problems

23.5.1 Lung-Related Disorders

Problems with the lungs and many lung-related disorders can cause a variety of types of CP. CP from respiratory causes is a common complaint and may indicate the presence of a serious or even life-threatening pathologic condition. Most CPs are the result of irritation or inflammation of the parietal pleura, as the visceral pleura is insensate, although the pain may arise from direct malignant invasion or trauma to the chest wall. Rapid recognition with appropriate understanding of the anatomy and physiology of CP from respiratory causes is vital to ensure timely and appropriate therapy.

Symptoms accompanying CP has often provided diagnostic clues. Cough or dyspnea suggests pulmonary disorders. Other possible etiologies include chest wall disorders, hyperventilation, or pulmonary disease, which are relatively common in some populations.

23.5.2 Pneumothorax

Pneumothorax is a leak of air from the lung into the thoracic cavity and causes a collapse of the lung [42]. CP associated with a collapsed lung typically begins suddenly and can last for hours. Pneumothorax can be often caused spontaneously, or by a traumatic event and an injury to the chest. Therefore, pneumothorax is defined as the abnormal presence of air within the pleural cavity that results in the partial or complete collapse.

Pneumothorax can cause acute CP that gets worse when the patient breathes as well as other symptoms, such as hypotension. Symptoms can vary from a non-descriptive complaint of shortness of breath or CP to complete cardiopulmonary collapse.

Pneumothorax is usually easy to diagnose. Diagnosis is based on a combination of clinical suspicion along with supporting imaging studies. The CP is characteristically unilateral and pleuritic. Chest X-ray will establish the diagnosis.

The condition of pneumothorax is considered a medical emergency and urgent care may be required. Lung re-inflation of the collapsed lung is performed by inserting the chest tube or related device. Treatment often involves surgical or non-surgical approaches with goal to alleviate symptoms and prevent recurrence.

23.5.3 Pulmonary Embolism (PE)

The cause of unexplained pleuritic CP, including sudden onset of difficulty breathing and rapid respiratory rate in PE occurs when a blood clot becomes lodged in a pulmonary artery, blocking blood flow to lung tissue [26, 43–45]. When a blood clot travels through the bloodstream and lodges in the lungs, this can cause acute pleuritis, dyspnea, and tachycardia. PE can damage part of the lung and other organs, and decrease oxygen levels in the blood. PE is more likely following deep vein thrombosis or after being immobile for several days following surgery or as a complication of cancer.

PE may also cause shock. PE is the most common potentially life-threatening cause, found in 5–20% of patients who present to the emergency department with pleuritic pain. The condition of PE is considered a medical emergency and urgent care may be required.

23.5.4 Pleuritis

If the membrane that covers the lungs becomes inflamed, it can cause CP that is made worse when the patient inhales or coughs. The condition of pleuritis is an inflammation or irritation of the lining of the lungs and the chest [6]. Pleurisy occurs when the tissues that line the lungs and chest wall become inflamed or infected, causing extreme pain. The patient likely feels a sharp pain when the patient breathes, coughs, or sneezes.

Pleuritic CP is a common presenting symptom and has many causes, which range from life threatening to benign, self-limited conditions. When the other significant causes of pleuritic CP have been excluded, the diagnosis of pleurisy can be made. There are numerous causes of pleurisy, with viral pleurisy among the most common. The most common causes of pleuritic CP are bacterial or viral infections, PE, and pneumothorax. Other less common causes include rheumatoid arthritis, lupus, and cancer.

Pleuritic CP includes MI, pericarditis, pneumonia, and pneumothorax [45]. An ECG is helpful, especially if there is clinical suspicion of MI, pericarditis, or PE.

Pleuritis is often treated with antibiotics. Treatment of pleurisy typically consists of pain management with non-steroidal anti-inflammatory drugs (NSAIDs), as well as specific treatments targeted at the underlying cause.

23.5.5 Pneumonia and Lung Abscess

Pneumonia is an infection of the lungs caused by fungi, bacteria, or viruses [46]. The lung infections can cause pleuritic and other types of CP, such as a deep chest ache. Pneumonia often comes on suddenly, causing fever, chills, cough, trouble breathing, and pus coughed up from the respiratory tract.

Pneumonia also causes acute CP, but these disorders are usually easy to diagnose. The pain is characteristically unilateral and pleuritic. Chest X-ray will establish the diagnosis. Life-threatening hemoptysis is the sole indication for emergency operation.

23.5.6 Empyema

Empyema is also called pyothorax or purulent pleuritis. Empyema is a condition in which pus gathers in the pleural space, which is the area between the lungs and the inner surface of the chest wall [47]. Empyema usually develops after pneumonia, which is an infection of the lung tissue. Pus is a fluid that is filled with immune cells, dead cells, and bacteria. Pus in the pleural space cannot be coughed out. Instead, it needs to be drained by a needle or surgery.

23.5.7 Tuberculosis (TB)

Tuberculosis (TB) is a highly infectious disease that primarily affects the lungs [48]. TB remains one of the most frequent causes of pleural effusions on a global scale, especially in developing countries [49]. TB pleural effusion is one of the most common forms of extrapulmonary TB and usually presents as an acute illness with fever, cough, and pleuritic CP.

23.5.8 Pulmonary Actinomycosis

Pulmonary actinomycosis is a rare bacterial lung infection and causes dyspnea and CP [50].

23.5.9 Viral Bronchitis

Acute bronchitis, which is an illness frequently encountered by primary-care physicians, is an inflammation of the tracheobronchial tree that results from a respiratory tract infection [51]. Acute bronchitis is characterized by a persistent cough and sputum production and is occasionally accompanied by fever or CP. Acute bronchitis may have a viral or bacterial origin and is often treated with antibiotics.

23.5.10 Legionnaires' Disease

Legionnaires' disease is a severe type of pneumonia or lung infection. Common symptoms included unproductive cough, dyspnea, CP, headache, confusion, nausea, vomiting, and diarrhea. However, respiratory symptoms are absent in 22% cases. Localizing chest signs were present in 95% cases [52].

23.5.11 Lung Cancer and Bronchial Carcinoma

Various pain syndromes frequently presented in lung cancer and bronchial carcinoma patients. CP is one of the most prevalent symptoms in patients diagnosed with lung cancer and bronchial carcinoma; it can arise from local invasion of the chest structures or metastatic disease invading bones, nerves, or other anatomical structures potentially painful [53].

CP can be a consequence of therapeutic approaches like surgery, chemotherapy, or radiotherapy. Conventional medical management of cancer pain includes prescription of opioids and coadjuvants at doses sufficient to control the symptoms without causing severe drug effects. When an adequate pharmacological medical management fails to provide satisfactory analgesia or when it causes limiting side effects, interventional cancer pain techniques may be considered. Interventional pain management is devoted to the use of invasive techniques such as joint injections, nerve blocks or neurolysis, neuromodulation, and cement augmentation techniques to provide diagnosis and treatment of pain syndromes resistant to conventional medical management. Advantages of interventional approaches include better analgesic outcomes without experiencing drug-related side effects and potential for opioid reduction thus avoiding central side effects.

23.5.12 Pulmonary Artery Sarcoma

Presenting symptoms of patients with pulmonary artery sarcoma are similar to those of patients with other pulmonary vascular disease, including progressive dyspnea, cough, hemoptysis, and CP [54–56].

23.5.13 Mediastinal Tumor

Mediastinal tumor causes with chronic CP [57] and worsening intermittent, chronic CP with recent progressive dysphagia, cough, and dyspnea [58].

23.5.14 Asbestosis

Asbestosis is a lung disease that develops when the patient inhales asbestos fibers and they cause scarring in the lungs. CP appears to be much more common in patients with benign asbestos diseases [59].

23.5.15 Sarcoidosis

Sarcoidosis with lung involvement is common and symptoms may include cough, dyspnea, and CP [60].

23.5.16 Asthma

Asthma is an inflammatory disorder of the airways. Asthma causes shortness of breath, wheezing, coughing, and sometimes CP. Bronchospasm or constriction of the air passages commonly occurs in the patients who have asthma and related disorders such as chronic obstructive pulmonary disease.

Asthma symptoms are broadly categorized as breathing symptoms such as difficulty breathing, shortness of breath, wheezing, and chest symptoms such as chest tightness, CP, and pressure or weight on chest, and cough symptoms such as cough and the presence of mucus or phlegm [61].

23.5.17 Goodpasture Syndrome

Goodpasture syndrome is a rare condition that occurs when the immune system attacks the walls of the lungs and the tiny filtering units in the kidneys. Lung symptoms usually antedate kidney symptoms and usually include coughing up blood, CP in less than 50% of cases overall, cough, and shortness of breath.

23.6 Digestive Causes

23.6.1 Gastrointestinal Problems

Gastrointestinal problems cause CP and include dysphagia, nausea, and vomiting suggest a gastrointestinal etiology. Of patients whose recurrent CP is not caused by CAD, approximately half have reflux esophagitis or esophageal contraction abnormalities.

23.6.2 Gastroesophageal Reflux Disease (GERD)

Esophageal disease is a common cause of recurrent CP. Heartburn and regurgitations are the typical symptoms of GERD [62]. Some patients with GERD present with typical symptoms such as heartburn and regurgitation and others with atypical symptoms such as CP [63]. Heart pain and heartburn from acid reflux feel similar partly because the heart and esophagus are located close to each other and share a nerve network. Among the non-cardiac CP patients, GERD is presented in 48.2% [64].

Reflux esophagitis causes pain by irritation of the esophageal mucosa. This painful, burning sensation behind the sternum occurs when stomach acid washes up from the stomach into the esophagus. Also known as acid reflux, GERD occurs when stomach contents move back into the throat. This may cause a sour taste in the mouth and a burning sensation in the chest or throat, known as heartburn. Esophagitis, usually secondary to acid reflux from the stomach, frequently causes esophageal pain.

Acid reflux symptoms are caused when stomach contents flow up from the stomach back into the esophagus, causing symptoms like heartburn, stomach pain, and burping. The acid causes chemical damage and inflammation of the mucosa, resulting in pain that often has a burning quality.

Clues to the presence of reflux esophagitis include a history of acid–peptic disease and symptoms of reflux, such as regurgitation or acid taste in the mouth. CP caused by esophageal reflux tends to occur after meals and may be related to body position. Episodes of pain can be induced by bending over at the waist. The pain often occurs at night, because the lateral position enhances reflux of acid into the esophagus. Factors that may trigger acid reflux include obesity, smoking, pregnancy, and spicy or fatty foods.

85.1% of the patients with microvascular angina reveals positive results of gastric or esophageal disease [65]. In spite of any existing evidence of microvascular angina or cardiac syndrome X, it will be more advisable to perform gastroesophageal studies to adequately manage CP.

Relief of pain by antacids, topical lidocaine, or by specific maneuvers to reduce reflux suggests the diagnosis. Proton pump inhibitor is used for acid reflux and heartburn.

23.6.3 Esophageal Motor Disorders (EMD)

Swallowing disorders related to disorders of the esophagus. Uncoordinated muscle contractions, i.e., spasms, and high-pressure contractions, i.e., nutcracker esophagus, are problems in the esophagus that can cause CP.

Esophageal motor disorders (EMD) commonly cause varying qualities of CP, which may be reported as heartburn, by contraction and spasm of the muscular wall of the esophagus. Dysphagia has been frequently a prominent symptom in patients with primary EMD. Esophageal spasm often occurs as a secondary manifestation of reflux esophagitis. As episodes of simple mucosal irritation and inflammation become more severe, the stimulation of local nerves leads to muscular spasm. The patients will report a pattern of pain similar to that seen in reflux esophagitis, occurring after meals and aggravated by body position.

EMD can be independent of acid reflux disease, as in patients with achalasia or diffuse esophageal spasm. The patients with EMD show a different pattern of episodes from the patients with acid reflux. The pain usually is unrelated to body position and may occur while eating instead of after meals.

EMD may be relieved by nitrates and calcium channel blockers, via relaxation of the smooth muscle wall of the esophagus. Because these agents relieve CP caused by CAD, the doctor may have difficulty using medication response as a clue to the cause of undiagnosed CP. The results of a therapeutic trial, particularly the rapidity of response must be carefully interpreted. Relief of pain within 3 min of a sublingual dose of nitroglycerin is more consistent with CAD than EMD. If relief occurs only after 10–15 min, esophageal disease is more likely. Nitrates and calcium channel blockers can relax the lower esophageal sphincter and aggravate esophageal reflux, thereby increasing symptoms of reflux esophagitis.

23.6.4 Esophageal Hypersensitivity

Esophageal hypersensitivity occurs when the esophagus becomes very painful at the smallest change in pressure or exposure to acid. The cause of the sensitivity is unknown.

23.6.5 Esophageal Rupture or Perforation

A sudden, severe CP following vomiting or a procedure involving the esophagus may be the sign of a rupture in the esophagus.

23.6.6 Achalasia

Achalasia occurs when the lower esophageal sphincter does not work properly. Some patients with achalasia complain of CP in addition to dysphagia and regurgitation. CP is said to be most common in young patients who have been symptomatic for a short time, and who often have vigorous achalasia.

23.6.7 Peptic Ulcers

A vague recurring discomfort of peptic ulcers may be the result of the painful sores in the mucosa of the stomach, esophagus, or duodenum. More common in people who smoke, drink a lot of alcohol, or take analgesics such as aspirin or NSAIDs such as ibuprofen, diclofenac, indomethacin, and loxoprofen, the pain often gets better when the patient eats or takes antacids. Among the patients with non-cardiac CP, peptic ulcer disease is presented in 17.0% [64].

23.6.8 Gastritis

Weakness in the stomach lining allows digestive fluids to damage and inflame it, causing gastritis. Among the patients with non-cardiac CP, gastritis is presented in 72.9% [64].

23.6.9 Hiatal Hernia

The common problem of hiatal hernia occurs when the top of the stomach pushes into the lower chest after eating [6, 66, 67]. This often causes reflux symptoms, including heartburn or CP. The pain tends to get worse when the patient lies down.

23.6.10 Gallbladder

CP may be due to a gallbladder problem [6, 68]. Gallstones or inflammation of the gallbladder can cause abdominal pain that radiates to the chest. After eating a fatty meal, the patient has a sensation of fullness or pain in the right lower chest area or the right upper side of the abdomen.

23.6.11 Pancreatitis

Chronic pancreatitis or inflammation of the pancreas can cause abdominal pain that radiates to the chest [69]. If the patient has pain in the lower chest due to pancreatitis, the pain is often worse when the patient lies flat and better when the patient lean forward.

23.7 Bone

23.7.1 Chest Wall Syndrome

Some types of CP may result from overuse or be associated with injuries to the chest area from a fall or accident and other problems affecting the structures that make up the chest wall [6].

The clinical diagnosis of chest wall syndromes has not been described well. The quality and location of chest wall pain vary greatly; precipitating factors are useful for diagnosis. Chest wall pain is often pleuritic and tends to be aggravated by moving the arms or torso. The pain can be reproduced by palpation or manipulation of the chest wall.

Mechanical chest wall pain is a common presenting complaint in the primary care office, ER, and specialty clinic [70]. Diagnostic testing is often expensive due to similar presenting symptoms that may involve the heart or lungs. Manual diagnostic and therapeutic skills can be learned to treat biomechanically complex rib-related chest wall pain in combination with interventional image-guided techniques.

23.7.2 Chest Wall Trauma

Chest wall trauma is common, and contributes significantly to morbidity and mortality of trauma patients [26]. Early identification of major chest wall and concomitant intrathoracic injuries is critical. Generalized management of multiple rib fractures and flail chest consists of adequate pain control including locoregional modalities; management of pulmonary dysfunction by invasive and non-invasive means; and, in some cases, surgical fixation. Patients with flail chest have substantial benefit which decreased ventilator and intensive care unit days, improved pulmonary function, and improved long-term functional outcome, when they undergo surgery compared with non-operative management [71].

23.7.3 Rib

Bruised or broken ribs cause CP. Pain from a rib fracture may worsen with deep breathing or coughing. CP is often confined to one area and may feel sore when the patient presses on it. The area where the ribs join the sternum may become inflamed. Rib metastases also cause CP.

23.7.4 Costochondritis

Patients with costochondritis frequently present with CP [72]. In the condition of costochondritis, the cartilage of the thorax, particularly the cartilage that joins the ribs to the sternum, becomes inflamed and painful. Sulfasalazine may be of additional long-term benefit.

23.7.5 Spine

Compression fractures of spine cause pressure on a nerve and CP. Spinal cord tumor should be considered among the possible causative factors of chronic CP [73]. Scoliosis, spinal spondylosis, ankylosing spondylitis are a form of arthritis that primarily affects the spine [74].

Ankylosing spondylitis causes severe inflammation of entheses and joints, especially those in and around the spine. The most widespread involvement of the respiratory system by this disease occurs when this pathological process gives rise to chest wall pain, diminished chest wall movement, and a dorsal stoop. As the healing of the inflammatory process takes place, calcification occurs which leads to rigidity of these structures, with consequent loss of chest expansion, which is exacerbated by the increasingly kyphotic spinal posture and intercostal muscle inefficiency. Treatment is by mobilizing physiotherapy coupled with a home exercise program encouraging mobility and improved cardiovascular fitness. The role of medication is to ease symptoms and hence enable exercise. As with many physical treatment methods, good quality controlled studies of efficacy are rare.

23.8 Muscle

23.8.1 Muscle-Related Problems

Muscle-related problems such as sore muscles from exertion cause CP [75]. The musculoskeletal system is a recognized source of CP. Despite the apparent benign origin, patients with musculoskeletal CP remain under-diagnosed, untreated, and potentially continuously disabled in terms of anxiety, depression, and activities of daily living. Several overlapping conditions and syndromes of focal disorders, including Tietze syndrome, costochondritis, chest wall syndrome, muscle tenderness, slipping rib, cervical angina, and segmental dysfunction of the cervical and thoracic spine, have been reported to cause pain.

23.8.2 Muscle Strain

Even really hard coughing can injure or inflame the muscles and tendons between the ribs and cause CP. CP tends to persist and it worsens with activity. Musculoskeletal causes of CP include costochondritis, rib pain caused by stress fractures, slipping rib syndrome, chest wall muscle injuries, fibromyalgia, and herpes zoster (HZ) [76].

23.8.3 *Fibromyalgia*

Chronic pain syndromes such as fibromyalgia can produce persistent muscle-related CP. Fibromyalgia remains an enigmatic and challenging clinical entity to manage, given its far-reaching spectrum of symptoms, including pain, chronicity, associated psychopathology, and lack of clinically available diagnostic tests [77].

23.9 Collagen Disease

23.9.1 *Systemic Lupus Erythematosus (SLE)*

Systemic lupus erythematosus (SLE), the most common form of lupus, is a chronic autoimmune disease that can cause severe fatigue and joint pain. Patients with SLE are at increased risk for the development of premature cardiovascular disease. Inflammation is thought to play an important role in both the pathogenesis of SLE and atherosclerotic vascular disease. Inflammatory processes that are shared by SLE and atherosclerotic disease include immune complex deposition and fixation, autoantibody binding, complement activation, and CD40-CD40 ligand interaction [78].

23.10 Nerve Problems

23.10.1 *Herpes Zoster (HZ)*

Viruses can cause chronic pain in the chest area. HZ is an infection of the nerves and skin that occurs after reactivation of the HZ virus, can cause chronic pain. The patient may develop pain along the back or chest before the shingles rash becomes apparent. Caused by a reactivation of the HZ virus, shingles can produce pain and a band of blisters from the back around to the chest wall. Caused by the HZ virus, shingles may prompt a sharp, band-like pain before a telltale appears several days later.

Chronic pain in the chest wall is a major complication after HZ infection of intercostal nerves. Post-herpetic neuralgia is usually difficult to control pain of such origin.

Many of the tender spots formed in the intercostal muscles after HZ are myofascial trigger points that respond to injection with referred pain, local twitch responses, and immediate pain relief [79].

23.11 Mental

23.11.1 Mental-Related Problem

CP and breathlessness are common somatic symptoms of emotional disorder in ambulatory care. Of patients with CP and breathlessness who are referred to a cardiac clinic, but subsequently shown not to have heart disease, the majority continue to report symptoms [6]. The patients with the worst outcome, in terms of continuing limitation of activity and use of medical resources, are those with CP but normal coronary arteries. A number of studies that fail to support a unitary theory of causation of non-cardiac CP are described.

A multifactorial, interactive model is proposed, with contributions from physical factors, such as palpitations and intercostal muscle pain, psychological factors, which include enhanced awareness and selective attention to bodily sensation; and environmental factors, such as previous exposure to cardiorespiratory disease in first-degree relatives or significant others. Although there have been few controlled intervention studies in patients with unexplained cardiorespiratory symptoms, there is evidence for the efficacy of both drug treatments and psychological treatment. The results of intervention studies in patients with CP and normal coronary arteries are eagerly awaited.

Atypical CP and breathlessness are common causes of office consultations and functional disability. The diagnoses should be established on the basis of positive evidence of psychiatric illness rather than by exclusion [7]. The etiology is multifactorial, and management is aimed at treating the underlying psychosocial problems or psychiatric illness. Cognitive-behavioral treatments are probably as effective as drug treatments in the short-term, and the care of these patients would be improved by a more detailed explanation of non-cardiac causes and a greater opportunity for patients to discuss their fears.

23.11.2 Panic Disorder

Panic disorder, which is a sudden episode of intense fear when there is no real danger or cause, can cause the CP [80]. Panic disorder can occur along with a chronic medical illness such as CAD and may lead to physiological worsening of that illness with more frequent episodes of CP [81]. Panic disorder is a prevalent psychiatric condition that often is chronic and rarely resolves without medical intervention. Many patients with panic disorder initially present with a variety of somatic symptoms, including CP, tachycardia, palpitations, tachypnea, profuse sweating, sensation of shortness of breath, nausea, dizziness, tingling sensations, trembling, or a fear of dying, and patients frequently seek care in ambulatory care settings. Panic disorder is a common cause of CP in patients with negative cardiac test results. Although panic disorder is classified as a single entity, it can have many dimensions and may be associated with significant morbidity. There have been significant advances in the treatment of panic disorder, and a range of therapeutic choices is now available. Four classes of medications, including the selective serotonin reuptake inhibitors (SSRIs), high-potency benzodiazepines, tricyclic anti-depressants, and monoamine oxidase inhibitors, may be considered for the management of patients with panic disorder. SSRIs as first-line treatment for patients with panic disorder, and paroxetine and sertraline have been approved by the U.S. Food and Drug Administration for use in panic disorder. The practicing doctors are choosing tailor therapy among the various pharmacotherapies for each patient's individual needs.

23.11.3 Hyperventilation Syndrome

Healthy breathing occurs with a healthy balance between breathing in oxygen and breathing out. Hyperventilation is a condition in which the patient starts to breathe very fast [82]. Hyperventilation can cause CP that is atypical of angina. CP may vary in location and may not be pleuritic. Respiratory alkalosis and sympathetic discharge may occur in both conditions. A useful clue is that the pain is often brought on by anxiety or emotions. The most useful tool for confirming hyperventilation is to demonstrate that CP can be reproduced by rapid breathing.

23.11.4 Non-Specific Chest Pain

Non-specific CP is common in primary care [83]. For most patients with non-specific CP, standard medical care does not offer sufficient help for symptom relief. One-tenth of patients with persistent CP underwent additional diagnostic testing of no known clinical benefit. Psychological referrals and psychosomatic medicine [84] are rarely given.

23.12 Special Persons

23.12.1 Children

CP is a common complaint among children of all ages [85–87]. The majority of the conditions causing CP are benign and self-limiting. CP rarely is due to cardiac disease, but deserves careful evaluation for this possibility. Chronic CP is a complaint that frequently prompts referral to pediatric cardiology clinics, although very few pediatric patients with this symptom will be found to have cardiac disease. The child and parents need to be assured that there is no heart defect and that there is no imminent danger of dying.

Almost all diagnoses can be made with a thorough history and physical examination. CP in the child who has a history of coin ingestion, trauma, previous cardiac disease, or conditions that put the child at risk for developing cardiac pathology deserves further study. Likewise, those who have a history of condition such as asthma, Marfan syndrome, or sickle cell disease warrant special consideration. The child who has CP of acute onset that interferes with sleep is precipitated by exercise, or is associated with dizziness, palpitations, syncope, or shortness of breath should be evaluated with the aid of laboratory tests. Most of those who have an abnormal physical examination such as fever, respiratory distress, abnormal breath sounds, cardiac murmur, abnormal rhythm or heart sounds, palpable subcutaneous air, or obvious trauma, require a chest X-ray and an ECG. Finally, the child who has chronic CP with no worrisome history and normal physical examination needs reassurance and careful follow-up rather than extensive studies.

23.12.2 Athletes

CP in the athlete may originate from structures within the thorax, such as the heart, lungs, or esophagus. Musculoskeletal causes of CP must be considered [88, 89]. CP in the athlete has a wide differential diagnosis. The doctors should diagnose chest wall pain in athletes by identifying the possible causes. Causes can be grouped due to the system involved musculoskeletal, cardiac, respiratory, gastrointestinal diseases, GERD, and exercise-induced asthma with more common causes including rib stress fractures, costochondritis, muscle strain. Psychogenic causes can be common.

Musculoskeletal problems of the chest wall can occur in the ribs, sternum, articulations, or myofascial structures. The cause is usually evident in the case of direct trauma. Athletes' bodies may be subjected to sudden large indirect forces or overuse, and stress fractures of the ribs caused by sporting activity have been extensively reported. These have been associated with golf, rowing, and baseball pitching in particular. Stress fractures of the sternum reported in wrestlers cause CP and tenderness of the sternum. Diagnosis is by bone scan and limitation of activity usually allows healing to occur. The slipping rib syndrome causes intermittent costal margin pain related to posture or movement, and may be diagnosed by the hooking maneuver, which reproduces CP and sometimes a click. Good results are possible with resection of the mobile rib. The painful xiphoid syndrome is a rare condition that causes pain and tenderness of the xiphoid and is self-limiting. Costochondritis is a self-limiting condition of unknown etiology that typically presents with pain around the second to fifth costochondral joints. The intercostal muscles may be injured, causing tenderness between the ribs. Other conditions that should be considered include epidemic myalgia, precordial catch syndrome, and referred pain from the thoracic spine.

Initial management of CP in athletes always should involve assessment for serious, life-threatening causes, such as MI. Atypical CP, or CP not due to myocardial ischemia, is a common presentation in the athletic population. Some conditions such as myocarditis warranting a long, at least 6 months, absence from training. Others, such as precordial catch require nothing more than reassurance. Corticosteroid injection may be useful in particularly troublesome cases.

23.13 Specific Treatments

23.13.1 Continuous Intercostal Nerve Blockade

Continuous intercostal nerve blockade by placing an intercostal catheter intraoperatively provides effective analgesia in patients undergoing single port, video-assisted thoracoscopic surgery anatomic resection [90]. Continuous intercostal nerve blockade by placing ICC may be considered a viable alternative for chronic CP management.

23.13.2 Spinal Cord Electrical Stimulation

Spinal cord stimulation (SCS) is the most commonly used implantable neurostimulation modality for the management of pain syndromes. The use of SCS suppressed intractable pain targeted at the T6 and T7 dermatomes of the chest wall in the manifestation of post-thoracotomy neuralgia [91]. SCS is one of the few therapeutic options in inoperable patients with chronic CP. SCS provides an effective, alternative treatment for selected patients with intractable cancer pain, cancer-related chest wall pain who have failed conservative treatment, and pain related to post-laminectomy syndrome who have failed conservative treatment [92, 93].

The current indications for SCS are refractory angina pectoris, peripheral vascular disease (PVD), failed-back surgery syndrome (FBSS), and complex regional pain syndrome (CRPS) Type I [94]. The use of SCS in patients with inoperable angina, that is, refractory angina pectoris, results in significant decreases in CP and hospital admissions as well as increased exercise duration, with less morbidity than with open procedures that are performed for pain control only. Patients with inoperable PVD also demonstrate significant improvements in pain relief, QOL, and limb mobility. Effective pain relief is obtained in 60–80% of patients with FBSS and CRPS Type I. These patients have significant improvements in QOL and a significantly greater chance of returning to work than patients who does not undergo SCS. SCS is useful as an effective treatment modality for pain associated with refractory angina pectoris, PVD, FBSS, and CRPS Type I.

Reported complications are mostly related to hardware and are relatively minor. SCS may provide pain relief with advantages over conservative treatments and more invasive techniques.

23.13.3 Cryoanalgesia

Cryoanalgesia, which is the use of cold to provide anesthesia or analgesia, is the oldest anesthetic and analgesic still in current clinical use [95]. Percutaneous cryoanalgesia is a safe and efficacious method of providing analgesia for chronic thoracic pain due to intercostal neuralgia.

References

1. Mant J, McManus RJ, Oakes RA, Delaney BC, Barton PM, Deeks JJ, et al. Systematic review and modelling of the investigation of acute and chronic chest pain presenting in primary care. Health Technol Assess. 2004;8(iii):1–158.
2. Higgins CB, Bettmann MA, Boxt LM, Gomes AS, Grollman J, Henkin RE, et al. Chronic chest pain--suspected cardiac origin. American College of Radiology. ACR Appropriateness Criteria. Radiology. 2000;215(Suppl):29–34.
3. Henkin RE, Levin DC, Bettmann MA, Gomes AS, Grollman J, Hessel SJ, et al. Chronic chest pain without evidence of myocardial ischemia/infarction. American College of Radiology. ACR appropriateness criteria. Radiology. 2000;215(Suppl):85–8.
4. Sox HC Jr, Margulies I, Sox CH. Psychologically mediated effects of diagnostic tests. Ann Intern Med. 1981;95:680–5.
5. Woodard PK, White RD, Abbara S, Araoz PA, Cury RC, Dorbala S, et al. ACR Appropriateness Criteria chronic chest pain-low to intermediate probability of coronary artery disease. J Am Coll Radiol. 2013;10:329–34. https://doi.org/10.1016/j.jacr.2013.01.018.
6. Hutter AM. Chest pain: how to distinguish between cardiac and noncardiac causes. Interview by Eric R. Leibovitch. Geriatrics. 1995;50:32–6, 39–40.
7. Bass C. Chest pain and breathlessness: relationship to psychiatric illness. Am J Med. 1992;92:12S–7S.
8. Tousoulis D, Androulakis E, Kontogeorgou A, Papageorgiou N, Charakida M, Siama K, et al. Insight to the pathophysiology of stable angina pectoris. Curr Pharm Des. 2013;19:1593–600.
9. Haasenritter J, Stanze D, Widera G, Wilimzig C, Abu Hani M, et al. Does the patient with chest pain have a coronary heart disease? Diagnostic value of single symptoms and signs--a meta-analysis. Croat Med J. 2012;53:432–41.
10. Caselli C, Rovai D, Lorenzoni V, Carpeggiani C, Teresinska A, Aguade S, et al. A new integrated clinical-biohumoral model to predict functionally significant coronary artery disease in patients with chronic chest pain. Can J Cardiol. 2015;31:709–16. https://doi.org/10.1016/j.cjca.2015.01.035.
11. Hussain M, Khan N, Uddin M, Al-Nozha MM. Duration analysis for coronary artery disease patients with chronic chest pain: an output from Saudi Arabia. J Cardiovasc Thorac Res. 2015;7:6–12. https://doi.org/10.15171/jcvtr.2015.02.
12. Achenbach S, Kramer CM, Zoghbi WA, Dilsizian V. The year in coronary artery disease. JACC Cardiovasc Imaging. 2010;3:1065–77. https://doi.org/10.1016/j.jcmg.2010.08.010.
13. Earls JP, White RD, Woodard PK, Abbara S, Atalay MK, Carr JJ, et al. ACR appropriateness criteria® chronic chest pain--high probability of coronary artery disease. J Am Coll Radiol. 2011;8:679–86. https://doi.org/10.1016/j.jacr.2011.06.022.
14. Wright RS, Monnahan RL, Kopecky SL, Jones CT, Holmes DR Jr. Cardiac catheterization reduces resource utilization in patients with chronic chest pain. Catheter Cardiovasc Interv. 2000;49:363–6.
15. Akers SR, Panchal V, Ho VB, Beache GM, Brown RKJ, Ghoshhajra BB, et al. ACR appropriateness criteria® chronic chest pain-high probability of coronary artery disease. J Am Coll Radiol. 2017;14:S71–80. https://doi.org/10.1016/j.jacr.2017.01.034.

16. Nance JW Jr, Bamberg F, Schoepf UJ. Coronary computed tomography angiography in patients with chronic chest pain: systematic review of evidence base and cost-effectiveness. J Thorac Imaging. 2012;27:277–88. https://doi.org/10.1097/RTI.0b013e3182631c5c.
17. Norum IB, Ruddox V, Edvardsen T, Otterstad JE. Diagnostic accuracy of left ventricular longitudinal function by speckle tracking echocardiography to predict significant coronary artery stenosis. A systematic review. BMC Med Imaging. 2015;15:25. https://doi.org/10.1186/s12880-015-0067-y.
18. Shimizu T, Umetani K, Murata Y, Harama T, Yano T, Makino A, et al. Acute myocardial infarction due to simultaneous spasm of 3 coronary arteries that worsened over time. Am J Emerg Med. 2017; https://doi.org/10.1016/j.ajem.2017.12.028.
19. Valgimigli M, Biscaglia S. Stable angina pectoris. Curr Atheroscler Rep. 2014;16:422. https://doi.org/10.1007/s11883-014-0422-4.
20. Risos L, Berkenboom G. Revascularization versus medical treatments in stable coronary artery disease: predicting the future of novel drug therapies for stable angina. J Cardiovasc Pharmacol. 2014;63:213–7. https://doi.org/10.1097/FJC.0000000000000051.
21. Cademartiri F, La Grutta L, Palumbo A, Maffei E, Martini C, Seitun S, et al. Computed tomography coronary angiography vs. stress ECG in patients with stable angina. Radiol Med. 2009;114:513–23. https://doi.org/10.1007/s11547-009-0388-4.
22. Siama K, Tousoulis D, Papageorgiou N, Siasos G, Tsiamis E, Bakogiannis C, et al. Stable angina pectoris: current medical treatment. Curr Pharm Des. 2013;19:1569–80.
23. Hung MJ, Hu P, Hung MY. Coronary artery spasm: review and update. Int J Med Sci. 2014;1:1161–71. eCollection 2014. https://doi.org/10.7150/ijms.9623.
24. Yeh YH, Su YJ, Liu CH. Acute aortic dissection (AAD) in the elderly. Arch Gerontol Geriatr. 2013;57:78–80. https://doi.org/10.1016/j.archger.2012.11.012.
25. Giunio L, Boric T, Bulat C, Dragicevic D, Lozo M. Cardiac Tamponade after Right Ventricular Perforation Caused by Screw-in Lead. Int J Angiol. 2016;25:e177–9. https://doi.org/10.1055/s-0036-1580700.
26. Gupta SK, Naheed Z. Chest pain in adolescent Japanese male mimicking acute coronary syndrome. Case Rep Crit Care. 2014;2014:176520. https://doi.org/10.1155/2014/176520.
27. Biesbroek PS, Beek AM, Germans T, Niessen HW, van Rossum AC. Diagnosis of myocarditis: current state and future perspectives. Int J Cardiol. 2015;191:211–9. https://doi.org/10.1016/j.ijcard.2015.05.008.
28. Basman C, Agrawal PR, McRee C, Saravolatz L, Chen-Scarabelli C, Scarabelli TM. Diagnostic approach to myocarditis mimicking myocardial infarction at initial presentation. Cardiol Res. 2016;7:209–13. https://doi.org/10.14740/cr485w.
29. Imazio M, Battaglia A, Gaido L, Gaita F. Recurrent pericarditis. Rev Med Interne. 2017;38:307–11. https://doi.org/10.1016/j.revmed.2016.12.006.
30. Kloos JA. Characteristics, complications, and treatment of acute pericarditis. Crit Care Nurs Clin North Am. 2015;27:483–97. https://doi.org/10.1016/j.cnc.2015.08.001.
31. Critoph C, Elliott P. Hypertrophic cardiomyopathy. Card Electrophysiol Clin. 2010;2:587–98. https://doi.org/10.1016/j.ccep.2010.09.010.
32. Shammas NW, Shammas GA, Keyes K, Duske S, Kelly R, Jerin M. Ranolazine versus placebo in patients with ischemic cardiomyopathy and persistent chest pain or dyspnea despite optimal medical and revascularization therapy: randomized, double-blind crossover pilot study. Ther Clin Risk Manag. 2015;11:469–74. https://doi.org/10.2147/TCRM.S82288.
33. Yeo KK, Low RI. Aortic stenosis: assessment of the patient at risk. J Interv Cardiol. 2007;20:509–16.
34. Aronow WS. Valvular aortic stenosis in the elderly. Cardiol Rev. 2007;15:217–25.
35. Woolf PK, Gewitz MH, Berezin S, Medow MS, Stewart JM, Fish BG, et al. Noncardiac chest pain in adolescents and children with mitral valve prolapse. J Adolesc Health. 1991;12:247–50.
36. Wigle ED, Rakowski H, Ranganathan N, Silver MC. Mitral valve prolapse. Annu Rev Med. 1976;27:165–80.
37. Aronow WS. Management of atrial fibrillation in the elderly. Minerva Med. 2009;100:3–24.
38. Aronow WS. Management of the older person with atrial fibrillation. J Am Geriatr Soc. 1999;47:740–8.

39. Diamond JA. Classic images in hypertension. Hypertensive heart disease in a patient admitted to hospital with dyspnea, chest pain, and severe hypertension. Am J Hypertens. 2001;14:969–70.
40. McDivitt JD, Barstow C. Cardiovascular disease update: pulmonary hypertension. FP Essent. 2017;454:24–8.
41. Turley AJ, McCarron B, de Belder MA. Acute rheumatic fever mimicking an acute coronary syndrome. Emerg Med J. 2006;23:e45.
42. Arshad H, Young M, Adurty R, Singh AC. Acute pneumothorax. Crit Care Nurs Q. 2016;39:176–89. https://doi.org/10.1097/CNQ.0000000000000110.
43. Vacca VM, Jehle J. Acute pulmonary embolism. Nursing. 2013;43:25–6. https://doi.org/10.1097/01.NURSE.0000427353.73708.9d.
44. Kline JA, Kabrhel C. Emergency evaluation for pulmonary embolism, part 1: clinical factors that increase risk. J Emerg Med. 2015;48:771–80. https://doi.org/10.1016/j.jemermed.2014.12.040.
45. Kass SM, Williams PM, Reamy BV. Pleurisy. Am Fam Physician. 2007;75:1357–64.
46. Adebonojo SA, Osinowo O, Adebo O. Lung abscess: a review of three-years' experience at the University College Hospital, Ibadan. J Natl Med Assoc. 1979;71:39–43.
47. Horio Y, Shiraishi Y, Watanabe N, Inoue S, Imanishi T, Asano K. Empyema associated with Campylobacter curvus infection. Respirol Case Rep. 2017;5:e00234. eCollection 2017 July. https://doi.org/10.1002/rcr2.234.
48. Sokolove PE, Rossman L, Cohen SH. The emergency department presentation of patients with active pulmonary tuberculosis. Acad Emerg Med. 2000;7:1056–60.
49. Zhai K, Lu Y, Shi HZ. Tuberculous pleural effusion. J Thorac Dis. 2016;8:E486–94. https://doi.org/10.21037/jtd.2016.05.87.
50. Jung HW, Cho CR, Ryoo JY, Lee HK, Ha SY, Choi JH, et al. Actinomyces meyeri Empyema: a case report and review of the literature. Case Rep Infect Dis. 2015;2015:291838. https://doi.org/10.1155/2015/291838.
51. Dere WH. Acute bronchitis: results of U.S. and European trials of antibiotic therapy. Am J Med. 1992;92:53S–7S.
52. Woodhead MA, Macfarlane JT. Legionnaires' disease: a review of 79 community acquired cases in Nottingham. Thorax. 1986;41:635–40.
53. Hochberg U, Elgueta MF, Perez J. Interventional analgesic management of lung cancer pain. Front Oncol. 2017;7:17. eCollection 2017. https://doi.org/10.3389/fonc.2017.00017
54. Parish JM, Rosenow EC 3rd, Swensen SJ, Crotty TB. Pulmonary artery sarcoma. Clinical features. Chest. 1996;110:1480–8.
55. Dursunoğlu N, Kiter G, Oztürk E, Tunç P, Colakoğlu N, Değirmencioğlu S, Yaren A. An old woman with weight loss and chest pain. Tuberk Toraks. 2010;58:85–8.
56. Martinelli G, Vianelli N, De Vivo A, Ricci P, Remiddi C, Testoni N, et al. Granulocytic sarcomas: clinical, diagnostic and therapeutical aspects. Leuk Lymphoma. 1997;24:349–53.
57. Boubacar E, Atsame-Ebang G, Rabiou S, Fatimazahra A, Mazti A, Sidibé IS, et al. Thymic large cell neuroendocrine carcinoma—a rare and aggressive tumor: a case report. J Med Case Rep. 2017;11:155. https://doi.org/10.1186/s13256-017-1331-2.
58. Webb AJ, Yassin AS, Saeed A, Yadav H, Utz JP. Mediastinal solitary fibrous tumor diagnosed by endobronchial ultrasound-directed biopsy. Am J Case Rep. 2017;18:549–52.
59. Allen RK, Cramond T, Lennon D, Waterhouse M. A retrospective study of chest pain in benign asbestos pleural disease. Pain Med. 2011;12:1303–8. https://doi.org/10.1111/j.1526-4637.2011.01209.x.
60. Heinle R, Chang C. Diagnostic criteria for sarcoidosis. Autoimmun Rev. 2014;13:383–7. https://doi.org/10.1016/j.autrev.2014.01.035.
61. Gater A, Nelsen L, Fleming S, Lundy JJ, Bonner N, Hall R, et al. Assessing asthma symptoms in adolescents and adults: qualitative research supporting development of the asthma daily symptom diary. Value Health. 2016;19:440–50. https://doi.org/10.1016/j.jval.2016.01.007.
62. Lemire S. Assessment of clinical severity and investigation of uncomplicated gastroesophageal reflux disease and noncardiac angina-like chest pain. Can J Gastroenterol. 1997;11:37B–40B.

63. Shapiro M, Simantov R, Yair M, Leitman M, Blatt A, Scapa E, et al. Comparison of central and intraesophageal factors between gastroesophageal reflux disease (GERD) patients and those with GERD-related noncardiac chest pain. Dis Esophagus. 2012;25:702–8. https://doi.org/10.1111/j.1442-2050.2011.01317.x.
64. Park SH, Choi JY, Park EJ, Lee JJ, Lee S, Na JO, et al. Prevalence of gastrointestinal diseases and treatment status in noncardiac chest pain patients. Korean Circ J. 2015;45:469–72. https://doi.org/10.4070/kcj.2015.45.6.469.
65. Nam CW, Kim KS, Lee YS, Lee SH, Han SW, Hur SH, et al. The incidence of gastroesophageal disease for the patients with typical chest pain and a normal coronary angiogram. Korean J Intern Med. 2006;21:94–6.
66. Palios J, Clements S Jr, Lerakis S. Chest pain due to hiatal hernia mimicking as cardiac mass. Acute Card Care. 2014;16:88–9. https://doi.org/10.3109/17482941.2014.889313.
67. Wanner GK, Nangeroni JP, Nisbet B. Large paraesophageal hiatal hernia in a patient with chest pain. J Am Osteopath Assoc. 2015;115:282. https://doi.org/10.7556/jaoa.2015.055.
68. Ferguson HJ, Bhalerao S. Gallbladder torsion presenting as chest pain. Ann R Coll Surg Engl. 2010;92:W25–6. https://doi.org/10.1308/147870810X12659688851357.
69. Lam S, Banim P. Massive loculated pleural effusion in a patient with pancreatic pseudocyst due to alcohol-related chronic pancreatitis. BMJ Case Rep. 2014; https://doi.org/10.1136/bcr-2014-204032.
70. Germanovich A, Ferrante FM. Multi-modal treatment approach to painful rib syndrome: case series and review of the literature. Pain Physician. 2016;19:E465–71.
71. Majercik S, Pieracci FM. Chest wall trauma. Thorac Surg Clin. 2017;27:113–21. https://doi.org/10.1016/j.thorsurg.2017.01.004.
72. Freeston J, Karim Z, Lindsay K, Gough A. Can early diagnosis and management of costochondritis reduce acute chest pain admissions? J Rheumatol. 2004;31:2269–71.
73. Marseglia GL, Savasta S, Ravelli A, Gaino TM, Burgio GR. Recurrent chest pain as the presenting manifestation of spinal meningioma. Acta Paediatr. 1995;84:1086–8.
74. Haslock I. Ankylosing spondylitis. Baillieres Clin Rheumatol. 1993;7:99–115.
75. Stochkendahl MJ, Christensen HW. Chest pain in focal musculoskeletal disorders. Med Clin North Am. 2010;9:259–73. https://doi.org/10.1016/j.mcna.2010.01.007.
76. Ayloo A, Cvengros T, Marella S. Evaluation and treatment of musculoskeletal chest pain. Prim Care. 2013;40:863–87, viii. https://doi.org/10.1016/j.pop.2013.08.007.
77. Almansa C, Wang B, Achem SR. Noncardiac chest pain and fibromyalgia. Med Clin North Am. 2010;94:275–89. https://doi.org/10.1016/j.mcna.2010.01.002.
78. Rhew EY, Ramsey-Goldman R. Premature atherosclerotic disease in systemic lupus erythematosus—role of inflammatory mechanisms. Autoimmun Rev. 2006;5:101–5.
79. Chen SM, Chen JT, Kuan TS, Hong CZ. Myofascial trigger points in intercostal muscles secondary to herpes zoster infection of the intercostal nerve. Arch Phys Med Rehabil. 1998;79:336–8.
80. Sheehan DV. Current concepts in the treatment of panic disorder. J Clin Psychiatry. 1999;60(Suppl 18):16–21.
81. Katon WJ. Chest pain, cardiac disease, and panic disorder. J Clin Psychiatry. 1990;51(Suppl):27–30, discussion 50-3
82. Greenberg DB, Murray GB. Hyperventilation as a variant of tardive dyskinesia. J Clin Psychiatry. 1981;42:401–3.
83. Glombiewski JA, Rief W, Bösner S, Keller H, Martin A, Donner-Banzhoff N. The course of nonspecific chest pain in primary care: symptom persistence and health care usage. Arch Intern Med. 2010;170:251–5.
84. Strasburger VC, Reeve A. The adolescent with chronic pains: basic principles of psychosomatic medicine. Adolesc Med. 1991;2:677–96.
85. Balfour IC, Rao PS. Chest pain in children. Indian J Pediatr. 1998;65:21–6.
86. Selbst SM. Consultation with the specialist. Chest pain in children. Pediatr Rev. 1997;18:169–73.
87. Feinstein RA, Daniel WA Jr. Chronic chest pain in children and adolescents. Pediatr Ann. 1986;15:685–6, 691–4

88. Sik EC, Batt ME, Heslop LM. Atypical chest pain in athletes. Curr Sports Med Rep. 2009;8:52–8.
89. Gregory PL, Biswas AC, Batt ME. Musculoskeletal problems of the chest wall in athletes. Author information. Sports Med. 2002;32:235–50.
90. Hsieh MJ, Wang KC, Liu HP, Gonzalez-Rivas D, Wu CY, Liu YH, et al. Management of acute postoperative pain with continuous intercostal nerve block after single port video-assisted thoracoscopic anatomic resection. J Thorac Dis. 2016;8:3563–71. https://doi.org/10.21037/jtd.2016.12.30.
91. Bagger JP, Jensen BS, Johannsen G. Long-term outcome of spinal cord electrical stimulation in patients with refractory chest pain. Clin Cardiol. 1998;21:286–8.
92. Yakovlev AE, Resch BE. Treatment of multifocal pain with spinal cord stimulation. Neuromodulation. 2012;15:210–3discussion 213. https://doi.org/10.1111/j.1525-1403.2012.00435.x.
93. Yakovlev AE, Resch BE, Karasev SA. Treatment of cancer-related chest wall pain using spinal cord stimulation. Am J Hosp Palliat Care. 2010;27:552–6. https://doi.org/10.1177/1049909110373240.
94. Lee AW, Pilitsis JG. Spinal cord stimulation: indications and outcomes. Neurosurg Focus. 2006;21:E3.
95. Green CR, de Rosayro AM, Tait AR. The role of cryoanalgesia for chronic thoracic pain: results of a long-term follow up. J Natl Med Assoc. 2002;94:716–20.

Chapter 24
Upper Abdominal Pain

Ju Mizuno and Kazuo Hanaoka

Abbreviations

AP	Abdominal pain
CPB	Celiac plexus block
CT	Computed tomography
FAPS	Functional abdominal pain syndrome
GES	Gastric electrical stimulation
H. pylori	Helicobacter pylori
IBS	Irritable bowel syndrome
NBS	Narcotic bowel syndrome
NSAID	Non-steroidal anti-inflammatory drug
OTC	Over-the-counter
SNB	Splanchnic nerve block

24.1 Organ

The upper abdomen houses several vital structures, including stomach, duodenum, liver, gallbladder, and pancreas. The liver, gallbladder, and pancreas which are three organs in the upper-right side of the abdomen work together to support digestion.

J. Mizuno
Department of Anesthesiology and Pain Medicine, Juntendo University Faculty of Medicine, Tokyo, Japan
e-mail: jmizuno@juntendo.ac.jp

K. Hanaoka (✉)
Department of Anesthesiology and Pain Relief Center, JR Tokyo General Hospital, Tokyo, Japan
e-mail: kazuo-hanaoka@jreast.co.jp

K. Shimoji et al. (eds.), *Chronic Pain Management in General and Hospital Practice*, https://doi.org/10.1007/978-981-15-2933-7_24

24.2 Diagnosis

One of the goals to diagnose abdominal pain (AP) is to rule out underlying conditions such as bowel perforation and obstruction.

The blood test can be performed. Using a sample of the patient's blood, a number of tests including complete blood count to look for signs of anemia and infections, electrolyte abnormalities, and liver and kidney function tests to examine electrolyte abnormalities, and liver and kidney issues, and albumin tests to assess the patient's nutritional status may be run.

The standard abdominal X-ray can be performed. An abdominal X-ray helps to find perforation and obstruction of small intestines or colon and any other abnormalities. The abdominal echocardiography and computed tomography (CT) scan can be performed. Using X-rays and special computer software create 2D and 3D images of the patient's stomach, intestines, and colon. Providing alternative views of the patient's abdominal organs, CT scan helps to examine details that might not be visible through other imaging tests.

The stool culture may be performed. A fecal occult blood test identifies microscopic amounts of blood, white blood cells, and evidence of food intolerances.

The upper endoscopy may be performed. With the help of an endoscope that pass through the patient's mouth and esophagus, the mucosa of the stomach and duodenum for ulcer, inflammation, infection, and cancer may be carefully examined. The colonoscopy or sigmoidoscopy may be performed. The entire length or just the lower part of the patient's colon with the help of a small flexible scope with tiny camera which insert into the rectum may be examined. Endoscopic ultrasound is successful in diagnosing a clinical etiology of chronic upper AP that is unrevealing for a definitive diagnosis with previous tests. The most frequent diagnoses included pancreaticobiliary tree abnormalities, chronic pancreatitis, and fatty liver disease [1].

24.3 Acute Upper Abdominal Pain (AP)

Causes of acute upper AP can include (1) gas, (2) acute gastritis, (3) stomach viruses, (4) peptic ulcer, (5) gallstones, (6) liver issues, (7) pancreas issues, (8) appendicitis, (9) constipation and bowel obstruction, (10) diverticular disease, and (11) muscle pain.

24.3.1 Gas

Gas occurs naturally in the intestines and digestive tract. When the gas accumulates, it can cause feelings of pressure, bloating, or fullness. An infection, virus, diarrhea, or constipation can cause gas pain to become very intense.

Gas pain is not usually serious, and over-the-counter (OTC) medicines can help. Gas usually goes away without specific treatment within a few hours.

24.3.2 Acute Gastritis

Weakness in the gastric mucosa allows digestive fluids to damage and inflame it, causing acute gastritis. Acute gastritis causes the gastric mucosa to become swollen and painful. Acute gastritis occurs in the short term and comes on quickly, usually because of a bacterial infection, such as with Helicobacter pylori (H. pylori) bacteria. Some conditions irritate the acute gastric mucosa, causing chronic gastritis.

For many patients, reducing gastric acid by eating a less acidic diet or taking medications can help. Analgesics can help with symptoms, while medicines that protect the gastric mucosa can prevent the symptoms from getting worse. Antibiotics can usually treat bacterial infections.

24.3.3 Stomach Viruses

Gastroenteritis is a stomach virus that can cause nausea, vomiting, and diarrhea, in addition to upper AP. The patients with a stomach virus may also have headaches, muscle pain, and low energy.

Avoiding heavy meals and drinking only clear liquids can help a patient stop vomiting. It is vital to avoid dehydration, so consider drinking something that restores electrolytes, such as a sports drink, until the symptoms pass. Symptoms usually go away on their own within a few days. Some patients may need medical treatment to avoid dehydration, including those with weakened immune systems, babies and young children, and the patients with serious health conditions, such as cancer.

24.3.4 Peptic Ulcer

A vague recurring discomfort of peptic ulcer may be the result of the painful sores in the mucosa of the esophagus, stomach, and duodenum. Peptic ulcer may cause dyspepsia. It is more common in people who smoke, drink a lot of alcohol, or take analgesics such as aspirin or non-steroidal anti-inflammatory drugs (NSAIDs) such as ibuprofen, diclofenac, indomethacin, and loxoprofen. The pain often gets better when the patient eats or takes antacids.

24.3.5 Gall Stones

Gallstones or inflammation of the gallbladder can cause the AP at the right upper side that is the most frequent presenting symptom [2]. Tenderness in the right upper quadrant is the most common sign [2].

Clinically, 29.4% of patients were categorized obese [2]. Gallstones are hard formations of cholesterol or bilirubin that can develop in the gallbladder. Majority of the stones are grossly cholesterol stones [2]. Gallstone by ultrasound is detected [2].

Gallstones do not always cause problems, but sometimes gallstones obstruct a biliary duct. A blockage from gallstones can cause intense pain, as well as vomiting, fatigue, and exhaustion. After eating a fatty meal, the patient has a sensation of fullness or pain. Untreated gallstones can sometimes obstruct biliary ducts, affecting the functioning of the liver and pancreas, and causing pain in the liver or pancreas. Therefore, gallstones may cause liver dysfunction. When liver dysfunction happens, a patient may experience jaundice, which is yellowing of the skin and eyes. Gallstones may also develop a serious inflammation of the pancreas.

Medication to dissolve the gallstones may be tried to prescribe. In most cases gallstones by surgical removal of the gallbladder are treated. Cholecystectomy is a safe and most effective procedure that provides ultimate cure for symptomatic gallstone disease [2]. The patient will be able to live a regular life without gallbladder.

24.3.6 Liver Issues

Liver diseases, such as acute hepatitis, can rarely cause upper AP. Additional symptoms of liver problems include yellow eyes or skin, dark urine, very pale or white bowel movements, nausea, vomiting, pain that gets progressively worse.

24.3.7 Pancreas Issues

If the patient has pain due to acute pancreatitis, the pain is often worse when the patient lies flat and better when the patient leans forward. Most cases of acute pancreatitis are related to gallstones. The diagnosis is based on upper AP, elevated lipase and amylase, and transabdominal ultrasound findings.

Management requires early aggressive hydration, pain control, nutritional support, and monitoring for progression [3]. Patients who develop hypovolemia, systemic inflammatory response, pancreatic necrosis, and organ failure have high mortality, risk of recurrence, and progression to chronic pancreatitis [3]. Management requires control of pain and exocrine and endocrine symptoms, plus reduction of risk factors, especially alcohol intake [3]. More than 80% resolve within a few days.

24.3.8 Appendicitis

Appendicitis is an infection of the appendix. In the early stages of appendicitis, the patient may notice dull ache around the navel, but this pain can radiate to the upper abdomen. As the infection gets worse, the pain moves to the lower-right side.

In most cases, appendicitis by surgical removal of the appendix is treated. Without treatment, it can cause the appendix to rupture, and the condition can become life-threatening.

24.3.9 Bowel Obstruction

A bowel obstruction makes difficult or impossible for anything to pass through. Bowel obstruction can cause intense pain, constipation, and difficulty digesting and absorbing food. In addition to AP, symptoms of bowel obstruction include vomiting bile, a greenish-yellow substance, a swollen stomach, an inability to pass gas, and intense cramping.

Medications, fluid, and analgesics often help. In some cases, an operation may need to remove the bowel obstruction. Bowel obstruction is a medical emergency, as the bowel can tear or become seriously infected.

24.3.10 Diverticular Disease

Small pouches called diverticula can appear in the colon. When diverticula become inflamed or infected, a patient can develop intense AP. The location of the pain depends on where the diverticula are. Probiotics and a high-fiber diet often help treat diverticulitis.

24.3.11 Muscle Pain

Pain from a mild muscle injury or spasms can cause temporary pain in the upper abdomen. The pain often gets better with gentle massage and rest. Some patients also find relief by using cold and hot packs.

24.4 Chronic Upper Abdominal Pain (AP)

When the patient has AP that lasts more than 3 months, the patient may have chronic AP. Chronic AP is defined as continuous or intermittent abdominal discomfort lasting for 3–6 months.

Chronic AP is divided into organic and functional pain. Organic chronic AP has clear anatomical, physiological, or metabolic causes and can also arise from the abdominal wall, nerve, or fascia. Functional chronic AP has common but more challenging condition when no clear source of pain, despite through investigation.

Chronic AP symptoms include difficulty describing and locating the patient's pain, dizziness, fatigue, headache, nausea, pain that is not affected by eating or physical activity. Symptoms sometimes appear with no known cause.

The incidence of unspecified AP is 22.9 per 1000 person-years. A cross-sectional survey among adult population reported as high as 25% have AP at one time. In a systemic review of chronic AP in children and adolescents, the prevalence rate ranged is 4–53%.

It is common for the patient with chronic AP to have normal test results. Diagnosis and management of patients with chronic AP is often challenging at primary care setting. Factors that contribute to chronic AP include poor sensitivity of the history and physical examination, a broad differential diagnosis that crosses several specialties, and an often negative diagnostic work. Chronic AP can be originated from any system, such as the gastrointestinal, genitourinary, and gynecological tracts. Emotions, life experiences, and other medical issues can affect the way. The patient's body interprets signals from the brain. This can cause the patient to be extra sensitive to pain, for example, visceral hypersensitivity.

The causes of chronic AP are many. Possible causes include inflammation of the patient's intestines, distention of an abdominal organ, and blood loss to an abdominal organ. Common differential diagnoses of chronic AP for adults that can be managed at primary care are (1) gastroparesis, (2) functional abdominal pain syndrome (FAPS), (3) functional dyspepsia, (4) narcotic bowel syndrome (NBS), (5) chronic gastroenteritis including inflammatory bowel diseases, (6) chronic pancreatitis, (7) cancer, gastroesophageal reflux disease, peptic ulcer, irritable bowel syndrome (IBS), chronic cholelithiasis, and chronic abdominal wall pain. Other possible causes may include urinary tract infection, nephrolithiasis, interstitial cystitis, painful bladder syndrome, primary dysmenorrhea, endometriosis, pelvic inflammatory disease, and stress or anxiety.

It may take time to fully understand the patient's condition, but there is plenty in the short term to help the patient feel better. An approach that has evolved based on clinical experience and review of the literature: identifying predominant bloaters and abdominal wall pain; exclusion of organic disease, including consideration of laparoscopy for diagnosis; consideration of functional chronic AP and the first and second line pharmacotherapies; and seeking specialist care in a pain clinic, psychiatry, or behavioral therapy [4].

The treatments for patients with chronic AP may include medication. Medicines including aspirin and NSAIDs may help the patients feel better. Medication including anti-depressants for anxiety is also needed to help the patients relieve symptoms.

Patients with chronic AP of undetermined etiology, 70% reported complete or substantial pain relief by the end of chronic pain management [5]. Pain character and location and the referring diagnosis are not predictors of pain relief. Long-term pain relief is reported by 35% of patients. A substantial group of patients with chronic AP of unknown etiology benefits from chronic pain clinic services.

24.4.1 *Gastroparesis*

Gastroparesis is a chronic and debilitating neuromuscular disorder of the upper gastrointestinal tract [6]. Gastroparesis is identified in clinical practice through the recognition of the clinical symptoms and documentation of delayed gastric emptying [7]. Gastroparesis may be related to a variety of underlying disorders, but diabetes mellitus is by far the most common cause [8].

Symptoms of gastroparesis include nausea, vomiting, epigastric pain, early satiety, postprandial fullness, bloating, upper AP, and weight loss [6–8]. Gastric scintigraphy with 99-technetium-labeled low-fat meal is the gold standard method of diagnosing delayed gastric emptying [8].

Pain management is essential, as nearly 90% of patients report symptoms of epigastric pain [6]. Dietary changes may improve symptoms in patients with mild disease [6]. Management of gastroparesis should include assessment and correction of nutritional state, relief of symptoms, improvement of gastric emptying and, in diabetics, glycemic control [7]. Patient's nutritional state should be managed by oral dietary modifications [7]. Parenteral nutrition is rarely required when hydration and nutritional state cannot be maintained [7]. If oral intake is not adequate, then enteral nutrition via jejunostomy tube needs to be considered [7].

Dietary measures and prokinetic drugs bring symptomatic relief in most patients [8]. Medical treatment entails use of prokinetic and anti-emetic therapies [7]. Anti-emetic medications have not been specifically tested in gastroparesis [7]. Some patients with severe nausea and vomiting will require anti-emetic medications [8]. Anti-emetics may relieve nausea and vomiting [7]. Other medications aimed at symptom relief include unapproved medications or off-label indications, and include domperidone, erythromycin primarily over a short term, and centrally acting anti-depressants used as symptom modulators [7].

As the treatment of gastroparesis is far from ideal, non-conventional approaches and non-standard medications are presented [8].

Few patients will fail medical therapy and will continue to have debilitating symptoms of gastroparesis. Such patients may benefit from a venting gastrostomy or a jejunostomy placed surgically, endoscopically, or fluoroscopically [8].

Current approved treatment options, including metoclopramide and gastric electrical stimulation (GES), which approved on a humanitarian device exemption, do not adequately address clinical need [7]. GES may relieve symptoms, including weekly vomiting frequency, and the need for nutritional supplementation, based on open-label studies [7]. GES can be an existing new approach in the management of gastroparesis.

24.4.2 *Functional Abdominal Pain Syndrome (FAPS)*

FAPS is one of the less common functional gastrointestinal disorders, yet FAPS is one with high health care impact [9]. FAPS presents continuously or nearly continuously for at least 3 months, with onset at least 6 months before diagnosis. FAPS is a debilitating disorder with constant or nearly constant AP [10]. FAPS is not feigned and causes some loss of daily functioning.

FAPS differs from the other functional bowel disorders. There is no or only occasional relationship of pain with physiologic events such as eating, defecation, and menstruation. FAPS is less common, symptoms largely are unrelated to physiologic events, and it has higher comorbidity with psychiatric disorders [11].

These criteria are geared to identify patients with severe symptoms as they require constant or nearly constant AP with loss of daily function and are differentiated from IBS based on their non-association with changes in bowel habit, eating, or other gut-related events [10].

FAPS has insufficient symptoms to meet criteria for another disorder of gastrointestinal function that would explain the pain. It is best understood from a biopsychosocial perspective as the interaction of biologic and psychosocial factors contributing to symptom experience and behavior [9].

No epidemiological studies have focused specifically on FAPS [10]. Estimates of prevalence range from 0.5 to 1.7% and tend to show a female predominance [10].

The pathophysiology is incompletely understood [11]. Because FAPS likely represents a heterogeneous group of disorders, peripheral neuropathic pain mechanisms, alterations in endogenous pain modulation systems, or both may be involved in any one patient [11]. The pain of FAPS relates primarily to dysfunction of central pain modulatory systems; however, disturbances in motility or visceral hypersensitivity may contribute [9]. The pathophysiology of FAPS appears unique in that the pain is caused primarily by amplified central perception of normal visceral input, rather than by enhanced peripheral stimulation from abdominal viscera [10].

There are characteristic clinical and behavioral features that typify patients with FAPS [9]. The medical evaluation must include the recognition through psychosocial assessment, physical examination, and a conservative, cost-effective effort to exclude other diseases [9].

The diagnosis of FAPS is symptom-based in accordance with the Rome III diagnostic criteria [10]. The diagnosis of FAPS is made on the basis of positive symptom criteria and a longstanding history of symptoms; in the absence of alarm symptoms, an extensive diagnostic evaluation is not required [11].

As cure is not feasible, the aims of treatment are reduced suffering and improved quality of life [10].Therapeutic options include central non-pharmacological and pharmacological modalities and peripheral modalities [10]. These can be combined to produce an augmentation effect [10]. Management is based on a biopsychosocial approach with a therapeutic patient-physician partnership at its base [10]. The empirical treatment algorithms use various classes of centrally acting drugs, including anti-depressants and anti-convulsants [11]. The treatment approach depends on establishing an effective physician-patient relationship, setting reasonable treatment goals, and using multicomponent medical and behavioral strategies that are individualized to patient needs [9]. The choice, dose, and combination of drugs are influenced by psychiatric comorbidities [11]. Psychological treatment options include psychotherapy, relaxation techniques, and hypnosis [11]. Patients with refractory FAPS may benefit from a multidisciplinary pain clinic approach [11]. In refractory cases, referral to a multidisciplinary pain treatment center might be helpful [9].

24.4.3 Functional Dyspepsia

Functional dyspepsia defined as chronic or recurrent pain or discomfort centered in the upper abdomen with no clinical or endoscopic evidence of known organic disease is very common and causes considerable morbidity and loss of productivity [12]. The other symptoms referable to the proximal gastrointestinal tract, such as nausea, early satiety, and bloating, may also be present [13]. Dyspepsia is a burning feeling in the upper abdomen, and sometimes in the mouth or throat. The pain may also feel like it stems from the chest. Patients with dyspepsia may present with associated complaints of AP, bloating, fullness, acid reflux, and epigastric tenderness on examination [14]. Mostly dyspepsia is a chronic relapsing problem [15]. Frequent dyspepsia that is very painful or occurs with unexplained weight loss could be a sign of a more serious concern. To be termed chronic, dyspepsia should have been present for 3 months or longer [13].

Dyspepsia is very common in western countries, where 10–40% of the population experience upper AP or discomfort over the course of 1 year [15]. Epidemiological studies have not convincingly demonstrated an association between H. pylori and non-ulcer dyspepsia [13].

Symptoms may or may not be meal related [13]. It usually appears when there is too much acid in the stomach, which can happen after eating highly acidic foods. Less commonly, dyspepsia can result from peptic ulcer, acid reflux, or even stomach cancer.

Over half the patients who present with chronic dyspepsia have no evidence of peptic ulceration, other focal lesions, or systemic disease and are diagnosed as having non-ulcer or functional dyspepsia [13]. Non-ulcer dyspepsia is a heterogeneous syndrome [13]. It has been proposed that this entity can be subdivided into a number of symptomatic clusters or groupings that suggest possible underlying pathogenetic mechanisms [13]. These groupings include ulcer-like dyspepsia, dysmotility-like dyspepsia, and reflux-like dyspepsia [13]. Ulcer-like dyspepsia shows typical symptoms of peptic ulcer. Dysmotility-like dyspepsia shows symptoms including nausea, early satiety, bloating, and belching that suggest gastric stasis or small intestinal dysmotility. Reflux-like dyspepsia shows heartburn or acid regurgitation with upper AP or discomfort.

The etiology of non-ulcer dyspepsia is not established, although it is likely a multifactorial disorder [13]. Motility abnormalities may be important in a subset of dyspepsia patients but probably do not explain the symptoms in the majority [13]. Other potential etiological mechanisms, such as increased gastric acid secretion, psychological factors, life-event stress, and dietary factors, have not been established as causes of non-ulcer dyspepsia [13].

Dyspepsia without an ulcer, non-ulcer dyspepsia, is diagnosed in patients at least twice as often as peptic ulceration [16]. Diseases that may present with similar symptoms include gastroesophageal reflux, biliary tract disease, chronic pancreatitis, and IBS [16]. A careful history and physical examination, supplemented by selected tests, usually lead to a correct diagnosis [16]. The pathogenesis of non-ulcer dyspepsia remains unknown. Gastric acid secretion, duodenogastric reflux, psychological factors, environmental exposures, and heredity probably do not play a major role [16].

Some patients may have motility disturbances, but whether these disturbances cause dyspepsia is unknown [16]. Campylobacter pylori infection and associated gastritis are common in non-ulcer dyspepsia, but their etiologic role is controversial, as is the importance of chronic duodenitis [16].

Patients with chronic dyspepsia lasting more than 1 month should be evaluated for the presence of alarm features [14]. The evaluation of patients with dyspepsia includes taking a comprehensive history and performing a physical examination [14]. Differential diagnoses of dyspepsia are best addressed using an anatomical approach [14]. Although taking a patient history has its limitations in making an accurate diagnosis, it is useful in guiding the selection of subsequent diagnostic tests. Alarm features mandate an upper gastrointestinal endoscopy examination, as these may be suggestive of a malignancy [14]. Prompt endoscopy is imperative in all patients with sinister symptoms including the first appearance of symptoms after the age of 50–55 [15]. In other patients, endoscopy is unlikely to contribute to medical management [15].

In patients who are symptomatic without an organic pathology, functional dyspepsia and other causes of AP need to be considered [14]. The physician involved in the care for dyspeptic patients needs to be aware of the current H. pylori prevalence [15]. In patients without alarm features, a H. pylori test-and-treat strategy is cost-effective if the prevalence of H. pylori infection is high [14]. Tests for H. pylori infection can be divided into non-invasive and minimally invasive tests [14]. A test-and-treatment strategy implies non-invasive testing for H. pylori and treatment of the infection if present seems to be the best approach under current conditions [15]. H. pylori prevalence among dyspeptics is 28–61% in recent studies [15]. With a continuing decrease in H. pylori prevalence the accuracy of the used non-invasive H. pylori test needs to be high and urea breath tests are to be preferred, the fecal antigen test being a reasonable alternative [15].

A first priority in management is reassuring patients that they do not have a serious disorder [12]. By recognizing the heterogeneity of patients who present with non-ulcer dyspepsia, more rational management may be possible [16]. OTC medicines are highly effective at managing temporary dyspepsia. Few drugs have established benefit and the choice depends on which symptoms predominate [12]. Many different antibiotic combination therapies such as triple therapy, quadruple therapy, levofloxacin-based therapy, sequential therapy, concomitant therapy, and probiotics with eradication therapy are now available for the eradication of H. pylori infection [14].

Management of non-ulcer dyspepsia is difficult because its pathogenesis is poorly understood and is confounded because of a high placebo response rate [13]. Until more data are available, it seems reasonable that treatment regimens target the clinical groupings described above [13]. Antacids are no more effective than placebo in non-ulcer dyspepsia, although a subgroup of non-ulcer dyspepsia patients with reflux-like or ulcer-like symptoms may respond to H_2-receptor antagonists [13]. Although an empiric trial of antacids or H_2 blockers has been recommended to treat dyspepsia, most controlled trials show that although these substances reduce severity of symptoms, they are no more effective than placebos in non-ulcer dyspepsia [16]. However, there is no significant benefit of these agents over placebo in many cases [13].

Prokinetic drugs may be most beneficial in those in whom discomfort rather than pain, bloating, or nausea is the most bothersome complaint and anti-secretory drugs in those with predominant epigastric pain [12]. Prokinetic drugs appear to be efficacious, and may be most useful in patients with dysmotility-like and reflux-like dyspepsia [13].

Bismuth has been shown to be superior to placebo in patients with H. pylori in a number of studies, but these trials had several shortcomings and others have reported conflicting findings [13]. Sucralfate was demonstrated in one study to be superior to placebo, but this finding was not confirmed by another group of investigators.

If the patient is H. pylori-negative and in case of persisting symptoms after successful H. pylori eradication, empirical treatment with an anti-secretory drug is justified [15]. At a very low prevalence of H. pylori in the dyspeptic population, i.e., below 10%, non-invasive testing for H. pylori loses its significance and empirical treatment with an anti-secretory drug becomes a rational first step [15]. Endoscopy is reserved for those patients in whom H. pylori eradication fails [15].

Functional dyspepsia is best managed using a multifaceted approach by establishing a good physician-patient relationship, dietary and lifestyle interventions, medical therapy, psychotherapy, and the use of psychotropic medications [14].

24.4.4 Narcotic Bowel Syndrome (NBS)

Chronic or frequently recurring AP can be treated with narcotics. There is marked worsening of pain when the narcotic dose wanes and improvement when narcotics are reinstituted. NBS is a subset of opioid bowel dysfunction that is characterized by chronic or frequently recurring AP that worsens with continued or escalating dosages of narcotics [17]. With increased prescription of opioids has come increased recognition of adverse consequences, including NBS [18]. There is a progression of the frequency, duration, and intensity of pain episodes. Patients with NBS have a high degree of comorbid psychiatric illness, catastrophizing, and disability; comorbid substance abuse must also be considered among this population [18].

The nature and intensity of the pain are not explained by a current or previous gastrointestinal diagnosis. NBS should be distinguished from opioid-induced bowel disorder, which results from the effects of opioids on gastrointestinal motility and secretion [18]. NBS can occur in patients with no prior gastrointestinal disorder who receive high dosages of narcotics after surgery or acute painful problems, and among patients with functional gastrointestinal disorders or other chronic gastrointestinal diseases who are managed by physicians who are unaware of the hyperalgesic effects of chronic opioids [17].

By contrast, the mechanisms of NBS are probably centrally mediated and include glial cell activation, bimodal opioid modulation in the dorsal horn, descending facilitation of pain, and the glutaminergic system [18]. The evidence for the enhanced pain perception is based on the following: (1) activation of excitatory anti-analgesic pathways within a bimodal opioid regulation system, (2) descending facilitation of pain at the rostral ventral medulla and pain facilitation via dynorphin and cholecystokinin activation, and (3) glial cell activation that produces morphine tolerance and enhances opioid-induced pain [17].

The syndrome is underrecognized and may be becoming more prevalent [17]. This may be the result of increases in using narcotics for chronic non-malignant painful disorders and the development of maladaptive therapeutic interactions around its use [17].

Characterized by incompletely controlled AP despite continued or increasing doses of opioids, NBS is estimated to occur in 4.2–6.4% of patients chronically taking opioids [18].

A trial of opioid detoxification resulted in complete detoxification for the vast majority of patients with reduction in pain symptoms [17]. However, despite improvement in pain, approximately half of patients returned to opioid use within 3 months [17]. Improved strategies are needed to identify patients who will respond to detoxification and remain off opioids [17]. Comorbid psychiatric and substance abuse disorders are barriers to durable response after detoxification and should be actively sought out and treated accordingly [17].

An effective patient-physician relationship is essential [17]. Treatment involves early recognition of the syndrome, an effective physician-patient relationship, graded withdrawal of the narcotic according to a specified withdrawal program, and the institution of medications to reduce withdrawal effects [18].

24.4.5 Chronic Gastroenteritis

Causes of chronic gastroenteritis include Crohn's disease, autoimmune diseases, sarcoidosis, allergies, and viruses in the patients with weakened immune systems. When acute gastritis is chronic, diagnosing and treating the underlying cause can help.

24.4.6 *Chronic Pancreatitis*

Chronic pancreatitis, which is inflammation of the pancreas, can cause upper AP [19]. Chronic pancreatitis is an irreversible fibroinflammatory disorder of the pancreas [20]. Genetic predisposition and repeated injury may be necessary for chronic pancreatitis [3].

Chronic pancreatitis presents with relapsing, remitting upper AP accompanied by features of malabsorption due to pancreatic exocrine insufficiency, and endocrine deficiency with the development of diabetes mellitus [20]. The associated increased hospitalization and high economic burden are related to chronic pancreatitis often presenting at advanced stage with irreversible consequences [20]. Diagnosing chronic pancreatitis at an early stage is still challenging and therefore chronic pancreatitis is believed to be under-reported [20].

Conservative management was feasible and effective in most patients with chronic pancreatitis [19]. Better recognition of the risk factors and conditions associated with chronic pancreatitis can lead to an earlier diagnosis and coupled with a multidisciplinary approach to treatment, ultimately reduce complications [20].

24.4.7 *Cancer Pain*

Pain can be encountered throughout every step of cancer treatment [21]. Opioids are the mainstay of cancer pain treatment [21]. However, a new group of therapeutics called coanalgesic drugs has been introduced to pain treatment [21]. These coanalgesics include gabapentinoids such as gabapentin, pregabalin, anti-depressants such as tricyclic anti-depressants, duloxetine, and venlafaxine, corticosteroids, bisphosphonates, N-methyl-D-aspartate antagonists, and cannabinoids [21].

24.5 Children

Many children report chronic AP that is severe and disruptive to normal lifestyle and schooling [22]. Assessment and management depend on identifying those with underlying organic disease, such as chronic infection, celiac disease, or inflammatory bowel disease, but avoiding unnecessary invasive investigations [22]. In those with a functional gut disorder, the aim of therapy is reassurance, a return to normal activity, and symptom control [22]. The recurrent AP is likely to be a functional disorder [22]. Psychological interventions such as cognitive behavioral and family therapy are effective, reducing symptoms and improving school attendance [22].

24.6 Nerve Block

The sympathetic nerve blocks are useful in many ways for relief of chronic pain.

24.6.1 Celiac Plexus Block (CPB)

Chronic upper AP occurs as a complication of various malignant and benign diseases including pancreatic cancer and chronic pancreatitis, and when present may contribute to lower quality of life and higher mortality [23]. Pain originating in upper abdominal viscera is transmitted through the celiac plexus, which is an autonomic plexus located in the retroperitoneum at the root of the celiac trunk [23]. Celiac ganglia play a major role in pain management for upper abdominal disorders, particularly chronic pancreatitis and pancreatic cancer [24].

Direct intervention at the level of the plexus, referred to as celiac plexus block (CPB) or neurolysis depending on the injectate, is a minimally invasive therapeutic strategy which has been demonstrated to decrease pain, improve function, and reduce opiate dependence [23]. CPB is indicated in pain due to intra-abdominal cancer, stemming from organs innervated by coeliac plexus.

Indications for CPB are acute pancreatitis, pancreatic cancer, and cancer pain from upper abdominal viscera [25]. The use of CPB to relieve intractable pain owing to upper abdominal malignancy is well established [26]. CPB and neurolysis are safe and effective treatments for chronic upper AP and should be considered early in patients experiencing such symptoms [23].CPB is also a treatment option to compliment splanchnicectomy in pain management [24].

Various percutaneous techniques have been reported that with appropriate preprocedural planning, use of image guidance by CT, and post-procedural care, the frequency and severity of complications are low and the success rate is high regardless of approach [23]. Endoscopic ultrasonography-guided celiac injection and percutaneous methods of CPB have been heavily studied and are two important methods used today [24].

The consecutive neurolytic CPB technique can provide analgesia and the alleviation of the secondary undesirable effects of analgesic drugs resulting from the decrease of morphine consumption in patients with upper abdominal terminal visceral cancer, mostly pancreatic cancer [27]. The main benefit of the intervention may be in reduced opiate dependence and opiate-associated side effects, which in turn improves quality of life [23]. Significant relief of pain is reported in 70–90% of patients, allowing a reduction in opioid use and in the occurrence of opioid-related side effects [26].

The reliability of its analgesic effect of CPB is high [27]. Duration of relief varies, but the majority of patients experience relatively pain-free deaths [26]. CPB is a relatively safe procedure, and although it is associated with common adverse effects such as diarrhea, hypotension, and local pain, these are mostly transient [26]. However, severe complications, including paraplegia, have been reported [26].

24.6.2 Splanchnic Nerve Block (SNB)

The thoracic splanchnic nerves play a major role in pain management for upper abdominal disorders, particularly chronic pancreatitis and pancreatic cancer [24]. Splanchnic nerve dissection and thermocoagulation are two common derivatives of splanchnicectomy that are commonly used today [24]. Splanchnic nerve block (SNB) via a transdiscal approach guided by CT is a technique that provides analgesia and the alleviation of the secondary undesirable effects of analgesic drugs resulting from the decrease of morphine consumption in patients with unresectable upper abdominal or lower esophageal neoplasms [28]. The reliability of its analgesic effect of SNB is high, with a low rate of severe complications.

24.7 Team Approach

By using a team approach, seamless care to help the patients get relief is delivered [29]. The treatments may include relaxation techniques, behavioral therapies, medical nutrition therapy, pain management, stress management, and alternative therapies, such as acupuncture. Special techniques including breathing exercises that the patients can perform on their own at home can help their abdominal muscles relax. Cognitive-behavioral therapy and psychotherapy can help reduce their anxiety. Therefore, the patients can focus on other things besides their pain. Working with experts from gastrointestinal nutrition services who specialize in gastrointestinal disorders, the patients are helped to find foods that are less likely to upset their stomach. By offering innovative approaches, experts at gastricintestine pain clinic address the source of the patient's pain. To provide the best treatment for cancer patients, cooperation of anesthesiologists with oncologists and surgeons becomes imperative [29]. It has been established that anesthetic techniques and drugs could minimize the perioperative inflammation.

References

1. Thompson MB, Ramirez JC, De La Rosa LM, Wood AS, Desai S, Arjunan A, Song J, Erickson RA. Endoscopic ultrasound in the evaluation of chronic upper abdominal pain of unknown etiology: a retrospective chart review examining the efficacy of EUS in determining a new diagnosis. J Clin Gastroenterol. 2015;49(2):e17–20. https://doi.org/10.1097/MCG.0000000000000174.
2. Ersumo T. Gallstone disease in a teaching hospital, Addis Ababa: a 5-year review. Ethiop Med J. 2006;44(1):49–59.
3. Walling A, Freelove R. Pancreatitis and pancreatic cancer. Prim Care. 2017;44(4):609–20. https://doi.org/10.1016/j.pop.2017.07.004.
4. Camilleri M. Management of patients with chronic abdominal pain in clinical practice. Neurogastroenterol Motil. 2006;18(7):499–506.

5. McGarrity TJ, Peters DJ, Thompson C, McGarrity SJ. Outcome of patients with chronic abdominal pain referred to chronic pain clinic. Am J Gastroenterol. 2000;95(7):1812–6.
6. Navas CM, Patel NK, Lacy BE. Symptomatic management of gastroparesis. Gastrointest Endosc Clin N Am. 2019;29(1):55–70. https://doi.org/10.1016/j.giec.2018.08.005.
7. Camilleri M, Parkman HP, Shafi MA, Abell TL, Gerson L; American College of Gastroenterology. Clinical guideline: management of gastroparesis. Am J Gastroenterol. 2013;108(1):18–37; quiz 38. https://doi.org/10.1038/ajg.2012.373.
8. Stanciu GO. Gastroparesis and its management. Rev Med Chir Soc Med Nat Iasi. 2001;105(3):451–6.
9. Drossman DA. Functional abdominal pain syndrome. Clin Gastroenterol Hepatol. 2004;2(5):353–65.
10. Sperber AD, Drossman DA. Review article: the functional abdominal pain syndrome. Aliment Pharmacol Ther. 2011;33(5):514–24. https://doi.org/10.1111/j.1365-2036.2010.04561.x.
11. Clouse RE, Mayer EA, Aziz Q, Drossman DA, Dumitrascu DL, Mönnikes H, Naliboff BD. Functional abdominal pain syndrome. Gastroenterology. 2006;130(5):1492–7.
12. Hu WH, Talley NJ. Functional (non-ulcer) dyspepsia: unexplained but not unmanageable. Med J Aust. 1998;168(10):507–12.
13. Talley NJ. Non-ulcer dyspepsia: myths and realities. Aliment Pharmacol Ther. 1991;5(Suppl 1):145–62.
14. Wee EW. Evidence-based approach to dyspepsia: from Helicobacter pylori to functional disease. Postgrad Med. 2013;125(4):169–80. https://doi.org/10.3810/pgm.2013.07.2688.
15. Thijs JC, Kleibeuker JH. The management of uninvestigated dyspepsia in primary care. Minerva Gastroenterol Dietol. 2005;51(3):213–24.
16. Talley NJ, Phillips SF. Non-ulcer dyspepsia: potential causes and pathophysiology. Ann Intern Med. 1988;108(6):865–79.
17. Kurlander JE, Drossman DA. Diagnosis and treatment of narcotic bowel syndrome. Nat Rev Gastroenterol Hepatol. 2014;11(7):410–8. https://doi.org/10.1038/nrgastro.2014.53.
18. Grunkemeier DM, Cassara JE, Dalton CB, Drossman DA. The narcotic bowel syndrome: clinical features, pathophysiology, and management. Clin Gastroenterol Hepatol. 2007;5(10):1126–39, quiz 1121–2.
19. Pongprasobchai S, Manatsathit S. Natural course of abdominal pain in chronic pancreatitis with intermittent (type A) pain after conservative treatment. J Med Assoc Thai. 2009;92(Suppl 2):S43–8.
20. Jalal M, Campbell JA, Hopper AD. Practical guide to the management of chronic pancreatitis. Frontline Gastroenterol. 2019;10(3):253–60. https://doi.org/10.1136/flgastro-2018-101071.
21. Esin E, Yalcin S. Neuropathic cancer pain: what we are dealing with? How to manage it? Onco Targets Ther. 2014;7:599–618. https://doi.org/10.2147/OTT.S60995.
22. Bremner AR, Sandhu BK. Recurrent abdominal pain in childhood: the functional element. Indian Pediatr. 2009;46(5):375–9.
23. Cornman-Homonoff J, Holzwanger DJ, Lee KS, Madoff DC, Li D. Celiac plexus block and neurolysis in the management of chronic upper abdominal pain. Semin Intervent Radiol. 2017;34(4):376–86.
24. Loukas M, Klaassen Z, Merbs W, Tubbs RS, Gielecki J, Zurada A. A review of the thoracic splanchnic nerves and celiac ganglia. Clin Anat. 2010;23(5):512–22. https://doi.org/10.1002/ca.20964.
25. Chaturvedi A, Dash HH. Sympathetic blockade for the relief of chronic pain. J Indian Med Assoc. 2001;99(12):698–703.
26. Chambers PC. Coeliac plexus block for upper abdominal cancer pain. Br J Nurs. 2003;12(14):838–44.
27. Yang FR, Wu BS, Lai GH, Wang Q, Yang LQ, He MW, Ni JX. Assessment of consecutive neurolytic celiac plexus block (NCPB) technique outcomes in the management of refractory visceral cancer pain. Pain Med. 2012;13(4):518–21. https://doi.org/10.1111/j.1526-4637.2012.01332.x.

28. Plancarte R, Guajardo-Rosas J, Reyes-Chiquete D, Chejne-Gómez F, Plancarte A, González-Buendía NI, Cerezo-Camacho O, Lee A, Medina-Santillan R. Management of chronic upper abdominal pain in cancer: transdiscal blockade of the splanchnic nerves. Reg Anesth Pain Med. 2010;35(6):500–6. https://doi.org/10.1097/AAP.0b013e3181fa6b42.
29. Gudaitytė J, Dvylys D, Šimeliūnaitė I. Anaesthetic challenges in cancer patients: current therapies and pain management. Acta Med Litu. 2017;24(2):121–7. https://doi.org/10.6001/actamedica.v24i2.3493.

Chapter 25
Central Pain

Marc Korn, Mary Leemputte, and Dost Khan

25.1 Causes of Pain

Central pain can result from a wide variety of CNS pathologies including vascular injury, infection, trauma, neoplasm, or demyelination; however, it most frequently occurs in the setting of stroke, multiple sclerosis, and spinal cord injury.

25.1.1 Stroke

Stroke has been identified as the most common cause of central pain. Each year, approximately 795,000 people experience a new or recurrent stroke [1]. It is estimated that 87% of these strokes are ischemic and 13% are hemorrhagic. While most cases of central poststroke pain (CPSP) occur after ischemic stroke, this may be due to the higher prevalence of ischemic strokes, it is estimated that the risk for CPSP is similar with ischemic and hemorrhagic strokes. Though chronic poststroke pain is seen in 8–14% of patients, it is one of the least recognized stroke related complications [2, 3].

A prospective population based study evaluated 297 stroke patients and identified severe pain in 32% of patients after 4 months and 21% after 16 months. Higher 16 month pain intensity was found to correlate with female sex, worse geriatric depression scale score, better mini-mental status examination score, and increased glycosylated hemoglobin [3].

In general, CPSP typically develops within 6 months of stroke onset. A review of CPSP after thalamic stroke identified that 36% of patients developed pain within

M. Korn · M. Leemputte · D. Khan (✉)
Northwestern University Feinberg School of Medicine, Department of Anesthesiology, Chicago, IL, USA
e-mail: dost.khan@gmail.com

K. Shimoji et al. (eds.), *Chronic Pain Management in General and Hospital Practice*, https://doi.org/10.1007/978-981-15-2933-7_25

1–3 months, 12% between 3 and 6 months, 6% between 6 and 12 months, and 11% after 12 months [4].

With regard to stroke location, thalamic (specifically right sided) and lateral medullary strokes have the highest incidence of CPSP. Dejerine–Roussy Syndrome was described in 1906 to refer specifically to a thalamic pain syndrome which manifests with severe contralateral pain [5]. Thalamic strokes account for 25–33% of all cases of CPSP [6]. Strokes of the lateral medulla impact the spinothalamic and trigeminothalamic tracts, resulting in changes in pain and temperature sensation in the ipsilateral face and contralateral body. The increased prevalence of CPSP from right-sided thalamic lesions may be due to a more prominent role of the right hemisphere with regard to pain processing.

25.1.2 Spinal Cord Injury

Spinal cord injury (SCI) is another common cause of central pain which is typically seen among younger patients (average age of 42 at time of injury). Patients are typically male (80%) with injuries often resulting from motor vehicle accidents, falls, or violent trauma. Annual incidence of SCI is approximately 17,000 new cases per year [7]. Pain related to SCI can be differentiated depending on location. Neuropathic pain below the level of the injury is classified as central pain. Pain which occurs at the level of the injury is classified as peripheral when it involves the nerve root and central when it involves the dorsal horn.

Studies suggest that the prevalence of post-SCI pain is 65–80% [8–10]. Further research suggested that at 12-month follow-up, 31% of patients had post-SCI pain at the level of the injury and 31% had pain below the level of the injury, although below-level pain may take up to 2 years to develop [11].

Musculoskeletal pain is the most commonly reported pain subtype among SCI patients; however, this pain is typically less severe. In a longitudinal study of SCI patients, 59 out of 73 patients (81%) reported pain at 5 years following SCI; 59% reported musculoskeletal pain, 41% at-level (segmental) neuropathic pain, 34% below-level neuropathic pain, and 5% visceral pain [9]. In this same study, patients ranked pain as the third most difficult complication related to their injury (behind decreased mobility and decreased sexual function) [9]. While neuropathic pain occurs less commonly, it is typically severe and results in significant limitations. It appears that SCI-related pain, specifically neuropathic pain, commonly worsens over time [11].

25.1.3 Multiple Sclerosis

Multiple sclerosis (MS) is an autoimmune demyelinating disease which results in brain and spinal cord dysfunction due to plaque accumulation. The disease has several distinct presentations among patients. The most common relapsing-remitting form presents with subacute neurologic deficits which intermittently improve and deteriorate.

Progressive MS manifests as a gradual worsening of neurologic deficit without distinct attacks. Regardless of disease subtype, disability from the disease is progressive and chronic pain is commonly seen with prevalence ranging from 29 to 80% [12, 13].

Several different types of pain are seen in MS patients. Pain, including trigeminal neuralgia and central pain, is one of the original presenting symptoms in some MS patients (5–23%). These patients have been shown to have a higher likelihood of developing chronic pain [14]. The Lhermitte sign, a paroxysmal shooting pain which occurs with neck flexion, is frequently experienced by MS patients. It is often associated with acute or subacute demyelinating plaques in the cervical spine. This hallmark symptom is related to dysfunction of the posterior column. Central neuropathic pain, on the other hand, involves dysfunction of the spinothalamic tract.

Among MS patients, central neuropathic pain is likely to occur in more than one location, depending on the locations of lesions throughout the CNS. Central pain is more common among patients with the relapsing-remitting form of MS. It is also more common among patients with higher degree of disability and longer duration of disease [14].

The pathophysiology of central pain is thought to occur due to changes from irritation and damage of central pain pathways, specifically the spinal-thalamic-cortical pathways. Lesions along this pathway lead to overactivity of the lateral thalamus.

CNS pathology results in denervation, along with sensitization and hyperexcitability of the surviving axons. In CPSP patients, lesions of the lateral thalamus can cause disruption of the GABAergic neurons of the ventral posterolateral thalamic nuclei. Painful sensation can result when input ascends to the cortex via surviving sensory neurons. Abnormal burst activity has been identified within the thalamus and is hypothesized to be a main cause of pain. In SCI, abnormal firing may also be seen, secondary to central sensitization from chronic nociceptive signaling from axons at the level of the injury.

Efficacy of intravenous lidocaine in the setting of SCI and CPSP suggests that central pain may be mediated, in part by sodium channels. MS lesions also result in increased sodium channel production. Excitatory amino acids like N-methyl-D-aspartate may also play an important role in transmission of input to thalamic nuclei [15]. As a result, intravenous ketamine infusions have been shown to reduce pain among these patients. Furthermore, norepinephrine originating from the locus ceruleus and the serotonergic pathway from the dorsal Raphe nuclei may have direct excitatory actions on thalamic nuclei[16]. Finally, a PET study demonstrated a significant decrease in opioid receptor binding among CPSP patients, in the thalamus, insula, anterior cingulate, and secondary sensory cortex. The authors hypothesized that this decrease in binding may be due to an increase in endogenous release, internalization or dysregulation of receptors or neuronal loss [17].

25.2 Signs and Symptoms

Patient with central pain may experience spontaneous or evoked symptoms. In the setting of spontaneous pain, symptoms can be continuous or paroxysmal. With regard to evoked pain, symptoms may be precipitated by nociceptive or non-nociceptive stimuli. Regarding the quality of the pain, patients often complain of aching, burning, lacerating, shooting, squeezing, and throbbing. Stimuli including touch, temperature, stress, or movement can all exacerbate the pain. Patients often experience allodynia, hyperalgesia, and dysesthesia.

Among CPSP, two-thirds of patients have impaired pinprick, temperature and touch sensation. Vibration and proprioceptive impairment are less common. Pain most commonly occurs in the arms, presenting less frequently in the leg, trunk, or face. Other neurologic deficits, including hemiparesis, ataxia, and choreoathetosis, may be present in up to 60% of patients [2]. Pain usually occurs contralateral to the stroke, although delayed ipsilateral symptoms have been seen [18]. Among patients with lateral medullary strokes, CPSP may be accompanied by hoarseness, dysphagia, ipsilateral Horner syndrome, and vestibular symptoms. These patients will often present with symptoms of the ipsilateral face and contralateral body [19].

25.3 Diagnosis

The diagnosis of central neuropathic pain should be considered in those patients with a known history of stroke, multiple sclerosis, and spinal cord injury. In particular, patients may note unusual cold, burning, tingling, pins-and-needles, stabbing, squeezing, shooting, and lancinating discomfort.

Neuropathic pain questionnaires have been developed and established in the screening of patients with such symptoms, including the Neuropathic Pain Questionnaire and Leeds Assessment of Neuropathic Symptoms and Signs. These tools exhibit sensitivities between 70 and 80% and attempt to evaluate patients based on both sensory descriptors and functional status. Patients with neuropathic pain may classically exhibit allodynia as well as hyperalgesia. Though affecting only 15–50% of patients with neuropathic symptoms, these findings are specific for a neuropathic etiology.

However, this approach is helpful only in diagnosing neuropathic pain in general. Because symptoms may overlap, it is important to differentiate central neuropathic pain from peripheral neuropathies as both etiology and treatment options may differ. To diagnose central neuropathic pain, symptoms must be consistent with the area of CNS injury. Because central neuropathic pain results from spinothalamic tract dysfunction, patients must also experience explicit sensory deficits. To do this, the clinician can assess pinprick and temperature alteration with everyday office instruments, including microfilaments and thermorollers. Differentiating this from generalized sensory deficits experienced after a T8 spinal cord injury, for example, can be especially difficult even for the most-skilled clinicians.

The process of determining an accurate diagnosis is complicated by the medley of concurrent pain conditions reported in patients who have experienced CNS insult. Those who have suffered stroke, spinal cord injury, or have been diagnosed with multiple sclerosis may experience symptoms which may closely mimic central neuropathic pain. These include musculoskeletal disorders, spasticity, as well as central sensitization following chronic pain.

Similarly, musculoskeletal disorders are also common in this patient population and may also present with burning pain in the affected extremity. This is especially common as these patients may suffer with immobility and chronic disuse of their extremities.

Spasticity resulting from CNS injury presents as a stiff resistance to movement in the affected limb. Pain may naturally ensue. Central neuropathic pain may similarly present with painful stiffness but necessitates disturbances in sensory processing as well. Thus, spasticity may be identified in a patient with tight, burning pain, and stiffness in a unilateral upper extremity after CVA, especially if physical examination indicates increased tone with rapid passive movement. However, to meet the definition of central neuropathic pain, the patient would need to demonstrate concurrent sensory and thermal alterations.

It is important to further differentiate central neuropathic pain from central sensitization. In the latter, peripheral nerve injury results in chronic afferent signaling. This repetitive nerve activity results in an upregulation of central nociceptive pathways, causing symptoms of allodynia and hyperalgesia. Symptoms may overlap considerably, and those patients with CNS injury may simultaneously endure peripheral neuropathies. Chronic lower extremity immobility, for example, may facilitate nerve compression as well as overuse injuries in the upper extremity. Accurate diagnosis thus requires detailed understanding of the patient's medical history, including a thorough analysis of radiographic evidence with CT scans and MRI reports.

25.4 General Treatments

Once a diagnosis of central neuropathic pain has been attained, comprehensive treatment options should be discussed with patients. No one medication or surgical intervention has been shown to treat symptoms exclusively. Appropriate treatment may include managing patient expectations, as full resolution may not be possible, even with multimodal therapy. However, studies have suggested that numerical pain rating scales may offer a measurement of clinical response, as even improvements of two points on a ten point scale may correlate with meaningful change. While clinical trials have been conducted in an attempt to delineate treatment algorithms for peripheral nerve disorders, the applicability of these results to central pain requires extensive extrapolation. This is especially risky as the pathophysiology and clinical course may differ based on the etiologies discussed. Interventions should be tailored to the etiology of the central neuropathic pain, as multiple studies suggest different results when stratifying for CNS insult.

25.4.1 Pharmacotherapy

Patients presenting with spinal cord injury, multiple sclerosis, and post-stroke syndromes alike have often experienced complicated hospital courses requiring numerous medications. With this in mind, a judicious approach to prescribing should be attempted, with the goal of avoiding mindless polypharmacy in patients at risk for psychological, physical, and cognitive complications.

That being said, careful consideration of the literature reveals that multimodal approaches are often required to decrease symptoms. Common treatment regimens often start with those medications well-established in the treatment of peripheral nerve disorders, including the anticonvulsants gabapentin, pregabalin, and lamotrigine. Antiepileptics are thought to decrease neuronal excitability by blocking sodium and calcium channels, by enhancing the inhibitory effects of gamma-aminobutyric acid inhibition and by decreasing the excitatory effects of glutaminergic transmission.

However, comprehensive studies suggest that etiology must be considered when choosing a regimen. For example, for central poststroke pain, studies suggest mixed results for pregabalin and gabapentin, but improvement in symptoms with lamotrigine and amitriptyline. After spinal cord injury, pregabalin and lamotrigine provide consistent improvement. For multiple sclerosis, antiepileptic regimens demonstrate mixed results.

Antidepressants have long been used for neuropathic pain. Generally speaking, tricyclic antidepressants have been theorized to modulate the pain response by inhibiting presynaptic uptake of norepinephrine and serotonin, in addition to enhancing N-methyl-D-aspartate receptor and ion channel blockade. They also may play a role in histamine, muscarinic, and opioid receptors. However, more research is required to determine which antidepressants are appropriate in central pain. Duloxetine has been shown to improve symptoms in multiple sclerosis. Many patients with central neuropathic pain experience concomitant mood disorders. Because of the complex interplay between psychiatric state and pain threshold, it is often difficult to parse the clinical effects in this way.

25.4.2 Surgical Interventions

More recently, neuromodulation has become increasingly more established as a possible intervention for patients experiencing refractory symptoms. Central neuropathic pain involves pathologic afferent signaling in addition to decreased inhibitory neuronal output. With this in mind, neuromodulation attempts to restore homeostasis by both blocking nociceptive signaling while stimulating those areas which once provided effective efferent inhibition.

Lesioning describes a group of interventions aimed at interrupting the pathologic afferent input necessary for central neuropathic pain. Historically it has included commissurotomy in which an incision is made which transects spinal cord fibers as they cross the midline. Dorsal root entry zone lesioning involves surgical interruption of spinal cord fibers using radiofrequency. With cordotomy, lesioning is completed at the level of the lateral spinothalamic tract pathways on the side contralateral to the affected painful areas. However, with these procedures, relief may be limited over time as pain often returns over years.

Neuromodulation allows for spinal cord stimulation by implanting electrodes in the epidural space adjacent to the posterior sensory columns of the spinal cord. With motor cortex stimulation, leads are placed parallel to the primary motor cortex. Deep brain stimulation has recently been implicated in the treatment of central neuropathic pain as well. With this, electrodes are used to modulate the supratentorial nuclei thought to regulate central pain signaling. These interventions have been especially effective post-spinal cord injury where leads can be placed adjacent to cervical or thoracic lesions, assuming there has been minimal disruption by mechanical fixation after the injury.

25.5 Case Reports

Multiple case reports of patients with central pain syndromes have been published which help to elucidate the presenting symptoms, diagnostic factors, and treatment options available.

25.5.1 Central Poststroke Pain (CPSP)

A 66-year-old female with a history of ischemic stroke to the bilateral basal ganglia and left thalamus presented with 3 years of severe lancinating pain on the right side of the face and hand. Pain progressed through the dorsum of her fingertips and the entire palmar surface of her hand. She also reported shooting pain on the right side of her face. By the time of presentation, the patient was being treated with amitriptyline, pregabalin, and gabapentin with minimal relief. A standard 0–10 point numerical pain scale was used and the patient consistently reported scores ranging 7–10. On physical examination decreased thermal sensation in the distribution of the right face was noted. Brief pain inventory (BPI) scores indicated that functional status, sleep and everyday activity were significantly impaired as a result. Anxiety and depression scores were likewise elevated. Repeat MRI confirmed findings consistent with ischemic changes in the left thalamus. While the care team discussed both motor cortex stimulation and deep brain stimulation with the patient, these were not possible for economic reasons. A stellate ganglion block was instead performed. The patient subsequently reported 3 days of 0/10 pain and scores of 3–4 for 1 month after the injection. With repeat injections at 1 and 3 months, the patient reported pain scores of 0–2 for 1 year. Amitriptyline was continued.

This case again highlights the importance of establishing a plausible central insult that is anatomically consistent with presenting symptoms. In this case, pain in the lateral hands and face were consistent with the recognized thalamic injury as seen on MRI. This is crucial as symptoms may overlap with other plausible etiologies. In this instance, symptoms closely mimicked trigeminal neuralgia which would have indicated different treatment options. Furthermore, symptoms resulted in impaired functional status and were seen with elevated anxiety/depression scores. Successful intervention resulted in decreased pain scores greater than 2 on a 10-point scale. Although further study is required, and this patient did not receive other interventions like motor cortex or deep brain stimulation, this suggests that stellate ganglion block may result in clinically significant outcomes once accurate diagnosis is made.

25.5.2 Spinal Cord Injury

A 54-year-old female with a history of incomplete T11 spinal cord injury due to electrocution presented with below-level pain described as electric and stabbing. She reported numeric rating scores (NRS) of 8/10. Her symptoms were nightly and constant, thus interfering with sleep on a nightly basis. She experienced moderate to severe pain in response to brushing (allodynia, as diagnosed with microfilament testing), as well as severe sharp pain in response to cold stimuli using thermorollers. The neuropathic pain symptom inventory (NPSI) was used to assess symptom severity and psychosocial impact with the multidimensional pain inventory-SCI version. The patient was started on pregabalin and opioids without relief. The patient was subsequently approved for participation in a clinical trial with plans to receive deep brain stimulation. Bilateral electrode leads were implanted into the anterolateral periaqueductal gray matter (PAG) while awake. One week later, the leads were connected to extension cables and tunneled to a generator. Electrode stimulation during first procedure resulted in near-immediate relief in symptoms. A blinded study was completed while stimulator settings were adjusted. The patient noted the most relief with a low mean pulse rate (0.67 Hz) and setting change required a few days for clinical effects.

This case suggests new indications for deep brain stimulation. While DBS has been successfully utilized in patients with peripheral neuropathies and phantom limb pain, this demonstrates its emerging role in the management of central neuropathic pain from the onset. Because the PAG receives afferent somatosensory input, it is possible that neuromodulation of this area results in improved homeostasis with regard to pain and temperature signaling. While further investigation is clearly required, the PAG receives input from the prefrontal cortex and amygdala, which may begin to explain its role in mood and function. It is important to note that, however, simultaneous medical management is also indicated in mitigating symptoms. In this case, the patient continued to receive pregabalin as well as intermittent opioid therapy.

25.5.3 *Multiple Sclerosis*

A 52-year-old Caucasian female was evaluated for 2 years of chronic left lateral hand pain. A diagnosis of multiple sclerosis had been made 15 years prior. She reported burning in her left index finger, as well as excessive cold in the area of discomfort. Physical examination was significant for allodynia (pain with light touch in the left hand). Known symptoms also included left foot weakness and spasticity. MRI of the cervical spine indicated a demyelinating lesion extending from C2 to C4 which involved the bilateral posterior columns. The rostral area of the lesion also included the left corticospinal and bilateral spinothalamic tracts. At the time of presentation, the patient was on Avonex (interferon beta-1a), pantoprazole, atorvastatin, sertraline, alendronic acid, baclofen, and gabapentin. Initial treatment included four stellate ganglion blocks. Gabapentin and sertraline were adjusted. The patient reportedly did not tolerate opioids. The patient experienced no relief and a spinal cord stimulator was trialed. A single octrode lead was placed left of the dorsal column, centered at C4–C5. It was left in place for 8 days. No relief was noted and the lead was removed. Acupuncture and physical therapy were attempted with little mitigation in symptoms. Pain was noted to affect her functional status and reported quality of life. A second trial, SCS trial was conducted in which the patient received one octrode in the lateral recess of the epidural space centered at C6–C7 with a second octrode medially adjacent. Because she noted analgesia with the leads in place and after removal, a permanent SCS was placed in the same location 1 month later. At follow-up the patient continued to report significant improvement in pain as quantified with BPI (brief pain inventory) scores.

This case highlights the importance of relating symptoms to the anatomic area of CNS injury. Here, there was radiologic evidence of spinothalamic involvement consistent with lateral hand discomfort. It also highlights the importance of differentiating central pain symptoms from other exam findings, including spasticity and weakness. Functionally-limited symptoms were present. Resolution of symptoms with lateral lead placement suggests that SCS assisted in normalizing afferent input to rostral CNS areas responsible for central pain.

25.6 Summary

Neuropathic pain of the peripheral nervous system is commonly encountered by clinicians, although diseases of the central nervous system can give rise to central pain. With a number of common neurologic conditions giving rise to this chronic pain syndrome, it is imperative that clinicians recognize common manifestations of the condition and respond with appropriate treatment strategies.

References

1. Benjamin EJ, Blaha MJ, Chiuve SE, Cushman M, Das SR, Deo R, de Ferranti SD, Floyd J, Fornage M, Gillespie C, Isasi CR, Jiménez MC, Jordan LC, Judd SE, Lackland D, Lichtman JH, Lisabeth L, Liu S, Longenecker CT, Mackey RH, Matsushita K, Mozaffarian D, Mussolino ME, Nasir K, Neumar RW, Palaniappan L, Pandey DK, Thiagarajan RR, Reeves MJ, Ritchey M, Rodriguez CJ, Roth GA, Rosamond WD, Sasson C, Towfighi A, Tsao CW, Turner MB, Virani SS, Voeks JH, Willey JZ, Wilkins JT, Wu JH, Alger HM, Wong SS, Muntner P, American Heart Association Statistics Committee and Stroke Statistics Subcommittee. Heart disease and stroke statistics-2017 update: a report from the American Heart Association. Circulation. 2017;135(10):e146–603. https://doi.org/10.1161/CIR.0000000000000485.
2. Kumar B, Kalita J, Kumar G, Misra UK. Central poststroke pain: a review of pathophysiology and treatment. Anesth Analg. 2009;108(5):1645–57.
3. Jonsson AC, Lindgren I, Hallstrom B, Norrving B, Lindgren A. Prevalence and intensity of pain after stroke: a population based study focusing on patients' perspectives. J Neurol Neurosurg Psychiatry. 2006;77:590–5.
4. Nasreddine ZS, Saver JL. Pain after thalamic stroke: right diencephalic predominance and clinical features in 180 patients. Neurology. 1997;48:1196–9.
5. Dejerine J, Roussy G. Le syndrome thalamique. Rev Neurol. 1906;12:521–32.
6. Andersen G, Vesteraard K, Ingeman-Nielsen M, Jensen TS. Incidence of central post-stroke pain. Pain. 1995;61(2):187–93.
7. National Spinal Cord Injury Statistical Center. Spinal cord injury (SCI) facts and figures at a glance. University of Alabama at Birmingham website, 2016. https://www.nscisc.uab.edu/Public/Facts%202016.pdf
8. Levi R, Hultling C, Nash MS, Seiger A. The Stockholm spinal cord injury study: 1. Medical problems in a regional SCI population. Paraplegia. 1995;33(6):308–15.
9. Siddall PJ, McClelland JM, Rutkowski SB, Cousins MJ. A longitudinal study of the prevalence and characteristics of pain in the first 5 years following spinal cord injury. Pain. 2003;103(3):249–57.
10. Rintala DH, Loubser PG, Castro J, Hart KA, Fuhrer MJ. Chronic pain in a community-based sample of men with spinal cord injury: prevalence, severity, and relationship with impairment, disability, handicap, and subjective Well-being. Arch Phys Med Rehabil. 1998;79(6):604–14.
11. Finnerup NB, Norrbrink C, Trok K, et al. Phenotypes and predictors of pain following traumatic spinal cord injury: a prospective study. J Pain. 2014;15(1):40–8.
12. Clifford DB, Trotter JL. Pain in multiple sclerosis. Arch Neurol. 1984;41(12):1270–2.
13. Svendsen KB, Jensen TS, Overvad K, Hansen HJ, Koch-Henriksen N, Bach FW. Pain in patients with multiple sclerosis: a population-based study. Arch Neurol. 2003;60(8):1089–94.
14. O'Connor AB, Schwid SR, Herrmann DN, Markman JD, Dworkin RH. Pain associated with multiple sclerosis: a systematic review and proposed classification. Pain. 2008;137(1):96–111.
15. McLean DE. Medical complications experienced by a cohort of stroke survivors during inpatient, tertiary-level stroke rehabilitation. Arch Phys Med Rehabil. 2004;85:466–9.
16. McCormick DA, Wang Z. Serotonin and noradrenaline excite GABAergic neurones of the guinea-pig and cat nucleus reticularis thalami. J Physiol. 1991;442:235–55.
17. Sprenger T, Berthele A, Platzer S, Boecker H, Tolle TR. What to learn from in vivo opioidergic brain imaging. Eur J Pain. 2005;9:117–21.
18. Kim JS. Delayed-onset ipsilateral sensory symptoms in patients with central poststroke pain. Eur Neurol. 1998;40:201–6.
19. Fitzek S, Baumgärtner U, Fitzek C, et al. Mechanisms and predictors of chronic facial pain in lateral medullary infarction. Ann Neurol. 2001;49(4):493–500.

Further Reading

Bennett M. The LANSS pain scale: the Leeds assessment of neuropathic symptoms and signs. Pain. 2003;19(5):306–214.

Benzon HT, et al. Central pain states. In: Essentials of pain medicine: Elsevier; 2018. p. 370–7.

Burkey A, Abla-Yao S. Successful treatment of central pain in a multiple sclerosis patient with epidural stimulation of the dorsal root entry zone. Pain Med. 2010;11(1):127–32.

Denkers MR, Biagi HL, O'Brien AM, Jadad AR, Gauld ME. Dorsal root entry zone lesioning used to treat central neuropathic pain in patients with traumatic spinal cord injury: a systematic review. Spine. 2002;27(7):177–84.

Farrar JT, Young JP Jr, LaMoreaux L, Werth JL, Poole RM. Clinical importance of changes in chronic pain intensity measured on an 11-point numerical pain rating scale. Pain. 2001;94(2):149–58.

Jensen TS, Finnerup NB. Allodynia and hyperalgesia in neuropathic pain: clinical manifestations and mechanisms. Lancet Neurol. 2014;13(9):924–35.

Jermakowicz W, Hentall I, Jagid J, Luca C, Adcock J, Martinez-Arizala A, Winerstrom-Noga E. Deep brain stimulation improves the symptoms and sensory signs of persistent central neuropathic pain from spinal cord injury: a case report. Front Hum Neurosci. 2017;11:177.

Krause SJ, Backonja MM. Development and preliminary validation of a pain measure specific to neuropathic pain: the neuropathic pain scale. Neurology. 1997;48(2):332–8.

Lee S, Zhao X, Hatch M, Chun S, Chang E. Central neuropathic pain in spinal cord injury. Crit Rev Phys Rehabil Med. 2013;25(3–4):159–72.

Liao C, Yang M, Liu P, Zong W, Zhang W. Thalamic pain alleviated by stellate ganglion block: a case report. Medicine. 2017;96(5):e6058.

Sindrup SH, Otto M, Finnerup NM, Jensen TS. Antidepressants in the treatment of neuropathic pain. Basic Clin Pharmacol Toxicol. 2005;96(6):399–409.

Watson JC, et al. Central neuropathic pain syndromes. Mayo Clin Proc. 2016;91(3):372–85.

Chapter 26
Management of Cancer Pain in Primary, Secondary, and Palliative Care

Emma Whitehouse and Nick Dando

26.1 Management of Cancer Pain Primary Care

Cancer is one of the most feared diseases in the UK, and for one in ten people receiving a cancer diagnosis is their biggest fear of all [1]. Pain is the most frequent complication of cancer [2]. Approximately a third of patients diagnosed with cancer report pain. This increases to 75–90% when the cancer becomes more advanced [3]. Patients often fear pain as a result of their cancer diagnosis, and it is often perceived as a sign that the cancer is becoming more advanced or more serious [4]. Pain results in a reduction in quality of life [5] and an increase in contact with health care professionals [6].

Unfortunately the management of cancer pain is frequently suboptimal despite a multitude of treatment options [7]. Results from the National Survey of Bereaved People in 2014 identified that 10% of people who died with cancer in 2014 had spent the last 48 h of their lives without adequate pain relief [8]. One-third of calls to out-of-hours (OOH) GP services in patients with a cancer diagnosis are about inadequate pain relief [9].

E. Whitehouse
Dr Lothe and Partners, Camberley, UK

N. Dando (✉)
Phyllis Tuckwell Hospice Care, Farnham, UK

University of Surrey, Surrey, UK
e-mail: Nick.Dando@pth.org.uk

K. Shimoji et al. (eds.), *Chronic Pain Management in General and Hospital Practice*, https://doi.org/10.1007/978-981-15-2933-7_26

26.1.1 Holistic, Whole-Person Assessment

When assessing pain in patients with cancer a holistic, whole person, or 'total pain' approach is required, incorporating the physical, psychological, spiritual, and emotional aspects of their pain. This approach is now widely adopted worldwide in community, acute hospital, and palliative care settings. It is important to ensure that, as much as is practicable, the setting allows for good open dialogue between the health care professional and the patient and their family or caregivers. Allowing sufficient time and privacy for open communication will aid planning and instil trust.

It is vital that both the patient and the family or carer(s) are asked about pain early in their disease trajectory and can express their thoughts, fears, and concerns. A good encounter with a health care professional can improve patient concordance with therapy and allows better adjustment to diagnosis [10].

Reassessment of their pain should be on a regular basis, as guided by the patient's symptom burden, response to treatment, and carer need. This should be documented and shared across the multidisciplinary team involved in the patient's care, subject to their approval for information sharing. In a community setting healthcare professionals should undertake an assessment of pain at each encounter. In an acute hospital or hospice setting, a pain assessment should be done on admission followed by daily reassessment [11]. An inadequate pain assessment and lack of documentation about pain are considered to be some of the greatest barriers to achieving effective pain relief [12]. Patients and their carers should be advised that most of the time pain can be controlled adequately with medication, minimising side effects and allaying their fears.

Key Summary Points: Holistic, Whole Pain Assessment

- Involve patient and their carers/family—exploring thoughts, fears, and concerns
- Allow sufficient time
- Acute/hospice—assess on admission and reassess daily
- Community—assess on each encounter
- Incorporate physical, psychological, emotional, and spiritual aspects
- Record and share patient's notes (subject to consent)

26.1.1.1 Detailed Assessment

As with the assessment of any pain, health care professionals should undertake a detailed multidimensional history (See Text Box 26.1) followed by relevant physical examination. Some of the pain the patient may be experiencing may not be related to their underlying cancer diagnosis. The resultant identification of the nature(s) of a patient's pain will guide management options: pharmacological and/or non-pharmacological, involving a multidisciplinary team approach where appropriate. Patient diaries are very useful in aiding these conversations, improving patient self-care and symptom reporting, but often need some guidance from healthcare professionals on initial introduction [13]. Example diaries are available online including Macmillan [14] and American Cancer Society [15], and these include brief guidance for patients on how to complete the pain diaries.

Box 26.1: Assessment of Pain—Adapted from SIGN Guideline 106 [16] and British Pain Society Guidelines [17]

- *Description of pain*
  - Site and number of pains
  - Intensity/severity of pains (consider using a pain tool)
  - Radiation of pain
  - Timing of pain
  - Quality of pain
  - Aggravating and relieving factors
- *Aetiology of pain*
  - pain caused by cancer
  - pain caused by treatment
  - pain associated with cancer-related debility (e.g., decubitus ulcers, dressing change)
  - pain unrelated to cancer or treatment
- *Breakthrough pain*—transitory flare of moderate-severe pain on background of stable chronic pain
  - predictable (incident), e.g., on movement
  - unpredictable (spontaneous)
- *Type of pain*
  - nociceptive
  - visceral
  - neuropathic
  - complex regional pain syndrome
  - mixed
- *Analgesic drug history*
  - Benefits
  - Side effects of medication, e.g., nausea, constipation, etc.
- *Impact of pain*
  - On function
  - On activities of daily living

  - On quality of life
  - On psychological well-being
    - assessment for clinically significant psychological disorder, e.g., anxiety and/or depression
- *Beliefs*
  - Meaning of pain
  - Effectiveness of its treatments
  - Consequences of drug therapies

Pain assessment tools are useful adjuncts to a detailed history taking; however, many different tools are used worldwide and there is no universally accepted tool. Cross-comparison between studies is then difficult and explains the varied outcomes of reported poor pain control in patients with cancer from 16% to 91% depending on the study and the pain tool used [18]. The European Association of Palliative Care recommends the use of standardised pain assessment tools in palliative care including visual analogue scales (VAS), numerical rating scales (NRS), and verbal rating scales (VRS) [19]. These tools are also valid for use in patients who are cognitively impaired, very frail, or in the dying phase.

26.1.1.2 Spirituality

Multiple studies and reports worldwide have assessed the impact of a cancer diagnosis on a patient, in the context of their belief system (including religion or faith) and how they and their families come to terms with a life-threatening illness, how it impacts on how they see themselves, their experiences, and their place in the world. Some studies have identified that psychological and social pains were worse than physical pains [20]. A report from Macmillan in 2017 identified that 23% of patients immediately thought that their cancer diagnosis meant their life was over; however, 85% reported that they did not want their cancer diagnosis to define them [21].

Acknowledging and exploring the impact of their cancer diagnosis on an individual's belief system needs to be part of the holistic or 'total pain' approach to cancer pain management. One tool to assess spirituality is HOPE. It identifies H: sources of hope, meaning, comfort, strength, peace, love, and connection, O: organised religion, P: personal spirituality and practices, E: effects on medical care and end-of-life care [22].

26.1.1.3 Psychosocial

The role of psychological factors in pain perception and an individual's response, both behaviourally and emotionally, is well documented for non-malignant pain [23]. This applies to cancer pain with an additional psychological component of what pain may indicate with regard to their disease progression, or beliefs around the use of strong opioids in advanced disease. Assessing patients for anxiety and depression is vital to management of their pain because the presence of these mental health conditions can alter their emotional and behavioural response to their pain, as well as the symptoms being masked by some aspects of their pain or side effects of their pain treatment [24, 25].

26.1.2 Principles of Pain Management

26.1.2.1 WHO Cancer Pain Ladder for Adults

This underpins the initial starting point of pharmacological management of adults with cancer pain. As shown in Fig. 26.1 it is a three-step process whereby patients are administered orally non-opioids (paracetamol, aspirin) followed by mild opioids (codeine, dihydrocodeine, tramadol), followed by strong opioids (morphine, oxycodone) until the patient has achieved a pain-free state. Other drugs, adjuvants, may be used alongside this, e.g., for neuropathic pain, etc.

If this approach is used 'by the clock', i.e., every 3–6 h rather than as required, then it is 80–90% effective at producing pain relief and is also inexpensive [26].

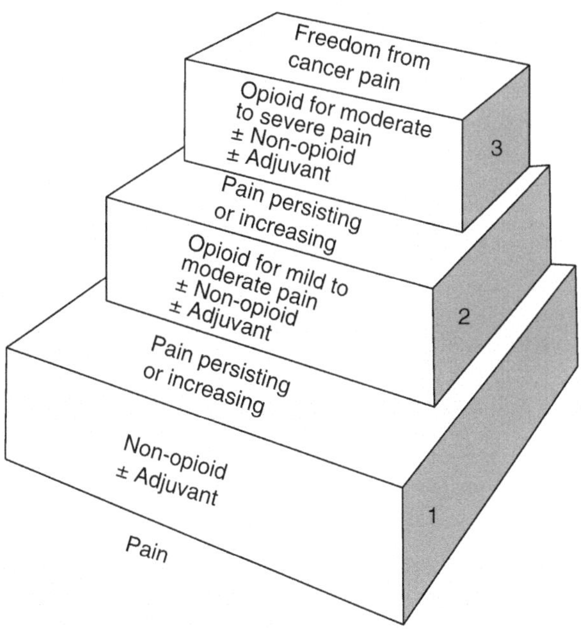

Fig. 26.1 WHO Cancer Pain ladder for adults [26]

Effective use of the pain ladder is based on a good initiation plan followed by regular reassessment of the patient both in terms of response to each stage and to side effects. Patients and their carers should have the rationale for regular therapy explained and breakthrough pain relief should also be provided.

26.1.2.2 Non-Steroidal Anti-Inflammatory Drugs (NSAIDs)

NSAIDs are used alongside the WHO analgesic ladder and are very effective in reducing pain related to inflammation and pain related to bony metastases [27]. These can be used orally and topically and no one specific agent has been shown to be superior to others. Awareness of, and assessment for, gastrointestinal and renal side effects must be followed, and management changed accordingly.

Key Summary Points: Oral Analgesic Control (Based on WHO Analgesic Ladder) [26, 28–30]

Step 1—Mild pain: Non-opioid +/− adjuvant

Drug choices paracetamol 1 g qds (max eight tablets in 24 h); NSAIDS

Step 2—Moderate pain: Weak opioid +/− non-opioid +/− adjuvant

Drug choices codeine 15–30 mg QDS (max 240 mg in 24 h); dihydrocodeine (max 240 mg in 24 h); tramadol (max dose 400 mg in 24 h)

Step 3—Moderate-severe pain: Opioids +/− non-opioid +/− adjuvant

Drug choices Oral: first line morphine; second line oxycodone

Subcutaneous: first line morphine/diamorphine; second line oxycodone.

Always consider prescribing an anti-emetic +/− laxative alongside step 2 and 3 and consider need for gastroprotection alongside NSAIDs. Warn patients about drowsiness when taking step 2 and 3 opioids.

Review regularly. Transdermal routes can be considered when pain is stable.

Subcutaneous routes can be used when oral routes are no longer an option.

Key Summary Point: Initiation of Step 3: Strong Opioids [28–30]

- Stop weak opioid
- Start oral morphine (first line strong opioid)
  - Immediate-release morphine: 2.5–5 mg every 4 h OR
  - Sustained-release morphine: total daily dose of 20 mg of oral morphine, e.g., 10 mg oral sustained-release morphine twice daily
- Breakthrough pain relief must also be prescribed at 1/6th of the total daily amount, e.g., 15 mg twice daily = 30 mg so breakthrough dose = 1/6th of 30 mg, i.e., 5 mg oral immediate-release morphine

- Review regularly to up-titrate the total daily amount balancing adequate pain control with side effects
- If patients have moderate or severe renal or hepatic impairment seek specialist palliative care advice
- If oral morphine is not tolerated or has adverse effects consider oxycodone as second line
  - Twice as potent as oral morphine, i.e., 40 mg oral morphine = 20 mg oral oxycodone

26.1.2.3 Transdermal Weak Opioids

Buprenorphine patches are useful in patients with stable pain; however, they should not be used first line unless oral options are not suitable [28, 29]. They are generally safe in renal impairment because it does not accumulate. Caution should be taken in patients with severe hepatic impairment because it is metabolised via the liver. Patches should be prescribed at the lowest acquisition cost [28, 29] and changed as per the BNF. This may vary from every 7 days to every 96 h depending on the dose and rotation of application sites is needed [31].

Key Summary Points: Initiation of Subcutaneous Opioids [17, 20, 28–30]

- Use when oral route is no longer an option
- Use morphine sulphate or diamorphine first line (depending on local preferences and doses needed. Diamorphine is highly soluble, so smaller volumes are needed to achieve higher doses)
- If patient is opioid naïve:
  - 10 mg morphine sulphate (10 mg/ml) over 24 h via CSCI
  - Breakthrough dose = 2.5 mg morphine sulphate (10 mg/ml) 2 hourly or as required
- OR convert oral opioid dose
  - Total oral morphine dose in 24 h: total morphine sulphate CSCI dose in 24 h = 2:1, e.g., 60 mg oral morphine = 30 mg CSCI morphine sulphate (10 mg/ml)

    Breakthrough dose = 5 mg morphine sulphate (10 mg/ml) 2 hourly or as required
  - Total oral morphine dose in 24 h: total diamorphine CSCI dose in 24 h = 3:1, e.g., 90 mg oral morphine = 30 mg CSCI diamorphine

    Breakthrough dose = 5 mg diamorphine 2 hourly or as required

26.1.2.4 Subcutaneous Administration

Consider subcutaneous opioids when oral options are no longer available [28, 29]. These can be provided as required or via continuous subcutaneous infusion (CSCI) via syringe driver.

26.1.2.5 Complementary Therapies

Evidence of most complementary therapies is limited or only shows short-term benefits. This should not mean that patients should be dissuaded from undertaking these therapies because they may promote short-term improvements in psychological well-being and resultant reductions in 'total pain' [32].

Massage and Aromatherapy

There is no evidence of long-term benefit from these therapies by they may confer short-term benefit and improve psychological well-being. [33–35].

Acupuncture

A systematic review of the evidence has not identified evidence for this approach [36]. However, one RCT of periauricular acupuncture demonstrated a pain reduction by 36% compared with 2% in the placebo group [37]. Another study did find a reduction in nausea and vomiting related to chemotherapy, which in turn may contribute to pain [38].

Music Therapy

There is mixed evidence for this with some benefit seen in small studies, but no convincing evidence from RCT data [39]. There was evidence of benefit in patients who were post-operative, where a small reduction in pain was seen [40].

Reflexology

There is limited evidence for this. One RCT found a 34% reduction in pain compared with placebo group from reflexology given by partners to their relatives with metastatic cancer pain [41]. The majority of other studies have not demonstrated convincing evidence but an improvement in overall psychological well-being may be noticed.

Reiki

There is limited evidence from one small study which found evidence of a modest reduction in cancer pain when reiki was combined with opioids compared with opioids and rest [42].

Hypnotherapy

There is limited evidence from a few small studies showing some benefit of hypnotherapy [43]. One year-long study found a reduction in pain in patients with metastatic breast cancer [44].

Physiotherapy

Physiotherapy assessment is part of the multidisciplinary approach of patients living with cancer. Physiotherapy can prevent and reduce disability [45]. Treatment consists of guidance on safe exercise levels as well as fascial release, postural correction, and muscle retraining. All of these can improve a patient's psychological and physical well-being, which could result in a reduction in 'total pain'.

Occupational Therapy

Occupational therapy assessment is part of the multidisciplinary approach of cancer pain management. The focus is on the assessment of the impact of the individual's pain on their functional performance in activities of daily living and its effect on quality of life. The interventions would include positioning (provision of appropriate seating and pressure relief); equipment (wheelchairs, dressing, and feeding aids); advice on activities of daily living and coping, and adaptations around the home, e.g., handrails, toilet aids, etc. All are likely to be helpful in the overall management and coping with pain at end of life [46].

Pain Education and Cognitive Behavioural Therapy

Cognitive behavioural therapy (CBT) is a proven intervention in the management of chronic non-malignant pain [23]. There is also some evidence that it can play a role in the management of cancer-related pain by improving quality of life and reducing distress. One large meta-analysis showed improvements in depression, objective physical and social outcomes, and quality of life [47].

Another meta-analysis of patients with breast cancer identified that CBT techniques showed a reduction in distress in two-thirds of the patients and 69% showed an improvement in pain levels. It showed that individual therapy had a better outcome for distress than group formats [48].

26.1.3 Case Example

Mr. AB, an 80-year-old man with metastatic prostate cancer, multiple bony metastases to ribs and spine, alongside lumbar degenerative disease, lives in a warden controlled flat with his wife.

On initial assessment he was identified as having bony pain at the site of the metastases, a generalised chronic ache in his lower back, and pain on rising from his chair and from his bed. He was unsteady on his legs with muscle wasting to his quadriceps and was losing weight. He had specific pain from his facet joints identified on examination. He struggled to get up in the night to pass urine and had a few near falls. He occasionally took a paracetamol or an ibuprofen when he was in pain. He disliked taking medications. He had a normal renal function.

He was started on regular paracetamol and an NSAID with gastrointestinal cover from a proton-pump inhibitor. This provided a modest improvement in his symptoms. He was referred to oncology for consideration of radiotherapy to his bony metastases—this took place but unfortunately failed to make a significant improvement in his symptoms. He was then reassessed, and a trial of a weak opioid was added. He was started on codeine 30 mg four times a day but unfortunately became very constipated and nauseous on this. On further reassessment he was keen to continue with the paracetamol and NSAID but was finding rising from chair and bed the most painful part of his day now. This was impacting on his activities of daily living and his sleep. He was referred to physiotherapy who gave him some chair exercises to strengthen his core and quadriceps. He was seen by occupational therapy and was provided with a bed rail to help him get up from a lying to sitting position and also a rollator frame to help him mobilise around his flat. He was also provided with some urine bottles, so he did not have to get up in the night to pass urine. He was trialled on morphine sulphate liquid for his incident pain related to certain movements. This regimen worked well and improved his function and sleep as a result.

26.2 Management of Cancer Pain in Secondary and Palliative Care

There is significant overlap in the management of cancer pain in primary, secondary, and palliative care phases of a patient's illness. There is no finite point when the model of pain management moves to a palliative approach. There should be a gradual evolution in the approach to symptom management as the patients' phase of illness moves from one focusing on active treatment of disease, to disease modifying anticancer treatment and then to a supportive and palliative approach. Patients may also present in primary and secondary care with advanced metastatic disease at the point of diagnosis and in this scenario, the primary focus of care may be on symptom management above anticancer treatment.

The key principles of cancer pain management in primary care remain central to the assessment and management of cancer pain in the setting of an acute hospital or cancer centre.

In secondary care, detailed assessment of pain should continue alongside active investigation and management of the underlying disease process. Routine investigations undertaken over regular outpatient attendances for anticancer treatment or during an admission will provide essential clinical information alongside history and examination findings. Renal function is important in guiding the choice of opioid analgesia in acute kidney injury secondary to complications including dehydration, sepsis, nephrotoxicity from other medications or obstructive uropathy. Radiological investigations, for example, diagnostic or restaging CT scans, can provide important additional information in interpreting a patient's description of pain in the context of physical examination findings.

Application of this essential diagnostic information, often rapidly available in the hospital setting, to the clinical assessment can help differentiate between different patterns of cancer pain, described as somatic (dull, aching, throbbing), visceral (gnawing, cramping) or neuropathic pain (burning, tingling, shooting). Cancer pain can also be characterised by predictable or unpredictable escalations in pain. Breakthrough pain has been defined as transitory exacerbations of pain that occur on a background of stable pain otherwise adequately controlled by around-the-clock opioid therapy [49, 50]. Breakthrough pain may occur spontaneously or may be described as incident pain which occurs in association with a predictable trigger such as movement or during a dressing change [20]. Understanding the origins of the pain and underlying pathophysiology can then guide the generation of management plans for cancer pain control.

Undergoing cancer treatment or an admission to hospital can be a time of significant uncertainty and fear for the individual and those close to them. Central to the provision of holistic palliative care is the concept of total pain originally described by Dame Cicely Saunders. She identified the complex interplay between physical, psychological, social, and spiritual elements of pain perception and the impact on the overall suffering of the individual [51]. Careful assessment of the patient's insight and emotional needs is also vital in understanding the impact of the physical pain on their ability to understand and manage the pain they are experiencing.

26.2.1 Approaches to Cancer Pain Control in Secondary and Palliative Care Opioids and the WHO Ladder

The principles of the WHO ladder applied in primary care remain a valid approach to the management of cancer pain in hospital and palliative care settings. However, it is also now accepted that opioid analgesia is of benefit to patients with cancer pain whose management has not followed the WHO ladder. A literature review exploring the evidence for use of step 2 opioids identified limited evidence that oral morphine at low doses could be used in opioid naïve cancer patients, resulting in a weak recommendation that patients whose pain is not adequately controlled on step 1 analgesia could be treated with either a regular step 2 opioid (e.g., codeine) or low doses of a step 3 opioid (e.g., morphine) [49]. Further evidence from an open-label, multicentre randomised trial of low dose morphine versus weak opioids (codeine or tramadol with paracetamol or tramadol alone) concluded that low dose morphine provided a more adequate level of control in moderate cancer pain with a reasonable tolerability profile, resulting in a positive impact on well-being [52].

A Cochrane review investigating the role for oral morphine in cancer pain undertaken in 2016 concluded that although the quality of the evidence was limited, oral morphine remains the gold standard for management of moderate to severe cancer pain [53]. NICE Guidelines for use of opioids in palliative care, developed in 2012 and updated in 2014 and 2016, also support the use of oral morphine for cancer pain control. The guidelines identify that titration of oral opioids can be undertaken with both immediate-release and sustained-release formulations and the choice should depend on patient preference [54].

Therefore, initial management of moderate to severe cancer pain in patients whose management is undertaken in secondary or palliative care settings should be with morphine sulphate as either immediate- or sustained-release preparations.

First Line Oral Strong Opioid for Cancer Pain [55]

- Morphine is the first line strong opioid for management of cancer pain.
- Titration to analgesic effect appears to be possible for both immediate-release (IR) and modified release (MR) formulations of oral morphine
- Titration of IR and MR formulations should be supplemented with oral immediate-release opioids as needed (PRN)

26.2.2 Alternative Opioids to Morphine

A Cochrane review of alternative opioids to morphine for the management of cancer pain supported the presence of opioids as the top rung of the WHO ladder but identified that some individual studies suggest that less than 80% of patients with cancer pain have satisfactory pain relief using the WHO ladder. Despite a limited evidence base the authors do, however, conclude that 19 out of 20 patients with moderate or severe cancer who are given and tolerate opioids should have pain reduced to mild or no pain within 14 days [56].

Opioid switching is the term given to the clinical practice of substituting one opioid with another when a satisfactory balance between pain relief and adverse effects is not achieved with appropriate titration of the first opioid [49]. A range of alternative opioids are available and could be considered in patients who do not achieve adequate pain relief with morphine and/or develop unmanageable side effects [49].

Oxycodone is a strong opioid analgesic which may be considered as an alternative first choice opioid for moderate or severe cancer pain [49] and also provides a second line option when considering opioid switching. A Cochrane review exploring the role for oxycodone in management of cancer-related pain concluded that although the quality of the evidence was low, oxycodone offers similar pain relief and adverse effects as other strong opioids including morphine [57].

Transdermal fentanyl is widely used in palliative care and, although the evidence base is limited [58], may be considered as an alternative first line treatment for patients with cancer pain whose analgesia requirements are stable and for whom the oral route is not appropriate [49, 54, 55]. Another potential benefit of the drug is that patients experience less constipation with fentanyl compared to oral morphine [54, 58]. It is recommended that the patient's pain control requirements are stable as the transdermal delivery means that achievement of a pharmacological steady state is slow [49] and does not, therefore, offer effective pain control in rapidly escalating or unstable pain.

Buprenorphine offers another transdermal option for management of cancer pain [49, 55]. Evidence suggests it is effective in cancer pain and neuropathic pain whilst being associated with less analgesic tolerance than some other opioids [59]. A 2016 Cochrane review concluded that there was insufficient evidence to support buprenorphine as a first line choice for cancer pain in comparison to morphine, oxycodone, or fentanyl but suggested that it could be considered as a later option for selected patients [60].

Methadone is a synthetic opioid which may also exert analgesic effect via antagonism of the N-methyl-D-aspartate (NMDA) receptor. There is experience of using methadone for severe cancer pain in the palliative care setting; however, the evidence base is small [61]. The drug has a complex pharmacological profile and there are concerns about the potential for prolongation of the QT interval with associated risk of cardiac arrhythmias. Therefore, methadone may have a role in the management of moderate to severe cancer pain, but careful consideration should be given to the risk of side effects and it should only be used by experienced professionals [49, 61].

Other potential opioid options with limited evidence for management of cancer pain include hydromorphone [62], tapentadol [63], and tramadol [64].

Alternative Strong Opioids for Management of Cancer Pain

- Oxycodone immediate release or modified release may be considered as a first line alternative to morphine or as a second line option
  - Oxycodone is twice as potent as oral morphine and therefore requires dose reduction compared to the oral morphine equivalent at a ratio of 2:1 (morphine to oxycodone) [65]

  - For example, oral morphine sulphate modified release 30 mg twice daily (60 mg in 24 h) is equivalent to oral oxycodone modified release 15 mg twice daily (30 mg in 24 h)
  - The breakthrough dose of oral oxycodone should be 1/6th of the 24 h dose. In this example, the breakthrough dose is therefore 5 mg of oral immediate-release oxycodone
- Transdermal fentanyl may be considered as a first line opioid for patients who do not have the oral route or as a second line option for patients with stable cancer pain. It should be avoided for management of unstable or acute pain
  - The transdermal fentanyl equivalent of oral morphine for patients on stable and well tolerated opioid therapy is 100:1 (fentanyl to morphine) [65, 66]
- Transdermal buprenorphine may be considered for patients whose pain does not respond to other opioid analgesics
  - The approximate transdermal buprenorphine equivalent of oral morphine is 100:1 (buprenorphine to morphine) [65, 66]
- *Please note the above conversions are guidelines and all opioid switches should be undertaken with caution. If opioid switches are undertaken in the context of toxicity, it is recommended that the dose of the new opioid is reduced by 25–50% then the new regimen re-titrated* [65]
- Opioid switches may be complex, and it is recommended that health care professionals also consult local guidelines or seek specialist advice from the palliative care team

26.2.3 Management of Breakthrough Cancer Pain

Episodes of breakthrough cancer pain occurring on the background of around-the-clock opioid analgesia should be treated with additional doses of immediate-release oral opioids [55]. For patients receiving around-the-clock oral morphine the breakthrough dose should be one-sixth of the 24 h around-the-clock morphine dose [20] and there should be appropriate up-titration of the around-the-clock opioid dose in response to uncontrolled background pain.

Predictable incident pain can be managed with oral immediate-release opioids; however, buccal or nasal preparations of trans-mucosal fentanyl offer a possible alternative. The potential advantage of these preparations relates to the more rapid speed of onset of pain relief and shorter duration of effect when compared to oral morphine, allowing anticipatory treatment of predictable pain prior to the event [20, 49]. The availability of a range of trans-mucosal and intranasal products provides good potential to tailor the choice of medication to the preferences of individual patient and the pattern of their incident pain. However, the dose titration can be complicated for some patients and requires upward titration independent of the background around the clock opioid, which should be equivalent to 60 mg of oral morphine. Although updated NICE guidelines [54] do not recommend offering fast acting fentanyl as a first line rescue medication for breakthrough cancer pain, they may offer an important option for selected patients with predictable incident pain on an appropriate dose of around-the-clock opioid.

26.2.4 Subcutaneous Opioid Administration

In addition to oral, transdermal, and trans-mucosal opioid administration, as in primary care, the subcutaneous route is an essential option for management of cancer pain in secondary and hospice care. Continuous subcutaneous infusion (CSCI) should be considered in clinical situations where patients temporarily lose the oral route (e.g., severe nausea or vomiting, head and neck cancer, prior to a procedure requiring the patient to be nil-by-mouth) or who lose the ability to swallow in the context of advanced, progressive disease.

The dose conversions from oral to subcutaneous morphine or diamorphine are the same as outlined for use in primary care; however, additional conversions are required if the patient requires switching to alternative opioids.

Example of a Conversion from Oral Morphine Sulphate to Subcutaneous Oxycodone

Step 1

- 60 mg oral morphine sulphate modified release twice daily (120 mg orally in 24 h) is equivalent to 30 mg oral oxycodone modified release twice daily (60 mg orally in 24 h) (2:1 morphine to oxycodone).

Step 2

- 30 mg oral oxycodone modified release twice daily (60 mg orally in 24 h) is equivalent to 30 mg oxycodone subcutaneously in 24 h (2:1 oral oxycodone to subcutaneous oxycodone) [65]
- These are example guidelines, it is recommended that health care professionals consult local guidelines or seek advice from the specialist palliative care team when considering opioid switches.

26.2.5 Management of Opioid Toxicity

Opioids play a vital role in the management of cancer pain; however, there may be concern amongst patients and health care professionals about the risks of opioid toxicity or overdose. Opioid toxicity in cancer pain management may occur as a result of accidental overdose by patients in the context of unstable pain, due to organ impairment as a complication of cancer (e.g., renal or hepatic impairment) or may develop iatrogenically from opioid prescription. Early signs of opioid toxicity may include effects on the central nervous system (CNS) including drowsiness or sedation or CNS hyperexcitability including myoclonus and hallucinations which may respond to management including dose reduction or opioid switching [49].

The main risk in severe opioid toxicity is that of respiratory depression which may be managed with naloxone. Regardless of the cause of the opioid toxicity, the urgent use of naloxone should only be considered when there is an immediate threat to life or diagnosed respiratory depression characterised by reduced respiratory rate with a corresponding decrease in oxygen saturation [67]. Concerns about the use of naloxone stem from two NHS England Patient Safety alerts [68, 69] which identified the risks associated with rapid or inappropriate reversal of opioid toxicity. The goal of management of opioid toxicity should be to reverse toxic side effects to ensure that the patient is not at risk of respiratory arrest [67]. The aim should not be to restore a normal level of consciousness as rapid reversal, particularly in long-term opioid use for cancer pain could result in a severe escalation in background pain.

A range of different definitions and guidelines for the management of opioid related respiratory depression exist [67] and clinical judgement should be used when assessing patients. However, in the context of opioid related cancer pain management, low doses of naloxone administered intravenously with careful monitoring should be considered (see Table).

26.2.6 Opioid Prescribing in Renal Impairment

Opioid metabolism is altered in renal impairment through reduced excretion and accumulation of metabolites, which is compounded by changes in hepatic metabolism [70]. Therefore, all opioids should be used with caution in renal impairment [71]. This will often entail starting at a lower than usual dose and increasing the dose interval. However, renal failure should not delay the use of opioids when necessary and the analgesic benefits must be balanced against potential side effects [70].

There is limited evidence regarding the safety of various opioids. Most of the research has been done in patients with cancer pain, and there is no absolute level of renal impairment at which caution is necessary [70, 72]. Evidence is of low quality with no RCT evidence; a recent systematic review [70] has largely echoed the findings of a previous systematic review [72]. Choice of opioid is therefore based on the presence or absence of active metabolites, risk of accumulation, and expert opinion [70–72].

Reversal of Opioid Induced Respiratory Depression (Adapted from [65, 67, 71, 73])

- If respiratory rate is greater than or equal to 8 breaths per minute and the patient easily rousable and not cyanosed, adopt a policy of 'wait and see'; consider reducing or omitting the next regular dose of opioid.
- If respiratory rate is less than 8 breaths per minute and the patient comatose/unconscious and/or cyanosed:
  - Give 100–200 µg naloxone IV stat
  - Give 100 µg IV every 2 min until respiratory function is stable
- OR
  - Dilute a standard ampoule containing naloxone (stock) 400 µg to 10 ml with 0.9% saline for injection
  - Administer 0.5 ml (20 µg) IV/IM/SC every 2–3 min until the patient's respiratory status is satisfactory, i.e., >8 breath/min. It may be necessary to repeat the naloxone injection as it is a shorter-acting drug than most opioid preparations.
- If multiple IV stat doses are required it may be appropriate to consider a continuous intravenous naloxone infusion.
- Ongoing monitoring may be required for up to or beyond 24 h, particularly if the patient has been treated with transdermal opioid preparations.

26.2.6.1 Use of Opioids in Mild to Moderate Renal Impairment (eGFR 30–89 ml/min)

Alfentanil and fentanyl do not have active metabolites and are therefore the safest choices in renal impairment. Opioids with active metabolites (Codeine, morphine, diamorphine, oxycodone) can be used with caution in mild to moderate renal impairment [71]. These drugs should be used at reduced dose and reduced frequency of administration [72]. Changes in renal function should be monitored, doses should be titrated cautiously, and patients should be monitored closely for signs or symptoms of opioid toxicity [72].

26.2.6.2 Use of Opioids in Severe Renal Impairment (eGFR <30 ml/min)

In severe renal impairment, the best available evidence suggests that alfentanil or fentanyl should be used first line as they do not have active metabolites and pharmacokinetics of these drugs are largely unaltered in renal impairment [49, 70, 72]. There is limited evidence for use of oxycodone in renal impairment [70, 72]. The outcome of a recent systematic review is inconclusive so the recommendation is that oxycodone should be used with caution in patients with renal impairment [70].

There is insufficient evidence regarding the use of buprenorphine in patients with eGFR <30 [70, 71]. However, there is a degree of clinical experience using buprenorphine in this setting and it is recommended in some guidelines [49, 59, 65]. Therefore, buprenorphine should be used with caution but may be an appropriate choice for patients requiring a transdermal opioid who do not meet the dose threshold for a fentanyl transdermal patch.

Options for Opioid Analgesia for Cancer Pain in Patients with Renal Impairment

The evidence base is limited so careful clinical assessment, individualisation, and monitoring are advised.

Oral opioids for cancer pain in renal impairment

- A pragmatic choice may be use of oxycodone immediate release (IR) at a reduced dose and no more than 2–4 hourly [65].
- Patients should be monitored closely for signs of opioid toxicity.
- There is no evidence to support use of oxycodone in preference to morphine in severe renal impairment [70, 72].
- Once pain is stable, consider switching to an opioid which is safer in renal impairment (e.g., a fentanyl transdermal patch).
- Buccal or sublingual fentanyl preparations may be used if clinically appropriate for incident pain.

Transdermal opioids for cancer pain in renal impairment

- For patients with stable pain, a fentanyl transdermal patch may be appropriate.
- Close monitoring and review are necessary to identify signs of opioid toxicity due to reduced clearance, and there is a risk of accumulation with transdermal preparations [65].
- If appropriate depending on the required dose, fentanyl should generally be used in preference to buprenorphine as outlined above.
- Transdermal opioids should not be used for patients with unstable pain requiring dose titration.

Parenteral Opioids for cancer pain in renal impairment

- Alfentanil should be considered as a first line option for subcutaneous administration.
- It is 30 times more potent than oral morphine (i.e., 30 mg PO morphine is equal to 1 mg alfentanil) [65].
- The PRN dose may be 1/sixth–1/tenth of the 24 h dose). Given the relatively short duration of action (plasma half-life 95 min), several doses may be needed for one episode of breakthrough pain [71].

- The short duration of action of alfentanil can make its use as a PRN opioid impractical in settings such as the community. In this situation, sub cutaneous oxycodone could be considered as an alternative at a reduced dose and no more than 2–4 hourly PRN; however, there should be close monitoring for signs of accumulation and toxicity.
- Clinical judgement should weigh up factors such as prognosis, availability of drugs, availability of staff, clinical expertise, risks of toxicity, and cost. It is recommended that advice is sought from the local specialist palliative care team.

The evidence for morphine and diamorphine in severe renal impairment is equivocal, with an unclear relationship between dose, degree of renal impairment, and opioid related side effects [70, 72]. Morphine and diamorphine should not be used routinely in patients with eGFR <30 as accumulation of metabolites is likely, with risks of side effects and opioid toxicity [72].

Use of Codeine in severe renal impairment should be avoided due to a significant increase in half-life and risk of metabolite accumulation [71, 72]. Methadone does not have active metabolites, so it is an option in severe renal impairment but should only be used by clinicians with experience in its use due to a long and unpredictable half-life with consequent risk of accumulation and opioid toxicity [70, 72].

26.2.7 Opioid Prescribing in Hepatic Impairment

Most drugs are metabolised via the liver, so hepatic impairment may lead to changes in pharmacokinetics and pharmacodynamics. This may include increased bioavailability, accumulation of drugs or metabolites, prolonged half-life, and disruption of the blood–brain barrier leading to higher CNS drug concentrations [71].

General Factors to Consider When Prescribing in Hepatic Impairment

- Hepatic encephalopathy—increased sensitivity to sedatives, hypnotics, and CNS depressants.
- Ascites—caution with drugs which cause salt and water retention (e.g., steroids, NSAIDS), and those which have a high sodium content (e.g., effervescent paracetamol).
- Coagulopathy—caution with anticoagulants and NSAIDS.
- Coexisting renal impairment (hepatorenal syndrome).
- Drug related factors—particularly metabolism and elimination.

26.2.7.1 General Principles of Opioid Prescribing in Hepatic Impairment

All opioids should be used with caution in patients with significant hepatic dysfunction as the risk of side effects and potential toxicity is increased and there is a risk of precipitating hepatic encephalopathy. These effects are unpredictable due to the complexity of opioid metabolism in hepatic impairment and the range of factors involved [74]. This, however, should not preclude their use when necessary for the management of pain and breathlessness in palliative care patients. There is very little available evidence regarding the choice of opioid in hepatic impairment; recommendations are therefore based on the presence or absence of active metabolites, risk of accumulation, and consensus opinion [74–76]. All opioids should be used at lower doses with longer intervals between doses. Titration should be cautious and ideally, modified release preparations and/or opioids with long half-lives should be avoided. Particular attention should be paid to prevention and management of constipation as this may worsen hepatic encephalopathy.

Options for Opioid Analgesia for Cancer Pain in Patients with Hepatic Impairment (Adapted from [65, 71, 74, 76])

- The evidence base is limited so careful clinical assessment, individualisation, and monitoring are advised.

Morphine

- Morphine is often used as the first line strong opioid for oral and parenteral use in patients with hepatic impairment.
- Due to decreased plasma clearance and prolonged elimination, morphine should be used at a reduced dose and with an increased dose interval [74, 76].
- With close monitoring on an inpatient unit, a dose interval of 2–4 hourly may be appropriate; in the community with less frequent assessment an appropriate dose interval would be 4 hourly.

Oxycodone

- Should be avoided in severe hepatic impairment due to severely impaired elimination and prolonged half-life [74]. It may be used with caution and at lower dose and increased dose interval in mild to moderate hepatic impairment.

Fentanyl

- The pharmacokinetics of fentanyl are not altered in severe hepatic impairment so it may be the opioid of choice in some situations [74, 76].

- However, caution should be used as transdermal preparations may lead to accumulation and require close monitoring, and should not be used for patients with unstable pain requiring dose titration.

Alfentanil

- Alfentanil is metabolised via oxidation, so hepatic impairment causes reduced drug clearance and therefore prolonged half-life. Alfentanil should therefore be used with caution.

Buprenorphine

- Buprenorphine should be used with caution in mild to moderate hepatic impairment, and use should be avoided in severe hepatic dysfunction.

Codeine and tramadol

- Codeine and tramadol require hepatic metabolism for conversion to active metabolites, and should therefore be avoided in moderate to severe hepatic impairment.

26.2.8 Adjuvant Analgesics

Whilst the WHO ladder and opioid analgesia play a vital role in the management of cancer pain, there are a number of adjuvant analgesics targeting other pain pathways which are important in the comprehensive management of cancer pain.

26.2.8.1 Antidepressants and Anticonvulsants

A systematic review exploring the role of antiepileptic or antidepressant drugs as adjuvants to opioid analgesia in cancer pain highlighted that neuropathic pain mechanisms may be present in up to 40% of patients with cancer pain. The review concluded that there is evidence of a moderate impact on neuropathic cancer pain following the addition of an antidepressant or anticonvulsant adjuvant; however, the reduction in pain intensity was unlikely to be more than 1 point on a 0–10 numerical rating scale and there was potential to increase adverse effects. It was particularly noted that there was significant adverse effects when an adjuvant was added to a stable opioid dose, suggesting that consideration is given to reducing the opioid dose when an adjuvant is started and titrating both drugs accordingly [77].

Antidepressant or Anticonvulsant Options for Management of Neuropathic Pain in Cancer (Adapted from [20, 49, 65, 77, 78])
Antidepressants

- Amitriptyline 10 mg nocte and titrate up every 5–7 days to maximum 75 mg daily. Do not use if there is a history of cardiac arrhythmias.
- Duloxetine 30–60 mg daily starting dose (clinical benefit at 60 mg) titrated up to 120 mg daily.

Anticonvulsants

- Gabapentin 100 mg three times a day titrated up to 600 mg three times a day (higher doses may be used under specialist advice). Dose reduce in renal impairment.
- Pregabalin 25–75 mg twice a day titrated up to 300 mg twice a day. Dose reduce in renal impairment.

Amitriptyline or gabapentin are recommended as options for management of neuropathic cancer pain that is only partially responsive to opioid analgesia [49]. Although not specific for cancer pain, NICE guideline CG173 [78] provides further evidence for the role of antidepressants and anticonvulsants in management of general neuropathic pain and could be considered, alongside clinical judgement, as part of clinical assessment and management of patients with cancer pain, particularly in the palliative context [65].

Other Pharmacological Adjuvant Options for Cancer Pain Management (Adapted from [20, 65])
Bisphosphonates

- Bisphosphonates should be considered as a therapeutic option in the management of cancer pain secondary to metastatic bone disease [20, 79]. The majority of the evidence relates to pain management in breast cancer, prostate cancer, and myeloma; however, the evidence is insufficient to recommend bisphosphonates as a first line therapy. The maximum response is likely to be observed by 4 weeks. [79].
- Hypocalcaemia and renal impairment are potential complications of bisphosphonate therapy and should be monitored for during treatment. Calcium and vitamin D supplementation should be considered [20].
- Bisphosphonate related osteonecrosis of the jaw (BRONJ) is a serious adverse event which causes osteonecrotic damage to the maxillary and

mandibular bone, resulting in development of non-viable, exposed bone which effects eating, speaking, and oral hygiene [80]. The incidence is 6–10% in cancer patients receiving bisphosphonates. It is recommended that patients have a dental review and complete any invasive dental work prior to commencing treatment and avoid any dental treatment during IV treatment.

Corticosteroids [81]

- The mechanism of action of corticosteroids in cancer pain is unclear but may include anti-inflammatory effects and reduction in local tissue oedema.
- There is weak evidence that corticosteroids may improve cancer pain for 1 week but the decision to undertake a steroid trial should be balanced against the potential risk of side effects.
- The impact of a trial of steroids should be carefully monitored, undertaken over a short period of time, and stopped promptly if there is no clinical benefit.

Ketamine [82]

- Dissociative anaesthetic which is thought to act by blocking NMDA receptors has been used under the supervision of specialists with experience in management of cancer pain.
- A recent Cochrane review concluded that there is insufficient evidence to draw conclusions regarding the use of ketamine in treatment of cancer pain and also noted that rapid dose escalation to 500 mg does not appear to have clinical benefit and may be associated with serious adverse events.

26.2.9 Interventional Options for Management of Cancer Pain

In secondary and hospice settings, interventional options for cancer pain management should always be considered alongside other non-pharmacological or pharmacological approaches. Options may include radiotherapy for pain relief in patients with bone metastasis [20], percutaneous cementoplasty for bone pain from pelvic bone metastases [20, 83], or vertebroplasty for malignant vertebral collapse [20, 84]. Anaesthetic options include local nerve blocks (e.g., coeliac plexus block [20]) or spinal administration of opioid analgesia [49, 85].

Acknowledgements Thank you to Dr. Amy Hawkins and Dr. Helen Burgess for their contribution to the sections on prescribing in renal and liver impairment. Thank you to Dr. Cate Seton-Jones and Mrs. Jayne Holland for permission to adapt the Phyllis Tuckwell Hospice Care Guidelines for Strong Opioids and Guidelines for the Use of Drugs in Renal and Liver Disease for use in this text.

References

1. Macmillan. Macmillan cancer support/ICM online survey of 2,096 UK adults. Fieldwork undertaken 22nd–24th (March 2017). Survey results are weighted to be representative of the UK population., s.l.: s.n; n.d.
2. van den Beuken-van Everdingen MH, de Rijke JM, Kessels AG, Schouten HC, van Kleef M, Patijn J. Prevalence of pain in patients with cancer: a systematic review of the past 40 years. Ann Oncol. 2007;18(9):1437–49.
3. Portenoy D. Cancer pain. Epidemiology and symptoms. Cancer. 1989;63(11 Suppl):2298–307.
4. Macmillan. Managing cancer pain [Online]. 2016. Available at: http://be.macmillan.org.uk/Downloads/CancerInformation/LivingWithAndAfterCancer/MAC11670ManagingPainE11lowrespdfALM20161214.pdf. Accessed 3 Dec 2017.
5. Daut C. The prevalence and severity of pain in cancer. Cancer. 1982;50(9):1913–8.
6. Kuo SS. The pharmacoeconomics of breakthrough cancer. Pain. 2013;27(2):167–75.
7. Fairchild A. Under-treatment of cancer pain. Curr Opin Support Palliat Care. 2010;4(1):11–5.
8. Office for National Statistics. National Survey of bereaved people (VOICES): 2014 (Q35). London: Office for National Statistics; 2015.
9. Adam WM. Why do patients with cancer access out-of-hours primary care? A retrospective study. Br J Gen Pract. 2014;619:e99–e104.
10. McLoughlin PA. Community specialist palliative care: experiences of patients and carers. Int J Palliat Nurs. 2002;8(7):344–53.
11. De Rond M, De Wit R, Van Dam F, Van Campen B, Den Hartog Y, Klievink R, Nieweg R, Noort J, Wagenaar M, Van Campen B. Daily pain assessment: value for nurses and patients. J Adv Nurs. 1999;29:436–44.
12. Herr K, Titler MG, Schilling ML, Marsh JL, Xie X, Ardery G, Clarke WR, Everett LQ. Evidence based assessment of acute pain in older adults: current nursing practices and perceived barriers. Clin J Pain. 2004;20(5):331–40.
13. Schumacher KL, Koresawa S, West C, Dodd M, Paul SM, Tripathy D, Koo P, Miaskowski C. The usefulness of a daily pain management diary for outpatients with cancer-related pain. Oncol Nurs Forum. 2002;29(9):1304–13.
14. Macmillan. Macmillan pain diary [Online]. 2013. Available at: https://www.macmillan.org.uk/ documents/cancerinfo/livingwithandaftercancer/macmillan-pain-diary.pdf. Accessed 5 Nov 2017.
15. American Cancer Society. Pain diary [Online]. 2016. Available at: https://www.cancer.org/content/dam/cancer-org/cancer-control/en/worksheets/pain-diary.pdf. Accessed 5 Nov 2017.
16. Scottish Intercollegiate Guidelines Network (SIGN) 106. Control of pain in adults with cancer. 2008. http://www.sign.ac.uk/sign-106-control-of-pain-in-adults-with-cancer.html. Accessed 21 Sept 2017.
17. British Pain Society. Cancer pain management [Online]. 2010. Available at: https://www.britishpainsociety.org/ static/uploads/resources/files/book_cancer_pain.pdf. Accessed 18 Nov 2017.
18. de Wit R, van Dam F, Abu-Saad HH, Loonstra S, Zandbelt L, van BuurenKarin A, van der Heijden K, Leenhouts G. Empirical comparison of commonly used measures to evaluate pain treatment in cancer patients with chronic pain. J Clin Oncol. 1999;17(4):1280–7.
19. Caraceni A, Cherny N, Fainsinger R, Kaasa S, Poulain P, Radbruch L, De Conno F. Pain measurement tools and methods in clinical research in palliative care recommendations of an expert working group of the European Association of Palliative Care. J Pain Symptom Manage. 2002;23(3):239–55.
20. Scottish Intercollegiate Guidelines Network. SIGN 106 Control of pain in adults with cancer. A national clinical guideline [Online]. 2008. Available at: http://www.sign.ac.uk/assets/sign106.pdf. Accessed 5 Nov 2017.
21. Macmillan. The C-word. How we react to cancer today. 2017. Available at: https://www.macmillan.org.uk/assets/1426915-the-c-word-macmillan-cancer-support-2017.pdf. Accessed 5 Nov 2017.

22. Anandarajah G, Ellen HE. 'Spirituality and medical practice: using the HOPE questions as a practical tool for spiritual assessment. Am Fam Physician. 2001;63:81–9.
23. Morley S, Eccleston C, Williams A. Systematic review and meta-analysis of randomized controlled trials of cognitive behaviour therapy and behaviour therapy for chronic pain in adults, excluding headache. Pain. 1999;80(1–2):1–13.
24. Passik SD, Dugan W, McDonald MV, Rosenfeld B, Theobald DE, Edgerton S. Oncologists' recognition of depression in their patients with cancer. J Clin Oncol. 1998;16(4):1594–600.
25. Spiegel D, Sands S, Koopman C. Pain and depression in patients with cancer. Cancer. 1994;74(9):2570–8.
26. WHO. WHO's cancer pain ladder for adults [Online]. 1986. Available at: http://www.who.int/cancer/palliative/painladder/en/. Accessed 5 Nov 2017.
27. McNichol E, Strassels SA, Goudas L, Lau J, Carr DB. NSAIDs or paracetamol, alone or combined with opioids, for cancer pain. Cochrane Database Syst Rev. 2006;1:CD005180.
28. NICE. Palliative care for adults: strong opioids for pain relief. Clinical Guideline 140 [Online]. 2016. Available at: https://www.nice.org.uk/guidance/cg140. Accessed Nov 2017.
29. NICE. Opioids in palliative care evidence update. 2016. Available from https://www.nice.org.uk/guidance/cg140?unlid=781078180201511261l725. Accessed 21 Sept 2017.
30. Guidelines and Audit Implementation Network. General palliative care guidelines for the management of pain at the end of life in adult patients. Belfast: Guidelines and Audit Implementation Network; 2011.
31. MedicinesComplete. BNF [Online]. 2017. Available at: https://www.medicinescomplete.com/mc/bnf/current/. Accessed Nov 2017.
32. Singh P, Chaturvedi A. Complementary and alternative medicine in Cancer pain management: a systematic review. Ind J Palliat Care. 2015;21(1):105–15.
33. Fellowes B, Barnes K, Wilkinson S. Aromatherapy and massage for symptom relief in patients with cancer. Cochrane Database Syst Rev. 2004;4:2004.
34. Post-White J, Kinney ME, Savik K, Gau JB, Wilcox C, Lerner I. Therapeutic massage and healing touch improve symptoms in cancer. Integr Cancer Ther. 2003;2(4):332–44.
35. Soden K, Vincent K, Craske S, Lucas C, Ashley S. A randomized controlled trial of aromatherapy massage in a hospice setting. Palliat Med. 2004;18(2):87–92.
36. Lee H, Schmidt K, Ernst E. Acupuncture for the relief of cancer-related pain—a systematic review. Eur J Pain. 2005;9(4):437–44.
37. Alimi D, Rubino C, Pichard-Léandri E, Fermand-Brulé S, Dubreuil-Lemaire ML, Hill C. Analgesic effect of auricular acupuncture for cancer pain: a randomized, blinded, controlled trial. J Clin Oncol. 2003;21(22):4120–6.
38. Ernst, E. Pittler, M. H., Wider, B. (2006) The desktop guide to complementary and alternative medicine. London: Elsevier/Mosby.
39. Ernst E, Pittler MH, Wider B. Complementary therapies for pain management. London: Elsevier/Mosby; 2007.
40. Cepeda MS, Carr DB, Lau J, Alvarez H. Music for pain relief. Cochrane Database Syst Rev. 2006;2:CD004843.
41. Stephenson NLN, Swanson M, Dalton J, Keefe FJ, Engelke M. Partner-delivered reflexology: effects on cancer pain and anxiety. Oncol Nurs Forum. 2007;34(1):127–32.
42. Olson K, Hanson J, Michaud M. A phase II trial of reiki for the management of pain in advanced. Cancer. 2003;26(5):990–7.
43. Rajasekaran M, Edmonds PM, Higginson IL. Systematic review of hypnotherapy for treating symptoms in terminally ill adult cancer patients. Palliat Med. 2005;19:418–26.
44. Nash T. The effectiveness of hypnosis in reducing pain and suffering among women with metastatic breast cancer and among women with temporomandibular disorder. Int J Clin Experiment Hypn. 2010;58(4):497–504.
45. Headley JA, Ownby KK, John LD. The effect of seated exercise on fatigue and quality of life in women with advanced breast cancer. Oncol Nurs Forum. 2004;31(5):977–83.
46. College of Occupational Therapists. Occupational therapy intervention in cancer. London: College of Occupational Therapists; 2004.

47. Graves KD. Social cognitive theory and cancer patients' quality of life: a meta-analysis of psychosocial intervention components. Health Psychol. 2003;22(2):210–9.
48. Sullivan MJ, Thorn B, Haythornthwaite JA, Keefe F, Martin M, Bradley LA, Lefebvre JC. Theoretical perspectives on the relationship between catastrophising and pain. Clin J Pain. 2001;17(1):52–64.
49. Caraceni A, et al. Use of opioid analgesics in the treatment of cancer pain: evidence-based recommendations from the EAPC. Lancet Oncol. 2012;13:e58–68.
50. Mercadante S, et al. Episodic (breakthrough) pain: consensus conference of an expert working group of the European Association for Palliative Care. Cancer. 2002;94:832–9.
51. Saunders C. The symptomatic treatment of incurable cancer. Prescribers J. 1984;4(4):68–73.
52. Bandieri E, Marilena M, Ripamonti CI, Artioli F, Sichetti D, Fanizza C, Santini D, Cavanna L, Melotti D, Conte PF, Roila F, Casinu S, Bruera E, Tognoni G, Luppi M. Randonmized trial of low dose morphine versus weak opioids in moderate cancer pain. Journal of Clin Oncol. 2016;34(5):436–42.
53. Wiffen P, Edwards JE, Barden J, McQuay HJM. Oral morphine for cancer pain. Cochrane Database Syst Rev. 2016;4:CD003868. https://doi.org/10.1002/14651858.CD003868.pub4.
54. NICE. Opioids in Palliative Care Evidence Update 58. 2014. Available from https://www.nice.org.uk/guidance/cg140/evidence/evidence-update-pdf-186447709. Accessed 10 Dec 2017.
55. NICE Clinical Guidance 140. Opioids in palliative care: safe and effective prescribing of strong opioids for pain in palliative care adults. 2012. Available from https://www.nice.org.uk/guidance/cg140. Accessed 10 Dec 2017.
56. Wiffen PJ, Derry S, Moore R. Tramadol with or without paracetamol (acetaminophen) for cancer pain. Cochrane Database Syst Rev. 2017;5:CD012508. https://doi.org/10.1002/14651858.CD012508.pub2.
57. Schmidt-Hansen M, Bennett MI, Arnold S, Bromham N, Hilgart JS. Oxycodone for cancer-related pain. Cochrane Database Syst Rev. 2017;8:CD003870. https://doi.org/10.1002/14651858.CD003870.pub6.
58. Hadley G, et al. Transdermal fentanyl in cancer pain. Cochrane Database Syst Rev. 2013;10:CD010270. https://doi.org/10.1002/14651858.CD010270.pub2.
59. Davis MP. Twelve reasons for considering buprenorphine as a frontline analgesic in the management of pain. J Support Oncol. 2012;10(6):209–19.
60. Schmidt-Hansen M, Taubert M, Bromham N, Hilgart JS, Arnold S. The effectiveness of buprenorphine for treating cancer pain: an abridged Cochrane review. BMJ Support Palliat Care. 2016;6:292–306.
61. Nicholson AB, Watson GR, Derry S, Wiffen PJ. Methadone for cancer pain. Cochrane Database Syst Rev. 2017;2:CD003971. https://doi.org/10.1002/14651858.CD003971.pub4.
62. Bao YJ, Hou W, Kong XY, Yang L, Xia J, Hua BJ, Knaggs R. Hydromorphone for cancer pain. Cochrane Database Syst Rev. 2016;10:CD011108. https://doi.org/10.1002/14651858.CD011108.pub2.
63. Wiffen P, Derry S, Naessens K, Bell RF. Oral tapentadol for cancer pain. Cochrane Database Syst Rev. 2015;9:CD011460. https://doi.org/10.1002/14651858.CD011460.pub2.
64. Wiffen P, Wee B, Derry S, Bell RF, Moore R. Opioids for cancer pain—an overview of Cochrane reviews. Cochrane Database Syst Rev. 2017;7:CD012592. https://doi.org/10.1002/14651858.CD012592.pub2.
65. Watson M, Armstrong P, Back I, Gannon C, Sykes N. Palliative adult network guidelines. 4th ed. Bedfordshire and Hertfordshire: London Cancer Alliance, Northern Ireland Clinical Networks; 2016.
66. British National Formulary. Prescribing in palliative care. 2017. Available from https://bnf.nice.org.uk/guidance/prescribing-in-palliative-care.html. Accessed 9 Dec 2017.
67. UK Medicines Information. What naloxone doses should be used in adults to reverse urgently the effects of opioids or opiates? 2017. Available from https://www.sps.nhs.uk/wp-content/uploads/2015/11/UKMi_QA-_Naloxone-dosing_Aug-17_FINAL.pdf. Accessed 9 Dec 2017.

68. NHS England Patient Safety Alert Stage 1. 2014. Available from https://www.england.nhs.uk/wp-content/uploads/2014/11/psa-inappropriate-doses-naloxone.pdf. Accessed 9 Dec 2017.
69. NHS England Patient Safety Alert Stage 2. 2015. Available from https://www.england.nhs.uk/patientsafety/wp-content/uploads/sites/32/2015/10/psa-naloxone-stage2.pdf. Accessed 9 Dec 2017.
70. Sande TA, Laird BJA, Fallon MT, et al. The use of opioids in cancer patients with renal impairment—a systematic review. Support Care Cancer. 2017;25:661–75.
71. Twycross R, Wilcock A, Howard P. Palliative care formulary 5. Nottingham: Palliativedrugs.com Ltd; 2014.
72. King S, et al. A systematic review of the use of opioid medication for those with moderate to severe cancer pain and renal impairment: a European palliative care research collaborative opioid guidelines project. Palliat Med. 2011;25:525–52.
73. Miaskowski C, et al. Principles of analgesic use in the treatment of acute pain and Cancer pain (6e). Skokie, IL: American Pain Society; 2008. p. 31.
74. Rhee C, Broadbent AM, et al. Palliation and liver failure: palliative medications dosage guidelines. JPSM. 2007;10(3):677–85.
75. Hanna M. The effects of liver impairment on opioids used to relieve pain in cancer patients. Palliat Med. 2011;25(5):604–5.
76. Larson AM, Curtis JR. (2006). Integrating palliative care for liver transplant candidates: "too well for transplant, too sick for life". JAMA. 2006;295(18):2168–76. https://doi.org/10.1001/jama.295.18.2168.
77. Bennett M. Effectiveness of antiepileptic or antidepressant drugs when added to opioids for cancer pain: systematic review. Palliat Med. 2010;25(5):553–9.
78. NICE Clinical Guidance 173. Neuropathic pain in adults: pharmacological management in non-specialist settings. 2013. Available from https://www.nice.org.uk/guidance/cg173. Accessed 21 Sept 2017.
79. Wong R, Wiffen P. Bisphosphonates for the relief of pain secondary to bone metastases. Cochrane Database Syst Rev. 2002;2:CD002068. https://doi.org/10.1002/14651858.CD002068.
80. Rollason V, Laverrière A, MacDonald L, Walsh T, Tramèr MR, Vogt-Ferrier NB. Interventions for treating bisphosphonate-related osteonecrosis of the jaw (BRONJ). Cochrane Database Syst Rev. 2016;2:CD008455. https://doi.org/10.1002/14651858.CD008455.pub2.
81. Haywood A, Good P, Khan S, Leupp A, Jenkins-Marsh S, Rickett K, Hardy JR. Corticosteroids for the management of cancer-related pain in adults. Cochrane Database of Syst Rev. 2015;4:CD010756. https://doi.org/10.1002/14651858.CD010756.pub2.
82. Bell RF, Eccleston C, Kalso EA. Ketamine as an adjuvant to opioids for cancer pain. Cochrane Database of Systematic Reviews. 2017;6:CD003351. https://doi.org/10.1002/14651858.CD003351.pub3.
83. NICE Interventional Procedures Guidance (IPG) 179. Percutaneous cementoplasty for palliative treatment of bony malignancies. 2006. Available from https://www.nice.org.uk/guidance/ipg179/resources/percutaneous-cementoplasty-for-palliative-treatment-of-bony-malignancies-pdf-1899863409460165. Accessed 10 Dec 17.
84. NICE Interventional Procedures Guidance (IPG) 12. Percutaneous vertebroplasty. 2003. Available from https://www.nice.org.uk/guidance/ipg179/resources/percutaneous-cementoplasty-for-palliative-treatment-of-bony-malignancies-pdf-1899863409460165. Accessed 10 Dec 2017.
85. British Pain Society. Intrathecal drug delivery for the management of pain and spasticity in adults: recommendations for best clinical practice. 2015. Available from https://www.britishpainsociety.org/ static/uploads/resources/files/itdd_2015_pro_v3.pdf. Accessed 10 Dec 2017.

Chapter 27
Arthritis Pain; Rheumatoid Arthritis, Osteoarthritis, and Fibromyalgia

Afsha Khan, João Calinas Correia, and David Andrew Walsh

27.1 Introduction

Rheumatoid arthritis (RA), osteoarthritis (OA), and fibromyalgia (FM) are common disabling and distressing conditions illustrating the production, amplification, and maintenance of pain by inflammation, tissue remodelling, and central pain mechanisms. The balance between different pain mechanisms determines the patient's experience, presentation to health care providers, and treatment response.

Musculoskeletal pain can continue over many years, punctuated by acute episodes or flares, although often with periods of relative or even absolute remission. Pain is usually experienced in multiple anatomical locations, but might present with a focus on one particular joint. The clinical picture might evolve rapidly, or over a period of years. Key mechanisms not only initiate pain, but also determine pain quality and severity, persistence or resolution, and lead to symptom complexity. Symptom relief and retarding structural change (disease modification) are the key therapeutic goals.

In this chapter we discuss RA, OA, and FM as representative diagnoses associated with inflammatory, structural, or central pain mechanisms, and how these

A. Khan · J. Calinas Correia
Department of Rheumatology and Back Pain Unit, Sherwood Forest Hospitals NHS Foundation Trust, Kings Mill Hospital, Sutton in Ashfield, UK

D. A. Walsh (✉)
Department of Rheumatology and Back Pain Unit, Sherwood Forest Hospitals NHS Foundation Trust, Kings Mill Hospital, Sutton in Ashfield, UK

Pain Centre Versus Arthritis and NIHR Nottingham Biomedical Research Centre, Division of Rheumatology, Orthopaedics and Dermatology, University of Nottingham Clinical Science Building, City Hospital, Nottingham, UK

Academic Rheumatology, Clinical Sciences Building, City Hospital, Nottingham, UK
e-mail: David.walsh@nottingham.ac.uk

K. Shimoji et al. (eds.), *Chronic Pain Management in General and Hospital Practice*, https://doi.org/10.1007/978-981-15-2933-7_27

mechanisms explain the clinical characteristics and inform optimal management of people presenting with musculoskeletal pain.

27.2 Musculoskeletal Diagnosis

RA is the commonest inflammatory arthritis, but other diagnoses (e.g., psoriatic arthritis, ankylosing spondylitis) might share pain mechanisms and respond to similar treatments. RA diagnosis requires inflammation in an appropriate clinical context. Evidence of inflammation might be clinical (soft-tissue swelling and tenderness), imaging (e.g., ultrasound, radiographic erosions) or laboratory (e.g., raised serum C-reactive protein, antibodies against citrullinated proteins) [1]. Systemic features or comorbidities such as interstitial lung disease, inflammatory bowel disease, or psoriasis might suggest inflammatory arthritis. OA diagnosis requires evidence of joint structural change; clinical (bony swelling, crepitus) or radiographic (osteophytes, subchondral sclerosis indicative of new bone formation, and joint space narrowing indicative of cartilage or meniscal damage) [2–4]. FM diagnosis is based on the presence of chronic widespread pain, affecting regions above and below the waist, on the right or left side of the body plus axial pain, with associated features of sleep, cognitive, or mood disturbance [5]. Blood tests and joint imaging are unaffected by FM.

Arthritis may present in a single joint [6], but characteristic patterns of joint involvement in established disease distinguish different diagnostic groups. RA is typically symmetric and commonly affects wrists, metacarpophalangeal, and proximal interphalangeal joints. OA can present in a single joint or group of joints, for example, affecting knees or hips, or small joints of the hands or feet. Differing joint distributions (e.g., generalised nodal OA) reflect discrete subgroups with different genetic predispositions and prognosis. People with OA in one knee are at above average risk of OA in the contralateral knee, producing a degree of symmetry in symptoms and radiographic change.

27.3 Mechanisms of Musculoskeletal Pain

Understanding the underlying mechanisms that initiate, augment, and maintain musculoskeletal pain is key to its optimal management [7].

Pain is a prominent feature of many rheumatological conditions, and is the result of a complex physiologic interactions that result in a highly individualised symptom pattern. Peripheral nociceptive input is processed by the central nervous system against a background of factors that also can enhance or diminish the pain experience. There are very large inter-individual differences in these central nervous system factors, such that some individuals with substantial peripheral nociceptive input (e.g., from joint damage or inflammation) will feel little or no pain, whereas others might experience pain with minimal or no identifiable tissue pathology.

Pain might be triggered by disease or by biomechanical factors. Sensitisation amplifies nociceptive inputs. Altered molecular expression and activity in peripheral nerves increases responses to mechanical stimuli and to the internal milieu (spontaneous pain). Central mechanisms, including temporal summation, descending facilitation, or impaired descending inhibition of spinal nociceptive transmission, each may contribute to musculoskeletal pain. Cognitive factors modulate pain, including placebo and nocebo effects, and affective mechanisms impact both pain processing and appraisal. There is often only a weak association between objective evidence of joint pathology and the severity of pain. Pain, despite a sparsity of objective evidence of ongoing disease, appears to increase psychological distress and disability.

RA, OA, and FM are prototypical diagnoses associated with inflammatory, structural, and centrally driven musculoskeletal pain, but musculoskeletal pain mechanisms might be shared between diagnostic groups. People with RA might also display erosive joint damage, and those with OA often have synovitis. Almost one-half of people presenting with new onset RA already have radiographic evidence of OA in their hands or feet [8]. People with RA or OA commonly display features also of FM [9, 10].

27.3.1 Musculoskeletal Nociception

The musculoskeletal system has a sophisticated sensory innervation that enables normal proprioception and alerts the individual to actual or threatened tissue damage (nociception). The articular capsule of the joint receives an extensive network myelinated nerve fibres with free complex or encapsulated nerve endings. Normal human synovium [11, 12] and subchondral bone [13] are also richly supplied with unmyelinated nerves. Similar innervations are found in tendons, ligaments, deep fascia, periosteum, and muscle. Myelinated Aβ fibres are activated by noxious stimuli (e.g., exceeding the normal range of joint movement), but also may play a role in normal proprioception. Small, unmyelinated sensory C fibres predominate in articular nerves and can be activated by noxious mechanical, thermal, or chemical stimuli. Fibres which normally are mechano-insensitive might react to mechanical stimuli in an inflamed joint (silent nociceptors). Articular cartilage in the normal adult joint is avascular and not innervated, as are the inner two-thirds of knee menisci [14]. These cartilaginous structures, although not being direct sources of pain, distribute and damp mechanical forces across the articular surface, thereby reducing activation of nociceptors in adjacent tissues.

Musculoskeletal pain is classically experienced on joint movement, in particular positions or during weight bearing, indicating mechanotransduction as a primary event in nociception. Shear stress causes conformational change and opening of mechano-gated ion channels in the nerve terminal membrane, and consequently nerve depolarisation [15]. Joint instability and altered joint shape, abnormal loading patterns, loss of the normal cushioning role of cartilage and menisci, and growth of nerve endings into structures that are normally not innervated (e.g., articular cartilage, menisci) each might contribute to mechanosensor activation in arthritis. Synovial effusion can increase intra-articular pressure from normally subatmospheric (−1.3 kPa [16]) to as high as +2.7 kPa in RA knees [17]. As intra-articular pressure increases, participants reported tightness around their knee and increasing pain. Raised intra-articular pressure in animals results in burst firing of articular afferents [18, 19].

Arthritis pain can also be constant and unremitting, continuing after mechanical stimulation has ceased [20]. This constant or background pain might be chemically mediated by factors which directly activate neurons, generated, for example, during inflammation. Low pH, ATP, and bradykinin activate ion channels (e.g., TRPV1) or G-protein coupled receptors on unmyelinated fibres within the joint. These unmyelinated fibres likely contribute to the inflammatory pain of RA, and subchondral nerve fibres might in part explain the association of bone marrow lesions (BMLs) observed on MRI with OA pain [21].

27.3.2 Peripheral Sensitisation

Pain during normal activity suggests sensitisation, and there is overwhelming evidence that sensory nerves within the joint are sensitised to mechanical and other stimuli in RA and OA. A greater understanding of the mechanisms and chemical mediators responsible for the generation and maintenance of peripheral sensitisation is leading to novel drugs that could alleviate arthritis pain. Inflammation of the joint lining (synovitis) is an early feature after joint injury, in RA, and also in OA. Inflammatory mediators orchestrate healing responses, but can also sensitise nerves. Small molecules such as histamine [22], 5-hydroxytryptamine [23], adenosine and nitric oxide [24], peptides including bradykinin [25, 26], lipid metabolites and ion channel ligands [27], cytokines (e.g., interleukin-1 (IL-1)β, IL-6, and tumour necrosis factor (TNF α), and chemokines (e.g., CCL2, also known as monocyte chemotactic protein-1) [28] each can sensitise peripheral nerves. These are well recognised to contribute to inflammation in RA [28] and many are also upregulated in OA [29]. Growth factors (in particular β-nerve growth factor (NGF), but also vascular endothelial growth factor) have attracted particular attention as possible mediators of peripheral sensitisation in arthritic joints [28].

Arachidonic acid metabolites contribute to the sensitisation of joint nociceptors by acute and chronic inflammation, which can be reduced by cyclooxygenase inhibitors (non-steroidal anti-inflammatory drugs, NSAIDs). Other lipid-derived factors (e.g., resolvins) might switch off inflammation, and also have potential to switch off pain by reducing sensitisation [30]. Resolution of pain might therefore be an active process, rather than an inevitable consequence of removing an injurious agent. Deficiencies in pain resolution mechanisms might explain how pain can persist even when arthritis is well controlled, and might point to novel therapeutic approaches.

Increases in ion channel expression, phosphorylation, and opening can contribute to peripheral sensitisation. The inflammatory mediators PGE_2, adenosine, and 5-hydroxytryptamine each augments sodium channel kinetics and TTX-resistant sodium currents [31, 32]. Several transient receptor potential (TRP) channels have been implicated in joint pain, including the TRPV (vanilloid), TRPA (ankyrin) [33], TRPC (canonical) [34], and TRPM (melanostatin) channel subfamilies. TRPV1 is activated by heat and by protons, and by the pungent component of chilli pepper, capsaicin. Activation may be followed by desensitisation, neurite retraction, and reduced nociception. TRPV1 inhibitors reduced pain behaviour in animal models of arthritis [35], but clinical development of TRPV1 inhibitors has proved difficult due to inadequate analgesic benefit at levels of TRPV1 inhibition not associated with adverse events. Repeated topical application of capsaicin can relieve OA pain [36].

Growth factors (in particular β-nerve growth factor (NGF), but also vascular endothelial growth factor) and the chemokine CCL2 (also known as monocyte chemotactic protein-1) have also attracted attention as possible mediators of peripheral sensitisation in arthritic joints [28]. NGF is a polypeptide produced within the joint by inflammatory and resident synoviocytes and chondrocytes [37]. NGF binds to cell surface receptors on the terminals of unmyelinated sensory nerves to cause peripheral sensitisation. NGF signalling can be inhibited either by biological agents that bind and neutralise NGF within the joint, or by inhibiting the tyrosine kinase activity of the high affinity NGF receptor, tropomyosin receptor kinase (Trk)A [38]. NGF blockade reverses peripheral sensitisation, while not inhibiting normal, protective nociceptive responses. Randomised controlled trials of NGF-blocking antibodies have demonstrated clinically important analgesic benefit in OA or low back pain [39], confirming a major contribution of peripheral sensitisation to arthritis pain. Antibodies that block NGF have rarely been associated with rapidly progressive OA, and ongoing clinical trials are better defining safety profiles to ensure that benefits and risks can be appropriately balanced.

27.3.3 Central Sensitisation

Central sensitisation, an increased responsiveness of neurons in nociceptive pathways in the central nervous system to their normal or subthreshold afferent input, represents a shift in the balance from inhibition to facilitation of nociceptive transmission. It is strongly associated with the development and maintenance of chronic musculoskeletal pain. Central sensitisation can lead to heightened sensitivities across all senses, not only mechanical sensitivity [40]. It is also associated with cognitive deficits, such as poor concentration and poor short-term memory [41], emotional distress, particularly anxiety [42], sleep disturbance, and fatigue [43, 44]. Clinical features of central sensitisation have been associated with adverse illness behaviours [45–47], pain catastrophising, and analgesic use [48]. Neural mechanisms underlying central sensitisation are complex, occur within both the spinal cord and brain, and can affect inputs from tissues and body regions distant from the affected joint [49–51].

Neurophysiological adaptation in the spinal cord includes windup, through which a series of nociceptive inputs results in progressively increased responsiveness of second-order neurons. A similar phenomenon of temporal summation is augmented in many people with OA, resulting in increased pain severity in response to repeated mechanical stimuli [52]. The time course of temporal summation is much longer (minutes) than windup, and the precise electrophysiological correlate of temporal summation is not fully defined.

Under many circumstances, nociceptive signalling is inhibited within the central nervous system, enabling people to take important defensive action (e.g., escape following acute injury). Descending inhibitory activity may result from another painful stimulus elsewhere in the body (a phenomenon experimentally exploited by testing of conditioned pain modulation (CPM)) and by exercise [53]. Some centrally acting analgesics might further augment these endogenous inhibitory pathways (e.g., duloxetine [54]). People with chronic pain, for example, OA [55] or FM [56], may have reduced capacity for CPM, and deficiencies in endogenous analgesic mechanisms might contribute to pain severity.

Central sensitisation might be driven by ongoing nociceptive input, but can also occur in the absence of any apparent tissue damage, or continue long after any such damage has fully repaired. It makes a major contribution to the pain of FM [57]. Central sensitisation is also, in part, genetically determined [58] and has been associated with high body mass index [59], comorbidities, and systemic inflammation [28], each of which may contribute to arthritis pain. Molecular mechanisms of central sensitisation might include increased neuropeptide and neurotrophin release by primary afferents, and cytokines such as IL-1 released by glial cells within the CNS [60].

27.3.4 Neuropathic Pain

Neuropathic pain results from damage or disease of the nervous system. Neuropathy can contribute to arthritis pain, for example, in RA where wrist synovitis can lead to median nerve entrapment neuropathy or where vasculitis can lead to a mononeuritis multiplex. Joint replacement surgery or arthroscopy can be associated with surgical nerve damage and consequent neuropathic pain. Sensory nerve terminals might be depleted in inflamed synovium [12], and markers of neuronal damage have been localised to dorsal root ganglia in animal models of OA [61].

Neuropathic pain from a variety of diagnoses might share qualities (e.g., burning, shooting), paraesthesiae, or sensory loss, some of which might be shared by musculoskeletal pain. This might reflect shared pain mechanisms rather than necessarily being indicative of actual neuropathy in RA, OA, or FM. Treatments developed for neuropathic pain might yet have benefit for people with arthritis if they target these shared pain mechanisms.

27.4 The Diagnosis of Arthritis Pain

Chronic musculoskeletal pain is defined in the World Health Organisation International Classification of Disease (ICD)-11 as chronic pain arising from a disease process affecting bone, joint, tendon, muscle, spine, or related soft tissue. This definition excludes neuropathic pain, and pain without probable musculoskeletal origin (e.g., FM) is coded as chronic primary pain. Diagnosis of musculoskeletal pain, therefore, depends on demonstrating a musculoskeletal disease process through history, examination, and investigation (Table 27.1).

The often weak relationship between pain and underlying musculoskeletal diagnosis supports the diagnostic classification of pain in its own right [62]. The distinction between arthritis pain due mainly to peripheral factors (nociception) and that due to changes in the nervous system (sensitisation) influences therapeutic recommendations. Active synovitis predicts responses to disease modifying anti-rheumatic drugs (DMARDs) such as methotrexate or TNFα blockers in RA,

Table 27.1 Summary of classification criteria for rheumatoid arthritis, osteoarthritis, and fibromyalgia

Arthritis	Patient history	Physical examination	Investigations
Rheumatoid arthritis [1]	Pain duration >6 weeks Morning stiffness >30 min Systemic symptoms, e.g., fatigue, anorexia	Synovitis Symmetrical joint Involvement Joint deformity (e.g., metacarpophalangeal joint ulnar subluxation) Extra-articular manifestations (e.g., subcutaneous nodules)	*Radiologic* Erosions on radiographs or MRI Synovitis noted by ultrasound or MRI *Serology* ESR or C-reactive protein Rheumatoid factor Anti-CCP antibodies
Osteoarthritis [2–4]	Localised joint pain. Age usually >50y. Morning stiffness <30 min	Palpable bony enlargement/ crepitus Reduced range of movement Joint deformity (e.g., knee varus)	*Radiologic* Joint space narrowing Osteophytes Subchondral cysts and sclerosis *Blood tests* unremarkable
Fibromyalgia [5]	Chronic widespread pain for at least 3 months Associated sleep disturbance, fatigue, poor cognition, depression, non-articular pain (abdominal, headache)	Physical signs not required for diagnosis, although widespread and non-articular tenderness may be present	Limited role mainly to exclude other diagnoses. Diagnosis of fibromyalgia is primarily based on history

and joint damage predicts response to joint replacement surgery, each acting in the periphery. Pain from sensitisation might better respond to treatment that targets the nervous system, including pharmacological and psychological interventions. Mistargeting treatments exposes people to unnecessary risk of adverse events, and displaces opportunities for more effective therapy.

Components of joint pathology and pain mechanisms might be shared between pathological disease categories. Pain due to synovitis, or pain due to subchondral bone pathology, might respond to similar treatments irrespective of whether the patient has RA or OA. Pain augmented by central sensitisation might respond equally to treatments that target central pain mechanisms, irrespective of rheumatological diagnosis. Arthroplasty can relieve joint pain, irrespective of whether the patient has an underlying diagnosis of RA or OA. Management of musculoskeletal pain, therefore, comprises approaches that are targeted to specific pathology, and also to pain mechanisms that are shared between diagnostic groups.

27.4.1 Pain Due to Inflammation

Increased warmth, soft-tissue swelling, and joint effusion each suggest synovitis. Joint stiffness which varies during the day and improves with movement is characteristic of inflammatory pain in RA [6]. Stiffness, may also be a feature of OA pain, although its relation to low level inflammation in OA is uncertain [63, 64]. The feelings of stiffness and swelling might be driven by the central nervous system. RA stiffness might be felt in an amputated limb [65], and people with FM describe joint stiffness and swelling in the absence of demonstrable joint pathology.

Blood tests might indicate systemic evidence of inflammation (e.g., raised erythrocyte sedimentation rate or C-reactive protein in RA), radiographs might demonstrate periarticular osteopenia or erosions in RA, and ultrasound or magnetic resonance imaging might confirm active synovitis. High Doppler signal on ultrasound or gadolinium enhancement of MRI indicate increased blood flow and have been associated both with vasodilation and angiogenesis [66], characteristics of acute and chronic inflammation, respectively. MRI evidence of synovitis may be strongly associated with pain severity even in OA [67], suggesting a direct involvement in pain pathology. Objective evidence of synovitis does not necessarily indicate that it is the current source of pain, although subclinical synovitis might predict subsequent symptomatic flares [68]. Empirical trials of anti-inflammatory treatment might be indicated when a contribution from inflammation to ongoing pain cannot otherwise be excluded.

27.4.2 Pain Due to Structural Changes

Pain on movement or weight bearing suggests biomechanical pain mechanisms. Signs of structural change can include bony swelling or deformity, limited joint mobility, and crepitus, a grating sensation between the joint surfaces, particularly in later stages of OA [64]. Current blood tests have limited value for identifying bone sources of arthritis pain, although raised alkaline phosphatase, evidence of increased osteoblast activity, is characteristic of active Paget's disease of the bone and predicts analgesic response to bisphosphonate treatment in this disease. Bone turnover in RA and OA occurs at a much lower rate than in Paget's disease, but novel bone biomarkers are showing promise for predicting OA pain prognosis [69].

Radiographs might reveal evidence of joint pathology (e.g., bone erosions in RA, osteophytes in OA, and cartilage loss, seen as joint space narrowing, both in RA and in OA). Radiographic erosions and joint-space narrowing are associated with disability in people with longstanding RA [70], although their contribution to reported RA pain might be small [71]. Radiographs are often normal in early disease despite joint pain. MRI can demonstrate internal joint derangements such as meniscal tears, or cartilage defects which are not apparent on plain radiographs. The changes seen in established disease might be more a result of previous repair processes rather than evidence of ongoing disease activity, and therefore often show only a weak association with pain. MRI features such as synovitis and bone marrow lesions, observed in both OA and RA, may be more strongly associated with pain severity than are other radiographic or MRI changes [72], suggesting a more direct involvement in pain mechanisms.

27.4.3 Sensitisation

Sensitisation often occurs alongside peripheral nociceptive drive, and focusing exclusively on synovitis or bone and cartilage changes risks denying people the benefits of treatments that might relieve pain by reducing sensitisation.

Sensitisation may alter the severity, quality, and distribution of pain. Symptoms other than pain might suggest changes within the central nervous systems. Joint pain may be accompanied by impaired body-perception, including reduced proprioceptive acuity [73, 74]. Depression and central sensitisation share biochemical mechanisms and therefore pharmacological approaches. Anxiety and bodily hypervigilance are common in FM, in which autonomic dysfunction and a predominance of sympathetic over parasympathetic function correlates with symptoms of anxiety, palpitations, sleep disturbance, and gastrointestinal disturbance [75, 76].

Questionnaires have been developed to help identify important contributions from central pain mechanisms. The Central Sensitization Inventory (CSI) is a questionnaire that brings together comorbid symptoms that are often associated with central sensitisation, including features of FM, headaches, and irritable bowel syndrome [77]. People with arthritis might have a significant contribution to their pain from central sensitisation even in the absence of comorbid diagnoses, and eight key clinical traits of anxiety, depression, catastrophising, neuropathic-like pain, sleep disturbance, fatigue, widespread pain distribution, and cognitive impact each predicts quantitative sensory testing evidence of central sensitisation in people with knee pain [78].

Tenderness (pain on innocuous light pressure) is characteristic of arthritis pain, and indicative of sensitisation. Peripheral sensitisation, perhaps resulting from inflammation in the joint, contributes to joint line tenderness. Central sensitisation might contribute to tenderness not only at the joint, but also at distant sites [51]. Rarely in arthritis, gentle brushing of the skin might be experienced as pain (dynamic allodynia) [50]. Discordance between joint line tenderness and clinician-observed features of inflammation might suggest central sensitisation in people with RA. Central sensitisation not only deserves treatment in its own right, but also confounds clinical assessment of RA inflammatory disease activity, potentially leading to under- or overestimation of the need for DMARD escalation [79]. Widespread tenderness at non-articular sites (trigger points) is characteristic of FM, although current FM classification and diagnostic criteria do not require the demonstration of positive FM trigger points [5]. The presence of joint line tenderness does not preclude a diagnosis of FM, and the detection of tenderness at non-articular sites does not preclude a diagnosis of OA or RA.

Tenderness is detected clinically using pressure sufficient to make the nail bed blanch. A more standardised stimulus can be provided through quantitative sensory testing. Pressure algometry, using a blunt, 1 cm^2, probe, measures with gradually increasing force when the sensation of pressure changes to that of pain. Pressure pain detection thresholds (PPTs) measured in this way might be reduced in people with RA, OA, or FM [51, 80, 81].

Additional measures of altered central pain processing are currently used in research more than in clinical practice. Other quantitative sensory testing modalities measuring temporal summation [82] or CPM [53] might indicate spinal or descending central sensitisation in people with musculoskeletal pain, although careful attention to methodological detail would be required for sufficient reliability to guide clinical decision making in an individual [82]. Neuroimaging measures of brain volume, function, or connectivity, also indicate changes in central processing [83] although their validity as measures of arthritis pain is uncertain. Brain regions active during arthritis pain also indicate pain localisation, saliency (pain's ability to grab attention), or emotional components, each of which can be shared with non-painful stimuli.

27.4.4 Neuropathic Pain

Questionnaire tools have been developed to aid clinical classification of neuropathic pain, including painDETECT [84]. PainDETECT uses Likert scales for severity of each pain characteristic, and so more severe pain is inevitably more likely to be classified as neuropathic, irrespective of its origin. Furthermore, descriptors such as intermittent or shooting might be interpreted by people with arthritis as the pain they experience on weight bearing or joint movement. Classification questionnaires do not, therefore, confirm the presence of neuropathy, but deserve further investigation as stratification or outcome tools for testing anti-neuropathic analgesics for musculoskeletal pain [85, 86]. Diagnosing neuropathic pain in people with musculoskeletal conditions may require extensive quantitative sensory testing, including sensory detection threshold assessment across a range of stimulus modalities, electrophysiological measurement of nerve conduction, imaging or tissue biopsy.

27.5 Pain Management

Arthritis treatment aims to control pain and maintain quality of life and function. Rapid pain relief may be achieved by directly acting analgesics, or, where inflammation or structural change drives pain, by suppressing inflammation or replacing a damaged joint.

RA, OA, and FM often co-exist [8–10], and comorbid musculoskeletal diagnoses might each contribute to arthritis pain. Treatment directed at only one pain mechanism might not necessarily provide clinically important analgesia. Oversimplifying arthritis pain to describe it as a single problem can result in unrealistic expectations from and consequent dissatisfaction with treatment. Intensive suppression of the immune system might expose people to unnecessary risk of infection, and divert attention from more effective treatments if apparent disease activity in people with RA is attributed to tenderness and pain driven predominantly by central sensitisation. However, the multiple mechanisms of arthritis pain also present multiple treatment opportunities. Multimodal treatments, where necessary, may provide superior benefit to any single treatment alone.

27.5.1 The Context of Effective Arthritis Pain Treatment

Despite the many available treatments, people with arthritis often do not access effective analgesia. Barriers to treatment include unfavourable beliefs about risks and benefits, and social or financial factors. Total hip or knee arthroplasties effectively relieve pain and disability in people with advanced OA, but there are large variations in provision between geographical regions despite similar prevalence of arthritis. The choice to undergo arthroplasty is based not only on symptoms and medical advice, but also on previous experiences of the individual, friends, and family [87]. Different individuals place varying importance on benefit and risks, and appropriate information can enable them to select treatments that match their particular values.

Beliefs about arthritis can influence treatment uptake. A misunderstanding of OA as a condition of 'wear and tear' and belief that chronic, like acute pain, is a 'warning signal' does not sit comfortably with recommendations to exercise. It might not be surprising if patients do not engage in activity if they believe that they are damaging their joints, and particularly if that belief is reinforced by short-term deterioration in pain with exercise. People may be hesitant to use analgesia if they worry it might mask their pain and lead to further damage.

Uncontrolled pain and reduced activity, however, are also harmful, not only causing distress, but deconditioning, social withdrawal, and increased risk of comorbidities, both local to the joint (e.g., weakness, loss of proprioception, contractures) and systemic (e.g., obesity, metabolic syndrome, cardiovascular risk). Exercise remains the cornerstone of evidence-based management for OA and FM, and also in RA can improve long-term pain outcomes [88]. Exercise needs to be sustainable and graded. Pain during exercise might be due to neuronal sensitisation or 'rewiring' of the joint, rather than any indication of ongoing joint damage. The words 'wear and tear' might correctly suggest to the patient a natural process, as opposed to fracture or cancer. However, the arthritic joint is constantly undergoing repair and does not simply wear out in the same way as might a car. Using analgesics to enable activity, far from causing further damage, might facilitate repair and compensatory adaptations.

Approximately one-half of benefit for musculoskeletal pain from any analgesic (pharmacological or non-pharmacological) results from context, rather than the specific properties of the treatment [89]. Contextual (or placebo) effects might be greater with more interventional treatments (e.g., injections compared to tablets), or those entailing contact with 'expert' clinicians. Positive patient expectation is a key mediator of contextual benefit. However, unrealistic expectations can also lead to dissatisfaction with treatment, and overemphasising risk can raise unwarranted concerns and thus undermine patient benefit. Expectations may be low if treatments are repeatedly ineffective or associated with adverse events.

Ideally tailored treatments should ensure that patients have the greatest likelihood of benefit as early in their care pathway as possible. Advice should be personalised, taking account of the individual's pain mechanisms, previous treatment experience, and individual risk. It should explain the underlying causes of arthritis pain, not only verbally, but also by confirmation when the patient experiences benefit from treatment. Treatments should address both immediate and long-term pain, rather than focusing exclusively on either short-term analgesic needs or long-term structural modification.

27.5.2 Pharmacological Management of Arthritis Pain

Pharmacological targets for improving arthritis pain aim to directly inhibit nociceptive transmission, reduce inflammation [90], dampen peripheral and central sensitisation [91, 92], or preserve joint integrity [90, 93]. The World Health Organisation analgesic ladder, although often appropriate for other conditions, should be interpreted with caution in musculoskeletal pain. Opioids might not be 'stronger' analgesics than non-steroidal anti-inflammatory drugs where synovitis is the main cause of pain. Stratification tools are being developed to help inform decisions on which treatments are most likely to offer useful analgesia, but lack sufficient reliability at present to be used in isolation.

27.5.2.1 Reducing Nociceptive Transmission

Nociceptive transmission might be suppressed at any point from the joint to the brain. Centrally acting treatments might have undesirable effects such as impaired cognitive function, nausea or, somnolence, and risk, in the case of opioids, dependency. Novel pharmacological agents targeting the primary nociceptors and unable to cross the blood brain might have advantages. Potential targets with some evidence in at least preclinical studies include sodium, TRPV1, and other ion channels and mechano-transducing molecules [94]. However, analgesics of this type have not has yet achieved key clinical endpoints in randomised controlled trials (RCTs) for musculoskeletal pain.

Nociceptive transmission can also be interrupted by chemical or physical disruption of peripheral nerves. Local anaesthetic can temporarily reduce joint pain when administered into the joint [95] or to local nerve trunks [96]. Benefits might outlive the expected duration of neuronal blockade, possibly in part due to placebo effects, but also perhaps by facilitating joint movement and rehabilitation, or by removing nociceptive drive to the maintenance of central sensitisation. Successful but temporary relief from local anaesthetic might provide diagnostic evidence of the source of musculoskeletal pain, and might predict more long-lasting nerve ablation, for example, by cryoneurolysis [97]. Radiofrequency denervation has been recommended where facet joints might be the source of low back pain [98], although back pain might originate from multiple structures and identification of isolated facet joint pain can be challenging. Unfortunately many joints have multiple, variable, and inaccessible innervations, making local denervation impracticable.

27.5.2.2 Targeting Inflammation

Pharmacological inhibition of inflammation may reduce both pain and joint damage in RA, but disease modification has not been demonstrated in OA. Glucocorticoids, delivered by intra-articular [99], oral [100], or parenteral [101] routes, may provide clinically meaningful and rapid pain relief in RA. Intra-articular glucocorticoid injection can substantially improve also OA pain [102]. Mechanisms by which intra-articular injection helps with OA pain remain uncertain. Benefit depends on accurate placement, but seems unrelated to clinical or imaging evidence of synovitis. Systemic glucocorticoids have not proven beneficial in OA, even in 'inflammatory' subgroups [103]. Benefit from intra-articular glucocorticoids might on average lasts 6 weeks. Repeated intra-articular injection raises concerns of impaired cartilage health, and associated risks of avascular necrosis or infection, as well as posing logistic issues for patients and health care delivery.

A variety of DMARDs can substantially reduce RA inflammation, reduce or prevent joint damage, preserve joint structure and function (Table 27.2). Combination therapies may have greater benefit than any single DMARD alone [104]. Peak analgesic benefit from DMARDs is typically 2–6 weeks after treatment initiation, and other analgesic strategies may be required during this period. DMARDs effective for RA pain have not reliably demonstrated benefit in OA [105].

Table 27.2 Disease modifying anti-rheumatic drugs (DMARDs) used for rheumatoid arthritis

Conventional synthetic DMARDs
Methotrexate
Sulphasalazine
Leflunomide
Hydroxychloroquine
Ciclosporin A
Azathioprine
Targeted Janus kinase inhibitors (e.g., tofacitinib)
Biologic DMARDs
Tumour necrosis factor inhibitors
Adalimumab
Golimumab
Certolizumab pegol
Etanercept
IL-1 receptor inhibitor
Anakinra
IL-6 receptor inhibitor
Tocilizumab
Anti-CD20 monoclonal antibody
Rituximab
CTLA-4-Ig fusion protein
Abatacept

Non-steroidal anti-inflammatory drugs (NSAIDs) inhibit prostaglandin biosynthesis by cyclooxygenases (COX), thereby reducing nociceptor activation and sensitisation, and also crossing the blood–brain barrier to inhibit COX within the central nervous system. NSAIDs might reduce synovitis to a small extent [106], but do not reduce inflammation-associated joint damage in human arthritis. NSAIDs have at least short-term analgesic benefits above placebo in RA [107] or OA [102], but not reliably in FM [108], possibly reflecting an absence of peripheral inflammation in FM. Topical NSAIDs may be useful for knee or hand OA pain [102]. Oral NSAIDs may be more effective than paracetamol for pain in RA [109] or OA [110]. Long-term benefit is difficult to confirm through RCTs, although withdrawal many years after commencing NSAIDs can result in increased pain which is ameliorated by reintroduction of NSAID to a greater extent than with placebo [111].

Adverse events from NSAIDs, in particular risks of gastrointestinal bleeding, cardiovascular events, or renal impairment are important but should not be overstated. Risks are higher with increasing age, and in those with additional risk factors such as comorbidities or use of other medications. In general, NSAID-associated risks persist but do not accumulate with increasing treatment duration. Indeed, risk of cardiovascular events might be highest shortly after NSAID initiation [112]. COX2 selective and non-selective NSAIDs appear equally effective for musculoskeletal pain, although propensity for gastrointestinal adverse events might differ. Gastrointestinal adverse events can be minimised by co-prescription of a proton pump inhibitor.

27.5.2.3 Reducing Sensitisation and Anti-neuropathic Analgesics

Antibodies have recently been developed that bind NGF and prevent its interaction with receptors and thereby inhibit sensitisation of peripheral nociceptors. RCTs of NGF-blocking antibodies have demonstrated consistent and sustained analgesic benefit above placebo in people with OA [39] or low back pain [113]. Rare but significant occurrence of rapidly progressive OA (RPOA) in anti-NGF treated patients has led to risk mitigation strategies being introduced in ongoing clinical trials. The mechanisms of RPOA in people treated with NGF blockers are not fully understood. Interaction with co-administered NSAIDs, and lack of correlation with analgesic potency suggests a possible specific biological effect, rather than an attribution to pain relief per se [37]. The potential for NGF blockade to relieve RA pain has not been explored in humans, although preclinical studies suggest that NGF drives peripheral sensitisation in inflammatory arthritis [38]. NGF is not reported to be upregulated in peripheral tissues in FM. Generalisation of RCT evidence between joint pathologies should be cautious and take account of possible disease-specific adverse events, as well as any benefits.

Several pharmaceuticals can improve neuropathic pain, working through a variety of mechanisms. Different drugs might have differing efficacy for different varieties of neuropathic pain. In the absence of clear demonstration of a neuropathic origin of musculoskeletal pain, empirical evidence of benefit is required for each class of anti-neuropathic analgesic. Negative trials recruiting unselected populations with OA do not necessarily exclude benefit in patient subgroups. Even so, it is unclear whether effective drugs work through the same mechanisms in both neuropathic and musculoskeletal pain. The primary mode of action of anti-neuropathic agents in musculoskeletal pain might be through reducing central sensitisation, for example, by augmenting descending inhibitory control.

Definitive trials of anti-neuropathic agents have not been reported in RA. Topical capsaicin and duloxetine have RCT evidence of analgesic efficacy in OA, although doses of topical capsaicin recommended for OA are lower than those effective for neuropathic pain. Duloxetine may also improve OA pain [114, 115]. Gabapentinoids were not superior to placebo in RCTs of OA hip and knee pain, although a recent study in hand OA suggested analgesic benefit [116]. Anti-neuropathic analgesics might have benefit in FM, including tricyclic antidepressants, selective serotonin, and noradrenaline reuptake inhibitors (e.g., duloxetine), and gabapentinoids [117]. Duloxetine- or tricyclic-induced analgesia is not dependent on their anti-depressant effects.

Central sensitisation might be reversed by removing peripheral nociceptive drive, for example, following joint replacement surgery [55]. The extent to which early suppression of inflammation in RA might prevent or reverse central sensitisation remains uncertain. Features associated with central sensitisation predict poor analgesic responses to DMARDs both in early and in established disease [118]. Evidence of central sensitisation also predicts poor response to total knee arthroplasty for OA [119].

27.5.2.4 Opioids for Musculoskeletal Pain

Despite their undoubted short-term benefits, opioids have not delivered on their promise for the long-term management of musculoskeletal pain. Mu opioid agonists such as morphine reduce the pain of RA or OA, but sustained benefit has been difficult to prove. Many patients do not gain important benefit above what would be achieved from placebo, and many discontinue treatment due to adverse events [120]. Increasing prevalence of medical opioid abuse, particularly reported in the USA, and increasing deaths from prescribed opioid overdose, have contributed to declining popularity as an analgesic strategy. Tolerance remains a possible explanation for an apparent discrepancy between short-term efficacy and long-term benefit. Clinical trials do not support the use of opioids for FM [117]. Several strategies are being explored to improve the benefit that can be achieved from opioid analgesia. Future preparations might have lower addictive or tolerance potential, and co-administration with peripherally-restricted opioid antagonists might lessen some adverse events such as opioid-induced constipation [121].

27.5.2.5 Other Analgesics

Paracetamol is commonly recommended for arthritis pain, although evidence is sparse from RCTs for any benefit [122]. Paracetamol was used long before the standardisation of RCT methodologies, it is extremely inexpensive, and it might be questioned what benefit would result from retrospectively developing the evidence base for its continued use. However, paracetamol has a narrow therapeutic window, risking hepatotoxicity only just above the recommended daily dose, and recent data suggest decreases in haemoglobin with paracetamol usage [123]. Paracetamol's widespread availability and low cost might reduce its potential for placebo analgesia.

Nefopam is a non-opioid analgesic with some evidence of benefit for musculoskeletal pain [124]. Its mechanism of action is uncertain, but might include inhibition of serotonin, norepinephrine, and dopamine reuptake, and might reduce glutamate signalling [125]. Its use can be limited by adverse events such as nausea, and caution should be exercised in people on antidepressant medications or susceptible to epilepsy. Cognitive adverse events are not uncommon, particularly in the frail and elderly.

Tramadol and tapentadol have opioid properties, but also inhibit norepinephrine reuptake. Initially noted to have greater analgesic efficacy at lower dose than mu opioid agonists, and thought to have less potential for abuse, tramadol is now the commonest prescribed drug of abuse in the USA. Cannabinoids have also been used for arthritis pain, although evidence for clinical benefit is weak [126].

27.5.3 Non-Pharmacological Arthritis Pain Management

Drugs alone are unlikely to cure arthritis pain, and multimodal, often multidisciplinary approaches are recommended. Exercise, orthotic, psychological or surgical approaches should be considered, alone or together with medications. Interdisciplinary working might improve access to multiple treatment modalities, particularly where specialists are scarce. CBT-informed treatments have been successfully delivered by physiotherapists or other allied health professionals. Non-pharmacological approaches may be considered 'complex interventions'. Careful selection of control interventions and attention to patient blinding are needed to avoid bias in RCTs.

27.5.3.1 Physical Therapies

Exercise remains the cornerstone of evidence-based management for OA and FM, and also in RA can improve long-term pain outcomes [88]. Direct comparisons in RCTs have not shown clear superiority for analgesia from any one exercise modality over another [127]. Physiotherapists combine multiple modalities matched to the individual patient's needs, ensuring that prescribed exercise is both acceptable and sustainable. Exercise might reduce mechanical factors that contribute to activity pain, for example, by balancing quadriceps strength and restoring normal patellar tracking in the femoral groove, or by restoring range of movement. Impaired proprioception and postural stability are common to RA [128], OA [73], and FM [129], and might in part be driven by changes in central processing of afferent signals associated with joint pain. Proprioceptive deficits might predispose to injury (for example, when the knee 'gives way') and can be ameliorated by physiotherapy. Loss of aerobic fitness can be associated with increased pain sensitivity [130], and aerobic exercise can reduce central sensitisation [131] and arthritis pain. Similar analgesic benefits between different exercise modalities might reflect large contributions from contextual factors, including more general lifestyle advice and cognitive reassurance.

Orthoses might reduce arthritis pain, by resting the affected joint or by adjusting biomechanical forces. Prolonged bed rest is not recommended, but resting splints might be helpful for active synovitis in the hands. Knee orthoses might facilitate optimal patellar tracking, or correct for valgus or varus instability. Shoe inserts might redistribute forces, for example, away from painful metatarsophalangeal joints (metatarsal bars), or prevent deformation during loading (e.g., medial longitudinal arch supports). Orthoses might aim to increase activity and be supplemented by strengthening and mobilisation exercises. Orthoses are not recommended for FM, where normal rather than abnormal biomechanical forces lead to musculoskeletal pain.

27.5.3.2 Psychological Approaches

A variety of psychological approaches can be helpful in the management of arthritis pain. In particular, cognitive behavioural therapy (CBT) may be useful in RA [107], OA [102], and FM [117]. CBT aims to change beliefs, build successful behaviours and coping strategies, and thereby improve quality of life. Psychological approaches address the wider impact of chronic pain, including anxiety, depression, cognitive function, sleep disturbance, and fatigue. Improvements during recent years in understanding the psychological factors in chronic pain have led to refinements in psychological approaches, addressing fear avoidance beliefs and developing acceptance and commitment therapy (ACT). Within such a fluid therapeutic environment, testing each protocol modification by RCT is not feasible. There is a widespread presumption of transferability of effectiveness from one diagnosis to another in the absence of specific RCT assessment of each modality in each disease. CBT may be of benefit irrespective of the duration of arthritis pain, although areas of concern to the patient might differ between early and established disease.

Psychological factors might be barriers to engagement with other effective treatments. Fear avoidance might reduce adherence with exercise recommendations, unhelpful beliefs might reduce analgesic use, and low mood and hopelessness may reduce motivation to engage in treatment. Accepting pain as an inevitable consequence of their diagnosis, or of getting older, might divert people unnecessarily from effective treatment. CBT does not directly change joint pathology, although adherence to disease modifying treatments might be a benefit.

Psychological interventions are appropriately developed by experts in the field, and initial evidence of benefit is often derived from RCTs in which treatment is delivered by specialists. Such stand-alone intervention might prove difficult to deliver, and might detract from other interventions that should be offered concurrently. Multidisciplinary intervention might be ideal but is resource intensive. Multidisciplinary working takes advantage of multiple practitioners, each specialist in their own area, but working in partnership as a coherent and synergistic team. Interdisciplinary working may be more feasible, and provision of psychologically based interventions by nurses or physiotherapists has become commonplace. Whether these approaches replicate (or even enhance) the benefit demonstrated for specialist-delivered psychological interventions remains to be proven.

27.5.3.3 Surgical Approaches

Arthroplasty is recommended for people with OA or RA with severe, persistent pain, and joint damage, pain that is not responsive to conservative measures. Other surgical approaches to relieve pain by altering joint biomechanics include fusion and tibial osteotomy. Possible analgesic benefits of tissue engineering, aiming to restore articular cartilage integrity, are the subject of ongoing clinical trials [132].

Total hip or knee replacement remains amongst the most effective of all treatments to improve quality of life. The benefits of total joint replacement for people with RA might exceed those even in OA [133]. How arthroplasty relieves pain remains incompletely understood. Bone, cartilage, and knee menisci are removed along with any nerve terminals in those tissues. The prosthetic joint transmits weight bearing forces directly to diaphyseal bone and provides a physical barrier preventing mediators from the synovial cavity accessing subchondral nerves.

Despite the overall success of arthroplasty, up to 20% of patients may have persistent disabling pain after total knee replacement [134]. Mechanisms of post-surgical pain might include problems with the joint (e.g., biomechanical factors, sepsis), or intra-operative nerve damage. Pain may be referred from outside the joint (e.g., from the back or hip). Central sensitisation might contribute to persistent post-surgical pain, even though for many people central sensitisation is ameliorated following joint replacement [135].

Risk factors for persistent post-arthroplasty pain include low mood, anxiety [136], and fear avoidance [137], possibly indicating barriers to effective post-surgical rehabilitation. Relative preservation of joint space on radiographs [138] and quantitative sensory testing evidence of central sensitisation [135] also predict poor outcomes, suggesting preoperative pain mechanisms not directly addressed by replacing the joint. Arthroplasty should not be offered for FM where joint structure is normal.

27.5.4 Addressing Comorbidities

Musculoskeletal diagnoses often co-exist. Attributing arthritis pain to a single mechanism can result in unrealistic expectations from and consequent dissatisfaction with treatment. Arthroplasty in OA, and DMARDs in RA may be less effective at relieving pain in people with comorbid FM, but are no less associated with adverse events. Non-musculoskeletal comorbidities also may exacerbate arthritis pain and be barriers to benefit from otherwise effective treatments. Effective weight reduction strategies, including behavioural, dietary, and surgical, might each reduce OA knee pain [139, 140]. Although often explained in terms of reduced biomechanical load on the affected joint, other mechanisms link weight and pain reduction, including changes in physical activity, psychosocial factors, and modulation of pain processing by adipokines. Diabetes mellitus is also associated with worse musculoskeletal pain [141]. People using anti-hypertensive agents other than beta blockers may report more severe pain [142], and comorbid conditions may preclude the use of specific analgesics. Treatments should ideally help both musculoskeletal pain and comorbid conditions. Treating comorbidities might affect pain processing, remove barriers to treatment, and reduce the personal impact of pain.

Joint hypermobility has been associated with musculoskeletal pain [143, 144], and comorbid hypermobility might moderate treatment recommendations. Hypermobility is attributable to genetic variation in connective tissue genes, for example, fibrillin-1 in Marfan syndrome [145], although specific genetic variants might not be identified in the more common joint hypermobility syndrome. Joint mobility can be increased by exercises, for example during ballet training. Hypermobility is often identified in childhood, and joint mobility tends to decrease with age. Hypermobility can be assessed using the Beighton score on clinical examination of nine joint regions; thumb apposition to the flexor aspect of the forearm, little finger, elbow and knee hyperextension, and palms to floor with knees extended. Specific investigations may seek specific clinical syndromes (e.g., Marfan or Ehlers–Danlos syndrome), particularly where monitoring may be indicated to reduce risk of serious medical complications such as aortic root dilatation. Genetic testing may be useful where there is a strong family history, although even Marfan syndrome may be caused by complex and multiple genetic variants. In hypermobility, excessive joint movement beyond the normal range may occur without initiating nociceptive pain, suggesting blunted mechanotransduction, perhaps attributable to altered interaction between sensory nerve terminals and connective tissues. Articular pain in hypermobility may share features with FM, with evidence of central sensitisation, and therefore might respond to treatments recommended for FM. However, exercise in people with hypermobility should not aim to further increase joint range of movement.

27.6 Prognosis

The prognosis of musculoskeletal disease has improved substantially during the past century, following, for example, the introduction of arthroplasty, and more recently for RA, biologic agents. People no longer necessarily expect disability and reduced participation to accompany advancing age. However, RA, OA, and FM do not have known cures, and treatment aims to control pain and pathology, whilst accepting that underlying disease persists and might reactivate. Musculoskeletal pain remains a major challenge.

Musculoskeletal pain has a variable course [146]. Early OA pain is characteristically intermittent, and people with RA, OA, or FM each reports periods of relative well-being interspersed with symptomatic flares [20]. Averaged pain scores across a disease population might suggest relentless pain progression, but conceal subgroups who do very well. Prognosis varies according to joint groups involved by OA, with hip or knee disease displaying often worse prognosis than hand OA, although nodal hand OA not infrequently causes persistent pain and disability [147]. Of people with RA who satisfy FM classification criteria at one time, 75% might no longer do so after a further year, although for many FM recurs [9].

Obesity may predict both OA incidence [148] and worse pain prognosis [149], but other risk factors for pain progression often differ from those predicting incident disease. Family history predicts increased risk of developing RA, OA, or FM, but family members with the same condition can display widely different disease courses. Age and sex seem to play a greater role in disease incidence than in pain prognosis. Psychological factors might not predict RA or OA disease incidence, but predict poor pain prognosis.

Predictors of pain might differ from those for structural damage. Seropositivity for rheumatoid factor or citrullinated peptides, and radiographic erosions at presentation each has predicted poor structural outcomes in RA, but not necessarily poor pain prognosis [118]. Radiographic OA heralds a worse pain prognosis in people with early knee pain [150], but improvement in OA pain is common even if joint structure does not change. Conversely, pain prognosis in FM is often poor, despite an absence of structural joint damage. Early, effective DMARD therapy in people with a poor structural prognosis might have reduced the predictive value of inflammatory biomarkers for pain in RA. Synovitis, however, might still predict poor pain prognosis in OA [67, 151], where disease modifying treatments are not yet available.

Pain prognosis is predicted by factors shared across RA, OA, or FM. Anxiety [152], depression [153], and high pain catastrophisation [154] each might predict persistent or worsening pain. Pain at multiple sites also heralds a worse functional prognosis, but not necessarily increasing pain in the index joint [155]. Quantitative sensory testing evidence of central sensitisation also predicts worse pain outcomes in people undergoing treatment [155–157].

Multiple biomarkers might need to be combined to accurately predict pain prognosis. Many risk factors are inter-correlated, and some factors might be more strongly associated with prognosis than are others. Structural change and ultrasound-detected synovitis each predicted knee pain prognosis in one community cohort after adjustment for each other, although structural change appeared to have the greater effect [150]. The strongest predictor of pain prognosis is often pain itself, but developing predictive algorithms that indicate treatable mediators of pain progression should better guide treatments to those who are most likely to gain long-term benefit.

27.7 Case Report 1

A female patient, 62 years of age, presented with worsening left knee pain over the past 4 months. She had had knee pain throughout the past 2 years. Her mother had suffered similar problems, so she took it as hereditary and until now had 'just put up with it'. She was known to suffer from longstanding anxiety, FM, and irritable bowel syndrome, as well as mild chronic obstructive pulmonary disease, which was well controlled at the time of presentation.

She was obese, with a BMI of 33, and worried about diabetes. She avoided exercise or vigorous physical activity because she was uncomfortable with her body appearance, she did not enjoy exercise, and she became short of breath with moderate exertion and had pain in her left knee, but also in the right knee and ankles, after only a short period of exercise. Knee pain significantly limited her walking, and when she tried to persevere she experienced muscle aches and fatigue. There had been no trauma that she could recall; the onset of the left knee pain was gradual. Her sleep was disturbed by pain. She was increasingly worried about how her pain was getting worse, and the impact this could have on her independence. Her anxiety had been poorly controlled over the few weeks before the consultation.

Physical Examination on presentation revealed mild bony enlargement and mild crepitus on passive flexion of her knees, each most marked on the left. She reported knee pain on single leg weight bearing and on mini-squat, again worse on the left. She displayed a full range of pain-free hip movements, near normal spinal examination, but some tenderness on palpation of paravertebral and major limb muscles.

The *impression* from the initial examination was of slowly progressing knee OA, worse on the left. The *treatment* plan included paracetamol, a topical non-steroidal anti-inflammatory cream, referral for physiotherapy, and advice on weight reduction. *Investigations* aimed to exclude an inflammatory arthritis; blood tests were unremarkable including a normal C-reactive protein.

At *review*, 2 months after the initial consultation, her knee pain had worsened. Her gastrointestinal symptoms, fatigue, and anxiety were equally worse. She had not continued with the physiotherapy because it was 'too painful the following day'. Her walking ability had decreased to 400 m before having to stop, feeling more breathless as well as more pain and fatigue. Findings on physical examination were unchanged from presentation.

Discussion Initial treatment followed best-practice guidelines for knee OA, but unfortunately this does not guarantee sustained benefit. Although her short-term response was good, a more long-term treatment plan was now required. A further injection might provide another window of opportunity for commencing exercise, but frequently repeated injections might risk harm, and a more sustained analgesic approach is important to enable exercise and activity. If she did not respond to conservative treatment over the following few months, surgery might be indicated.

Management She chose to have her knee injected, and her topical NSAID was changed to naproxen with a proton pump inhibitor as gastroprotection. Knee radiography was arranged to inform future discussion on possible surgery, and showed small osteophytes and some medial tibiofemoral joint space narrowing, similar in both knees.

Progress Symptoms improved for the ensuing 6 months, and she engaged with community physiotherapy and with paced exercise. Her left knee pain resolved and she noticed limited, although significant, improvements in gastrointestinal symptoms, dyspnoea, anxiety, and sleep. Her weight remained stable. She was engaging in similar social activities as at presentation, but now able to enjoy them. The improvement gave her confidence in the diagnosis and treatment of knee OA.

Six months later her pain deteriorated again, as did her anxiety, sleep disruption, and gastrointestinal symptoms, and she requested a repeat injection. She was well motivated to remain active if her pain could be settled.

Discussion included the relative potential for benefit from and risks of different treatment modalities: repeat glucocorticoid injection, surgery, and multidisciplinary pain management. Frequent injections might risk compromising joint health, and this should be balanced against the temporary benefit which she had experienced with the previous injection. She displayed several potentially adverse prognostic factors for knee arthroplasty, including anxiety, widespread pain and other features suggesting central sensitisation, high BMI, and preserved joint space on recent radiographs, although these would not necessarily preclude benefit from surgery. The patient herself had noticed the links between her symptoms of OA, FM, irritable bowel syndrome, and anxiety and was keen to understand this more to help her to manage her symptoms.

27.8 Case Report 2

A 33-year-old teacher presented with a 12- week history of pain and swelling affecting wrists, second and third metacarpophalangeal joints of both hands and her left knee. Regular ibuprofen, obtained from the chemist, had provided only limited relief. Her maternal aunt had RA. Examination revealed 7 swollen and 17 tender joints from a 28-joint count, and she rated the impact of her arthritis on her general well-being during the past week as 78 mm on a 100 mm scale from 'best imaginable' to 'worst imaginable' health. Her joint symptoms were making her feel low, she was anxious about her future, and reported that her joint pain was making it difficult to sleep and she was feeling tired all day. Blood tests provided by her GP demonstrated normal full blood profile except for a slightly raised platelet count. C-reactive protein (56 mg/l) and erythrocyte sedimentation rate (75 mm/h) were both substantially raised. She had a strongly positive rheumatoid factor and anti-citrullinated peptide antibodies, but negative anti-nuclear antibodies. Radiographs of hand and feet demonstrate the soft-tissue swelling plus juxta-articular osteopenia. A diagnosis of early RA was made.

Management She was treated with an intramuscular injection of methylprednisolone (120 mg) to provide rapid symptom relief, and started on combination therapy with methotrexate (increasing to 20 mg orally once per week), sulphasalazine (increasing to 1 g twice daily) plus hydroxychloroquine (initially 400 mg daily).

Discussion This patient had severe symptoms and several poor prognostic indicators for outcome of her RA in that she was strongly seropositive, had high inflammatory markers, and a large number of involved joints. Radiographic erosions at presentation would also have indicated a poor prognosis, but are not uncommonly absent within the first few weeks since the symptom onset.

At *review* in the hospital clinic 12 weeks later, she reported that she had felt better after the steroid injection and was able to get back to work, but after 3 weeks the pain had again deteriorated and she had by then been on sick leave for the past 8 weeks. She described joint stiffness lasting 2 h in the morning, she had been arguing with the children who did not understand why she could not do the things she used to with them, and requested a further steroid injection. On examination, the doctor found her knee to be still swollen, and 19 of the 28 joints examined were tender. She rated the impact of her arthritis on her general health over the past week as 82 mm on the 100 mm scale. C-reactive protein was 10 g/l and ESR 23 mm/h. Sulphasalazine and hydroxychloroquine were discontinued, and anti-TNF therapy commenced in combination with her methotrexate. She received a further intramuscular injection of 120 mg methylprednisolone.

At *review* 12 weeks later, she complained of being severely affected by joint pains, morning stiffness lasting 2 h with lack of energy, and difficulty doing even light tasks. Her sleep was disturbed and she needed to rest during the day. She reported that she felt worse than when she was first given the diagnosis of RA. Work had proved impossible and she therefore had given up her job. Examination, however, did not reveal any swollen joints, although her tender joint count remained high (26/28), with tenderness at non-articular sites. ESR and CRP were now normal, but her arthritis was still having a major impact on her life.

Discussion This lady is describing features consistent with central sensitisation and satisfies classification criteria for FM. Indeed she already displayed features of FM at presentation (a substantial excess of tender over swollen joints, fatigue, sleep, and mood disturbance), although she and her clinician interpreted these as being a natural consequence of inflammatory disease activity. These clinical features suggested a poor pain prognosis with treatments that suppress inflammation alone and a more holistic approach might have been indicated earlier in the care pathway. Management should aim to maintain normal physical and social function, and early changes to employment may be difficult to reverse.

27.9 Summary

RA, OA, and FM are common disabling and distressing conditions illustrating the production, amplification, and maintenance of pain by inflammation, altered joint structure, and central pain mechanisms. Nociception, peripheral sensitisation and central sensitisation determine pain quality and severity, persistence or resolution, and the discordance sometimes apparent between reported pain and observed evidence of disease. Pain mechanisms are shared between diagnostic groups, and pain diagnosis complements disease diagnosis to inform management. Addressing joint pathology might not alone resolve pain, and analgesia should complement treatments that might retard structural disease progression. Multimodal approaches are recommended to achieve both short- and long-term pain relief, each intervention delivered within an optimised therapeutic context. Systemic or locally administered pharmaceuticals might reduce nociceptive transmission, inflammation, sensitisation, or future structural damage. Non-pharmacological interventions include exercise, orthotics, psychological and surgical approaches. Addressing comorbidities can improve pain and remove barriers to effective treatment. Musculoskeletal pain prognosis is highly variable and difficult to predict. Pain can continue over many years, punctuated by acute episodes or flares, although often with periods of relative or even absolute remission. With optimal treatment, pain progression is not inevitable.

References

1. Neogi T, Aletaha D, Silman AJ, Naden RL, Felson DT, Aggarwal R, et al. The 2010 American College of Rheumatology/European League Against Rheumatism classification criteria for rheumatoid arthritis: phase 2 methodological report. Arthritis Rheum. 2010;62(9):2582–91.
2. Altman R, Asch E, Bloch D, Bole G, Borenstein D, Brandt K, et al. Development of criteria for the classification and reporting of osteoarthritis. Classification of osteoarthritis of the knee. Diagnostic and therapeutic criteria committee of the American Rheumatism Association. Arthritis Rheum. 1986;29(8):1039–49.
3. Altman R, Alarcon G, Appelrouth D, Bloch D, Borenstein D, Brandt K, et al. The American College of Rheumatology criteria for the classification and reporting of osteoarthritis of the hip. Arthritis Rheum. 1991;34(5):505–14.
4. Altman R, Alarcon G, Appelrouth D, Bloch D, Borenstein D, Brandt K, et al. The American College of Rheumatology criteria for the classification and reporting of osteoarthritis of the hand. Arthritis Rheum. 1990;33(11):1601–10.
5. Wolfe F, Clauw DJ, Fitzcharles MA, Goldenberg DL, Hauser W, Katz RL, et al. 2016 Revisions to the 2010/2011 fibromyalgia diagnostic criteria. Semin Arthritis Rheum. 2016;46(3):319–29.
6. Rindfleisch JA, Muller D. Diagnosis and management of rheumatoid arthritis. Am Fam Physician. 2005;72(6):1037–47.
7. Phillips K, Clauw DJ. Central pain mechanisms in the rheumatic diseases: future directions. Arthritis Rheum. 2013;65(2):291–302.
8. McWilliams DF, Marshall M, Jayakumar K, Doherty S, Doherty M, Zhang W, et al. Erosive and osteoarthritic structural progression in early rheumatoid arthritis. Rheumatology (Oxford). 2016;55(8):1477–88.
9. Wolfe F, Hauser W, Hassett AL, Katz RS, Walitt BT. The development of fibromyalgia–I: examination of rates and predictors in patients with rheumatoid arthritis (RA). Pain. 2011;152(2):291–9.
10. Brummett CM, Urquhart AG, Hassett AL, Tsodikov A, Hallstrom BR, Wood NI, et al. Characteristics of fibromyalgia independently predict poorer long-term analgesic outcomes following total knee and hip arthroplasty. Arthritis Rheumatol. 2015;67(5):1386–94.
11. Gronblad M, Konttinen YT, Korkala O, Liesi P, Hukkanen M, Polak JM. Neuropeptides in synovium of patients with rheumatoid arthritis and osteoarthritis. J Rheumatol. 1988;15(12):1807–10.
12. Mapp PI, Kidd BL, Gibson SJ, Terry JM, Revell PA, Ibrahim NB, et al. Substance P-, calcitonin gene-related peptide- and C-flanking peptide of neuropeptide Y-immunoreactive fibres are present in normal synovium but depleted in patients with rheumatoid arthritis. Neuroscience. 1990;37(1):143–53.
13. Suri S, Walsh DA. Osteochondral alterations in osteoarthritis. Bone. 2012;51(2):204–11.
14. Ashraf S, Wibberley H, Mapp PI, Hill R, Wilson D, Walsh DA. Increased vascular penetration and nerve growth in the meniscus: a potential source of pain in osteoarthritis. Ann Rheum Dis. 2011;70(3):523–9.
15. Heppelmann B, McDougall JJ. Inhibitory effect of amiloride and gadolinium on fine afferent nerves in the rat knee: evidence of mechanogated ion channels in joints. Exp Brain Res. 2005;167(1):114–8.
16. Levick JR. An investigation into the validity of subatmospheric pressure recordings from synovial fluid and their dependence on joint angle. J Physiol. 1979;289:55–67.
17. Jayson MI, St Dixon AJ. Intra-articular pressure in rheumatoid arthritis of the knee. I. Pressure changes during passive joint distension. Ann Rheum Dis. 1970;29(3):261–5.
18. Andrew BL, Dodt E. The deployment of sensory nerve endings at the knee joint of the cat. Acta Physiol Scand. 1953;28(4):8287–96.
19. Ferrell WR, Nade S, Newbold PJ. The interrelation of neural discharge, intra-articular pressure, and joint angle in the knee of the dog. J Physiol. 1986;373:353–65.

20. Hawker GA, Davis AM, French MR, Cibere J, Jordan JM, March L, et al. Development and preliminary psychometric testing of a new OA pain measure–an OARSI/OMERACT initiative. Osteoarthr Cartil. 2008;16(4):409–14.
21. Lo GH, McAlindon TE, Niu J, Zhang Y, Beals C, Dabrowski C, et al. Bone marrow lesions and joint effusion are strongly and independently associated with weight-bearing pain in knee osteoarthritis: data from the osteoarthritis initiative. Osteoarthr Cartil. 2009;17(12):1562–9.
22. Herbert MK, Just H, Schmidt RF. Histamine excites groups III and IV afferents from the cat knee joint depending on their resting activity. Neurosci Lett. 2001;305(2):95–8.
23. Birrell GJ, McQueen DS, Iggo A, Grubb BD. The effects of 5-HT on articular sensory receptors in normal and arthritic rats. Br J Pharmacol. 1990;101(3):715–21.
24. Kelly DC, Asghar AU, Marr CG, McQueen DS. Nitric oxide modulates articular sensory discharge and responsiveness to bradykinin in normal and arthritic rats in vivo. Neuroreport. 2001;12(1):121–5.
25. Kanaka R, Schaible HG, Schmidt RF. Activation of fine articular afferent units by bradykinin. Brain Res. 1985;327(1-2):81–90.
26. Neugebauer V, Schaible HG, Schmidt RF. Sensitization of articular afferents to mechanical stimuli by bradykinin. Pflugers Arch. 1989;415(3):330–5.
27. Brouwers H, von Hegedus J, Toes R, Kloppenburg M, Ioan-Facsinay A. Lipid mediators of inflammation in rheumatoid arthritis and osteoarthritis. Baillieres Best Pract Res Clin Rheumatol. 2015;29(6):741–55.
28. Walsh DA, McWilliams DF. Mechanisms, impact and management of pain in rheumatoid arthritis. Nat Rev Rheumatol. 2014;10(10):581–92.
29. Malfait AM, Schnitzer TJ. Towards a mechanism-based approach to pain management in osteoarthritis. Nat Rev Rheumatol. 2013;9(11):654–64.
30. Huang J, Burston JJ, Li L, Ashraf S, Mapp PI, Bennett AJ, et al. Targeting the D Series resolvin receptor system for the treatment of osteoarthritis pain. Arthritis Rheumatol. 2017;69(5):996–1008.
31. England S, Bevan S, Docherty RJ. PGE2 modulates the tetrodotoxin-resistant sodium current in neonatal rat dorsal root ganglion neurons via the cyclic AMP-protein kinase A cascade. J Physiol. 1996;495(Pt 2):429–40.
32. Gold MS, Reichling DB, Shuster MJ, Levine JD. Hyperalgesic agents increase a tetrodotoxin-resistant Na+ current in nociceptors. Proc Natl Acad Sci U S A. 1996;93(3):1108–12.
33. Horvath A, Tekus V, Boros M, Pozsgai G, Botz B, Borbely E, et al. Transient receptor potential ankyrin 1 (TRPA1) receptor is involved in chronic arthritis: in vivo study using TRPA1-deficient mice. Arthritis Res Ther. 2016;18:6.
34. Alawi KM, Russell FA, Aubdool AA, Srivastava S, Riffo-Vasquez Y, Baldissera L Jr, et al. Transient receptor potential canonical 5 (TRPC5) protects against pain and vascular inflammation in arthritis and joint inflammation. Ann Rheum Dis. 2017;76(1):252–60.
35. Varga A, Nemeth J, Szabo A, McDougall JJ, Zhang C, Elekes K, et al. Effects of the novel TRPV1 receptor antagonist SB366791 in vitro and in vivo in the rat. Neurosci Lett. 2005;385(2):137–42.
36. Laslett LL, Jones G. Capsaicin for osteoarthritis pain. Prog Drug Res. 2014;68:277–91.
37. Jayabalan P, Schnitzer TJ. Tanezumab in the treatment of chronic musculoskeletal conditions. Expert Opin Biol Ther. 2017;17(2):245–54.
38. Ashraf S, Bouhana KS, Pheneger J, Andrews SW, Walsh DA. Selective inhibition of tropomyosin-receptor-kinase A (TrkA) reduces pain and joint damage in two rat models of inflammatory arthritis. Arthritis Res Ther. 2016;18(1):97.
39. Schnitzer TJ, Marks JA. A systematic review of the efficacy and general safety of antibodies to NGF in the treatment of OA of the hip or knee. Osteoarthr Cartil. 2015;23(Suppl 1):S8–17.
40. Phillips K, Clauw DJ. Central pain mechanisms in chronic pain states–maybe it is all in their head. Best Pract Res Clin Rheumatol. 2011;25(2):141–54.
41. Yunus MB. Role of central sensitization in symptoms beyond muscle pain, and the evaluation of a patient with widespread pain. Best Pract Res Clin Rheumatol. 2007;21(3):481–97.

42. Curatolo M, Arendt-Nielsen L, Petersen-Felix S. Central hypersensitivity in chronic pain: mechanisms and clinical implications. Phys Med Rehabil Clin N Am. 2006;17(2):287–302.
43. Campbell CM, Buenaver LF, Finan P, Bounds SC, Redding M, McCauley L, et al. Sleep, pain catastrophizing, and central sensitization in knee osteoarthritis patients with and without insomnia. Arthritis Care Res (Hoboken). 2015;67(10):1387–96.
44. Lee YC, Lu B, Edwards RR, Wasan AD, Nassikas NJ, Clauw DJ, et al. The role of sleep problems in central pain processing in rheumatoid arthritis. Arthritis Rheum. 2013;65(1):59–68.
45. Wieseler-Frank J, Maier SF, Watkins LR. Immune-to-brain communication dynamically modulates pain: physiological and pathological consequences. Brain Behav Immun. 2005;19(2):104–11.
46. Meeus M, Nijs J. Central sensitization: a biopsychosocial explanation for chronic widespread pain in patients with fibromyalgia and chronic fatigue syndrome. Clin Rheumatol. 2007;26(4):465–73.
47. Melzack R, Coderre TJ, Katz J, Vaccarino AL. Central neuroplasticity and pathological pain. Ann N Y Acad Sci. 2001;933:157–74.
48. Valdes AM, Warner SC, Harvey HL, Fernandes GS, Doherty S, Jenkins W, et al. Use of prescription analgesic medication and pain catastrophizing after total joint replacement surgery. Semin Arthritis Rheum. 2015;45(2):150–5.
49. Hochman JR, Davis AM, Elkayam J, Gagliese L, Hawker GA. Neuropathic pain symptoms on the modified painDETECT correlate with signs of central sensitization in knee osteoarthritis. Osteoarthr Cartil. 2013;21(9):1236–42.
50. Hochman JR, French MR, Bermingham SL, Hawker GA. The nerve of osteoarthritis pain. Arthritis Care Res (Hoboken). 2010;62(7):1019–23.
51. Suokas AK, Walsh DA, McWilliams DF, Condon L, Moreton B, Wylde V, et al. Quantitative sensory testing in painful osteoarthritis: a systematic review and meta-analysis. Osteoarthr Cartil. 2012;20(10):1075–85.
52. Arendt-Nielsen L, Yarnitsky D, Arendt-Nielsen L, Yarnitsky D. Experimental and clinical applications of quantitative sensory testing applied to skin, muscles and viscera. J Pain. 2009;10(6):556–72.
53. Fingleton C, Smart KM, Doody CM. Exercise-induced hypoalgesia in people with knee osteoarthritis with normal and abnormal conditioned pain modulation. Clin J Pain. 2017;33(5):395–404.
54. Bannister K, Patel R, Goncalves L, Townson L, Dickenson AH. Diffuse noxious inhibitory controls and nerve injury: restoring an imbalance between descending monoamine inhibitions and facilitations. Pain. 2015;156(9):1803–11.
55. Kosek E, Ordeberg G. Lack of pressure pain modulation by heterotopic noxious conditioning stimulation in patients with painful osteoarthritis before, but not following, surgical pain relief. Pain. 2000;88(1):69–78.
56. Lautenbacher S, Rollman GB. Possible deficiencies of pain modulation in fibromyalgia. Clin J Pain. 1997;13(3):189–96.
57. Sluka KA, Clauw DJ. Neurobiology of fibromyalgia and chronic widespread pain. Neuroscience. 2016;338:114–29.
58. Hermans L, Van Oosterwijck J, Goubert D, Goudman L, Crombez G, Calders P, et al. Inventory of personal factors influencing conditioned pain modulation in healthy people: a systematic literature review. Pain Pract. 2016;16(6):758–69.
59. de Kruijf M, Peters MJ, L CJ, Tiemeier H, Nijsten T, Hofman A, et al. Determinants for quantitative sensory testing and the association with chronic musculoskeletal pain in the general elderly population. Pain Pract. 2016;16(7):831–41.
60. Nieto FR, Clark AK, Grist J, Hathway GJ, Chapman V, Malcangio M. Neuron-immune mechanisms contribute to pain in early stages of arthritis. J Neuroinflammation. 2016;13(1):96.
61. Thakur M, Rahman W, Hobbs C, Dickenson AH, Bennett DL. Characterisation of a peripheral neuropathic component of the rat monoiodoacetate model of osteoarthritis. PLoS ONE. 2012;7(3):e33730.

62. Treede RD, Rief W, Barke A, Aziz Q, Bennett MI, Benoliel R, et al. A classification of chronic pain for ICD-11. Pain. 2015;156(6):1003–7.
63. Hinton R, Moody RL, Davis AW, Thomas SF. Osteoarthritis: diagnosis and therapeutic considerations. Am Fam Physician. 2002;65(5):841–8.
64. Punzi L, Oliviero F, Plebani M. New biochemical insights into the pathogenesis of osteoarthritis and the role of laboratory investigations in clinical assessment. Crit Rev Clin Lab Sci. 2005;42(4):279–309.
65. Haigh RC, McCabe CS, Halligan PW, Blake DR. Joint stiffness in a phantom limb: evidence of central nervous system involvement in rheumatoid arthritis. Rheumatology (Oxford). 2003;42(7):888–92.
66. Taylor PC. VEGF and imaging of vessels in rheumatoid arthritis. Arthritis Res. 2002;4(Suppl 3):S99–107.
67. Hill CL, Hunter DJ, Niu J, Clancy M, Guermazi A, Genant H, et al. Synovitis detected on magnetic resonance imaging and its relation to pain and cartilage loss in knee osteoarthritis. Ann Rheum Dis. 2007;66(12):1599–603.
68. Han J, Geng Y, Deng X, Zhang Z. Subclinical synovitis assessed by ultrasound predicts flare and progressive bone erosion in rheumatoid arthritis patients with clinical remission: a systematic review and metaanalysis. J Rheumatol. 2016;43(11):2010–8.
69. Nwosu LN, Allen M, Wyatt L, Huebner JL, Chapman V, Walsh DA, et al. Pain prediction by serum biomarkers of bone turnover in people with knee osteoarthritis: an observational study of TRAcP5b and cathepsin K in OA. Osteoarthr Cartil. 2017;25(6):858–65.
70. Drossaers-Bakker KW, Zwinderman AH, Vliet Vlieland TP, Van Zeben D, Vos K, Breedveld FC, et al. Long-term outcome in rheumatoid arthritis: a simple algorithm of baseline parameters can predict radiographic damage, disability, and disease course at 12-year followup. Arthritis Rheum. 2002;47(4):383–90.
71. Sokka T, Kankainen A, Hannonen P. Scores for functional disability in patients with rheumatoid arthritis are correlated at higher levels with pain scores than with radiographic scores. Arthritis Rheum. 2000;43(2):386–9.
72. Neogi T. Structural correlates of pain in osteoarthritis. Clin Exp Rheumatol. 2017;35(Suppl 107(5)):75–8.
73. Knoop J, Steultjens MP, van der Leeden M, van der Esch M, Thorstensson CA, Roorda LD, et al. Proprioception in knee osteoarthritis: a narrative review. Osteoarthr Cartil. 2011;19(4):381–8.
74. Nishigami T, Mibu A, Tanaka K, Yamashita Y, Yamada E, Wand BM, et al. Development and psychometric properties of knee-specific body-perception questionnaire in people with knee osteoarthritis: the Fremantle Knee Awareness Questionnaire. PLoS ONE. 2017;12(6):e0179225.
75. Martinez-Lavin M. Biology and therapy of fibromyalgia. Stress, the stress response system, and fibromyalgia. Arthritis Res Ther. 2007;9(4):216.
76. Reyes Del Paso GA, Garrido S, Pulgar A, Martin-Vazquez M, Duschek S. Aberrances in autonomic cardiovascular regulation in fibromyalgia syndrome and their relevance for clinical pain reports. Psychosom Med. 2010;72(5):462–70.
77. Neblett R, Cohen H, Choi Y, Hartzell MM, Williams M, Mayer TG, et al. The central sensitization inventory (CSI): establishing clinically significant values for identifying central sensitivity syndromes in an outpatient chronic pain sample. J Pain. 2013;14(5):438–45.
78. Akin-Akinyosoye K, Frowd N, Marshall L, Stocks J, Fernandes G, Valdes A, et al. Traits associated with central pain augmentation in the knee pain in the community (KPIC) cohort. Pain. 2018; in press.
79. McWilliams DF, Ferguson E, Young A, Kiely PD, Walsh DA. Discordant inflammation and pain in early and established rheumatoid arthritis: latent class analysis of early rheumatoid arthritis network and British society for rheumatology biologics register data. Arthritis Res Ther. 2016;18(1):295.

80. Joharatnam N, McWilliams DF, Wilson D, Wheeler M, Pande I, Walsh DA. A cross-sectional study of pain sensitivity, disease-activity assessment, mental health, and fibromyalgia status in rheumatoid arthritis. Arthritis Res Ther. 2015;17:11.
81. Carli G, Suman AL, Biasi G, Marcolongo R. Reactivity to superficial and deep stimuli in patients with chronic musculoskeletal pain. Pain. 2002;100(3):259–69.
82. Kvistgaard Olsen J, Fener DK, Waehrens EE, Wulf Christensen A, Jespersen A, Danneskiold-Samsoe B, et al. Reliability of pain measurements using computerized cuff algometry: a DoloCuff reliability and agreement study. Pain Pract. 2017;17(6):708–17.
83. Cagnie B, Coppieters I, Denecker S, Six J, Danneels L, Meeus M. Central sensitization in fibromyalgia? A systematic review on structural and functional brain MRI. Semin Arthritis Rheum. 2014;44(1):68–75.
84. Freynhagen R, Baron R, Gockel U, Tolle TR. PainDETECT: a new screening questionnaire to identify neuropathic components in patients with back pain. Curr Med Res Opin. 2006;22(10):1911–20.
85. Moreton BJ, Tew V, das Nair R, Wheeler M, Walsh DA, Lincoln NB. Pain phenotype in patients with knee osteoarthritis: classification and measurement properties of painDETECT and self-report Leeds assessment of neuropathic symptoms and signs scale in a cross-sectional study. Arthritis Care Res (Hoboken). 2015;67(4):519–28.
86. Rifbjerg-Madsen S, Waehrens EE, Danneskiold-Samsoe B, Amris K. Psychometric properties of the painDETECT questionnaire in rheumatoid arthritis, psoriatic arthritis and spondyloarthritis: Rasch analysis and test-retest reliability. Health Qual Life Outcomes. 2017;15(1):110.
87. Hawker GA, Guan J, Croxford R, Coyte PC, Glazier RH, Harvey BJ, et al. A prospective population-based study of the predictors of undergoing total joint arthroplasty. Arthritis Rheum. 2006;54(10):3212–20.
88. Baillet A, Zeboulon N, Gossec L, Combescure C, Bodin LA, Juvin R, et al. Efficacy of cardiorespiratory aerobic exercise in rheumatoid arthritis: meta-analysis of randomized controlled trials. Arthritis Care Res (Hoboken). 2010;62(7):984–92.
89. Zhang W, Robertson J, Jones AC, Dieppe PA, Doherty M. The placebo effect and its determinants in osteoarthritis: meta-analysis of randomised controlled trials. Ann Rheum Dis. 2008;67(12):1716–23.
90. Keystone EC, Kavanaugh AF, Sharp JT, Tannenbaum H, Hua Y, Teoh LS, et al. Radiographic, clinical, and functional outcomes of treatment with adalimumab (a human anti-tumor necrosis factor monoclonal antibody) in patients with active rheumatoid arthritis receiving concomitant methotrexate therapy: a randomized, placebo-controlled, 52-week trial. Arthritis Rheum. 2004;50(5):1400–11.
91. Andratsch M, Mair N, Constantin CE, Scherbakov N, Benetti C, Quarta S, et al. A key role for gp130 expressed on peripheral sensory nerves in pathological pain. J Neurosci. 2009;29(43):13473–83.
92. Russell FA, Fernandes ES, Courade JP, Keeble JE, Brain SD. Tumour necrosis factor alpha mediates transient receptor potential vanilloid 1-dependent bilateral thermal hyperalgesia with distinct peripheral roles of interleukin-1beta, protein kinase C and cyclooxygenase-2 signalling. Pain. 2009;142(3):264–74.
93. Nishimoto N, Hashimoto J, Miyasaka N, Yamamoto K, Kawai S, Takeuchi T, et al. Study of active controlled monotherapy used for rheumatoid arthritis, an IL-6 inhibitor (SAMURAI): evidence of clinical and radiographic benefit from an x ray reader-blinded randomised controlled trial of tocilizumab. Ann Rheum Dis. 2007;66(9):1162–7.
94. Malfait AM, Miller RJ. Emerging targets for the management of osteoarthritis pain. Curr Osteoporos Rep. 2016;14(6):260–8.
95. Creamer P, Hunt M, Dieppe P. Pain mechanisms in osteoarthritis of the knee: effect of intraarticular anesthetic. J Rheumatol. 1996;23(6):1031–6.

96. Shanahan EM, Ahern M, Smith M, Wetherall M, Bresnihan B, FitzGerald O. Suprascapular nerve block (using bupivacaine and methylprednisolone acetate) in chronic shoulder pain. Ann Rheum Dis. 2003;62(5):400–6.
97. Radnovich R, Scott D, Patel AT, Olson R, Dasa V, Segal N, et al. Cryoneurolysis to treat the pain and symptoms of knee osteoarthritis: a multicenter, randomized, double-blind, sham-controlled trial. Osteoarthr Cartil. 2017;25(8):1247–56.
98. Ward S, Arvin B, Blowey S, Hill P, Mason M, MacFarlane G, et al. Low back pain and sciatica in over 16s: assessment and management. London: National Institute for Health and Care Excellence; 2016.
99. Blyth T, Hunter JA, Stirling A. Pain relief in the rheumatoid knee after steroid injection. A single-blind comparison of hydrocortisone succinate, and triamcinolone acetonide or hexacetonide. Br J Rheumatol. 1994;33(5):461–3.
100. Kirwan JR, Hallgren R, Mielants H, Wollheim F, Bjorck E, Persson T, et al. A randomised placebo controlled 12 week trial of budesonide and prednisolone in rheumatoid arthritis. Ann Rheum Dis. 2004;63(6):688–95.
101. Choy EH, Kingsley GH, Corkill MM, Panayi GS. Intramuscular methylprednisolone is superior to pulse oral methylprednisolone during the induction phase of chrysotherapy. Br J Rheumatol. 1993;32(8):734–9.
102. Conaghan PG, Dickson J, Grant RL, Guideline Development G. Care and management of osteoarthritis in adults: summary of NICE guidance. BMJ. 2008;336(7642):502–3.
103. Wenham CY, Hensor EM, Grainger AJ, Hodgson R, Balamoody S, Dore CJ, et al. A randomized, double-blind, placebo-controlled trial of low-dose oral prednisolone for treating painful hand osteoarthritis. Rheumatology (Oxford). 2012;51(12):2286–94.
104. Hazlewood GS, Barnabe C, Tomlinson G, Marshall D, Devoe D, Bombardier C. Methotrexate monotherapy and methotrexate combination therapy with traditional and biologic disease modifying anti-rheumatic drugs for rheumatoid arthritis: abridged Cochrane systematic review and network meta-analysis. BMJ. 2016;353:i1777.
105. Dimitroulas T, Lambe T, Klocke R, Kitas GD, Duarte RV. Biologic drugs as analgesics for the management of osteoarthritis. Semin Arthritis Rheum. 2017;46(6):687–91.
106. Brandt KD, Mazzuca SA, Buckwalter KA. Acetaminophen, like conventional NSAIDs, may reduce synovitis in osteoarthritic knees. Rheumatology (Oxford). 2006;45(11):1389–94.
107. (NICE) NIoCE. Clinical Guideline 789. Rheumatoid arthritis: The management of rheumatoid arthritis in adults. NICE. 2009.
108. Derry S, Wiffen PJ, Hauser W, Mucke M, Tolle TR, Bell RF, et al. Oral nonsteroidal anti-inflammatory drugs for fibromyalgia in adults. Cochrane Database Syst Rev. 2017;3:CD012332.
109. Wienecke T, Gotzsche PC. Paracetamol versus nonsteroidal anti-inflammatory drugs for rheumatoid arthritis. Cochrane Database Syst Rev. 2004;1:CD003789.
110. Bannuru RR, Schmid CH, Kent DM, Vaysbrot EE, Wong JB, McAlindon TE. Comparative effectiveness of pharmacologic interventions for knee osteoarthritis: a systematic review and network meta-analysis. Ann Intern Med. 2015;162(1):46–54.
111. Trijau S, Avouac J, Escalas C, Gossec L, Dougados M. Influence of flare design on symptomatic efficacy of non-steroidal anti-inflammatory drugs in osteoarthritis: a meta-analysis of randomized placebo-controlled trials. Osteoarthr Cartil. 2010;18(8):1012–8.
112. Bally M, Dendukuri N, Rich B, Nadeau L, Helin-Salmivaara A, Garbe E, et al. Risk of acute myocardial infarction with NSAIDs in real world use: Bayesian meta-analysis of individual patient data. BMJ. 2017;357:j1909.
113. Katz N, Borenstein DG, Birbara C, Bramson C, Nemeth MA, Smith MD, et al. Efficacy and safety of tanezumab in the treatment of chronic low back pain. Pain. 2011;152(10):2248–58.
114. Chappell AS, Ossanna MJ, Liu-Seifert H, Iyengar S, Skljarevski V, Li LC, et al. Duloxetine, a centrally acting analgesic, in the treatment of patients with osteoarthritis knee pain: a 13-week, randomized, placebo-controlled trial. Pain. 2009;146(3):253–60.

115. Abou-Raya S, Abou-Raya A, Helmii M. Duloxetine for the management of pain in older adults with knee osteoarthritis: randomised placebo-controlled trial. Age Ageing. 2012;41(5):646–52.
116. Sofat N, Harrison A, Russell MD, Ayis S, Kiely PD, Baker EH, et al. The effect of pregabalin or duloxetine on arthritis pain: a clinical and mechanistic study in people with hand osteoarthritis. J Pain Res. 2017;10:2437–49.
117. Macfarlane GJ, Kronisch C, Dean LE, Atzeni F, Hauser W, Flus E, et al. EULAR revised recommendations for the management of fibromyalgia. Ann Rheum Dis. 2017;76(2):318–28.
118. McWilliams DF, Walsh DA. Factors predicting pain and early discontinuation of tumour necrosis factor-alpha-inhibitors in people with rheumatoid arthritis: results from the British society for rheumatology biologics register. BMC Musculoskelet Disord. 2016;17:337.
119. Petersen KK, Arendt-Nielsen L, Simonsen O, Wilder-Smith O, Laursen MB. Presurgical assessment of temporal summation of pain predicts the development of chronic postoperative pain 12 months after total knee replacement. Pain. 2015;156(1):55–61.
120. Noble M, Treadwell JR, Tregear SJ, Coates VH, Wiffen PJ, Akafomo C, et al. Long-term opioid management for chronic noncancer pain. Cochrane Database Syst Rev. 2010;(1):CD006605.
121. Mehta N, O'Connell K, Giambrone GP, Baqai A, Diwan S. Efficacy of methylnaltrexone for the treatment of opiod-induced constipation: a meta-analysis and systematic review. Postgrad Med. 2016;128(3):282–9.
122. Machado GC, Maher CG, Ferreira PH, Pinheiro MB, Lin CW, Day RO, et al. Efficacy and safety of paracetamol for spinal pain and osteoarthritis: systematic review and meta-analysis of randomised placebo controlled trials. BMJ. 2015;350:h1225.
123. Roberts E, Delgado Nunes V, Buckner S, Latchem S, Constanti M, Miller P, et al. Paracetamol: not as safe as we thought? A systematic literature review of observational studies. Ann Rheum Dis. 2016;75(3):552–9.
124. Richards BL, Whittle SL, Buchbinder R. Neuromodulators for pain management in rheumatoid arthritis. Cochrane Database Syst Rev. 2012;1:CD008921.
125. Girard P, Chauvin M, Verleye M. Nefopam analgesia and its role in multimodal analgesia: a review of preclinical and clinical studies. Clin Exp Pharmacol Physiol. 2016;43(1):3–12.
126. Fitzcharles MA, Baerwald C, Ablin J, Hauser W. Efficacy, tolerability and safety of cannabinoids in chronic pain associated with rheumatic diseases (fibromyalgia syndrome, back pain, osteoarthritis, rheumatoid arthritis): a systematic review of randomized controlled trials. Schmerz. 2016;30(1):47–61.
127. Uthman OA, van der Windt DA, Jordan JL, Dziedzic KS, Healey EL, Peat GM, et al. Exercise for lower limb osteoarthritis: systematic review incorporating trial sequential analysis and network meta-analysis. BMJ. 2013;347:f5555.
128. Bearne LM, Scott DL, Hurley MV. Exercise can reverse quadriceps sensorimotor dysfunction that is associated with rheumatoid arthritis without exacerbating disease activity. Rheumatology (Oxford). 2002;41(2):157–66.
129. Jones KD, King LA, Mist SD, Bennett RM, Horak FB. Postural control deficits in people with fibromyalgia: a pilot study. Arthritis Res Ther. 2011;13(4):R127.
130. Jones MD, Booth J, Taylor JL, Barry BK. Limited association between aerobic fitness and pain in healthy individuals: a cross-sectional study. Pain Med. 2016;17(10):1799–808.
131. Naugle KM, Fillingim RB, Riley JL 3rd. A meta-analytic review of the hypoalgesic effects of exercise. J Pain. 2012;13(12):1139–50.
132. Makris EA, Gomoll AH, Malizos KN, Hu JC, Athanasiou KA. Repair and tissue engineering techniques for articular cartilage. Nat Rev Rheumatol. 2015;11(1):21–34.
133. Judge A, Arden NK, Cooper C, Kassim Javaid M, Carr AJ, Field RE, et al. Predictors of outcomes of total knee replacement surgery. Rheumatology (Oxford). 2012;51(10):1804–13.
134. Beswick AD, Wylde V, Gooberman-Hill R, Blom A, Dieppe P. What proportion of patients report long-term pain after total hip or knee replacement for osteoarthritis? A systematic review of prospective studies in unselected patients. BMJ Open. 2012;2:e000435.

135. Izumi M, Petersen KK, Laursen MB, Arendt-Nielsen L, Graven-Nielsen T. Facilitated temporal summation of pain correlates with clinical pain intensity after hip arthroplasty. Pain. 2017;158(2):323–32.
136. das Nair R, mhizha-Murira JR, Anderson P, Carpenter H, Clarke S, Groves S, et al. Home-based pre-surgical psychological intervention for knee osteoarthritis (HAPPiKNEES): a feasibility randomized controlled trial. Clin Rehabil. 2018;32:777–89.
137. Filardo G, Merli G, Roffi A, Marcacci T, Berti Ceroni F, Raboni D, et al. Kinesiophobia and depression affect total knee arthroplasty outcome in a multivariate analysis of psychological and physical factors on 200 patients. Knee Surg Sports Traumatol Arthrosc. 2017;25(11):3417–23.
138. Valdes AM, Doherty SA, Zhang W, Muir KR, Maciewicz RA, Doherty M. Inverse relationship between preoperative radiographic severity and postoperative pain in patients with osteoarthritis who have undergone total joint arthroplasty. Semin Arthritis Rheum. 2012;41(4):568–75.
139. Messier SP, Loeser RF, Miller GD, Morgan TM, Rejeski WJ, Sevick MA, et al. Exercise and dietary weight loss in overweight and obese older adults with knee osteoarthritis: the arthritis, diet, and activity promotion trial. Arthritis Rheum. 2004;50(5):1501–10.
140. Richette P, Poitou C, Garnero P, Vicaut E, Bouillot JL, Lacorte JM, et al. Benefits of massive weight loss on symptoms, systemic inflammation and cartilage turnover in obese patients with knee osteoarthritis. Ann Rheum Dis. 2011;70(1):139–44.
141. Magnusson K, Hagen KB, Osteras N, Nordsletten L, Natvig B, Haugen IK. Diabetes is associated with increased hand pain in erosive hand osteoarthritis: data from a population-based study. Arthritis Care Res (Hoboken). 2015;67(2):187–95.
142. Valdes AM, Abhishek A, Muir K, Zhang W, Maciewicz RA, Doherty M. Association of beta-blocker use with less prevalent joint pain and lower opioid requirement in people with osteoarthritis. Arthritis Care Res (Hoboken). 2017;69(7):1076–81.
143. Velvin G, Bathen T, Rand-Hendriksen S, Geirdal AO. Systematic review of chronic pain in persons with Marfan syndrome. Clin Genet. 2016;89(6):647–58.
144. Syx D, De Wandele I, Rombaut L, Malfait F. Hypermobility, the Ehlers-Danlos syndromes and chronic pain. Clin Exp Rheumatol. 2017;35(Suppl 107(5)):116–22.
145. Canadas V, Vilacosta I, Bruna I, Fuster V. Marfan syndrome. Part 1: pathophysiology and diagnosis. Nat Rev Cardiol. 2010;7(5):256–65.
146. Bastick AN, Wesseling J, Damen J, Verkleij SP, Emans PJ, Bindels PJ, et al. Defining knee pain trajectories in early symptomatic knee osteoarthritis in primary care: 5-year results from a nationwide prospective cohort study (CHECK). Br J Gen Pract. 2016;66(642):e32–9.
147. Green DJ, Jordan KP, Protheroe J, van der Windt DA. Development of hand phenotypes and changes in hand pain and problems over time in older people. Pain. 2016;157(3):569–76.
148. Reyes C, Leyland KM, Peat G, Cooper C, Arden NK, Prieto-Alhambra D. Association between overweight and obesity and risk of clinically diagnosed knee, hip, and hand osteoarthritis: a population-based cohort study. Arthritis Rheumatol. 2016;68(8):1869–75.
149. Wesseling J, Bastick AN, ten Wolde S, Kloppenburg M, Lafeber FP, Bierma-Zeinstra SM, et al. Identifying trajectories of pain severity in early symptomatic knee osteoarthritis: a 5-year followup of the cohort hip and cohort knee (CHECK) study. J Rheumatol. 2015;42(8):1470–7.
150. Sarmanova A, Hall M, Fernandes GS, Bhattacharya A, Valdes AM, Walsh DA, et al. Association between ultrasound-detected synovitis and knee pain: a population-based case-control study with both cross-sectional and follow-up data. Arthritis Res Ther. 2017;19:281.
151. Zhang Y, Nevitt M, Niu J, Lewis C, Torner J, Guermazi A, et al. Fluctuation of knee pain and changes in bone marrow lesions, effusions, and synovitis on magnetic resonance imaging. Arthritis Rheum. 2011;63(3):691–9.
152. Mallen CD, Peat G, Thomas E, Lacey R, Croft P. Predicting poor functional outcome in community-dwelling older adults with knee pain: prognostic value of generic indicators. Ann Rheum Dis. 2007;66(11):1456–61.

153. Collins JE, Katz JN, Dervan EE, Losina E. Trajectories and risk profiles of pain in persons with radiographic, symptomatic knee osteoarthritis: data from the osteoarthritis initiative. Osteoarthr Cartil. 2014;22(5):622–30.
154. Alschuler KN, Molton IR, Jensen MP, Riddle DL. Prognostic value of coping strategies in a community-based sample of persons with chronic symptomatic knee osteoarthritis. Pain. 2013;154(12):2775–81.
155. Carlesso LC, Niu J, Segal NA, Frey-Law LA, Lewis CE, Nevitt MC, et al. The effect of widespread pain on knee pain worsening, incident knee osteoarthritis (OA), and incident knee pain: the multicenter OA (MOST) study. J Rheumatol. 2017;44(4):493–8.
156. Edwards RR, Dolman AJ, Martel MO, Finan PH, Lazaridou A, Cornelius M, et al. Variability in conditioned pain modulation predicts response to NSAID treatment in patients with knee osteoarthritis. BMC Musculoskelet Disord. 2016;17:284.
157. Wylde V, Sayers A, Lenguerrand E, Gooberman-Hill R, Pyke M, Beswick AD, et al. Preoperative widespread pain sensitization and chronic pain after hip and knee replacement: a cohort analysis. Pain. 2015;156(1):47–54.

Chapter 28
Vascular Pain

Kellie Gates and Pegah Safaeian

28.1 Prevalence and Risk Factors

As the mean age of the population increases, it can be anticipated that the prevalence of peripheral vascular disease (PVD) will also trend in that direction. Patients who suffer from chronic vascular disease are often afflicted with several other medical comorbidities, which can make their care both difficult and costly [1]. In the population of patients over 40 years of age, it is estimated that almost 8.5 million Americans have some degree of peripheral vascular disease [2]. Many of these patients often go undiagnosed, due to the absence of and the unpredictable nature of symptoms [3].

There are many risk factors that can predispose a patient to peripheral vascular disease. Some of the more notable risk factors include current or former smoking history, hypertension, diabetes, hyperlipidemia, chronic kidney disease, and advanced age (>60 years of age) [4]. Many of these risk factors overlap with those that predispose patients to cardiovascular disease and it has been observed that patients with PVD are at a significantly higher risk of cardiovascular and cerebrovascular morbidity and mortality [5].

Given the high rate of associated serious comorbidities, patients with PVD often experience frequent hospital admissions and, depending on the severity, can require multiple surgical interventions for management of their disease. During a hospital stay or in the perioperative period, these patients struggle with acute worsening of their baseline pain, which can often be difficult to treat due to associated advanced age or renal impairment which make the use of certain medications unfavorable [6]. Uncontrolled pain promotes the stress response and heightened activity of the auto-

K. Gates
Illinois Bone and Joint Institute, Chicago, IL, USA

P. Safaeian (✉)
Virginia Mason Medical Center, Seattle, Washington, USA
e-mail: Pegah.Safaeian@VirginiaMason.org

K. Shimoji et al. (eds.), *Chronic Pain Management in General and Hospital Practice*, https://doi.org/10.1007/978-981-15-2933-7_28

nomic nervous system, which is consequential in patients with underlying cardiovascular and cerebrovascular disease [7]. Additionally, poorly controlled pain can lead to impaired respiratory effort, dampened immune function, ileus, and decreased wound healing in a perioperative setting, all of which are catastrophic to a patient's postoperative course.

Patients with ischemic disease often suffer from painful symptoms, ranging from intermittent claudication, to acute pain with an occlusive event, to chronic pain and central sensitization over time. Most commonly, in the initial stages of this disease, patients experience intermittent claudication with activities. There is a subset of patients with PVD who are asymptomatic, but they often have multiple associated risk factors which can raise suspicion for concomitant PVD prior to official diagnosis [8]. Worsening pain is often associated with disease progression and pain at rest can reflect severely compromised circulation and critical limb ischemia. In patients suffering from critical limb ischemia, over 25% require major amputation, with many others undergoing reconstructive arterial surgery [9]. Along with the need for high-risk surgical intervention, critical limb ischemia itself is predictive of poor patient outcomes. The risk of mortality for newly diagnosed patients is up to 20% within 1 year of initial diagnosis and up to 40–75% within 5 years [10].

A wide range of conditions exist that can fall under the category of "vascular disease." These are a frequent and significant source of pain for patients and include vasculitis, thromboembolic disease, Reynaud's phenomenon, and varicose veins which can adversely affect a patient's function and quality of life [11]. There are also a number of syndromes that also occur due to an alteration in the regulation or the structure of the vascular system, including complex regional pain syndrome, thoracic outlet syndrome, and phantom limb pain [12, 13]. Given the wide breadth of these illnesses and the extreme variation in associated pathology, this chapter will primarily focus on ischemic peripheral vascular disease and the pain associated with this.

28.2 Diagnosis

When addressing the peripheral vascular disease, categories have been created based off of the presenting state of the patient. The American College of Cardiology/American Heart Association categorizes PVD into asymptomatic PVD, claudication, critical limb ischemia, and acute limb ischemia [14]. As previously discussed, critical limb ischemia is often linked to pain at rest, but can also often be correlated to pathologic skin changes including ulcers or even gangrene [15]. Acute limb ischemia occurs in the scenario of an abruptly occluded vessel producing significant symptoms, often described as the "six Ps." These include paresthesia, pain, pallor, pulselessness, poikilothermia (meaning impaired temperature regulation resulting in a cool extremity), and paralysis.

The primary diagnostic tool used to assess peripheral vascular disease is the ankle-brachial index (ABI). This test has a high sensitivity and specificity in identifying lower-extremity stenosis, but can also be used to identify arterial injury or damage in a trauma patient. This is accomplished by initially taking the upper extremity blood pressure, then using a Doppler to assess the lower extremity pressure. By inflating the sphygmomanometer until the arterial signal disappears on Doppler (either the dorsalis pedis or posterior tibial, either can be used), the lower extremity systolic pressure can be identified. To calculate the ABI, divide the lower extremity systolic pressure by the upper extremity systolic pressure [16]. Normal ranges are from 0.9 to 1.3, while moderate PVD is seen at levels from 0.41 to 0.9. Anything less than 0.4 is deemed severe and anything above 1.3 indicates a vessel with such significant calcification that it is unable to be compressed [17].

Given the risk factors of PVD and the patient population that suffers from this disease, it has been shown that there can be an improvement in identification of patients at high risk for cardiovascular adverse events when incorporating the ABI into their evaluation [18]. Up to 60% of myocardial infarctions (MIs) occur within patients without identified coronary artery disease [19], while 60–80% of acute MIs affect patients who are in the low to intermediate risk group using the Framingham Risk Scores, a commonly used scoring system to estimate the 10-year cardiovascular risk of an individual [20]. A meta-analysis of 16 studies including 48,344 patients noted that the inclusion of patients with a low ABI helped to identify more patients at risk of cardiovascular morbidity and mortality, and those patients with a low ABI were at double the risk of 10-year total mortality, cardiovascular mortality, and major coronary event [21].

28.3 Grading

Grading of the disease is also an important aspect of the management and treatment. The main grading tool utilized for diagnosis is the Fontaine classification, which stages the disease based on patient symptoms (Table 28.1). A more elaborate grading system is the Rutherford classification, which takes into account the chronicity of the disease, such as acute vs. chronic pathologies, and also incorporates objective findings such as arterial brachial indices, pulse volume recordings, and Doppler [22]. The more surgically oriented classification system is the Trans-Atlantic Inter-Society Consensus Document (TASC) II, which discusses the anatomy of the disease location, treatment, and surgical management including open vs. endovascular repairs [23].

Table 28.1 Fontaine classification [24]

Grade	Symptoms
Stage I	Asymptomatic, incomplete blood vessel obstruction
Stage II	Mild claudication pain in limb
Stage IIA	Claudication at a distance >200 m
Stage IIB	Claudication at a distance of <200 m
Stage III	Rest pain, mostly in the feet
Stage IV	Necrosis and/or gangrene of the limb

28.4 Pathophysiology

There are many risk factors associated with the formation of peripheral vascular disease. As listed above, the most significant of these include hypertension, hyperlipidemia, diabetes, chronic kidney disease, and smoking. At a cellular level, this promotes endothelial injury which initiates the cascade of vascular promotion of atherosclerosis. Via the proliferation of smooth muscle cells, the development of foam cells, platelet activation, and localized inflammation, vascular narrowing and occlusion occur.

Endothelial injury can cause retention and incorporation of low-density lipoproteins (LDLs) within the wall of the vasculature. These LDLs are often predisposed to oxidation by reactive oxygen species, which leads to a pro-inflammatory state and activation of the superficial endothelium. Recruitment of macrophages and monocytes that are responsible for the build-up of foam cells is often at the center of this atherosclerotic state. Foam cells are macrophages that have ingested LDLs, which tends to give them a foamy appearance and thus, their name. At the onset of atherosclerosis formation, this macrophage function may be beneficial, however the lack of negative feedback can compromise immune function and cause an accumulation of foam cells at the site due to their diminished ability to migrate [25]. Also occurring during this time is the release of inflammatory cytokines which can lead to smooth muscle cell proliferation and pain. Finally, a fibrous plaque is formed that has the propensity to destabilize, leading to thrombosis and acute vascular occlusion [26].

28.5 Pain Caused by Vascular Ischemia

Pain linked to peripheral vascular disease is multi-faceted and seems to include input from multiple sources. Primarily, the pain can be linked to inflammatory, nociceptive, and neuropathic input. The combination of these insults is what creates the debilitating pain state that many of these patients experience daily [27].

28.5.1 Inflammatory Pain

As discussed in the pathology of atherosclerosis formation, multiple pro-inflammatory cytokines and other noxious mediators are released in the response to endothelial injury. At a localized level, these can promote nociceptor activity and can increase excitation of these nociceptors. These metabolites can include bradykinin, serotonin, histamine, eicosanoids, and the cytokines include interleukin-1β, tumor necrosis factor-α, and interleukin-6 [28]. Individually and combined, these act to excite and sensitize nociceptive afferent fibers to stimuli. Nerve growth factor is also secreted by macrophages and can directly alter the A-δ pain fibers, causing a greater proportion of these to have nociceptor properties via a heightened expression of substance P [29].

Poor circulation in the affected limb often leads to a build-up of toxic metabolites that cannot be cleared, while areas distal to the occlusion become hypoxic and acidotic. A larger amount of free H+ ions can cause hyperalgesia and pain. There are H+-gated cation channels expressed in the brain and dorsal root ganglion that contribute to pain associated with acidotic conditions within tissues. These include the rapid on-off ASIC channel and the sustained-acting DRASIC channel, which can promote pain states and sensitization [30].

28.5.2 Neuropathic Pain

Neuropathic pain occurs when there is damage to neuronal tissue itself. With PVD and chronic limb ischemia, neuropathies can form from damage to the nerves and surrounding tissues. Whether or not this damage occurs primarily to motor or sensory nerves is a topic of debate; however, it seems that nerve fibers of all sizes and degrees of myelination can be affected [31, 32]. Studies on the histologic changes of human nerves showing that large, myelinated fibers are more prone to ischemia than the small, unmyelinated axons in patients that suffer from chronic vasculitis [33]. It has also been noted that ischemic extremities experience an altered threshold for temperature sensation, suggesting that A-delta fibers are more significantly impacted [16].

Neuropathic pain seems to be associated more heavily with critical limb ischemia and the formation of chronic pain states. This can be observed in patients who have persistent pain after surgical intervention was performed to alleviate mechanical occlusion. Peripheral sensitization can occur from a number of pro-inflammatory mediators at the area of ischemia, while central sensitization occurs through chronically stimulated nociceptors. Both of these mechanisms contribute to chronic, often difficult to treat pain. Along with sensitization, it has been shown that there is a degree of pain which may occur through reperfusion injury, during which there can be increases in interleukin 1-β and its receptor in the dorsal root ganglia which directly excite and sensitize nociceptive afferent fibers [34]. The characteristics of pain in patients with critical limb ischemia may indicate that the pain is more neuropathic in nature, given the descriptive factors of the pain as "burning, shooting, and stabbing" [35].

28.5.3 Nociceptive Pain

Nociceptive pain occurs via activation of peripheral nociceptive fibers, particularly A-δ and C-fibers. A-δ fibers are thinly myelinated and are responsible for the rapid-onset, sharp intense pain, while C-fibers are unmyelinated and are more involved in the slow-onset, burning pain. This is not linked to actual neuronal damage, unlike neuropathic pain. Nociceptive pain can be linked to pain caused by intermittent claudication and less likely to pain caused by critical ischemia and localized neuron destruction [30]. Chronic ischemia in PVD affects nerve fibers of all size, including Aβ, Aδ, and C-fibers [37].

Outside of the realm of atherosclerotic vascular disease, patients who suffer from lower extremity pain due to vasospasm or from distal arterial occlusive disease, particularly Reynaud's, can benefit from lumbar sympathetic blocks. These serve to decrease the overactive sympathetic input to the vascular system of the given extremity and thus, diminish the vascular spasms producing pain [36]. The efficacy of these injections speaks to the involvement of the autonomic nervous system to certain vascular pathologies and how this should be considered in the management of certain vascular pain.

28.6 Formation of Chronic Pain States

There has been noted to be a link between severe PVD and central sensitization, which often leads patients to a state of chronic pain [37]. Central sensitization can be caused from prolonged nociceptor input and overstimulation, inducing hypersensitivity and a persistent state of high reactivity. Central sensitization includes hyperalgesia and allodynia, which is often secondary to changes in electrophysiologic and neurohormonal activity in the brain [38]. Specifically, this may be linked to ongoing input from C-fibers, which are activated in ischemic states by inflammatory mediators and also potentially by continuous muscle contraction caused by ischemia [39]. C-fibers are subject to the phenomenon of windup, which leads to a decrease in feedback inhibition on C-fibers which can promote central sensitization. Increases in sensory changes also correlate with worsening severity of PVD. Previous studies have demonstrated that the destruction of both large (Aβ) and small (Aδ and C) nerve fibers is involved in the pathology of ischemia; however, it may be the impaired small-fiber function that more significantly contributes to complications associated with PVD. Often small injuries to an affected ischemic limb can lead to greater consequences, including skin ulcers and infections due to poor localized perfusion [37].

28.7 Treatment

28.7.1 Risk Factor Modification

As discussed above, critical limb ischemia (CLI) is most commonly the result of arterial occlusive disease from atherosclerosis, often in association with diabetes, hypercholesterolemia, and hypertension [40]. Thus, risk factor modification should be customized to address the individual's risk factors, often involving use of a comprehensive program including lifestyle modification, exercise, and medical management.

Control of blood glucose in diabetics is important in risk factor modification as it is associated with more severe and rapidly progressive PAD. Atherosclerosis in diabetic patients has a propensity for affecting the distal vessels, which are ultimately less amenable to revascularization [41]. In addition to appropriate glycemic control, weight management, foot care, and wound prevention are required. With regard to foot care, daily evaluation of the lower extremities is important to prevent skin cracking and breakdown ultimately resulting in wound formation and infection. Appropriate protective foot wear must be used, such as shoes with a wide toe box.

Smoking cessation must also be addressed with patients. The risk of PAD progression almost doubles with tobacco use and can accelerate disease progression. The combination of nonpharmacologic and pharmacologic approaches has been shown to have the greatest efficacy in smoking cessation [42].

28.8 Pharmacologic Management

28.8.1 Antiplatelet Therapy

Antiplatelet therapy is prescribed in PAD to prevent major adverse cardiovascular events including MI, stroke, or vascular death. Antiplatelet therapy with aspirin alone or clopidogrel alone is recommended in patients with symptomatic PAD [43]. These patients, when treated with antiplatelet therapy, had a 22% odds reduction for cardiovascular events [43]. However, there is no consensus regarding which antiplatelet agent to be used. In a trial comparing clopidogrel versus aspirin, clopidogrel was more effective than aspirin in cardiovascular risk reduction in patients with symptomatic PAD [44].

Data is limited regarding use of dual antiplatelet therapy; however, it is often prescribed in patients following revascularization. A literature review revealed two small randomized control trials showing decrease in need for repeat revascularization in patients with PAD following initial revascularization [45]. Dual antiplatelet therapy with Clopidogrel and aspirin was the only treatment associated with a significant reduction of major amputations following leg revascularization [46, 47]. The benefits of dual therapy must be weighed against the increased risk of bleeding, and should thus be used judiciously.

28.8.2 Anticoagulant Therapy

The COMPASS trial, a large, multicenter, double blind, placebo controlled study, evaluated the role of rivaroxaban, an oral factor Xa inhibitor, in patients with PAD of the lower extremities, of the carotid or coronary arteries. Patients were randomized to receive rivaroxaban, at a low dose twice daily, rivaroxaban low dose twice daily in addition to low dose aspirin, or low dose aspirin once daily alone.

The primary outcomes evaluated included major cardiovascular events or major adverse limb events such as amputation. Dual therapy with low dose rivaroxaban twice daily in addition to aspirin had a 28% reduction in cardiovascular events. Major adverse limb events, including limb ischemia leading to revascularization and amputation, were reduced by 46% in the dual therapy group when compared to aspirin alone. While dual therapy did result in an increased risk of major bleeding, there was no reported increase in fatal or critical organ bleeds. Rivaroxaban twice daily when compared to aspirin alone did not decrease cardiovascular or limb events [48].

The use of warfarin in conjunction with aspirin has also been evaluated, and was not found to be more effective than antiplatelet therapy alone in preventing cardiovascular events. Additionally, there was a substantial increase in risk of life-threatening bleed [49].

28.8.3 Statins

In addition to recommendation for dietary modification, treatment with a statin is indicated for all patients with PAD. In one statins when compared to placebo, reduced the rate of major vascular events by 22% [43]. Cholesterol reduction with the use of a statin has also been shown to improve pain free walking distance when compared to placebo, in symptomatic patients with PAD [50].

28.8.4 Antihypertensive Agents

Treatment of hypertension (HTN) with antihypertensive therapy is recommended regardless as to whether the patient has a concurrent diagnosis of PAD, to reduce risk of cardiovascular events. There is no class of antihypertensive medication that is believed to be superior in management of HTN in patients with PAD [43]. In November of 2017, the American College of Cardiology/American Heart Association Task Force published updated guidelines with regard to evaluation and management of blood pressure, with the goal of treatment to be less than 130 mm Hg systolic/80 mm Hg diastolic [51]. Of note, normotensive patients with PAD treated with the use of ACE inhibitors were found to have a 25% reduced risk of cardiovascular events when compared to placebo [52].

Pharmacologic recommendations	Class of recommendation	Level of evidence
Single antiplatelet therapy in symptomatic PAD	I	A
Statins in all patients with PAD	I	A
Antihypertensives in all with hypertension and PAD	I	A
ACEIs in all with hypertension and PAD	IIa	B

28.8.5 *Treatment of Intermittent Claudication*

Symptoms of intermittent claudication (IC), classically of calf aching, fatigue, and cramping, occur during physical activity when the metabolic demands of the muscle are not met by the available circulation, and are alleviated during rest. If the activity level does not surpass this threshold, the patient will remain asymptomatic [53].

Cilostazol targets phosphodiesterase and inhibits platelet aggregation, but unlike other antiplatelet agents, it also improves endothelial cell function. Cilostazol has shown symptomatic improvement when compared with placebo or when compared to other antiplatelet agents [54]. Pentoxifylline has also been evaluated in the treatment of IC, the mechanism of action of which is through reduction in blood viscosity, improving erythrocyte flexibility and promoting microcirculatory flow. However, the effectiveness in treatment is unclear. In one multicenter RTC there was no difference when compared to placebo when examining maximal walking distance [55].

28.9 Alternative Therapies

28.9.1 *Hyperbaric Oxygen*

While there is no clear evidence for the use of hyperbaric oxygen treatment (HBOT) in the treatment of critical limb ischemia (CLI), it is an established treatment for chronic non healing wounds. In a Cochrane review of HBOT for diabetic foot ulcers, the authors found that HBOT improved healing at 6 weeks, and additionally, may reduce the number of major amputations in that patient population [56]. Despite the lack of evidence, HBOT may be considered in patients with CLI who have not responded to or are not candidates for revascularization [57].

28.9.2 *Angiogenesis*

Therapeutic angiogenesis may have the potential to treat ischemic lesions through the proliferation of collateral blood vessels, thus enhancing tissue perfusion. The use of growth factors, specifically fibroblast growth factor [58], vascular endothelial growth factor [59], and hepatocyte growth factor [60], have been used in patients with CLI via injection and gene transfer. Phase I trials have shown that these treatments are safe but large RCTs are needed to evaluate efficacy. Additionally, stem cell therapy has also been used to induce angiogenesis. In one meta-analysis of 37 trials, the use of intramuscular autologous bone marrow cell therapy specifically was safe and potentially effective in improving ischemia, ulcer healing, and amputation [61]. In another meta-analysis of 13 clinical trials significant improvements were seen in the rate of amputations, ulcer healing and ABI for stem cell therapy when compared to controls [62]. While there may be promise in stem cell therapy in the future, there remains a need for large, multicenter, RCTs.

28.10 Rehabilitation

A supervised, structured exercise regimen is a first line treatment for intermittent claudication (IC), the goals of which are to reduce symptoms, improve physical disability, and decrease cardiovascular events [63]. In one meta-analysis, supervised exercise programs increased pain free walking distance by 180% [64]. Furthermore, improvement in ambulation has been shown to improve the patient's perceived quality of life [65]. When comparing the combination of a home walking regimen and cilostazol, versus aortoiliac stenting versus a structured exercise program, the supervised exercise cohort had superior improvement in treadmill walking performance, walking distance, as well as an associated increase in high density lipoprotein and decrease in fibrinogen, when compared to the other two groups [66]. In another RTC, patients with claudication were randomized to endovascular revascularization in addition to supervised exercise or supervised exercise alone. At 1 year, both groups had significant improvement in walking distance and quality of life measures. The greatest improvement however was in the combination group [67].

A supervised exercise program begins with an initial assessment to evaluate walking capacity and limitations. The patient will then exercise, most commonly by treadmill walking, until they experience onset of claudication, continue until ischemic leg pain is near maximal, then stop until the pain subsides, following which they resume exercise again. They continue this routine throughout the course of the session, usually 1 h in length. The exercise prescription may include three weekly sessions for a total of 12 weeks [68]. Following completion of the program, patients are transitioned to exercising independently. Adherence to a program, whether supervised or unsupervised, may be challenging.

28.11 Pain Management

28.11.1 Pharmacologic Management

The ideal treatment for vascular ischemic pain is achieved through reperfusion. Patients who are pending revascularization, or, in whom revascularization has failed or is not an option, pharmacologic pain control is needed. While attempts should be made to manage pain with acetaminophen or nonsteroidal anti-inflammatories, often, opioids are required. In patients with concurrent hypertension or renal insufficiency the use of nonsteroidal anti-inflammatories should be avoided or used judiciously. It is also important to evaluate for signs or symptoms of depression and treat accordingly [57].

28.11.2 Spinal Cord Stimulation (SCS)

While neuromodulation has been predominantly evaluated in the treatment of neuropathic or sympathetically mediated pain, there has been research evaluating the use of spinal cord stimulation (SCS) in ischemic pain. The mechanism of action in ischemic pain is likely due to stimulation of sensory fibers which activate a cascade, ultimately resulting in release of vasodilators that stimulate smooth muscle relaxation. Subsequent improvements in microcirculation act to reduce tissue ischemia and thus, reduce pain [69].

In one prospective study, patients with inoperable limb ischemia were randomized to SCS with analgesic treatment vs. analgesic treatment alone and followed over an 18-month period. Long-term pain relief was seen only in the SCS group. At the study endpoint, limb salvage rates between groups were equal. On subgroup analysis, patients without arterial hypertension had significantly lower rates of amputation in the SCS group [70]. In a separate retrospective review of 260 patients who underwent SCS, 98 were diagnosed with PAD, with a mean follow-up 43 months. In the PAD cohort, 11% reported poor pain control (defined as 30–49% improvement in pain), while 87% reported good relief (50–79% improvement). Complications rates were over 17% [71].

The role of transcutaneous oxygen measurements (TcPO2) in patient selection for SCS in PAD has been reviewed. TcPO2 can be used to predict severity of vascular disease as well as in assessment of outcomes. Normal TcPO2 is approximately 60 mm Hg and levels below 20 mm Hg are an indication for revascularization [72, 73]. In a large, multicenter European prospective study, patients diagnosed with CLI were further categorized into those with baseline TcPO2 <30 mm Hg, or baseline <10 mm Hg that increased to >20 mm Hg after stimulation trial and compared to controls. Patients with improvement in TcPO2 during the stimulation trial had significant improvement in microcirculation, pain relief, and limb preservation. The authors concluded that TcPO2 screening should play a role in patient selection for SCS [74].

In a Cochrane review nearly 450 patients with PAD either received standard of care alone or SCS in addition to standard of care. At 12-month follow-up, amputation was required less often in the SCS group. Additionally, the SCS group required less pharmacologic pain management. No difference was found with regard to the rate of ulcer healing. The conclusion made was in favor of SCS, with regard to reduction in rates of amputation, when compared to standard of care. With regard to complications, 12% required repeat surgical intervention for electrode or lead failure and an infection rate of approximately 3% was reported [75]. The benefits and potential complications and added costs of SCS must be weighed.

While potentially promising, SCS is limited to patients who are not surgical candidates and have failed conservative management or in whom there is persistent pain or ischemia despite previous attempts at revascularization.

28.12 Revascularization

28.12.1 Surgical Revascularization

Surgical revascularization is used in cases of acute or critical limb ischemia (CLI) as well as with claudication following failure with medical management [53]. Lower extremity bypass grafting and endarterectomy are the main surgical techniques used, the goal of which is to establish pulsatile flow distally [76]. Generally speaking, endarterectomy is most suited for proximal arteries including the aorta, iliac, common femoral and profunda arteries, while bypass grafting is preferred for distal, long, or diffuse disease [76]. When choosing the appropriate approach, one must take into account the site of the lesion, severity of disease, anastomoses, and availability of venous material for bypass grafting [77].

28.12.2 Endovascular Revascularization

Endovascular techniques have provided an alternative to open surgical revascularization and their use has been increasing in the last two decades [76]. Generally, short stenotic or occlusive lesions can be treated with endovascular techniques, while long lesions may require surgical treatment. Percutaneous transluminal balloon angioplasty (PTA) was the first nonsurgical strategy used [78]. To address the concern of residual stenosis, as well as to improve long-term patency of the vessel, stenting is performed [68]. However, PTA, with or without stenting, can cause vessel trauma and injury which can result in vessel recoil and development of neointimal hyperplasia, over time leading to formation of in-stent restenosis [79]. The use of drug eluting stents (DES), drug coated balloons (DCB), and laser atherectomy have been developed to address this [76, 80]. Atherectomy, another endovascular procedure, is an ablative process using a laser which was developed to debulk and remove atherosclerotic plaque and restore patency [78]. In the EXCITE ISR trial, the efficacy of excimer laser atherectomy in addition to PTA versus PTA alone for in-stent restenosis found that laser atherectomy showed superiority when compared to PTA alone, for reduction in lesion revascularization at 6 months and also had significantly fewer procedural complications [81].

While endovascular treatments are associated with decreased procedural morbidity and mortality, there continue to be concerns regarding cost, durability, and appropriate application [76]. The most common complications of endovascular techniques include bleeding, pseudoaneurysm, perforation, dissection, embolization, and infection [78].

To date, there has been one RCT directly comparing surgical and endovascular approaches, the BASIL trial, in which 452 patients with CLI were randomized to lower extremity bypass or balloon PTA. The authors found that at 2 years, there was no significant difference with regard to amputation free survival between the two approaches. After 2 years, bypass was associated with improved survival (7 months on average) and amputation free survival (6 months) [82]. Of note, this study did not use some of the more recent endovascular approaches available.

28.13 Amputation

It is estimated that over a 5-year period, approximately 5% of patients with intermittent claudication will progress to lower extremity amputation [83]. Following failure of conservative management and attempts at revascularization, lower extremity amputation may be necessary. Generally it is a last resort and used when significant tissue loss has occurred [84]. Of note, in the literature amputations can be referred to based on the level, for instance, metatarsal, transtibial (commonly, below knee), and transfemoral (above knee), or by minor and major classification. Minor amputations refer to those amputations occurring below the ankle and typically have minor consequences on mobility [84]. Major amputations are defined as being at the level of the ankle or above and performed in patients with extensive necrosis or infectious gangrene, to prevent further complications [77]. In a patient with symptomatic PAD, if revascularization is not an option, the rate of major amputation is 20–25%. Following amputation, the mortality rate at 1 year is estimated to be 48% and 3 years, 70%. However this is variable dependent on the extent of amputation, for instance, the 3-year mortality following above knee amputation is 76%, compared to 63% in patients with below knee amputations [85]. Early recognition of tissue loss is needed to improve limb salvage.

28.14 Summary

The prevalence of peripheral vascular disease (PVD) and critical limb ischemia (CLI) is anticipated to increase with an aging population. Patients with ischemic disease often have chronic and worsening pain associated with disease progression. Pain at rest can reflect severely compromised circulation and CLI. While there are multiple causes of vascular pain including vasculitis, thromboembolic disease, Reynaud's phenomenon, and varicosities, as well as diseases that alter regulation of the vascular system including CRPS, thoracic outlet syndrome, and phantom limb pain, all of which adversely affect function and quality of life, this chapter primarily focuses on ischemic PVD. Pain associated with PVD is multi-faceted and may include inflammatory, nociceptive, and neuropathic components. Management thus involves a multi-faceted approach as well, including risk factor modification of comorbid conditions, medical management with phosphodiesterase inhibitors such as Cilostazol and rehabilitation with a structured and supervised exercise program. Ultimately, treatment must include attempts at revascularization, with an endovascular or surgical approach, the ultimate goal being reperfusion and improvement in arterial circulation to resolve ischemia. In patients that have failed conservative management and revascularization or in whom there are contraindications to revascularization, then consideration should be made for spinal cord stimulation as well as further measures at pain management and alternative therapies.

References

1. Mahoney EM, Wang K, Keo HH, Duval S, Smolderen KG, Cohen DJ, Steg G, Bhatt DL, Hirsch AT. Vascular hospitalization rates and costs in patients with peripheral artery disease in the United States. Circ Cardiovasc Qual Outcomes. 2010;3:642–51.
2. Allison MA, Ho E, Denenberg JO, Langer RD, Newman AB, Fabsitz RR, Criqui MH. Ethnic-specific prevalence of peripheral arterial disease in the United States. American Journal of Preventive Medicine 2007;32(4):328–33. Am J Prevent Med. 2014;47:103.
3. Hirsch AT. Peripheral arterial disease detection, awareness, and treatment in primary care. JAMA. 2001;286:1317.
4. Roger VL, Go AS, Lloyd-Jones DM, et al. Heart disease and stroke statistics--2012 update: a report from the American Heart Association. Circulation. 2011;125(1):e2–e220.
5. Criqui MH, Langer RD, Fronek A, Feigelson HS, Klauber MR, Mccann TJ, Browner D. Mortality over a period of 10 years in patients with peripheral arterial disease. N Engl J Med. 1992;326:381–6.
6. Talsma J. Pain control in the elderly. Drug Topics. 2013;157(8):p42.
7. Custodis F, Schirmer SH, Baumhäkel M, Heusch G, Böhm M, Laufs U. Vascular pathophysiology in response to increased heart rate. J Am Coll Cardiol. 2010;56:1973–83.
8. Mcdermott M, Guralnik J, Ferrucci L. Asymptomatic peripheral arterial disease is associated with more adverse lower extremity characteristics than intermittent claudication. J Vasc Surg. 2008;48:1063.
9. Jensen S, Vatten L, Myhre H. The prevalence of chronic critical lower limb ischaemia in a population of 20,000 subjects 40–69 years of age. Eur J Vasc Endovasc Surg. 2006;32:60–5.
10. Wolfe JHN. Defining the outcome of critical ischaemia. A one year prospective study. Br J Surg. 1986;73:321.
11. Ahumada M, Vioque J. Prevalence and risk factors of varicose veins in adults. Medicina Clinica (Barcelona). 2004;123:647–51.
12. Sanders RJ, Hammond SL, Rao NM. Diagnosis of thoracic outlet syndrome. J Vasc Surg. 2007;46(3):601–4.
13. Jänig W, Baron R. Complex regional pain syndrome: mystery explained? Lancet Neurol. 2003;2:687–97.
14. Rooke TW, Hirsch AT, Misra S, et al. American College of Cardiology Foundation Task Force; American Heart Association Task Force. Management of patients with peripheral artery disease (compilation of 2005 and 2011 ACCF/AHA Guideline Recommendations): a report of the American College of Cardiology Foundation/American Heart Association Task Force on Practice Guidelines. J Am Coll Cardiol. 2013;61(14):1555–70.
15. Creager MA, et al. Acute Limb Ischemia. N Engl J Med. 2012;366(23):2198–206.
16. Ponka D, Baddar F. Ankle-Brachial Index. Can Fam Physician. 2013;59(3):P270.

17. Park C (2017) Ankle-brachial index measurement. In: Overview, periprocedural care, technique. http://emedicine.medscape.com/article/1839449-overview. Accessed 4 Jan 2018.
18. Baena-Díez JCAM, Alzamora MT, Forés R, Pera G, Torán P, Sorribes M. Ankle-brachial index improves the classification of cardiovascular risk: PERART/ARTPER study. Revista Española de Cardiología (English Edition). 2011;64:186–92.
19. Kannel WB, Doyle JT, Mcnamara PM, Quickenton P, Gordon T. Precursors of sudden coronary death. Factors related to the incidence of sudden death. Circulation. 1975;51:606–13.
20. Brindle P. Predictive accuracy of the Framingham coronary risk score in British men: prospective cohort study. BMJ. 2003;327:1267.
21. Ankle Brachial Index Collaboration, Fowkes FG, Murray GD, et al. Ankle brachial index combined with Framingham risk score to predict cardiovascular events and mortality. JAMA. 2008;300:197.
22. Mcclurken ME. Suggested standards for reports dealing with lower extremity ischemia. J Vasc Surg. 1987;5:501.
23. Norgren L, Hiatt WR, Dormandy JA, et al. TASC II working group. Inter-society consensus for the management of peripheral arterial disease. Int Angiol. 2007;26(2):81–157.
24. Fontaine R, Kim M, Kieny R. Surgical treatment of peripheral circulation disorders [in German]. Helv Chim Acta. 1954;21(5–6):499–533.
25. Moore KJ, Sheedy FJ, Fisher EA. Macrophages in atherosclerosis: a dynamic balance. Nat Rev Immunol. 2013;13:709–21.
26. Siracuse JJ, Chaikof EL. The pathogenesis of diabetic atherosclerosis. In: Diabetes and peripheral vascular disease. Totowa: Humana Press; 2012. p. 13–26.
27. Seretny M, Colvin L. Pain management in patients with vascular disease. Br J Anaesth. 2016;117:ii95–ii106.
28. Benzon HT, et al. Neurochemistry of somatosensory and pain processing. In: Essentials of pain medicine. Philadelphia: Elsevier; 2008.
29. Neumann S, Doubell TP, Leslie T, Woolf CJ. Inflammatory pain hypersensitivity mediated by phenotypic switch in myelinated primary sensory neurons. Nature. 1996;384:360–4.
30. Waldmann R, Lazdunski M. H -gated cation channels: neuronal acid sensors in the NaC/DEG family of ion channels. Curr Opin Neurobiol. 1998;8:418–24.
31. England JD, Ferguson MA, Hiatt WR, Regensteiner JG. Progression of neuropathy in peripheral arterial disease. Muscle Nerve. 1995;18:380–7.
32. Weinberg DH, Simovic D, Isner J, Ropper AH. Chronic ischemic monomelic neuropathy from critical limb ischemia. Neurology. 2001;57:1008–12.
33. Fujimura H, Lacroix C, Said G. Vulnerability of nerve fibres to ischaemia. Brain. 1991;114:1929–42.
34. Ross JL, Queme LF, Lamb JE, Green KJ, Ford ZK, Jankowski MP. Interleukin 1β inhibition contributes to the antinociceptive effects of voluntary exercise on ischemia/reperfusion-induced hypersensitivity. Pain. 2017;159(2):380–92.
35. Rüger LJ, Irnich D, Abahji TN, Crispin A, Hoffmann U, Lang PM. Characteristics of chronic ischemic pain in patients with peripheral arterial disease. Pain. 2008;139:201–8.
36. Gevirtz C. Pain management in peripheral vascular disease. Semin Cardiothorac Vasc Anesth. 1999;3:182–90.
37. Lang PM, Schober GM, Rolke R, Wagner S, Hilge R, Offenbächer M, Treede R-D, Hoffmann U, Irnich D. Sensory neuropathy and signs of central sensitization in patients with peripheral arterial disease. Pain. 2006;124:190–200.
38. Woolf CJ. Central sensitization: implications for the diagnosis and treatment of pain. Pain. 2011;152(3 Suppl):S2–15. https://doi.org/10.1016/j.pain.2010.09.030.
39. Mense S. Nociception from skeletal muscle in relation to clinical muscle pain. Pain. 1993;54:241–89.
40. Gordon T, Kannel WB. Predisposition to atherosclerosis in the head, heart, and legs. The Framingham study. JAMA. 1972;221(7):661–6.
41. Rice TW, Lumsden AB. Optimal medical management of peripheral arterial disease. Vas Endovas Surg. 2006;40(4):312–27.

42. Jonason T, Bergström R. Cessation of smoking in patients with intermittent claudication: effects on the risk of peripheral vascular complications, myocardial infarction and mortality. Acta Med Scand. 1987;221(3):253–60.
43. Gerhard-Herman M, et al. 2016 AHA/ACC guideline on the management of patients with lower extremity peripheral artery disease: executive summary. A report of the American College of Cardiology/American Heart Association task force on clinical practice guidelines. Circulation. 2016;135(12):1–273.
44. Gent M, et al. A randomised, blinded, trial of clopidogrel versus aspirin in patients at risk of ischaemic events (CAPRIE) CAPRIE Steering Committee. Lancet. 1996;348(9038):1329–39.
45. Burdess A, et al. Randomized controlled trial of dual antiplatelet therapy in patients undergoing surgery for critical limb ischemia. Ann Surg. 2010;52(6):37–42.
46. Belch JJ, et al. Results of the randomized, placebo-controlled clopidogrel and acetylsalicylic acid in bypass surgery for peripheral arterial disease (CASPAR) trial. J Vasc Surg. 2010;52(4):825–33.
47. Tepe G, Bantleon R, et al. Management of peripheral arterial interventions with mono or dual antiplatelet therapy--the MIRROR study: a randomised and double-blinded clinical trial. Eur Radiol. 2012;22(9):1998–2006.
48. Anand S, Bosch J, Eikelboom J, Connolly S, et al. Rivaroxaban with or without aspirin in patients with stable peripheral or carotid artery disease: an international, randomised, double-blind, placebo-controlled trial. Lancet. 2017;391(10117):219–29.
49. Anand S, Yusuf S, Xie C, et al. Oral anticoagulant and antiplatelet therapy and peripheral arterial disease. N Engl J Med. 2007;357(3):217–27.
50. Mohler E, Hiatt WR, et al. Cholesterol reduction with atorvastatin improves walking distance in patients with peripheral arterial disease. Circulation. 2003;108(12):1481–6.
51. Whelton PK, Carey RM, et al. 2017 ACC/AHA/AAPA/ABC/ACPM/AGS/APhA/ASH/ASPC/NMA/PCNA guideline for the prevention, detection, evaluation, and management of high blood pressure in adults. JACC. 2017;71(19):e127–248.
52. Yusuf S, Sleight P, et al. Effects of an angiotensin-converting-enzyme inhibitor, ramipril, on cardiovascular events in high-risk patients. N Engl J Med. 2000;342(3):145–53.
53. Vartanian S, Conte MS. Surgical intervention for peripheral arterial disease. Circ Res. 2015;116:1614–28.
54. Bedenis R, Stewart M, Cleanthis M, Robless P, Mikhailidis DP, Stansby G. Cilostazol for intermittent claudication. Cochrane Database Syst Rev. 2014;10:CD003748.
55. Salhiyyah K, Senanayake E, Abdel-Hadi M, Booth A, Michaels JA. Pentoxifylline for intermittent claudication. Cochrane Database Syst Rev. 2015;1:CD005262.
56. Kranke P, Bennett M, Roeckl-Wiedmann I, Debus S. Hyperbaric oxygen therapy for treating chronic wounds. Cochrane Database Syst Rev. 2015;2:CD004123.
57. Norgren L, Hiatt WR, et al. Inter-society consensus for the management of peripheral arterial disease (TASC II). J Vasc Surg. 2007;45(Suppl S):S5–S67.
58. Belch J, Hiatt WR, et al. Effect of fibroblast growth factor NV1FGF on amputation and death: a randomized placebo-controlled trial of gene therapy in critical limb ischemia. Lancet. 2011;377(9781):1929–37.
59. Muona K, Mäkinen K, et al. 10-year safety follow-up in patients with local VEGF gene transfer to ischemic lower limb. Gene Ther. 2012;19(4):392–5.
60. Morishita R, Makino H, et al. Phase I/IIa clinical trial of therapeutic angiogenesis using hepatocyte growth factor gene transfer to treat critical limb ischemia. Arterioscler Thromb Vasc Biol. 2011;31(3):713–20.
61. Fadini GP, Agostini C. Autologous stem cell therapy for peripheral arterial disease meta-analysis and systematic review of the literature. Atherosclerosis. 2010;209(1):10–7.
62. Liu Y, Xu Y, Fang F, Zhang J, Guo L, Weng Z. Therapeutic efficacy of stem cell-based therapy in peripheral arterial disease: a meta-analysis. PLoS One. 2015;10(4):e0125032.
63. Hamburg N, Balady GJ. Exercise rehabilitation in peripheral artery disease: functional impact and mechanisms of benefits. Circulation. 2011;123(1):87–97.

64. Gardner AW, Poehlman ET. Exercise rehabilitation programs for the treatment of claudication pain. A meta-analysis. JAMA. 1995;274(12):975–80.
65. Tsai JC, Chan P, et al. The effects of exercise training on walking function and perception of health status in elderly patients with peripheral arterial occlusive disease. J Intern Med. 2002;252(5):448–55.
66. Murphy T, et al. Supervised exercise versus primary stenting for claudication resulting from aortoiliac peripheral artery disease, six-month outcomes from the claudication: exercise versus endoluminal revascularization (CLEVER) study. Circulation. 2013;125:130–9.
67. Fakhry F, Spronk S, et al. Endovascular revascularization and supervised exercise for peripheral artery disease and intermittent claudication: a randomized clinical trial. JAMA. 2015;314(18):1936–44.
68. Frontera W, DeLisa JA. DeLisa's physical medicine & rehabilitation, practices and principles. Philadelphia: Lippincott, Williams & Wilkins; 2010.
69. Naoum J, Arbid EJ. Spinal cord stimulation for chronic limb ischemia. Methodist Debakey Cardiovasc J. 2013;9(2):99–102.
70. Jivegård LE, Augustinsson LE, et al. Effects of spinal cord stimulation (SCS) in patients with inoperable severe lower limb ischemia: a prospective randomized controlled trial. Eur J Vasc Endovasc Surg. 1995;9(4):421–5.
71. Reig E, Abejón D. Spinal cord stimulation: a 20-year retrospective analysis in 260 patients. Neuromodulation. 2009;12(3):232–9.
72. Andersen C. Noninvasive assessment of lower extremity hemodynamics in individuals with diabetes mellitus. J Vasc Surg. 2010;52(3 Suppl):76–80.
73. Byrne P, Provan JL, et al. The use of transcutaneous oxygen tension measurements in the in the diagnosis of peripheral vascular insufficiency. Annals of Surg. 1984;26(3):159–65.
74. Amann W, Berg P, Gersbach P, Gamain J, Raphael JH, Ubbink DT, European Peripheral Vascular Disease Outcome Study SCS-EPOS. Spinal cord stimulation in the treatment of non-reconstructable stable critical leg ischaemia: results of the European peripheral vascular outcome study (SCS-EPOS). Eur J Vasc Endovasc Surg. 2003;26(3):280–6.
75. Ubbink DT, Vermeulen H. Spinal cord stimulation for non-reconstructable chronic critical leg ischaemia. Cochrane Database of Syst Rev. 2013;2:CD004001. https://doi.org/10.1002/14651858.CD004001.pub3.
76. Farber A, Eberhardt RT. The current state of critical limb ischemia. JAMA Surg. 2016;151(11):1070–7.
77. Aboyans V, Ricco JB, et al. 2017 ESC guidelines on the diagnosis and treatment of peripheral arterial diseases, in collaboration with the European Society for Vascular Surgery (ESVS): document covering atherosclerotic disease of extracranial carotid and vertebral, mesenteric, renal. Eur Heart J. 2017;39(9):1–71.
78. Shishehbor M, Jaff MR. Percutaneous therapies for peripheral artery disease. Circulation. 2016;134:1–33.
79. Inoue S, Koyama H, et al. Pathogenetic heterogeneity of in-stent lesion formation in human peripheral arterial disease. J Vasc Surg. 2002;35(4):672–8.
80. Krankenberg H, Tubler T, et al. Drug-coated balloon versus standard balloon for superficial femoral artery in-stent restenosis: the randomized femoral artery in-stent restenosis (FAIR) trial. Circulation. 2015;132(23):2230–6.
81. Dippel E, Makam P, et al. Randomized controlled study of excimer laser atherectomy for treatment of femoropopliteal in-stent restenosis: initial results from the EXCITE ISR trial (EXCImer laser randomized controlled study for treatment of FemoropopliTEal in-stent restenosis). JACC Cardiovasc Interv. 2015;8(1 Pt A):92–101.
82. Bradbury AW, Adam DJ, et al. Bypass versus Angioplasty in Severe Ischaemia of the Leg (BASIL) trial: an intention-to-treat analysis of amputation-free and overall survival in patients randomized to a bypass surgery-first or a balloon angioplasty-first revascularization strategy. J Vasc Surg. 2010;51:5–17.

83. Hooi JD, Kester A, et al. Asymptomatic peripheral arterial occlusive disease predicted cardiovascular morbidity and mortality in a 7-year follow-up study. J Clin Epidemiol. 2004;57(3):294–300.
84. Swaminathan A, Sreekanth V, et al. Lower extremity amputation in peripheral artery disease: improving patient outcomes. Vasc Health Risk Manag. 2014;10:417–24.
85. Jones WS, Patel MR, et al. High mortality risks after major lower extremity amputation in Medicare patients with peripheral artery disease. Am Heart J. 2013;165(5):809–15.

Index

K. Shimoji et al. (eds.), *Chronic Pain Management in General and Hospital Practice*, https://doi.org/10.1007/978-981-15-2933-7

D

O

U

V

The manufacturer's authorised representative in the EU is Springer Nature Customer Service Centre GmbH, Europaplatz 3, 69115 Heidelberg, Germany. If you have any concerns regarding our products, please contact ProductSafety@springernature.com

Printed and bound by CPI Group (UK) Ltd, Croydon, CR0 4YY
30/09/2026
02225241-0017